D1440941

RESPIRATORY DEFENSE MECHANISMS

LUNG BIOLOGY IN HEALTH AND DISEASE

Executive Editor: **Claude Lenfant**
Director, Division of Lung Diseases
National Institutes of Health
Bethesda, Maryland

VOLUME 1 IMMUNOLOGIC AND INFECTIOUS REACTIONS IN THE LUNG, *Edited by Charles H. Kirkpatrick and Herbert Y. Reynolds*

VOLUME 2 THE BIOCHEMICAL BASIS OF PULMONARY FUNCTION, *Edited by Ronald G. Crystal*

VOLUME 3 BIOENGINEERING ASPECTS OF THE LUNG, *Edited by John B. West*

VOLUME 4 METABOLIC FUNCTIONS OF THE LUNG, *Edited by Y.S. Bakhle and John R. Vane*

VOLUME 5 RESPIRATORY DEFENSE MECHANISMS (in two parts), *Edited by Joseph D. Brain, Donald F. Proctor, and Lynne M. Reid*

VOLUME 6 DEVELOPMENT OF THE LUNG, *Edited by W. Alan Hodson*

Other volumes in preparation

PATHOGENESIS AND THERAPY OF LUNG CANCER *Edited by Curtis Harris*

CHRONIC OBSTRUCTIVE PULMONARY DISEASE *Edited by Thomas L. Petty*

EXTRAPULMONARY MANIFESTATIONS OF RESPIRATORY DISEASE, *Edited by Eugene D. Robin*

LUNG WATER AND SOLUTE EXCHANGE, *Edited by Norman C. Staub*

RESPIRATORY DEFENSE MECHANISMS

(IN TWO PARTS)

PART II

Edited by

Joseph D. Brain

Harvard University School of Public Health
Boston, Massachusetts

Donald F. Proctor

The Johns Hopkins University
Schools of Hygiene and Public Health, and Medicine
Baltimore, Maryland

Lynne M. Reid

Harvard Medical School
Boston, Massachusetts

MARCEL DEKKER, INC. New York and Basel

Library of Congress Cataloging in Publication Data
Main entry under title:

Respiratory defense mechanisms.

(Lung Biology in health and disease; v. 5)
Includes bibliographies.
1. Respiratory organs. 2. Natural immunity.
3. Mucous membrane. 4. Cilia and ciliary motion.
I. Brain, Joseph D. II. Proctor, Donald F.
III. Reid, Lynne. IV. Series.
RC756.L83 vol. 5 [QP121] 616.2'4'008s
ISBN 0-8247-6532-X [612'.2] 76-29567

MARCEL DEKKER, INC.
270 Madison Avenue, New York, New York 10016

Current printing (last digit):
10 9 8 7 6 5 4 3 2 1

PRINTED IN THE UNITED STATES OF AMERICA

CONTRIBUTORS

Jean D. Acton, Ph.D. Associate Professor, Department of Microbiology and Immunology, The Bowman Gray School of Medicine of Wake Forest University, Winston-Salem, North Carolina

A. C. Allison, D.Phil., D.M., F.R.C. Path. Head of Cell Pathology Division, Clinical Research Centre, Harrow, Middlesex, England

Joseph A. Bellanti, M.D. Professor of Pediatrics and Microbiology, Director, International Center for Interdisciplinary Studies of Immunology at Georgetown, Georgetown University Medical Center, Washington, D.C.

Joseph D. Brain, Sc.D. in Hyg. Associate Professor of Physiology, Harvard University School of Public Health, Boston, Massachusetts

J. Bernard L. Gee, M.D. Associate Professor of Medicine, Department of Internal Medicine, Yale University School of Medicine; Director, Winchester Chest Clinic, Yale-New Haven Hospital, New Haven, Connecticut

John J. Godleski, M.D. Assistant Professor, Department of Pathology, Medical College of Pennsylvania, Philadelphia, Pennsylvania

Gary L. Huber, M.D. Chief, Division of Respiratory Diseases, Department of Medicine, Harvard Medical School, Boston, Massachusetts

W. G. Johanson, Jr., M.D. Associate Professor of Medicine, University of Texas, Health Science Center at San Antonio, San Antonio, Texas

Atul S. Khandwala, Ph.D.† Assistant Professor of Biochemistry and Medicine, Department of Internal Medicine, Yale University Lung Research Center, New Haven, Connecticut

---

Present Affiliation

†Senior Biochemist, Department of Biochemistry and Drug Metabolism, USV Pharmaceutical Corporation, Tuckahoe, New York

F. Marc LaForce, M.D.† Chief of Medical Service, Veterans Administration Hospital, Denver, Colorado

Lee V. Leak, Ph.D. Professor and Chairman, Department of Anatomy, The Ernest E. Just Laboratory of Cellular Biology, Howard University College of Medicine, Washington, D.C.

David E. Leith, M.D. Associate Professor, Department of Physiology, Harvard University School of Public Health, Boston, Massachusetts

Robert J. Mason, M.D. Assistant Professor of Medicine in Residence, Department of Medicine, Cardiovascular Research Institute, University of California, San Francisco, California

Paul E. Morrow, Ph.D. Professor, Departments of Radiation Biology and Biophysics, and Pharmacology and Toxicology, The University of Rochester School of Medicine and Dentistry, Rochester, New York

Quentin N. Myrvik, Ph.D. Professor and Chairman, Department of Microbiology and Immunology, The Bowman Gray School of Medicine of Wake Forest University, Winston-Salem, North Carolina

Eveline E. Schneeberger, M.D. Associate Professor, Department of Pathology, Harvard Medical School, Boston Massachusetts; Department of Pathology, The Children's Hospital Medical Center, Boston, Massachusetts

Sorell L. Schwartz, Ph.D. Professor, Department of Pharmacology, Georgetown University School of Medicine, Washington, D.C.

Sergei P. Sorokin, M.D. Associate Professor of Cell Biology, Department of Physiology, Harvard University School of Public Health, Boston, Massachusetts

J. G. Widdicombe, D.M. Professor and Chairman, Department of Physiology, St. George's Hospital Medical School, London, England

---

Present Affiliation

†Associate Professor of Medicine, University of Colorado School of Medicine, Denver, Colorado

FOREWORD

I would be hard put to say whether the expansion of research on the lung and on respiratory disease is a precursor or a result of increasing public awareness of the importance of pulmonary illness. Whatever the case, we have undoubtedly witnessed both phenomena within a relatively short period of time, and with them a rather sobering realization of the limitations in both scientific and general public knowledge of lung disease. New concerns about the impact of environmental and occupational hazards on lung function–impacts that may only manifest themselves in frank disease after decades of seemingly innocuous exposure–serve to remind us all that society pays a heavy price when knowledge lags behind action, and moreover that society looks to science for solutions.

This series of monographs is, therefore, most timely and important. The substantial increase in the number and variety of scientific reports on respiratory and pulmonary topics makes it all the more critical that work in this field be subjected to thorough and comprehensive review as a service to the scientist and the physician who find it virtually impossible to "keep up," let alone to assimilate and evaluate a rapidly growing body of knowledge in an area of human health that is of mounting importance.

Chronic and acute lung diseases are among the major causes of disability and death in all age groups. From a public health standpoint, prevention of these diseases is a goal that amply justifies an increased commitment of research resources. For it is clear that the most effective paths toward prevention will emerge out of disciplined study in many fields, from the physiology and biochemistry of the respiratory system to the pathology and therapy of respiratory disorders.

I feel sure that this series of publications will continue to make a substantial contribution to the science and practice of medicine and to the hopes we have for more effective concepts and methods of preventing a major segment of human disease.

Theodore Cooper, M.D.
Former Assistant Secretary for Health
Department of Health, Education,
and Welfare

PREFACE

The lungs have a unique proximity to the environment. The same thinness and delicacy that qualify the air-blood barrier for the rapid exchange of oxygen and carbon dioxide reduce its effectiveness as a barrier to inhaled microorganisms, allergens, carcinogens, toxic particles, and noxious gases. Adults, depending on their size and physical activity, breathe from 10,000 to 20,000 liters of air daily. Contaminating particles and gases which enter the body with this air are potentially hazardous. The purpose of the following chapters (in two parts) is to explore the diverse physiological mechanisms which prevent the accumulation and deleterious action of inhaled particles and gases. Thus, both the modification of the inspired air prior to its access to the lungs as well as the forces brought to bear against noxious influences reaching the respiratory surfaces are discussed.

The prevalence of airborne disease provides ample evidence that this formidable array of respiratory defenses is not invulnerable. Perhaps a better understanding of the exact nature of these physiological mechanisms may lead to ways of defending them against injury or even enhancing them and, thus, decreasing human susceptibility to respiratory disease.

Unit One is devoted to the respiratory air conditioning system. In these chapters, the overall objective is to describe the anatomical nature of the upper air passages as it influences the flow of inspiratory air, and to consider how this results in modification of the ambient air prior to access to the lungs. Unit Two describes our knowledge of airway secretions and the cilia which move them. The mucous membranes of the respiratory tract and the nature and action of respiratory tract cilia are examined. This unit also covers the biochemical and rheological properties as well as the pharmacological and physiological control of airway secretions. Unit Three then integrates cilia and secretions and treats the question of mucociliary transport. Basic mechanisms, environmental influences, and the impact of mucosal injury and repair are considered.

Unit Four describes other major factors involved in the removal of inhaled deposited materials. Following a discussion of the overall clearance kinetics usually seen, the importance of respiratory reflexes and cough is considered. The unit concludes with a discussion of the pulmonary lymphatic system and the nature and properties of the air-blood barrier. The final group of chapters, Unit

Five, emphasizes the role of phagocytic cells in defending the lung with special emphasis on the physiological and pathological roles of pulmonary macrophages.

After careful consideration of each subject area, the editors attempted to recruit authors who could summarize each topic and anticipate new directions of study. Each contributor has raised pressing questions against the background of a hard core of experimental facts. No obligation was felt to review all of the existing sprawling literature; rather, each author was encouraged to be selective. Inevitably, there is occasional overlap among some chapters; yet where this serves to preserve continuity in the development of each author's ideas, it has been considered important to maintain it.

Although the focus of these chapters is usually the adult human, we encouraged inclusion of comparative and developmental aspects of each topic. Similarly, although the series is not intended to be a handbook for clinicians, both pathological and clinical dimensions are included whenever appropriate. Overall, it is our hope that these chapters will be a chronicle of significant past contributions, a stimulus for their rapid and thoughtful application, and a guide for future work.

Joseph D. Brain
Donald F. Proctor
Lynne M. Reid

ACKNOWLEDGMENTS

Respiratory Defense Mechanisms is part of the Lung Biology in Health and Disease series. Dr. Claude Lenfant, Director of the Division of Lung Diseases at the National Heart,Lung, and Blood Institute, is the Executive Editor for the series. We thank him for serving as a catalyst for our efforts and for his guidance. We thank the many reviewers who critically examined the chapters and made countless valuable suggestions. We thank Ms. Judith Richards and Ms. Betty Hauser for their essential role as editorial assistants. They orchestrated the review process, made frequent suggestions regarding content and form, reviewed page proofs, and generally provided an invaluable unifying influence. Finally, and most important, the editors wish to thank the contributors for their heroic efforts in writing and revising their chapters.

INTRODUCTION

The lung, an organ continuously exposed to the environment, has been recognized for almost five centuries to be susceptible to damage by substances carried in the air. As pointed out in Chapter 1, Leonardo da Vinci observed nearly 500 years ago that "inspired air could carry dust into and damage the lung." Thus, the integrity of the lung depends upon effective protective mechanisms against airborne hazards.

Many outstanding scientists have contributed to our knowledge of the Respiratory Defense Mechanisms. In 1953, Julius Comroe emphasized the "self-protective or defense mechanisms" of the lung in his Harvey Lecture on "The Function of the Lung." This, undoubtedly, was the beginning of a new wave of research that benefitted from advances in morphology, biophysics, and biochemistry.

This monograph provides an in-depth review and analysis of the defense mechanisms of the lung. It is a comprehensive report that includes a discussion of all known mechanisms. The authors represent many disciplines; hence, this most important function of the lung is considered from the viewpoint of the physiologist, the ultramicroscopist, the biochemist, the biophysicist, the microbiologist, the immunologist, and also the clinician. Although incomplete, this list points to a breadth of coverage that could only be accomplished through the extraordinary cooperation and enthusiasm of the editors who, although representing different disciplines, had a common goal.

As a personal note, I would like to acknowledge the dedicated and tireless efforts of Joseph D. Brain, Donald F. Proctor, and Lynne M. Reid, and to express my gratitude to them for editing such an original and excellent volume.

Claude Lenfant, M.D.
Bethesda, Maryland

CONTENTS

CONTENTS OF PART I

RESPIRATORY DEFENSE MECHANISMS

Unit Four

PULMONARY CLEARANCE OF INHALED MATERIALS

Despite continuing deposition of inhaled particles, the lungs are remarkably clean and sterile. Even the diseased and blackened lungs of miners succumbing to coal workers' pneumoconiosis contain less than 5% of the mine dust originally deposited there. The younger, healthy lung exhibits even greater potency in the pursuit of cleanliness.

When describing the mechanisms of pulmonary clearance, we always discuss the mucociliary transport system and the macrophage system. Some of the topics discussed in this unit are less frequently part of the "textbook" explanation of lung cleansing. However, they are no less substantial. In fact, in the pathogenesis of some lung diseases, the pathways discussed here may assume paramount importance.

Considered first are the quantitative aspects of clearance and the effects of particle size, solubility, and site of deposition. The role of cough is followed by a discussion of respiratory reflexes and their contribution to lung defense. Chapter 14 describes interstitial fluid movement and the involvement of the lymphatics in particle clearance. Classically, lymphatic removal of particulates from the lower respiratory tract was often thought to be the major route. Its importance was probably exaggerated for several reasons. Early judgments were usually based on morphological studies in which histological procedures washed away many particles and cells being cleared via the airways; thus, the importance of the airway route was underestimated. Drawing quantitative conclusions about dynamic processes from static observations can also be misleading. A pathway's importance is a function of the transport speed as well as the number of particles present. For example, if the same quantity of particles are present but are moving 100 times as fast along an airway as through a lymph node, then the airway is clearing 100 times as many particles. Certainly the average speed of particles in lymph nodes is very low.

Yet, although our estimates of the percentage of particles cleared via the lymphatics have dropped, our appreciation of the importance of those particles entering the lymphatics has greatly increased. Precisely because particles are slowly cleared, they attain great significance in the pathogenesis of many lung diseases. Months and years after exposure to particles, these connective tissue burdens may constitute the major reservoir of retained particles.

Chapter 18 focuses on the properties of the air-blood barrier and its potential for particle penetration. The extent to which the pulmonary capillary bed serves as a protective filter eliminating debris, pathogens, and cells from the circulating blood is also discussed.

Convincing evidence for the existence of all the clearance pathways discussed in this unit is presented. Yet, little is known about them quantitatively; their relative importance in health and disease is virtually unknown. Elaborate experimental protocols would be necessary to accurately quantitate fractions that traversed the different clearance pathways. Theoretically clearance by the various routes could be measured by monitoring the final pathways for the airways, the blood vessels, and the lymphatics, using various ingenious approaches. Such preparations would be very difficult and complications would persist. Allowance must be made for the possibility of crossover from one clearance path to another. It is also likely that the extent to which each pathway is used depends on the sizes, solubilities, and other chemical properties of the deposited particles, as well as the time after the exposure and the degree of disease present.

Other questions are raised by topics in this unit. Although considerable evidence indicates that particles and cells move along the alveolar surface to the beginnings of the mucociliary transport system, practically nothing is known about the forces or mechanisms responsible for alveolar-bronchiolar transport. Tropisms, such as chemotropism, do not seem to account for a purposeful migration of macrophages mouthward. A "sucking" force created by the cilia has been proposed but seems to have little physical basis. The continual production of surfactant and its tendency to remain as a monolayer might provide a moving surface for macrophages and dust.

The existence of a surface-tension gradient along the fluid surface is also probable and may be important in the movement of the fluid surface. Respiratory excursions seem to play a part in the movement of fluid, particles, and cells from the alveoli. Perhaps shape and area changes coincident with ventilation move particles, cells, and lining fluids. As lung volume changes, alveoli change shape and crevices and folds may appear and disappear. Finally, the random movement of macrophages may account for some of their removal.

Thus, although Unit Four demonstrates a considerable expansion of our knowledge of clearance mechanisms, key issues remain unsolved.

Joseph D. Brain

14

Clearance Kinetics of Inhaled Particles

PAUL E. MORROW

The University of Rochester School of Medicine and Dentistry
Rochester, New York

I. Introduction

A. Rationale for Kinetic Descriptions

There are two principal reasons why quantitative descriptions of the removal processes of particulate matter from the respiratory system are important: (a) they provide a prospective and retrospective basis for toxicological evaluations, both chemical and radiologic; (b) they provide an insight into the status of several important functions of the respiratory system and thereby permit the procurement of "norms" and the development of appropriate physiological evaluation methods.

In elaboration of the first point, it is evident that the amount of inhaled, extrinsic material present in specific respiratory regions and the respective persistence times of the material therein determine the dose to and the action(s) on the associated respiratory structures; in other words, dose-effect estimates are directly determined by the retention characteristics of the material. These retention functions can be incorporated into predictive models and serve in planning and control, or they can be used for analyses of individual exposure situations.

To the second point, one needs only to acknowledge that virtually all quantitative estimations of mucociliary transport in the human respiratory tract have utilized measurements of particles [1,23,33,45]. Either airborne or after deposition, the use of aerosolized materials as physiological markers has been increasingly widespread in respiratory research, especially since radioisotopes have become available. Applications have included the study of macrophage activity, airway patency, and distinctions in regional clearance mechanisms and pathways [17,32,72,107,114,115]. Also, it has been possible to extend these applications to health effect assessments, e.g., the effect of drugs, air pollutants, smoking, and disease states on mucociliary transport [15,73,75,106,123,125, 129]. In experimental animals, many of these approaches have included other "untraditional" evaluations of pulmonary functions such as alveolar cell proliferation, pulmonic lymphatic drainage, and permeability at the level of the alveolar membrane [12,17,20,28,29,32,53,81,94].

From the general standpoint of analyzing transport phenomena, a great variety of mathematical descriptions are available to express changing events. In more specific terms, descriptions must be chosen in the light of the following operational alternatives: precise mathematical descriptions usually of specific data designed to provide the "best fit"; mathematical descriptions directed at generalizing most or all of the available data on a given process; or formulations constructed at the biomechanistic level wherein some identifiable relationships are synthesized into a coherent entity. Each of these approaches has a rational objective—the first presumably provides the least erroneous mathematical description, and within the rules implicit in this pursuit, simplicity wins in case of "tie." In the second case, the objective is most likely the procurement of a pragmatic description which unifies myriad findings into a single utilitarian statement; however, the mathematical formulation evolved may be far less precise than in the former case. The third approach is that of the scientific realist who is not content with empiricism, but builds his description from fundamental relationships so that the end-product is solid scientifically. Without question, the third approach should produce the most appropriate and reliable kinetic model(s). With complex systems, e.g., intact animals, it is also the most difficult approach to accomplish.

Mathematical descriptions undoubtedly occur whereby all three of these objectives are served simultaneously, and equally well, but in the real world of biomedical research it is rare that even two of these three objectives are achieved. In terms of dust clearance phenomena, this is unfortunately the case. The reason is simply the dearth of quantitative information on even the most thoroughly studied system of particulate clearance we can identify, e.g., mucociliary transport from the tracheobronchial region; therefore, we are forced to rely upon mathematical generalizations of a semiempirical nature to accomplish and justify the task of developing kinetic formulations for experimental data.

It will facilitate presentation of the kinetic descriptions to follow if a few basic principles are reviewed. Imagine a compartment which contains either intrinsic material or material rapidly introduced as a single "instantaneous" intake, and assume this compartment is under the influence of a single removal process. Diagrammatically, the model has the following form:

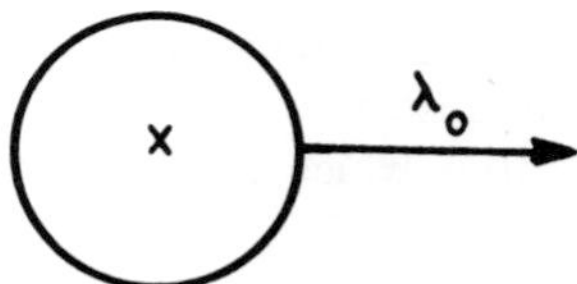

where X represents the amount of material in the compartment and λ_0 denotes a one-way elimination process. If the fractional removal rate (dX/dt)/X from the compartment is constant, the elimination process is first order and can be expressed by

$$\frac{dX}{dt} = -\lambda_0 X \tag{1}$$

Multiplying both sides of the equation by $\exp(\lambda_0 t)$ (exp is the base of the natural logarithm and t is time) and setting the equation equal to 0 gives

$$\frac{dX}{dt} \exp(\lambda_0 t) + X\lambda_0 \exp(\lambda_0 t) = 0 \tag{2}$$

The left term is the time derivative of the product $X \exp(\lambda_0 t)$, therefore, by substitution

$$\frac{d}{dt} [X \exp(\lambda_0 t)] = 0 \tag{2a}$$

and by integration

$$X(t) = X(o) \exp(-\lambda_0 t) \tag{3}$$

Equation (3) is the familiar exponential description which indicates that at time t the amount remaining X(t) of the original amount X(0) (i.e., the amount at time zero) is determined by the product $X(0) \exp(-\lambda_0 t)$. From Eq. (3) one can also see that

$$\ln X(t) = \ln X(o) - \lambda_0 t \tag{3a}$$

and when X(t) = X(o)/2 (i.e., 50% clearance has occurred), then $t = T_{1/2}$.

$T_{1/2} = \ln 2/\lambda_0 = 0.693/\lambda_0$ where $T_{1/2}$ is the retention half-time in units of t. Substituting this expression for λ_0 in Eq. (3) leads to Eq. (3b). Specifically,

$$X(t) = X(o) \exp\left(-\frac{0.693}{T_{1/2}} t\right) \tag{3b}$$

When two parallel processes are removing material from the compartment instead of one and they both cause X to decrease at constant fractional rates λ_{01} and λ_{02}, we have a condition which is an extension of the first exponential model where now

$$-\frac{dX}{dt} = \lambda_{01}X + \lambda_{02}X = (\lambda_{01} + \lambda_{02})X \tag{4}$$

and from which it follows that the predicted amount retained at time t is

$$X(t) = X(o) \exp[-(\lambda_{01} + \lambda_{02})t] \tag{5}$$

Equation (5) would apply to the following diagrammatic model

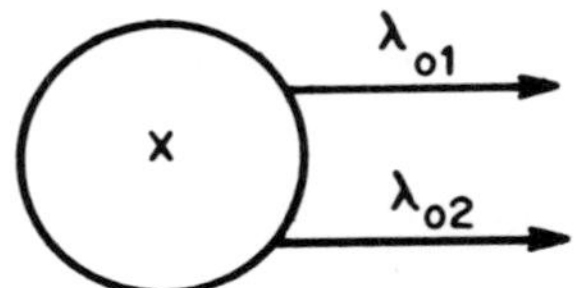

which depicts a simple open system with parallel removal processes. If λ_{01} is a biological elimination rate and λ_{02} a radioactive decay rate, this would be a modification of the first model wherein the compartment was uniformly labeled with a radioisotopic form of X.

When this simple case is encountered in practice, measurements of the change in X with time due to λ_{01} and λ_{02} will always appear to follow a rate λ_e which is numerically equal to the sum of λ_{01} and λ_{02}. Coefficient λ_e, therefore, can be termed the effective decay rate and is equal to $0.693/T_{1/2}$(eff) where $T_{1/2}$(eff) is the effective half-time. Since the investigator normally knows the physical half-life of the radioisotope, hence λ_{02}, the biological removal rate can easily be calculated either by $\lambda_{01} = \lambda_e - \lambda_{02}$ or $1/T_{1/2}(\text{biol}) = 1/T_{1/2}(\text{eff}) - 1/T_{1/2}(\text{phys})$.

A major variation of the foregoing exponential models involves continuous or repetitive intake, where r(t) is the intake rate, which can be diagramed as follows

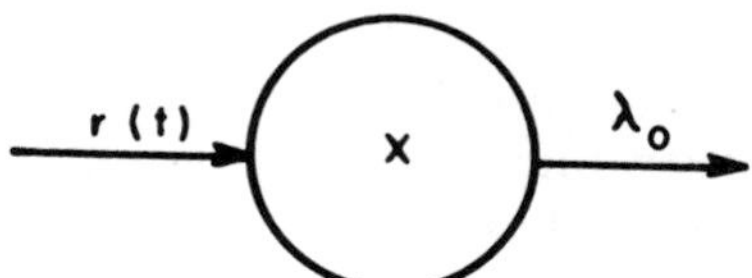

For this model we have

$$\frac{dX}{dt} = -\lambda_0 X + r(t) \tag{6}$$

Multiplying by exp(λt) as before and integrating between $\tau = 0$ and $\tau = t$ gives

$$X(t) = X(o)\exp(-\lambda_0 t) + \int_0^t r(\tau)\exp[-\lambda_0(t-\tau)]\,d\tau \tag{7}$$

If the value of r(t) is constant and equal to r, then

$$X(t) = X(o)\exp(-\lambda_0 t) + \frac{r}{\lambda_0}[1 - \exp(-\lambda_0 t)] \tag{7a}$$

where all the other symbols have the same meaning as before.

In many instances the quantity of interest is not the clearance rate or the retained fraction, but the dose. The dose is proportional to the time integral of the retained material. From Eq. (5) one may obtain

$$\int_{t_1}^{t_2} X(\tau)\,d\tau = \frac{X(o)}{\lambda_e}[\exp(-\lambda_e t_1) - \exp(-\lambda_e t_2)] \tag{8}$$

from which it follows that

$$\int_0^t X(\tau)\,d\tau = \frac{X(o)}{\lambda_e}[1 - \exp(-\lambda_e t)] \tag{9}$$

and

$$\int_0^\infty X(\tau)\,d\tau = \frac{X(o)}{\lambda_e} \tag{10}$$

where λ_e is either the biological or effective removal coefficient.

The final example concerns the case where removal rate is not a constant fraction of X, i.e., when $\frac{dX/dt}{X} \neq \lambda$. A commonly used example of this condition is when $\frac{dX/dt}{X} = -\lambda/t$, i.e., the rate of removal varies inversely with time.

Raabe [103] pointed out that this can be interpreted as either a decreasing rate constant or as a case where a decreasing amount of material is available for clearance. Clearance under this circumstance is described by a power function.

Power function clearance is usually described by the equation

$$X = \frac{X(\tau)}{\tau^{-\lambda}} t^{-\lambda} \tag{11}$$

where $X(\tau)$ is the amount retained at $t = \tau$, generally the earliest sample time, and λ is some power. The negative sign, as in the exponential formulations, connotes a decay or removal process.

For the case of a constant input into an initially empty compartment, the compartmental content of a power function model increases linearly with time according to

$$X = \frac{rt}{\lambda + 1.0} \tag{11a}$$

where r is the constant input rate. If the input is turned off at time t_E, the subsequent clearance is given by

$$X = \left(\frac{rt_E^{\lambda + 1.0}}{\lambda + 1.0}\right) t^{-\lambda} \quad \text{where } t \geqslant t_E \tag{11b}$$

Although power function clearance often provides an adequate description of experimental data, its prediction of a linear buildup during a constant input for protracted periods makes it suspect, since one generally observes a leveling off to a steady-state value in most cases of prolonged, constant input.

Other features of the power function model, including its integration, are discussed in Sec. II.B. For further reading on the subject of kinetic analyses appropriate to this chapter, publications by Raabe, [103], Wagner [130], Jacques [55], and Rescigno and Segre [104] are recommended.

B. Review of Respiratory Clearance Mechanisms

Particulate clearance from the respiratory system can be viewed simplistically as occurring in three ways: absorptive transport, nonabsorptive transport, and a combination of the two. In reality, the circumstance of combined transport is probably the most frequent case, with the others representing the extreme conditions where one or the other transport phenomenon becomes small enough to be neglected. However, the problem is complicated by the lack of a rigorous basis for classifying a process as absorptive or nonabsorptive, notwithstanding numerous examples where the alveolar permeation of inhaled materials has been described according to these general working definitions. As normally used, it is clear that these definitions are based on an interpretation of a sequence of events; for example, if a material promptly appears in the blood after having been inhaled, it is evidence, a priori, of absorptive transport, never mind the extant evidence that some ions or monomeric forms are "slowly" absorbed, while some macromolecules and colloidal materials may be transported relatively quickly [12,53,79,85]. Although the working definitions are imprecise, they are useful in conveying the general order and importance of events.

This effort to account for particulate behavior in vivo can be refined to include some specific clearance mechanisms and their predominant sites of action. Absorption occurs throughout the respiratory system, although mechanistic information is fragmentary. The fact that the nasal mucosa can be a significant absorption site is often overlooked, but this must be appreciated without information on specific transport mechanisms [25]. Nonabsorptive transport mechanisms and pathways have received far more attention. The two major processes for clearing particles from the respiratory system are endocytosis, serving principally the alveolar region, and mucociliary transport, serving mainly the conducting airways. These processes have been the object of many studies [15,17,107,124] and recent reviews [58,59,79] and are dealt with in Chaps. 11, 12, 19, 20, and 21 in considerable detail. Nevertheless, it is useful to emphasize that little or no quantification has been made for the transport of a single inhaled material by either endocytosis or absorption. Mucociliary transport, particularly in the tracheobronchial tree, has been quantified, although some of the techniques used in, and the interpretations made from, such studies are open to question [80,83] (see Sec. II.B).

Viewing the respiratory clearance of particles in terms of absorptive and nonabsorptive transport mechanisms and pathways leads us to explore the possibility of a predictive classification of particulate matter into similar categories on some physicochemical basis or bases. Indeed this effort has met with some success. For example, the Task Group on Lung Dynamics [11] drew heavily upon the periodic classification of the elements in order to predict the behavior of different substances within the biochemical milieu of the lungs. Mercer [77] proposed that physical parameters of the aerosol distribution and a nonequilibrium solubility measurement (in vitro) of the material could provide quantitative retention predictions. Others [85,88] have shown the value of special ultrafiltration and solubility studies.

C. Methods and Limitations of Clearance Measurements

Ideally, the measurement of retention depends upon determining the persistence of an inhaled material at its deposition site as a function of time. The temporal changes in retention are expressed as a fraction of the initial value either on an absolute or relative scale. Since there is ample evidence that the clearance rates from a given functional area and by a given removal process are not greatly influenced by the absolute amounts of particulate matter present, it would appear that either basis of expression can be justified [14,35,86]; some important exceptions have been noted, however [64,79].

Most of the modern studies of particulate clearance in man have depended upon radioactively tagged "inert" particles. This approach has the singular advantage of providing many measurements in the same subject. In laboratory animals, a greater variety of inhaled materials has been used, but radioisotopes were generally involved. In some studies of experimental animals, especially where nonradioactive materials were utilized, the standard retention procedure is serial sacrifice and analytical recovery of the inhaled material. This approach normally requires many animals and, accordingly, provides highly variable data.

Technically, external measurements of gamma photons from radioactive isotopes within the lungs are relatively simple and these can be expressed quantitatively when the initial deposition pattern is reasonably well known or determinable, i.e., can be reproduced with known amounts of radioactivity in an appropriate chest phantom.

As a practical matter in human retention measurements, it is necessary to rely heavily upon the time course of clearance events for their identification and interpretation. As will be discussed more fully in Secs. II.B,C, it is an accepted practice to separate tracheobronchial and alveolar clearance events purely on the basis of the observed clearance rates. In Fig. 1, this practice is portrayed by a hypothetical set of data from two subjects exposed to a radioactive monodisperse aerosol having aerodynamic diameters, d_a, of 6 μm and 3 μm, respectively.

The prolonged retention phases, which have become clearly evident by 24 hr postexposure, can be extrapolated to zero time and the intercept values utilized as estimates of the initial alveolar deposition. For separation of the "tracheobronchial" portion of the curves, the alveolar component must be "stripped" from the net curve. This has been accomplished graphically in the case of the 3 μm data; the exponential alveolar clearance phase is thereby described by an intercept value of 55% and a slope with an effective half-time of $\geqslant$76 hr. It should be noted, however, that this illustrative case is based on data collected over a period of time entirely too brief for an accurate estimation of alveolar (or lung) clearance.

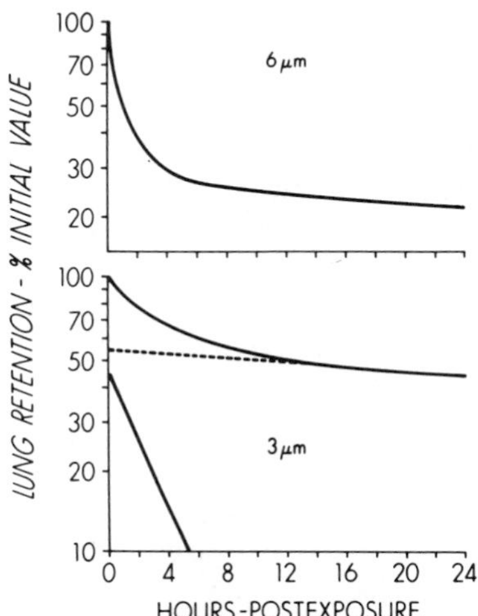

FIGURE 1 Clearance curves. The upper graph depicts a typical exponential retention curve obtained by serial measurements of thoracic activity subsequent to the oral breathing and deposition of uniformly sized particles of 6 μm aerodynamic diameter (d_a) labeled with a gamma-emitting radiosotope. Alveloar retention can be estimated from such data by the technique indicated in the lower graph based on particles of 3 μm d_a. Here, the alveolar retention phase is extrapolated back to zero time to obtain the initial alveolar deposition. Values from the resulting straight line are subtracted from those on the measured curve to obtain the initial clearance phase. In this example, the rapid TB phase has a half-time of 2.5 days and an intercept of 45%; the alveolar retention X(t) can be expressed by the following equation:

$$X(t) = 0.55 \exp(-0.00912t)$$

where t is in days. Using the same procedure on the 6 μm data would reveal only 26% of the initial deposition in the alveolar region.

All such retention measurements invariably reflect differential rates of radioisotopic removal and the time course of radioactive measurements may be made more complex by rearrangements of radioactivity within the thoracic volume, as well as by multiple processes affecting clearance. Consequently, two types of external counting systems have been developed: one makes use of one large detector or a number of small (e.g., 2 in. diam) scintillation detectors set in a planar array so that zonal clearance may be measured; these may be part of a gamma camera or have collimated detectors and individual outputs. The second system generally utilizes a multidetector array arranged circumferentially about the thorax so that the combined output of the detectors is relatively insensitive to the distribution of radioactivity within the thorax. The two systems have distinctive merits and limitations [4,87]. Analogous detection systems have been developed for the nasal airways [71,100,125].

Recently, two new approaches for measuring retention have been examined in intact experimental animals and these may prove to be increasingly important to human studies. Specifically, the use of serial radiography to examine the tracheobronchial retention of radiopaque materials has been reported [13,14] and at least one report pertains to human subjects [34]. Another possibility is suggested by recent studies of x-ray fluorescence [44], but so far a specific application to lung clearance has not been reported.

Whatever the measurement technique, there is little reason to believe that anatomically precise retention measurements have been or can be achieved. There are many limitations, but perhaps the largest and most convincing is that of simply ascertaining and delimiting the deposition site. This is an especially vexing problem in the intact subject, and only in certain areas is it simplified by working with dissected structures. Superficially, it may seem straightforward to remove the major bronchi and trachea from the lung lobes, but what of the balance of the bronchial tree? Is it possible to obtain either a bronchial or an alveolar tissue sample which is quantitatively meaningful on a practical basis? Apparently not. But, returning to the excised trachea and major bronchi—does this constitute a simple sample where the cleared or clearing material is within the mucus of the luminal surface? Possibly, but certainly there could be appreciable material within lymphoid tissue and in the perivascular and peribronchial lymphatics [81,127]. Without belaboring the point, it is necessary to appreciate the heterogeneity and intimacy of lung structures and the practical difficulties of isolating pure anatomical areas.

Given the possibility of harvesting alveolar tissue exclusive of the bronchial and bronchiolar airways, how definitive would the retention data become? Measurements of alveolar tissue en masse would fail to answer some questions; for example, if inhaled material is found interstitially, it has certainly been removed from the alveolar-air interface, but has it been "cleared"? Descriptions of particulate clearance are only slightly more tenuous and ambiguous when a gross analysis is undertaken, e.g., as by external counting, than when some of these "microscopic" problems are partially solved, e.g., as by dissection. We must woefully conclude that at most levels of anatomical organization and by any practical method known, the retention of inhaled materials within the respiratory system is crudely determined.

II. Kinetic Descriptions of Particulate Clearance According to Respiratory Region

A. Nasal Passages

1. Representative Studies and Clearance Descriptions

Two experimental approaches for studying particulate clearance in the nasal airways have been reported. The first, typified by the studies of Andersen and coworkers and Proctor and coworkers (6-8,100), is restricted to the measurement of mucociliary velocities (transit times) in those anatomical areas of the nasal airways which are ciliated, and the movement of mucus-borne particles is in a posterior direction (see Chap. 11). These investigations specifically avoided the more anterior regions, e.g., the vestibular area and external nares, wherein the mucosa is either transitional or devoid of cilia. These areas were avoided by manual placement of the radioactive particles into discrete locations and then following the particle movement by collimated, external, radiation detectors. Nevertheless, as a study of Andersen et al. [7] clearly reveals, there is a large variability in particle transit times despite the effort to place the particles initially at the same anatomical sites. These workers concluded that in the largest percentage of subjects (~60%), there was a prompt and continuous posterior migration of the test particles (0.5 mm diam) with an average mucous velocity of 0.84 cm/min (0.23-2.36 cm/min). The remaining subjects manifested slower and more erratic transport velocities with approximately 15% of the individuals exhibiting either very slow velocities or no effective particle motion at all [7].

A more recent analysis by Andersen et al. [8] designed to reveal the action of relative humidity on the flow of nasal mucus showed that in a group of normal subjects, the means determined for the mucociliary velocities were apparently log-normally distributed. The estimations of means were very consistent in three studies and could be described by a log-normal distribution with an overall median mucous velocity of 0.5 cm/min and a geometric standard deviation of ~2.0.

The second experimental method for measuring nasal clearance utilizes the study of particulate transport following deposition from an aerosol. In the main, these studies have made use of radioactive, monodisperse particles between 2 and 7 μm aerodynamic diameter [15,33,47,71]. These results, based on the initial pattern of deposition which is due largely to inertial impaction, give considerably different clearance information from the former studies since the principal deposition sites of such particles are in the more anterior nasal areas; consequently, most of these particles experience no mucociliary transport toward the naso- and oropharynx and must be cleared by extrinsic means. Depending upon the particle size, a lesser fraction of the particles deposits somewhat more posteriorly and these generally manifest transport rates characterized by biological half-times from minutes to hours. For example, in the study of Fry and Black [33], most of the posterior zone cleared exponentially with a half-time of 20 min or less, whereas the anterior zone manifests a half-time uniformly exceeding 3 hr. In the majority of subjects, the clearance of the anterior zone was even more protracted (>12 hr); these subjects, nevertheless, were generally found to be free of the radioactive particles on the day following exposure indicating that some extrinsic means of removal was invoked, e.g., nose wiping and blowing. It is appropriate to note here that mucous transport can occur in nonciliated areas. Hilding [42], Sadé et al. [105] and Taylor [116] describe this in terms of the traction exerted by cilia in adjacent areas.

2. *Kinetic Generalizations and Their Mechanistic Relationships*

At present, it seems premature to attempt a serious generalization of nasal clearance data. The available data are very limited and suggestive of a complex relationship between aerodynamic particle sizes, areal deposition sites within the nasal airways, and the resulting clearance patterns.

On the basis of the data of Black and coworkers [15,33], which are probably the most appropriate, it is possible to foresee a diphasic exponential description in which the anterior nose, probably corresponding to Landahl's areas 1 and 2, and evidently the most important deposition site for particles greater than 1 μm aerodynamic size, could be served by a single biological half-time of around 0.2 days. Despite the information on protracted retention, this clearance value is suggested by the fact that dust removal from the anterior zone is normally complete in 24 hr despite inconsequential mucociliary removal. The more posterior areas, which will cope with less aerosol mass are cleared by mucociliary transport and could be assigned a half-time of between 0.01 and 0.02 days. The data of Andersen et al. [6-8], Proctor and Wagner [101], and Quinlan et al. [102] suggest a value closer to 0.01 days. The relative weighting, given these two phases, will favor greatly the anterior zone and its slower clearance rate, and this would be probably a function of the aerodynamic particle size. For example, the data of Fry and Black [33] indicate a 0.85:0.15 relationship might apply to the retention functions obtained with the 2-7 μm d_a range of particle size. Thus, a general exponential expression

$$X(t) = 0.15 \exp(-69.30t) + 0.85 \exp(-3.465t) \tag{12}$$

is indicated, where t is expressed in days and the other symbols are the same as before.

The Task Group on Lung Dynamics created by the International Commission for Radiological Protection (ICRP) published its model for particulate clearance from the human respiratory system in 1965 [11]. The model was intended for use in radiological protection to control or limit the exposure of radiation workers. It can be applied, however, to many other areas of pulmonary research. That portion of the model which pertains to the nasal passages (NP) recognizes two clearance pathways working in parallel, an absorptive one termed a and the other, a nonabsorptive pathway termed b. A tripartite classification scheme based on the chemistry of inhaled materials was utilized to allocate a given substance to these two pathways [11]. For example, a material composed of dimensionally stable, "insoluble" particles, denoted class Y by the Task Group, is fractionated such that $f_a = 0.01$ and $f_b = 0.99$. Both clearance pathways were deemed exponential in character and assigned clearance coefficients λ_a and λ_b, respectively (Fig. 2).

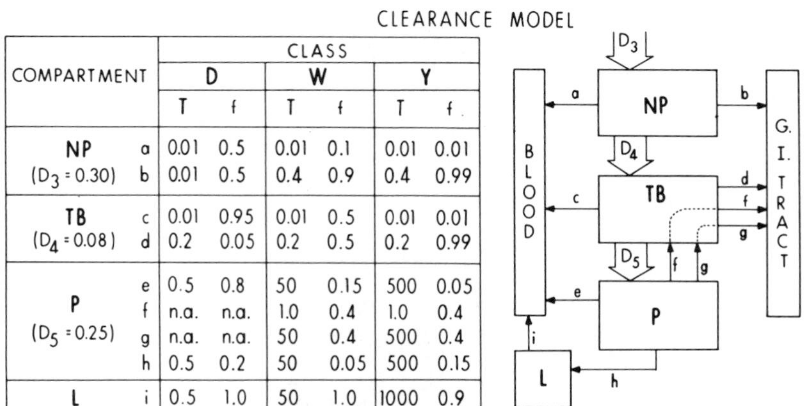

COMPARTMENT		CLASS D T	D f	W T	W f	Y T	Y f
NP	a	0.01	0.5	0.01	0.1	0.01	0.01
(D_3 = 0.30)	b	0.01	0.5	0.4	0.9	0.4	0.99
TB	c	0.01	0.95	0.01	0.5	0.01	0.01
(D_4 = 0.08)	d	0.2	0.05	0.2	0.5	0.2	0.99
P	e	0.5	0.8	50	0.15	500	0.05
	f	n.a.	n.a.	1.0	0.4	1.0	0.4
(D_5 = 0.25)	g	n.a.	n.a.	50	0.4	500	0.4
	h	0.5	0.2	50	0.05	500	0.15
L	i	0.5	1.0	50	1.0	1000	0.9

FIGURE 2 ICRP clearance model. The schematic diagram at the right depicts three respiratory compartments: nasal passages, NP; tracheobronchial airways, TB; and pulmonary parenchyma, P, and their clearance pathways, a-h. The lymph nodes are portrayed as compartment L with clearance pathway i. The tabular portion of the figure indicates the biological half-times, T and compartmental fractions, f, for each pathway and for materials in either of three classifications, D. W. and Y. The notation n.a. signifies "not applicable." This classification pertains to the relative retention behavior of the inhaled material, especially in the P compartment, i.e., biological half-times of days, weeks, and years, respectively. For planning purposes, a standard aerosol with a 1 μm mass median aerodynamic diameter is used, hence the deposition fractions D_3, D_4, and D_5 given in the left column.

The ICRP general retention equation for a single intake [Eq. (13)]:

$$X(t) = X(o) \sum_{n} f_n \exp(-\lambda_n t) \tag{13}$$

is utilized for the determination of the time integral of radioactivity in a compartment served by n clearance pathways. The specific form of Eq. (13) applicable to the nasal passages (NP), is

$$X(t) = X(o) \left\{ f_a \exp[-(\lambda_a + \lambda_r)t] + f_b \exp[-(\lambda_b + \lambda_r)t] \right\} \tag{13a}$$

where $X(0) = D_3$ of Fig. 2, i.e., the deposition fraction in the NP compartment. To the ICRP, the determination of dose is the paramount consideration, therefore the following form is used when integrating the exposure to some time t.

$$I(t) = X(o) \left(\frac{f_a}{\lambda_a + \lambda_r} \left\{ 1 - \exp[-(\lambda_a + \lambda_r)t] \right\} + \frac{f_b}{\lambda_a + \lambda_r} \left\{ 1 - \exp[-(\lambda_b + \lambda_r)t] \right\} \right) \tag{14}$$

when $t \gg 1/(\lambda_n)$, Eq. (14) simplifies to

$$I(t) = X(o) \left(\frac{f_a}{\lambda_a + \lambda_r} + \frac{f_b}{\lambda_b + \lambda_r} \right)$$

For ICRP applications, this is the customary circumstance since t is normally taken to be 18,250 days or 50 years, the assumed occupational lifetime of a worker.

As revised and presently utilized by the ICRP, the decay coefficients for the nasal passages λ_a and λ_b are based on half-times of 0.01 and 0.4 days, respectively. According to the model, f_a represents the fractional deposit following all absorptive processes in the nose, whereas f_b represents the fraction following the particulate transport pathways, viz., those associated with mucociliary activity.

Equation (13a) and Fig. 2 draw attention to the fact that the decay coefficients λ_a, λ_b and λ_r do not determine the magnitude of the compartmental fractions, f_a and f_b in the ICRP model. Were this the case, λ_a and λ_b would produce greatly different f values than those set aside for the NP region in Fig. 2. For example, with class W. and Y materials, the fraction of the deposited material following pathway f_a will be determined by $\lambda_a/(\lambda_a + \lambda_b)$ and that following f_b by $\lambda_b/(\lambda_a + \lambda_b)$; the respective compartmental fractions would be, therefore,

0.976 and 0.024, for both classes of materials. In the case of Class D materials, there would be a 0.50:0.50 partitioning among f_a and f_b since λ_a is equal to λ_b. By contrast, the values for f_a and f_b in Fig. 2 for Class W substances are 0.1 and 0.9, respectively, while those for Class Y are 0.01 and 0.99, respectively. Only with the Class D materials are the values of f_a and f_b the same as the clearance rate coefficients would determine.

The ICRP clearance model manifests two major concerns: (a) that the partitioning of material reflects the nature of inhaled material, and (b) that the rates of absorption and particulate transport reflect to a practical extent what is known about the overall removal process. These concerns ostensibly provide the basis for specifying the values of both the pathway fractions and their rate coefficients in the Fig. 2 model. Nevertheless, it is evident there is a workable alternative. Since the value of λ_r is constant for a given radionuclide and the value of a representative mucociliary transport rate, λ_b, can be assigned (and easily meet the needs of NP dosimetry), λ_a could be varied to accommodate various classes of materials and produce the proper fractionation of the material deposited within the NP compartment according to pathways a and b. For example, if Class Y materials were cleared by pathway f_a with a 40-day biological half-time ($\lambda_a = 0.0173$) and by pathway b with a 0.4-day biological half-time ($\lambda_b = 1.73$), this produces the desired results of negligible absorption and the 0.01 (f_a) to 0.99 (f_b) compartmentalization. For Class W, f_a could be governed by a 4-day biological half-time if the value of λ_b were kept the same, and for Class D the values for λ_a and λ_b would both be based on a 0.4-day biological half-time (or any other combination where $\lambda_a = \lambda_b$) provided the time integral was not found to be excessive for rapidly transported substances. Perhaps this alternative was not attractive to the ICRP in view of its slightly greater complexity, but it should be considered by those interested in physiological modeling.

Brain and Valberg [18] published a mathematical interpretation of the Lung Dynamics Task Group retention model (see Fig. 2). They adjusted the basic retention equation utilized by the Task Group, for conditions of *continuous exposure,* and applied it to all respiratory regions including the nasal passages (NP). Their general expression is as follows:

$$X_i(t) = r_i \sum_n \frac{f_{in}}{\lambda_{in}} [1 - \exp(-\lambda_{in} t)] + X_i(o) \sum_n f_{in} \exp(-\lambda_{in} t) \qquad (15)$$

The summation over n implies summing over all of the pathways clearing the ith compartment, λ_n are the biological (or effective) clearance rates for pathways carrying fraction f_n of the contained material, r_i denotes the deposition rate in compartment i, and the other symbols have the same meaning as before. When Eq. (15) is applied specifically to the NP compartment, it has the following form

$$X(t) = r_i \left(\frac{f_a}{\lambda_a + \lambda_r} \left\{ 1 - \exp[-(\lambda_a + \lambda_r)t] \right\} + \frac{f_b}{\lambda_b + \lambda_r} \left\{ 1 - \exp[-(\lambda_b + \lambda_r)t] \right\} \right) + X(o) \left\{ f_a \exp[-(\lambda_a + \lambda_r)t] + f_b \exp[-(\lambda_b + \lambda_r)t] \right\} \tag{15a}$$

where the symbols are the same as before.

The ICRP nasal model for single, pulse intakes, as well as the Brain-Valberg version for continuous intake, utilizes exponentials to describe both the absorptive and nonabsorptive clearance processes. Absorption from the respiratory mucosa, especially diffusive transport, is expected to be a first-order process [20,53] ; on the other hand, information on mucociliary transport within the nose provides little support for an exponential model. The available information suggests that, although the mucous transport is directed posteriorly, the more anterior and posterior portions of the nose exhibit very slow clearance rates compared to the central zone [9,71,126] . Treating these compartmental divisions as an entity would be expected to result in variable clearance rates according to the deposition pattern. Occasionally, on a happenstance basis, a deposition pattern might occur which would lead to a clearance pattern seemingly exponential in character.

A new ICRP task group under the chairmanship of T. T. Mercer [78] , after careful review of nasal deposition and clearance studies, attacked the problem by utilizing a nasal compartment consisting of four segments, basically those of Landahl [65] , and then calculating nasal deposition patterns at various mean airflow rates in the four segments for particles between 1 and 10 μm aerodynamic diameter.

The Task Group concluded that no continuing clearance of the deposited material occurred from segment 1 (the most anterior segment), although it was subject to clearance at the individual's discretion as noted in Sec. II.A.1. Segments 2, 3, and 4 were envisioned as being in a series arrangement so that, for example, the deposited material cleared from segment 2, with its transitional epithelium, would pass to segment 3 where it would be cleared according to the intrinsic, mucociliary transport velocity of that segment to segment 4. By assigning appropriate mucous transport rates to the various segments and stipulating their anatomical lengths, the transit time τ for material crossing each segment was estimated. For example, the value for τ_2 of 600 min is based on a pathlength of 2 cm. It is interesting to note here that the Task Group considered most of the available information on mucociliary transport in the nasal airways as pertinent specifically to segments 3 and 4.

Since inertial impaction is the major deposition process in their nasal clearance model, the Task Group assumed that particulate deposition within a segment was confined initially to the anterior edge of the segment. The subsequent posterior movement of the deposit was determined by that segment's transit time τ. Consequently, the exposure of a given segment j to a radioactive dust deposited at its origin will be

$$(\text{exposure})_j = X_j \left[\frac{1 - \exp(-\lambda\tau_j)}{\lambda}\right] \tag{16}$$

where X_j is the total activity deposited at the jth segment, λ is the radioactive decay constant, and τ_j is the appropriate transit time. This model assumes the exponential nature of the exposure is entirely vested in λ and the total exposure is governed by τ_j, provided the radioactive decay is not extremely rapid as compared to τ_j.

Similarly, subsequent ("downstream") segments will receive a radiation exposure from deposit X_j as will the jth segment from any deposit in preceding segments. Thus exposure for the jth segment can be expressed as follows:

$$X_j = \frac{1}{\lambda}(1 - e^{-\lambda\tau_j})\left[X_j + \sum_{i=1}^{j-1} X_i \exp\left(-\lambda \sum_{k=1}^{j-1} \tau_k\right)\right] \tag{17}$$

This newly proposed nasal model recognizes those subcompartments of the nose which have been identified in relation to deposition and clearance phenomena associated with "insoluble," uniform particles. Such a mucous clearance model based on an interacting series of three "escalators" running in the same direction each at an independent, fixed velocity seems to be supported by the collective experimental data. However, no single study has analyzed clearance events in all segments. For instance, the data of Quinlan et al. [102] and Tremble [126] were among those used by the Task Group for evaluating the transit times in segments 3 and 4; the work of Hilding [41] and Tremble [126] are cited as typical of the studies used to estimate τ_2. Thus the model produces some difficulties for the experimentalist who is interested in testing or exploiting the implicit aerosol and functional relationships of the model. For radiological protection, especially in the use of a model to control radiation exposures, the validity of the deposition predictions, the assumed invariability of segmental transit times and the universality of the anatomical dimensions chosen, are not points of contention, nor is there a technical problem of measuring the clearance events in the 4 segments of a human nose. Coping with segment 1 dosimetrically is undoubtedly a much more important concern.

B. Tracheobronchial Airways

1. Representative Studies and Clearance Descriptions

Several decades have passed since Findeisen [31] and Landahl et al. [65,66] developed their models for dust deposition in the respiratory system. Their efforts in relation to tracheobronchial (TB) deposition necessitated development of a systematic description of the airways of the lungs from which mean airflow velocities, particle transit times, branching angles and other necessary parameters could be estimated and generalized. Morphometric descriptions of the TB region continue to be objects of intensive study and frequently appear as bases for new analyses of airflow patterns, particulate deposition and related matters [40,46,95,98,131].

The functional aspects of the TB region, especially as regards mucosal absorption and mucociliary transport, were not studied and developed simultaneously with the deposition models; in fact, it has been due mainly to aerosol studies within the past decade that we have our present understanding of TB clearance in man. In roughly chronological order, some of the significant human studies on dust removal from the tracheobronchial region include: Albert and Arnett [1], Toigo et al. [125], Wagner et al. [129], Luchsinger et al. [75], Albert et al. [2-4], Morrow et al. [80,86,87], Booker et al. [16], Sanchis et al. [106], Camner and Philipson [21], Camner et al. [22], Newhouse et al. [90], and Barton and Lourenco [10]. In the past few years numerous studies of constitutional, pharmacological, and environmental factors affecting TB clearance in man have also been reported [22,37,73,108,121,123].

The earliest clearance studies cited utilized heterodisperse aerosols, and certain aspects of these studies are discussed in Sec. III.A. Suffice to say that the later studies of TB clearance largely utilizing monodisperse aerosols, provided simpler interpretations of clearance events and clarified the relationships between particle size, deposition site and clearance behavior in the TB region. Even so, most of these studies were reported without any attempt at a mathematical formulation of the retention data. In contrast to the treatment of deposition data [72,78], most authors have been content to provide graphic presentations of their retention measurements utilizing a semilogrithmic plot and implying the general suitability of the exponential clearance description.

Aside from the studies cited, a wealth of supportive data on tracheobronchial functions has been obtained from studies on experimental animals, and, while these are too numerous to cite, several reviews and books consider many of them [72,107,114,115,129], as well as Chaps. 7-11 of this volume.

Another important source of information fundamental to tracheobronchial clearance has been the specialized studies of radon dosimetry [5,39,54,117].

Interest in this topic arose from the suspected association between atmospheric radon and a high incidence of lung cancer among miners. The important radiation sources in these exposures are believed to be the first several decay products of radon, which are both nongaseous and alpha particle-emitting. The dosimetric models developed were forced to consider, among other things, the thickness and motion of the mucous layer, since that was believed to affect the residence time of the daughter products in relation to the bronchial cells at risk. Although those specialized models are no longer accepted for radon dosimetry, they made a contribution to our knowledge of tracheobronchial clearance.

The constitutional or intrinsic variability of tracheobronchial clearance in man has been admirably described by Albert et al. [2] and Camner and Philipson [21]. Under what must be regarded as well-controlled conditions of exposure to uniformly sized aerosols, Albert et al. showed that the "90% clearance time" (the time for 90% of the overall bronchial clearance to be completed following the administration of a test aerosol) generally had a standard deviation (σ) of about 30% among subjects of different smoking habits and sex. Within more uniform groups, e.g., female, cigarette smokers, the variability was substantially reduced, but σ generally exceeded 17%. Their data summaries also suggest that an individual's variability is substantially smaller than the variability within a group of individuals of similar smoking habits and sex.

Another interesting relationship demonstrated by Albert et al. [2] was one between the 24 hr clearance values, tracheobronchial deposition, and an impaction parameter, $\rho d^2 Q$ (this parameter is derived from the particle mass and the average airflow velocity during inspiration). In this study two particle sizes were breathed sequentially and the amount of each retained 24 hr after deposition was measured. To the authors, this indicated that the *relative* dimensions of the bronchial tree with respect to generation level were constant except for proportional differences in airway caliber among subjects. This conclusion necessitates that different clearance rates apply to different generation levels in a consistent way. The concept that mucociliary transport is a physiological process having different rates at different levels of bronchial organization so that differences in the rates of clearance of "insoluble particles" within the bronchial tree can be related to their site of deposition [72,78,80,82] is of major significance. That more than one rate of clearance is manifest after inhaling particles of a specific and uniform size, reflects the fact that particulate deposition is never precisely limited to a single generation level.

On the basis of clearance measurements from subjects exposed either to monodisperse or heterodisperse radioactive aerosols, Morrow [82] described the resulting measurements of thoracic retention by the sum of four exponentials, three of these pertained to the tracheobronchial airways. It was evident from the treatment of their data and also that done by others, especially

Newhouse et al. [90] and Sanchis et al. [106], that zonal clearance constants could be assigned the hilar, central, and peripheral areas of the thoracic field. With aerosols of small size, ~2 μm MMAD, (mass median aerodynamic diameter), the hilar deposition was so limited as to reduce the number of exponential terms required to describe the overall TB clearance to two. Similarly, with 10-15 μm particles (oral breathing), deposition in the hilar and midzone regions was found to be so dominant that often only one term was needed to describe the totality of clearance. While it was recognized that the TB zones were somewhat arbitrary and determined by the external detector configuration, and that they lacked uniformity and uniqueness with respect to anatomical structures, they did apparently provide an adequate demarcation of the large, medium, and fine bronchial structures.

The multiexponential expression for TB retention alluded to has the same basic form as Eq. (13), i.e.,

$$X(t) = a \exp(-\lambda_1 t) + b \exp(-\lambda_2 t) + c \exp(-\lambda_3 t) + d \exp(-\lambda_4 t) \qquad (18)$$

where λ_{1-3} can be imagined as either the intrinsic removal coefficients of the TB zones or their effective coefficients when a radionuclide is concerned. The parameter λ_4 applies only to alveolar retention. The values assigned to λ_1, λ_2, and λ_3 were 1.4 hr^{-1}, 0.28 hr^{-1}, and 0.14 hr^{-1}, respectively, and these are considered constant under normal conditions. With either a heterodisperse or monodisperse aerosol, the relative fractions a-d will vary according to the size of the aerosol MMAD), but their sum is always 1.0. In practice, a given thoracic clearance curve can be analyzed in the manner of Fig. 1 and zonal depositions computed retrospectively.

Another description of tracheobronchial clearance suggested by Morrow [82,83] is the simple power function. This was reported as appropriate to describe clearance events in most subjects for up to 24 hr postexposure, the duration of clearance events generally accepted as tracheobronchial. The basic equation has already been discussed in Sec. I.A, viz.,

$$X(t) = X(1)t^{-\lambda} \qquad (19)$$

where X(1) is the amount present (retained) 1 hr postexposure, t is the subsequent time in hours, and λ is a constant. In all the studies analyzed, the exposure durations were less than 5 min and the monodisperse aerosols were administered by mouth breathing. In analyses reported earlier [80,82] it was proposed that the values of X(1) and λ depended upon the aerodynamic particle size, d_a. On the basis of a few limited comparisons with heterodisperse aerosols, the parameter MMAD was found similarly relatable to X(1) and λ.

The data from another group of important studies of dust clearance in man have relied entirely on single exponential descriptions. Camner et al. [23]

reported on the tracheobronchial clearance of 6-7 μm, d_a, fluorocarbon particles labeled with ^{18}F. These studies were limited to about 2 hr postexposure during which 80% or more of the activity was eliminated. Measurements were made on the same individuals on two separate occasions a day or more apart and the patterns were found to be highly reproducible in a given subject. Between-subject variations were substantially larger: in six male subjects the biological half-time of this early clearance ranged between 11 and 60 min with a geometric mean of 24.3 min. Astonishingly, two female subjects manifest clearance half-times ranging between 3.0 and 7.3 min with the same aerosol and conditions of exposure, again emphasizing the remarkable variability encountered among subjects.

In a study with Philipson, Camner reported measurements on ^{99m}Tc-labeled plastic spheres at different breathing rates and different particle sizes [21]. This study showed that as the particle size increased from 4.0 to 7.8 μm, the TB clearance half-times decreased substantially. Increasing the mean airflow velocity during inspiration of a constant aerosol size produced a similar decrease in clearance half-times. Both of these demonstrations clearly implicate shifts to earlier (more central) deposition sites within the tracheobronchial tree.

Measurements of mucociliary velocities in the tracheobronchial tree of human subjects were recently reported by Santa Cruz et al. [108]. These investigators employed a fiberoptic bronchoscope and filmed the movement of disks of Teflon sheet approximately 0.7 mm diam. In 16 normal subjects, the average velocity was 21.5 mm/min (σ 5.5) and the average maximal velocity noted was 35.6 mm/min (σ 12.4). These velocities are in marked distinction to those in patients with obstructive lung disease where the same measurements were 1.7 mm/min (σ 0.8) and 4.3 mm/min (σ 2.4), respectively. Such data add to the credibility of current models and strongly indicate the value of kinetic analyses in the diagnosis and therapy of lung disease.

Recent studies by Lourenco et al. [74], Goldberg and Lourenco [36], Thomson and Pavia [122], Barton and Lourenco [10], and Matthys et al. [76] do not contribute quantitative data on TB transport per se, but like earlier studies by Thomson and Pavia [121] and Morrow et al. [87], they demonstrate that assessments of tracheobronchial clearance in normal subjects and in patients with respiratory disease depend upon changes in the rate and the regularity of clearance which are largely secondary to altered TB deposition patterns rather than to mucociliary dysfunction. Recognition of this fact has led Dolovich et al. [26] to propose a special index to assist in the analysis of tracheobronchial clearance data in certain clinical conditions.

Recent studies by Iravani [51,52] of mucociliary function in rats challenge the present view of a continuous mucous coating on the airway epithelium. It is unclear if this condition is unique to the rat; consequently its impact on kinetic interpretations of tracheobronchial clearance in man is completely obscure.

2. Kinetic Generalizations and Their Mechanistic Relationships

The mathematical description of tracheobronchial clearance in man proposed by the Task Group on Lung Dynamics [11] is based largely on animal experimentation. It envisioned tracheobronchial clearance as two "parallel" processes, each describable by a single exponential expression. For example, with materials of limited solubility (the Task Group's Class Y), a small fraction (0.01) of the particles deposited in the tracheobronchial region will be removed by an absorptive pathway (f_c) with a biological half-time of 0.01 days ($\lambda_c = 69.3$), while most of the material (0.99) is depicted as following a nonabsorptive process f_d equivalent to mucociliary transport. The removal rate of the f_d pathway, λ_d, is based on a 0.2 day biological half-time.

The value of 3.46 day^{-1} for λ_d was selected so as to provide a conservative, simplifying substitute for the several constants usually needed to describe mucociliary clearance in the bronchial tree [48]. For dosimetric purposes, the ICRP utilizes the following form in which the time integral of activity following a single brief intake is calculated for t = 50 years:

$$I(t) = X(o)\left(\frac{f_c}{\lambda_c + \lambda_r} + \frac{f_d}{\lambda_d + \lambda_r}\right) \tag{20}$$

where X(0) is the same as D_4 of Fig. 2 and denotes the fraction of the intake deposited initially in the TB compartment.

It should be noted that the decay coefficients λ_c and λ_d do not determine the compartmental fractions f_c and f_d. A similar constraint was discussed in Sec. II.A.2 for the ICRP model of the NP compartment and an alternative strategy was pointed out.

Since in all inhalation exposures, some fraction of the inhaled material will be deposited in the alveolated areas of the lung (D_P), it is necessary to account for the clearance of this material which utilizes the tracheobronchial tree. Portions of D_P which follow pathways f_f and f_g are subject to alveolar clearance rates λ_f and λ_g, respectively, and both result in material being conducted through the TB region by nonabsorptive transport having a transit time determined by λ_d (refer to Fig. 2). Thus, alveolar deposition brings about a second expression of TB exposure which must be added to Eq. (20), viz.,

$$I(t) = D_P\left(\frac{f_f\lambda_f}{\lambda_f + \lambda_r} + \frac{f_g\lambda_g}{\lambda_g + \lambda_r}\right)\frac{1}{\lambda_d + \lambda_r} \tag{21}$$

In the foregoing expression, the term within brackets is the amount of the alveolar deposit following removal processes $f_f\lambda_f$ and $f_g\lambda_g$, respectively, while the unbracketed term is the effective transport time through the tracheobronchial tree. The translocated material, which produces the TB exposure according to Eq. (21), is recognized in most tracheobronchial studies. One of the major difficulties with the interpretation of tracheobronchial data is to differentiate between these two deposits and their subsequent tracheobronchial clearance which undoubtedly overlap in time and vary in prominence.

According to the present version of the ICRP lung model [50] λ_f is based on a biological half-time of 1.0 day, but the value of λ_g is determined by the clearance classification of the inhaled material. For example, with most "poorly soluble" materials, λ_g will be based on a biological half-time from weeks to years. This conforms to the generally accepted viewpoint that alveolar retention of inert, "insoluble" particles (the usual test system employed in human studies) is orders of magnitude more protracted than retention in the tracheobronchial tree.

Brain's and Valberg's analysis of the Lung Dynamics model has been cited [Sec. II.A, Eq. (15)]. Their general retention equation for continuous intake can be expressed for the TB compartment as follows:

$$X(t) = r\left(\frac{f_c}{\lambda_c + \lambda_r}\left\{1 - \exp[-(\lambda_c + \lambda_r)t]\right\} + \frac{f_d}{\lambda_d + \lambda_r}\left\{1 - \exp[-(\lambda_d + \lambda_r)t]\right\}\right)$$
$$+ X(o)\left\{f_c \exp[-(\lambda_c + \lambda_r)t] + f_d \exp[-(\lambda_d + \lambda_r)t]\right\} \tag{22}$$

and the corresponding integrated form is

$$I(t) = rt\left[\frac{f_c}{\lambda_c + \lambda_r}\left(1 + \frac{\exp[-(\lambda_c + \lambda_r)t] - 1}{(\lambda_c + \lambda_r)t}\right)\right.$$
$$\left. + \frac{f_d}{\lambda_d + \lambda_r}\left(1 + \frac{\exp[-(\lambda_d + \lambda_r)t] - 1}{(\lambda_d + \lambda_r)t}\right)\right]$$
$$+ X(o)\left(\frac{f_c}{\lambda_c + \lambda_r}\left\{1 - \exp[-(\lambda_c + \lambda_r)t]\right\}\right.$$
$$\left. + \frac{f_d}{\lambda_d + \lambda_r}\left\{1 - \exp[-(\lambda_d + \lambda_r)t]\right\}\right) \tag{23}$$

where rt is the amount deposited by deposition rate r during exposure time t, and $x(0)$, λ_c, λ_d, λ_r, f_c, and f_d have the same notational meanings as in Eq. (20).

When the exposure is evaluated for 50 years, one obtains

$$I(t) = [rt + X(o)]\left(\frac{f_c}{\lambda_c + \lambda_r} + \frac{f_d}{\lambda_d + \lambda_r}\right) \tag{24}$$

These equations and Eq. (20) all neglect the contribution of the D_P fraction cleared by pathways f_f and f_g described by Eq. (21) and may significantly underestimate the TB exposure since the magnitude of this D_P fraction can exceed that of the tracheobronchial deposit. For example, with a 1 μm MMAD aerosol, 80% of the D_P deposit, which constitutes 25% of the mass inhaled will be translocated by pathways f and g; tracheobronchial deposition is only 8% of the mass inhaled, so in this instance direct deposition accounts for only one-third of the total TB exposure.

The ICRP model for tracheobronchial clearance depicts a single absorptive (f_c) and nonabsorptive (f_d) pathway, both being exponential in character. This obvious oversimplification can only be supported partially by basic mechanisms. As previously noted, absorptive transport often follows exponential kinetics (Sec. II.A.2). Nonabsorptive transport in the TB compartment differs substantially from that of the NP compartment in that there is a regular gradient of transport velocities in the TB compartment with the slowest found in the peripheral airways (~0.01 mm/min) and the most rapid found in the trachea (~1 cm/min); therefore, each subdivision of the TB tree can be considered as having a single linear or exponential transport rate, since over short periods of time they are virtually indistinguishable and equally useful for describing subdivisional clearance. When retention in the entire tracheobronchial tree is measured, the overall change with time is a conglomerate of subdivisional rates. In such a case, the rate-limiting areas of the TB tree are progressively more distal with time; therefore, the overall clearance rate becomes progressively slower. This changing clearance rate with time has been described satisfactorily by a multiexponential expression [80,82], but it lacks a mechanistic basis.

The power function description, while inadequate in matters of protracted exposures and often complicated in matters of integrated dose and initial conditions, provides a succinct description of tracheobronchial clearance. Implicitly, the power function equation indicates that either the clearance rate will change with time or that the amount of material within a compartment which is available for clearance will change with time. In the case of the tracheobronchial tree, the removal rate is time-dependent.

The appropriateness of the power function is further demonstrated by an analysis of recent data by Albert et al. [2] on normal subjects exposed while breathing at 14 respirations/min (Table 1).

The measured values of $\overline{\lambda}$ were obtained from graphic plots of the clearance data reported on normal subjects. The mean coefficient of determination $(\overline{r})^2$ for each group of measurements, indicates the goodness-of-fit of the experimental data to the respective power function equation computed therefrom using the basic form

TABLE 1 Relationship Between Power Function Exponent, λ, and the Aerodynamic Particle Size

d_a (μm)	$\overline{\lambda}$ (measured)	$\overline{\lambda}$ (estimated)	$\overline{(r)}^2$
<2	0.08 (0.06-0.09)	0.10	0.92
>2<3	0.13 (0.12-0.14)	0.25	0.84
>3<4	0.20 (0.15-0.23)	0.35	0.90
>4<5	0.39 (0.31-0.47)	0.45	0.95
>5<6	0.56 (0.41-0.74)	0.55	0.94
>6<7	0.65 (0.60-0.68)	0.62	0.97

$$X(t) = X(1)t^{-\lambda} \tag{19}$$

where X(t) is the retention at time t, X(1) is the amount retained at time 1 and λ is a constant. The relationship of $\overline{\lambda}$ to the particle size, d_a is found to be nonlinear but can be approximated by setting $\lambda = 0.1\ d_a$. Using this relationship, the estimated values of $\overline{\lambda}$ in Table 1 are based on the midsize of the respective d_a ranges used in the study. A relationship between X(1) and d_a can also be established, e.g., as d_a increases, X(1) decreases, but it is more complex and less reliable.

A potentially useful variation of the foregoing models comes from their amalgamation. For example, a form suggested by Tyler [128] permits the following retention equation

$$X(t) = \epsilon^{\lambda_1}(\epsilon + t)^{-\lambda_1} \exp(-\lambda_2 t) \tag{25}$$

where ϵ is a small time, t is the real time since exposure, λ_1 is a positive exponent, and λ_2 is the exponential decay rate. Committee 4 of ICRP [49] has suggested a similar form:

$$X(t) = X(1)(\epsilon + t)^{-\lambda_1} \cdot \exp(-\lambda_2 t) \tag{26}$$

where X(1) is the retention at $\epsilon + t = 1$. Both of these formulations provide a power function initially and exponential clearance at later times and thereby eliminate some of the problems associated with a simple power function, e.g., integrating from $t = 0$ to $t = \infty$. Nevertheless, neither of these expressions offers an improved mechanistic basis over the power function and both are untested in respiratory system applications.

C. Alveolated Structures

1. Representative Studies and Clearance Descriptions

There are two types of human studies of special appropriateness to this topic. The first was alluded to in the earlier discussion of airway clearance studies (refer to Fig. 1 and to Secs. I.C and II.B.1), wherein a demarcation in compartmental deposition and clearance was made by considering the initial rapid clearance phase to be tracheobronchial and the later, more protracted retention phase to be alveolar. Studies in which this technique was employed characteristically involved single, brief exposure to relatively "inert, insoluble" aerosol materials, mainly of value to investigations of mucociliary transport, airway patency, etc. In fact, most of these studies were directed at airway physiology and only incidentally included alveolar retention measurements. Nevertheless, this method can be applied to other exposures, e.g., the terminating exposure in a multiple exposure series, but compartmentalizing the deposition pattern may prove more difficult. If the alveolar clearance rate is the major research interest, the usual course of action is to avoid the initial clearance phase by waiting 24 hr post-exposure, or thereabout, to commence measurements.

Representative of the studies using temporal distinctions for determining alveolar deposition and clearance are those of Albert and Arnett [1], Albert et al. [3], Thomson and Short [124], Booker et al. [16], Morrow et al. [87], Newhouse et al. [90], and Lippmann and Albert [72]. Although most of these studies were only a few days duration, an alveolar phase is distinguishable; when it was described, a single exponential term was adequate. In most cases, no mathematical formulation was offered, only graphic depictions of the data on linear or semilogarithmic plots; occasionally, the percentage retention at specific postexposure times was tabulated and used for comparisons. In all cases, exponential clearance was either identified or implicit in the treatment of the data, but clearly, it was only regarded as a basis for describing empirically the measurements and was not concerned with either exploiting or elucidating clearance mechanisms.

The second type of human study has provided, in general, fewer exposure data but far more kinetic measurements pertinent to the alveolar compartment, specifically, the study of occupational exposure cases, especially those from radiation industries. Many such cases are tabulated in the report of the Task Group on Lung Dynamics [11], but more contemporary examples are available in such reports as Newton and Rundo [91] and Gupton and Brown [38], both concerned with ^{60}Co oxide. These two studies can be regarded as exceptional in terms of the exposure and retention data presented, but both are typical in the sense that the kinetic descriptions bear an uncertain relationship to the compartmentalization of the inhaled cobalt. The Gupton and Brown paper is interesting in its utilization of the ICRP model by which an analysis is made assuming that the total chest activity equals the sum of the lung and lymph node ^{60}Co burdens. The reports of both studies used multiexponential terms to describe ^{60}Co clearance over several postexposure years. In those studies, as in the others cited, clearance has been described by single or multiexponentials purely on the ground that it provided an adequate description of the lung retention measurements.

Human autopsy data should also be mentioned, although they have been generally disappointing in their contribution even to qualitative aspects of alveolar retention. However, a recent paper by Lewis and Coughlin [70] is comparitively outstanding. They reported the average recovery of acid-insoluble dust, termed "soot," from 146 lungs of male subjects was 1.2 mg g^{-1} fresh tissue, which is equivalent to ~1.7 g of soot per individual set of lungs. This value concurs closely with that reported by King et al. [61] also for the lungs of adult males not involved in the dusty trades. The mean age of the subjects analyzed by Lewis and Coughlin was 61.3 years and most had a history of smoking. While the lung content of soot in smokers did not differ significantly from that in either non- or ex-smokers, a positive dependence was evident between the dust content and age. A linear regression analysis of the retained concentration of soot in fresh tissue vs. age yielded a slope of 0.0172 mg g^{-1} $year^{-1}$ of life.

Unfortunately, there was no appropriate aerosol exposure, intake, or clearance information accompanying these autopsy data. The exclusion of large bronchial airways and the drainage lymph nodes from the recovery analyses may have caused an underestimation of the total retained soot. In any case, there is probably little to be gained from speculating about the atmospheric levels of soot, the deposition fractions, etc. which may have prevailed. The assumption of a constant rate of intake to the P compartment seems reasonable, however, so if we wish to presume the P compartment was subject to first-order clearance, as most short-term clearance data in man seem to suggest, then we can ask: Is a linear cumulative retention logical?

The question raised is a general one for differentiating zero and first-order processes since there are common circumstances in which a first-order process seems linear. As the soot retention kinetics are not subject to experimental manipulations, we must tentatively conclude that the linear buildup of lung soot will gradually change with time and approach a steady-state retention value (perhaps at age 150?). Phrased another way, if the P compartment clearance half-time for "soot" was 50 years or longer in these subject(s), the autopsy data would hardly be expected to reveal its nonlinearity over the life span of the average subject, taking into account the statistical variabilities manifest; thus the autopsy data are compatible with exponential clearance.

Information from nonhuman sources has also contributed to our present understanding of alveolar retention. A very valuable resource has been experimental data from inhalation studies in laboratory animals, especially since the patterns of clearance are often found to be similar in several species. Also, because it has been recognized that the physicochemical nature of the inhaled material is often the primary determinant of alveolar clearance, an increased use of animal and in vitro studies concerned with physicochemical processes has ensued. These include demonstrations of consistent alveolar clearance kinetics for a given material [35], similarities between intramuscular and alveolar retention times [85,120], correlations between clearance half-times and nonequilibrium solubility measurements [77,84], and correlations between clearance half-times and other properties of the inhaled materials [24,57,88,112].

As in the other cases discussed, the kinetic descriptions which have been associated with the physicochemical studies have been largely empirical. For example, Morrow et al. [88] demonstrated a parallelism between the alveolar clearance and an ultrafiltration test of the same aerosol materials, viz., mercuric oxide, manganese dioxide, ferric oxide, and uranium dioxide. The alveolar clearance coefficients, λ_{alv}, determined for the different materials in dogs were as follows:

$$H_gO(\lambda_{alv}) = 0.021 \text{ day}^{-1}; \qquad MnO_2(\lambda_{alv}) = 0.017 \text{ day}^{-1};$$

$$Fe_2O_3(\lambda_{alv}) = 0.011 \text{ day}^{-1}; \qquad UO_2(\lambda_{alv}) = 0.0038 \text{ day}^{-1}$$

whereas the fractions of the respective materials suspended in bovine serum, which passed through an ultrafilter under specified conditions were: H_gO-0.70; MnO_2-0.30; Fe_2O_3-0.15; and UO_2-<0.01. A comparison of clearance coefficients and ultrafiltration fractions yields a variable ratio, but the respective rankings are identical and supportive of "solubilization" as a dominant clearance mechanism. After studying 20 additional aerosol materials by the same techniques, a partially successful attempt to organize this information was made (Fig. 11 in Ref. 85). An analogous investigation of uranium compounds by Steckel and West [112] also established a presumptive relationship between solubilities ("half-dissolving times") and lung retention times.

Other studies of relevance to particulate removal mechanisms in the lung parenchyma include those directed at specific clearance mechanisms such as endocytosis, macrophage mobilization, lymphatic uptake, and alveolar permeability, but since major sections of this monograph consider these topics (see Parts IV and V), these will only be briefly alluded to and in the light of their potential value to kinetic analyses. For example, estimates of the output of "alveolar free cells," which are presumably alveolar macrophages, by Spritzer et al. [111] and Brain [17] of approximately 2×10^6 cells/hr are vitally important data, as is the information on cytodynamics of the respiratory tract typified by the work of Shorter et al. [109] and the recent studies of Normann [92,93] on the kinetics of phagocytosis. Normann's analysis of phagocytic uptake of particulate matter injected intravenously provides another interesting case of zero- and first-order kinetics [92].

2. *Kinetic Generalizations and Their Mechanistic Relationships*

The ICRP model (Fig. 2), describes particulate clearance from the pulmonary parenchyma (P) as a three-component process: transport into the blood across the alveolar membrane (f_e); transport into the blood via the pulmonic lymphatic drainage (f_h); and particulate transport based on the alveolar macrophage coupled to the mucociliary transport within the tracheobronchial tree. The latter pathway is envisioned as consisting of two components, f_f and f_g, which differ in magnitude and in their associated clearance coefficients λ_f and λ_g. In such a model, the rate constants $\lambda_{e\text{-}h}$ cannot be utilized to determine the compartmental fractions, $f_{e\text{-}h}$, as suggested for the simpler cases of the tracheobronchial and nasal compartments. The P compartment must be considered subcompartmentalized in order to provide for the equal and substantial fractions, f_f and f_g, which are depicted as having very different clearance rates, 0.693 day^{-1}, and to favor lymphatic transport (f_h) over direct absorption into the blood (f_e) where the applicable λ's are the same.

As previously noted, λ_f is constant and equal to 0.693/0.4 day = 1.73 day^{-1}, but λ_g varies with the classification of the deposited material. Justification for the f_f and f_g fractions is based primarily on studies of the macrophage response to inhaled dust [17,32,64] and possibly reflects differences in resident and recruited macrophage populations. An exception is made for materials which manifest prompt absorption; for these particulate transport pathways f_f and f_g are considered inappropriate and the total alveolar deposit is assigned to absorptive pathways f_e and f_h.

Alveolar dust retention persisting for months and years is well-established. On intuitive grounds, endocytosis might be assumed the dominant clearance mechanism, but systemic distribution studies and the success of certain "solubility" models [77,85] in explaining alveolar retention, contradict this viewpoint. Thus, the ICRP model in assigning a 500-day biological half-time to Class Y materials indicates that the alveolar deposit is fractionated as follows: 0.05 represents absorption to blood, f_e; nonabsorptive clearance via the tracheobronchial tree, f_g, is 0.40; and lymphatic removal, f_h, accounts for 0.10. The balance of the alveolar clearance is by the more rapid macrophage removal, f_f. The alveolar clearance rates denoted by λ_e, λ_g, and λ_h are assigned the same value (0.693/500 day = 0.014 day^{-1}) as there was not adequate information available to assign independent rate constants to these pathways. The rationale of the P compartment model is based on the recognition of major pathways and the creation of reasonable compartmental fractions so that the correct amount of retention occurs in the tracheobronchial lymph nodes, fecal elimination is of the right order, systemic absorption and urinary excretion are of the expected magnitudes, and the overall pulmonary retention time is appropriate for dosimetry. Obviously these criteria are based on animal and human studies of many substances, from which distributional patterns have been broadly identified and categorized without the benefit of direct information on specific clearance mechanisms and pathways.

For the P region, the ICRP retention equation for a "pulse" intake is an appropriate restatement of Eq. (13), viz.,

$$X(t) = X_0 \Big\{ f_e \exp[-(\lambda_e + \lambda_r)t] + f_f \exp[-(\lambda_f + \lambda_r)t] + f_g \exp[-(\lambda_g + \lambda_r)t] + f_h \exp[-(\lambda_h + \lambda_r)t] \Big\} \qquad (27)$$

where all of the symbols have the same meanings as before.

Expressing the time integral of activity in the P region is completely analogous to the descriptions for the airways, viz., Eqs. (14) and (21). The 50-year integral is therefore

$$I(t) = D_P \left(\frac{f_e}{\lambda_e + \lambda_r} + \frac{f_f}{\lambda_f + \lambda_r} + \frac{f_g}{\lambda_g + \lambda_r} + \frac{f_h}{\lambda_h + \lambda_r} \right) \qquad (28)$$

Additional equations pertaining to lymphatic uptake (see Sec. III.C), total translocation of inhaled material to the gastrointestinal tract, total absorption into the blood, and the special case of daughter products, are available [18, 50]. While the ICRP model is simplistic, many of these translocation phenomena have rather complex descriptions so that a computer program is helpful. Committee 2 of ICRP has facilitated the use of the model in its new report [48] by computing the time integral of activity for hundreds of specific radionuclides in all respiratory compartments, and for each of the three clearance classifications which apply. For these calculations a standard particle size of 1 μm MMAD is used to determine the compartmental fractions and a single intake of 1 μCi is assumed. All calculations are listed along with a procedure which can be used to adjust the values for other aerosol distributions and intakes. Brain and Valberg have also created a useful nomogram for estimation of integrated exposure times using the ICRP model [18].

A unique alveolar clearance model, proposed by Mercer [77], is based entirely on physicochemical parameters: those determining the particle size distribution of the deposited aerosol, and a nonequilibrium solubility rate constant for the aerosol material determined in an appropriate biological medium. For describing the aerosol distribution, the mass median diameter and the geometric standard deviation (σ_g) are required. The solubility coefficient is determined in terms of the mass (grams) dissolved per unit time when standardized by the specific surface area of the aerosol (cm^2/g).

Mercer assumed that a particle of mass m would dissolve at a rate proportional to its surface area s according to the equation

$$\frac{dm}{dt} = -ks \tag{29}$$

where k is a proportionality constant having dimensions of mass per unit area per unit time. Since $s \propto m^{2/3}$, the dissolution equation may be written as

$$\frac{dm}{dt} = -\alpha_s k \left(\frac{m}{\alpha_v \rho}\right)^{2/3} \tag{30}$$

where the shape factors, $\alpha_s = s/D^2$ and $\alpha_v = m/\rho D^3$, are assumed to have a constant ratio, D is the particle diameter, and ρ is the particle's density. This equation may be integrated and arranged to give the mass of the particle at any time prior to complete dissolution as

$$m = m_0 \left(1 - \frac{\alpha_s kt}{3\alpha_v \rho D_0}\right)^3 \tag{31}$$

where m_0 and D_0 are the particle's initial mass and diameter, respectively.

The especially important and unique contribution of Mercer's approach is manifest when the solubility model is applied to a particulate population which initially possesses a log-normal size distribution, i.e., a distribution in which the logarithms of the particle diameters are normally distributed rather than the actual diameters. Such a distribution is frequently encountered with both natural and synthetic aerosols and has the general form

$$f_0(x) = \frac{1}{\sigma\sqrt{2\pi}} \exp\left(\frac{-(\ln x - \ln m)^2}{2\sigma^2}\right) \tag{32}$$

where x is a random variable whose logarithm is normally distributed with a mean m and a variance of σ^2 [19]. For an aerosol, x will be expressed as in some form of the particulate diameter, i.e., D (frequency), D^2 (surface), or

D^3 (volume); for clearance, the mass or volume distribution is normally considered. Mercer used Eqs. (31) and (32) to determine the total mass dissolution for a log-normally distributed group of particles and found that the mass fraction M/M_0 was an expression requiring numerical evaluation, where M_0 is the initial mass of the distribution and M is the undissolved mass at any time t. After calculating M/M_0 as a function of a dimensionless parameter β (= $\alpha_s kt/\alpha_v \rho D_m$, where D_m is the mass median diameter of the distribution) for several values of σ, he found the predicted dissolution curves could be described by a simple sum of exponentials of the form

$$\frac{M}{M_0} = f_1 \exp(-\lambda_1 \beta) + f_2 \exp(-\lambda_2 \beta) \tag{33}$$

in which $\lambda_1 \beta$ and $\lambda_2 \beta$ are exponents which govern the dissolution rate and f_1 and f_2 are the associated mass fractions. The values of f and λ are only functions of the geometric standard deviation of the distribution. Since β is a dimensionless function of time, when the physical parameters of the particles and the distribution are known, Eq. (33) expresses M/M_0 simply as a function of time.

Mercer noted that when $M/M_0 = 0.5$, all distributions have essentially the same value of β, namely, 0.6, so that a simple estimation of the clearance half-time for the initial long-term component is provided, viz.,

$$t_{1/2} = \frac{0.1 \rho D_m}{k} \tag{34}$$

when the appropriate units are expressed in grams · centimeter · days, and the particles are assumed to be compact spheres ($\alpha_s/\alpha_v = 6$).

Experimental verification of Mercer's solubility model has depended upon the foregoing equation correlating the solubility coefficient k and the biological half-time $t_{1/2}$ for alveolar clearance. The studies of Kanapilly et al. [57], Phalen and Morrow [99], and Morrow et al. [84] can be cited in addition to several studies described by Mercer. The methods used in these studies are similar. A sample of aerosol was obtained approximating that portion of the distribution which would deposit in the P compartment. Some of this material is then placed in a system with a simulant of interstitial or lung fluid, present either in large excess or continuously renewed. By sampling the fluid periodically, the mass of material dissolved per unit time (usually per day) is measured. Part of the selected aerosol sample was also subjected to a specific surface area determination by gas adsorption; thus k was expressed in g day^{-1} cm^{-2}.

Drawing upon the example of Kanapilly et al. [57], they determined that ^{90}Sr-labeled clay particles have a k (in vitro) equal to 3.2×10^{-8} g day^{-1} cm^{-2}.

When these clay particles were studied after inhalation, the alveolar clearance half-time was found to be 385 days, suggesting that the total fraction removed per day by all clearance mechanisms was 1.8×10^{-3}. Using other experimental information, they estimated that 9×10^{-4} and 1×10^{-4} were the respective daily fractions removed from the alveolar compartment by particulate transport to the GI tract and by translocation to the regional lymph nodes. The difference, $1.8 \times 10^{-3} - (9 \times 10^{-4} + 1 \times 10^{-4}) = 8 \times 10^{-4}$, was, therefore, assumed to be the daily fraction removed by dissolution.

Using the same basic development of Mercer, i.e., Eq. (29), they stated it in terms of the fraction of the mass dissolved per day, F, where

$$F = \frac{1}{m} \cdot \frac{dm}{dt} = \frac{1}{m} ks \tag{35}$$

with spherical particles, it follows that

$$F = \frac{k\pi D_m{}^2}{\frac{\pi}{6} \rho D_m{}^3} = \frac{6k}{\rho D_m} \tag{36}$$

where D_m is the diameter of the particle expressed in centimeters. For the experiment in point, ρ was 2.3 g/cm^3 and D_m was 1.1×10^{-4} cm. To obtain an estimate of the k (in vivo), we rearrange Eq. (36) and substitute as follows:

$$k = \frac{\rho D_m F}{6} = 0.383(1.1 \times 10^{-4})(8 \times 10^{-4}) = 3.37 \times 10^{-8} \tag{36a}$$

This value of k is quite similar to that obtained by in vitro measurements.

The foregoing case is more complicated than some in which Eq. (34) is used simply with the experimentally determined (in vitro) value for k; the predicted and measured half-times are then compared. This comparison presumes that essentially all of the alveolar deposit follows dissolution. This was apparently the case with uranium dioxide experiments, i.e., the actual lung clearance was quite closely predicted by Mercer's half-time equation [77], while tissue analyses taken at sacrifice revealed substantial amounts of uranium in the lymph nodes, and other analyses revealed preferential elimination of the uranium was via the gastrointestinal tract, inferring particulate transport via the bronchial tree [68, 88]. This paradox may be interpreted several ways: assuming that our view of the facts is correct, then the lymph node burden in absolute terms, might be regarded as too small or at least within the allowable error of the half-time estimate; the GI elimination could be presumed as biliary or to reflect the clearance

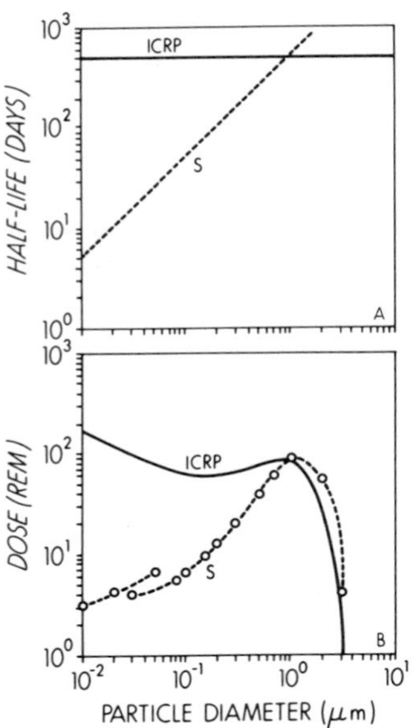

FIGURE 3 The surface area model of Parsont et al. [97]. (A) Comparison of the clearance half-times for $^{238}PuO_2$ particles as predicted by the surface area model (S) and the ICRP model. It can be seen that the S model predicts a P compartment retention half-time which varies with particle size, whereas the ICRP designation of a Y class substance places a 500-day biological half-time on PuO_2 in the P compartment, irrespective of particle size. (b) Comparison of the 50-year dose by the same models. In effect, the S model requires that the clearance classification for $^{238}PuO_2$ change according to the predicted solubility of the various particle sizes. The shape of the ICRP curve reflects only the deposition pattern in the P compartment. (Reproduced with the permission of the authors and the publisher.)

of lung secretions in which the dissolved uranium was continuously sequestered. An even more intriguing possibility is that the solubility concept somehow predicts the totality of alveolar clearance for certain materials when solubilization is not the only removal process or even the dominant one. Perhaps k is an index of the surface-free energy of the particle and that this is a key determinant in other removal processes, e.g., endocytosis.

Recently, Parsont et al. [97] compared Mercer's solubility model with the ICRP clearance model in terms of pulmonary retention and dosimetry. Their approach is illustrated by Fig. 3A.

The ICRP half-time for class Y material in the P compartment is 500 days; the variable dissolution half-times associated with particles of different sizes are also depicted for a class Y material, viz., ^{238}Pu, for which the k was determined as 10^{-7} g day^{-1} cm^{-2}, α_s/α_v was assumed to equal 10, and ρ equalled 10 g/cm^3.

For calculation of lung dose by the two models, a time-integrated air concentration of 1 mCi-sec/m^3 was assumed. As seen in Fig. 3B, the two models provide striking differences in the 50-year dose predictions when particles smaller than 0.5 μm are concerned, whereas for particles greater than 0.5, the lung doses are quite comparable. The dose calculations were based on monodisperse particles of different size rather than the more complex case of different MMADs associated with heterodisperse aerosols, each with different geometric standard deviations. While this demonstration with uniform aerosol particles dramatizes the size-effect inherent in the solubility model, it overestimates the effect which would be anticipated with heterodisperse aerosols, since increasing σ_g at a given mass median diameter will reduce the dissolution rate, i.e., increase the dissolution half-time. Nevertheless, the authors have made a valuable contribution in bringing these complementary concepts together.

Another important feature of the presentation of Parsont et al. was their emphasis on the indirect consequences of the small particle-effect. In the case of plutonium dioxide, the estimated bone, liver, and kidney doses were substantially increased, pointing to the possibility that a plutonium dioxide aerosol consisting of ultrafine particles might be so much more mobile than more conventional PuO_2 dust, as to change the organ receiving the greatest dose, for example, to shift it from lungs to skeleton. A similar effect would be expected with high specific activity forms of plutonium. Biological data comparing the retention of $^{238}PuO_2$ and $^{239}PuO_2$ in animals at a constant microcurie intake fully supports their contention [96]. Also, a study by Johnson et al. [56] with extremely fine $^{239}PuO_2$ gave short lung retention and high skeletal values compared to other PuO_2 data, again confirming their general thesis.

Too few data are available on alveolar clearance mechanisms and pathways to provide a detailed defense for the exponential descriptions advocated, e.g., Eqs. (27) and (33). In the ICRP model, several alveolar clearance processes are represented by a single rate coefficient which is intimately linked to the chemical nature of the inhaled material. We can support the assumption that exponential clearance is reasonable by a consideration of the underlying mechanisms; for example, the dissolution of a particulate distribution has been shown to be indistinguishable from an exponential process; it is known that absorption from the alveolar spaces often follows exponential kinetics [20,28]; and a probablistic model for macrophage-dust-particle interaction could give rise to similar kinetics [92]. Whether these processes are viewed as coexistent or one or another is dominant with a given dust, an exponential clearance description is clearly rational and has mechanistic bases. Unfortunately, at the present time we have no way of unambiguously measuring and quantifying these several clearance processes, nor can we assume they are exclusive in type and character, nor can we assign them to different materials in an enlightened manner.

If our view of several exponential clearance mechanisms in the alveolar region is correct, it is surprising that so many experimentally determined clearance curves, involving man and several other species, can be described by single exponentials [11,79]. Dominance on the part of one clearance mechanism might be plausible in isolated instances if, for example, it were determined entirely by the physicochemical nature of the material. In this regard, we might also challenge the ICRP values for the various pathway fractions in the P region; if we assume they are unrealistic, e.g., macrophage function might always be small or even trivial compared to absorption, then an alternative explanation for dominance might be available. Also, it is conceivable the complex nature of alveolar clearance is overlooked or misinterpreted by the assumption that the early, rapid, clearance phase is tracheobronchial.

Other uncertainties and examples of our inability to measure and interpret particulate clearance events have been discussed in Sec. I.C. Nevertheless, the fact that at least six orders of magnitude are needed to describe alveolar clearance half-times, viz., 10^{-3} to 10^{3} days must be stressed, and this fact should be appreciated in the context of known biological processes and their time scale. Obviously, much more basic information is needed on alveolar clearance mechanisms before these seemingly inexplicable matters can be understood. In the meantime, kinetic descriptions of clearance from the alveolar region will remain empirical and presumptive.

III. Special Clearance Considerations

A. Studies with Heterodisperse Aerosols

The discussion of clearance kinetics has emphasized data from investigations of monodisperse aerosols in the human respiratory system, especially the lower airways, because simpler interpretations of both deposition and retention measurements are provided in comparison to heterodisperse aerosols. Nevertheless, two models, whose raison d'être are heterodisperse aerosols encountered in the work place and the atmosphere, have been discussed in this paper, specifically, the ICRP model and the "solubility" model of Mercer. With the ICRP model, the mass median aerodynamic diameter of the aerosol distribution is used to determine the mass deposited in the NP, TB, and P compartments. Once this and the classification of the material is established, the clearance model is then applied (see Fig. 2 and Ref. 11). In Mercer's model, several parameters of the aerosol distribution are required including the mass median diameter, particle density, and geometric standard deviation. These physical parameters are utilized directly to predict the subsequent clearance behavior of the alveolar deposit.

The nasal and tracheobronchial models under development by a new task group of ICRP (see Secs. II.A,B, and Ref. 78) are also designed for use in the control of occupational exposures to heterodisperse particles. Consequently, they too must attempt to correlate deposition and retention phenomena with parameters of the aerosol distribution. The inertial properties of uniform particles may be used to estimate the deposition pattern, which, in turn, determines the appropriate removal pathways and rates. However, an additional step will be required to apply these concepts to heterodisperse aerosols. How this will be done is unclear, but it may be accomplished in a manner similar to that used in the present ICRP model in which the mass median aerodynamic diameter of the aerosol distribution serves as a singular deposition parameter, and the index of heterodispersity, σ_g, is ignored, since both a σ_g of 1.0 (ideally monodisperse) or of 3.5 (widely heterodisperse) are equally well described insofar as their mass deposition is concerned by the MMAD [11].

Any multiexponential expression useful for either compartmental or general clearance descriptions of monodisperse aerosols should be suitable for heterodisperse aerosols, although the probability of obtaining clearance data from a given compartment, e.g., the tracheobronchial tree, which are as characteristic and reproducible with respect to different particle sizes, is greatly diminished. However, in the clearance studies of Sanchis et al. [106] and Newhouse et al. [90] which utilized heterodisperse aerosols, the clearance patterns associated with a given aerosol distribution were sufficiently typical with respect to zonal deposition and clearance rates that notable differences could be established between normal and abnormal subjects. A successful application of heterodisperse aerosols to functional evaluations was also demonstrated by another earlier study [87].

The use of monodisperse aerosols must be preferred for the study of respiratory clearance functions, but kinetic analyses and descriptions which are applicable to heterodisperse aerosols are far more useful and relevant to environmental scientists, health physicists, and toxicologists. As a practical matter, well-controlled studies of carefully characterized, heterodisperse aerosols must be encouraged. At present, there are too few studies available in which the necessary degree of care has been taken; as a consequence, the assessments of the resulting clearance data as to consistency, mechanistic bases, etc., must be considered tentative. This experience could conceivably lead to an increased reliance upon heterodisperse aerosols in functional evaluation and to an increased awareness of the salient parameters which must be controlled and measured when experiments are correctly undertaken.

B. Single Versus Multiple Exposure Kinetics

The general equation from Brain and Valberg for the ICRP "lung" model [Eq. (15)] was referred to as appropriate to multiple or continuous intakes. Kotrappa [63] and Snyder [110] suggested slightly different formulations also directed at the ICRP applications. For example, in Kotrappa's version for continuous intake, the NP retention at time t would equal

$$rD_{NP}\left(\frac{f_a}{\lambda_a + \lambda_r}\left\{1 - \exp[-(\lambda_a + \lambda_r)t]\right\} + \frac{f_b}{\lambda_b + \lambda_r}\left\{1 - \exp[-(\lambda_b + \lambda_r)t]\right\}\right) \quad (37)$$

where r is the intake rate, e.g., μCi/day, and the other symbols are the same as before. This equation, unlike Eq. (15a) assumes that the NP compartment is empty when the continuous intake commences, and therefore the second term of Eq. (15a) is omitted. In addition, it should be noted that these equations for continuous intake are based on the concept that continuous-exposure kinetics are determinable from single-exposure kinetics, i.e., the systems are linear.

To check the validity of this assumption, it is useful to consider certain evidence on the two types of exposure. In a uranium dioxide study involving single and chronic exposures [68,69] there was a consistent finding in three species that the long-term (alveolar) retention half-times were a function of the duration of the exposure (see Fig. 4). With dogs and rats, a doubling of the post-exposure retention time was seen as the lung burden of UO_2 increased with exposure duration. This general finding has been reported by several other investigators [11]; it is to be contrasted with the negligible effect reported on retention despite enormous differences in absolute lung burdens and following different multiple exposure regimens when comparable postexposure times are compared [30]. It is also noteworthy that in both the acute and chronic exposure studies cited, no lung pathology was detected. Where investigators have reported a "mass" effect on retention after a single exposure, the exposure levels and lung deposits were extraordinarily high [62].

It is unfortunate that so few comparative data exist on the effects of different exposure regimens so that the general concept of postexposure retention time increasing with exposure time could be accepted, properly qualified, or rejected. Where it is known to apply, several kinds of factors may be operating [89] and most of these are mass related. For example, it is generally believed that some clearance mechanisms can be "overwhelmed" especially if the deposited material is cytotoxic [27]. An even more likely mass effect, and one possibly appropriate to UO_2 is that implicit in Mercer's solubility model. Mercer showed that if a given aerosol distribution was breathed continually and the rate of deposition was r (grams per unit β), then the undissolved mass M accumulated at some value of β is

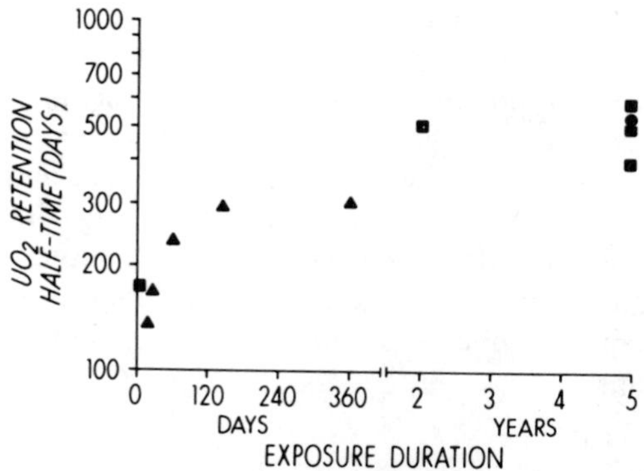

FIGURE 4 Lung retention half-times for uranium dioxide in relation to the exposure duration. In this graphic summarization, rat, dog, and monkey data are depicted by the symbols, ▲, ■, and ●, respectively. It can be seen that the post-exposure retention half-times for UO_2 more than double when single and prolonged exposure measurements are compared. The several dog values at five years are from different groups within the same study (see Refs. 68 and 69).

$$M = r \int_0^{\beta} [f_1 \exp(-\lambda_1 \beta) + f_2 \exp(-\lambda_2 \beta)] \, d\beta$$

$$= r \left\{ \frac{f_1}{\lambda_1} [1 - \exp(-\lambda_1 \beta)] + \frac{f_2}{\lambda_2} [1 - \exp(-\lambda_2 \beta)] \right\} \tag{38}$$

where the terms are the same as those in Eq. (33) from which this relationship is derived. At large values of β, M approaches an equilibrium value M_e given by

$$M_e = r \left(\frac{f_1}{\lambda_1} + \frac{f_2}{\lambda_2} \right) \tag{39}$$

The "solubility" model also predicts that the rate R at which mass M is dissolved equals

$$R = r [1 - f_1 \exp(-\lambda_1 \beta) - f_2 \exp(-\lambda_2 \beta)] = r - \frac{dM}{d\beta} \tag{40}$$

We see that the predicted rate of dissolution is affected by the amount of undissolved mass in the lungs although the parameters of the freshly deposited or inhaled aerosol remain unchanged. If and when M_e is reached, then R becomes constant.

Thus, we have substantial theoretical and experimental bases for rejecting the generalization that single- and multiple-exposure kinetics are linear. In the absence of an established systematic relationship between exposure duration and lung retention, the biomedical researcher should consider each case independently. There will probably be no impetus to overthrow the simple, linear concept as a tenet of toxicologic and radiologic protection, since it seems presently that the change in retention time induced by different exposure regimens might only involve a factor of 2 or 3. Also, the usual expectation, occupationally, is for irregular, acute or intermittent exposure conditions. However, in this era of increasing concern about public health, it is easy to foresee the need for developing continuous exposure models to contend with air pollution and other environmental problems.

C. Lymph Node Clearance

Chapters 3 and 17 of this monograph are devoted to the lymphatic system of the lungs. In addition, several reports [119,127] and reviews [37,67,81] have been published which are concerned mainly with the role of pulmonic lymphatics in particulate matter clearance. This apparent wealth of information belies our understanding of this clearance function, especially in any quantitative terms. There is more than ample evidence to establish the lymphatic drainage of the lungs as a primary clearance pathway. What circumstances cause its role to vary is unclear. There are those who consider any lymphatic transport of inhaled material as evidence a priori of cytotoxicity and the associated incapacitation of normal clearance mechanisms serving the alveolar region, thereby permitting the penetration of some inhaled material into the alveolar membrane [62]. In view of many demonstrations of both prompt and prolonged lymphatic uptake of "physiologically inert" colloids and particles, cytotoxicity seems untenable as a generalizing concept [81].

Whatever the mechanistic bases, lymphatic uptake of particulate matter has been evaluated mainly by nodal retention data, a dubious criterion, since nodal retention is not absolute, and quantitative harvests of lymph nodes are difficult, if not impossible, to achieve. Moreover, histological examination of lung tissue often reveals substantial amounts of retained dust in the subpleural, peribronchial, and perivascular lymphatics, and intrapulmonary lymphoid tissue so that correlations involving alveolar and lymph node levels of a material may be incorrectly based. Despite these uncertainties and shortcomings, there are numerous studies in which more than 10% of the initial alveolar deposit was subsequently recovered in the drainage nodes [119].

Several lymph node models have been described which are uniquely appropriate to the drainage nodes of the lungs. Collectively, they are of three general types: (a) purely empirical descriptions of the lymph node content with time; (b) mathematical formulations relating the lymph node content (or concentration) of a material to its alveolar content (or concentration); (c) the same approach as (b) except that the correlation is dependent upon a subcompartmental fraction of the alveolar material. In all of these pursuits, the principal objective has been to determine the lymph node dose. The apparent lack of interest in the buildup and clearance kinetics of the nodes is due to the technical difficulties of obtaining such data and the limited amount of mechanistic information which exists on the lymphatic permeation and transport of inhaled materials.

Recently a serial radiographic procedure was described by Kilpper et al. [60] and an innovative method of utilizing a solid state radiation detector within the esophagus in order to measure the radioactivity of the hilar lymph nodes was reported [113]. These new techniques portend increased interest in and procurement of nodal kinetic data.

A long-term, chronic exposure study of uranium dioxide was the basis of one of the earliest reported empiric descriptions of lymph node concentration as a function of exposure conditions [43]. These investigators noted that the logarithm of the buildup of the lymph node concentration of UO_2 with time, at a given exposure concentration, resembled a rectangular hyperbola, so they chose the following form to describe this relationship:

$$\log(LN_{conc} + 1) = \frac{t}{a + bt} \tag{41}$$

where LN_{conc} is the micrograms UO_2/g of fresh lymph node tissue, t is the exposure time in days, and a and b are empirically determined constants which were different for different aerosol concentrations and species. For example, the data obtained in dogs from a 5-year exposure (5 hr/day, 5 days/week) to a concentration of 5 mg U/m^3 could be described by setting a equal to 21.9 and b equal to 0.195. This formulation predicted a steady-state concentration in the lymph nodes of about 135 mg U; approximately one-half of this steady-state value was actually achieved in the 5 years [68].

These data and additional data from other UO_2 studies [69,89] were utilized by Mercer [77] for adapting his solubility model to the problem of lymph node buildup. For this, Mercer assumed that the rate at which mass is transferred to the lymph nodes is small compared to the rate the lung is cleared by dissolution. Following a single intake, the buildup rate for the lymph nodes would have the following form:

$$\frac{dX_{LN}}{d\beta} = k_n X_{lung} - \lambda_3 X_{LN} \tag{42}$$

where X_{LN} is the amount of material in the nodes, k_n is the fraction of the lung burden X_{lung} which is transferred per unit β, and λ_3 is the fraction of X_{LN} cleared from the nodes per unit β (refer to Sec. II.C.2 for a description of β). From this basic equation, the lymph node content resulting from a single intake can be derived, viz.,

$$X_{LN} = k_n X_{lung}(o) \sum_{i=1}^{2} \frac{f_i}{\lambda_i - \lambda_3} [\exp(-\lambda_3\beta) - \exp(-\lambda_i\beta)] \tag{43}$$

and for the continuous exposure circumstance, Mercer expressed the amount of material in the lymph nodes as follows:

$$X_{LN} = k_n X^E_{lung} \sum_{i=1}^{3} a_i [1 - \exp(-\lambda_i\beta)] \tag{44}$$

where X^E_{lung} is the equilibrium value for lung content [see Eq. (39)], a_i pertains to various functions of f_i and λ_i (see Ref. 77), and β is determined either experimentally or estimated from certain physicochemical measurements (Sec. II.C.1). In both Eqs. (43) and (44), the range of i is determined by the heterogeneity of the distribution (σ_g). For highly persistent materials, Mercer assumed the lymph node clearance coefficient λ_3 was essentially zero, i.e., nodal retention was infinitely long; this assumption provided a good fit to the experimental data on uranium dioxide. Mercer's model for the lymph nodes is unique in that it predicts that the buildup kinetics will be influenced by the particle size distribution within the alveolar deposit as well as the magnitude of the deposit.

Thomas [119] examined lymph node retention in experimental animals in relation to the postexposure time and the lung content of material. He assumed exponential lung clearance and proposed that the rate of lymph node buildup would be proportional to the lung content X(t) at time t, i.e., $dX_{LN}/dt \propto X(t)$.

The distinction between single and chronic exposure kinetics was in the values assigned the lung clearance fraction(s) and coefficient(s) which determine X(t). Thomas' model and the biological data cited in his development, tend to support the relationship expressed by the following equation:

$$\frac{[X_{LN}]}{[X_{lung}]} = 0.01066t^{1.095} \tag{45}$$

where $[X_{LN}]$ and $[X_{lung}]$ are the concentrations of material in the nodes and lungs respectively, at time t when t is expressed in days. This relationship presumably holds for materials which manifest prolonged alveolar and nodal retention times, e.g., +4 actinide oxides.

Thomas [118] also proposed an interspecies model for lung and lymph node buildup kinetics. The crux of the approach was a four-compartment lung from which the lymph node uptake was controlled by three of those compartments, each having vastly different λ's (day^{-1}), viz., 0.46 ~ 0.002 and 0.00007, respectively. Different species were envisioned, furthermore, to have different initial allocations to these compartments presumably reflecting certain species-specific characteristics of lung and lymph node retention. For example, dog lung retention (X_{lung}) was described at time t by the general expression

$$X_{lung}(t) = A_0 \exp(-\lambda_A t) + C_0 \exp[-(\lambda_C + k)t] + F_0 \exp[-(\lambda_F + k)t] \qquad (46)$$

where A_0, C_0, and F_0 are the initial amounts present in the respective lung compartments A, C and F; λ_A, λ_C, and λ_F are the respective compartmental clearance rates which transport material to other sites than the lymph nodes, and k is a clearance rate constant describing lung to lymph node transport exclusively. Lymph node (X_{LN}) buildup was described by

$$\frac{dX_{LN}}{dt} = kC + kF - \lambda_F X_{LN} \qquad (47)$$

where $\lambda_F X_{LN}$ describes the concomitant nodal clearance. Thus, only three of the four lung compartments are assigned to dogs and determine lung retention; only two of the three compartments affect lymph node buildup, however. In distinction, rodents are assigned four lung compartments; lymph nodal uptake depends on three of the four compartments [118].

Although Thomas suggests a possible structural and functional basis for each of the four lung compartments, they are more intuitive than real. Equipped with such a multiplicity of compartments and clearance coefficients, it is not remarkable that the model can reproduce "typical" lung and lymph node retention patterns and concentration ratios. However, in order to use the interspecies model, clearance data are needed which can be expressed quantitatively in terms of three or four lung compartments. Additionally, information is needed on interspecies distinctions implicit in this model, especially those which will enhance extrapolations from laboratory animals to man.

The ICRP model for the lymph nodes differs from those of Thomas and Mercer in that it develops from a subcompartment of the alveolar region (P); accordingly, the lymph node (L) content is determined by $f_h \int_0^t P\,dt$; thus the amount of material having entered L after a single intake is

$$D_P f_h \int_0^t \exp[-(\lambda_h + \lambda_r)t]\,\lambda_h\,dt = \frac{D_P f_h \lambda_h \{1 - \exp[-(\lambda_h + \lambda_r)t]\}}{\lambda_h + \lambda_r} \tag{48}$$

When $t >> 1/\lambda_h$, the foregoing equation simplifies to

$$\frac{D_P f_h \lambda_h}{\lambda_h + \lambda_r} \tag{48a}$$

It can be seen that only pathway h governs the transport of material from compartment P to the lymph nodes; the fraction of the P deposit, $f_h D_P$, is fixed for a given classification of material and independent of pathways e, f, and g which also clear P.

The ICRP model describes lymph node clearance in a simplistic fashion. Clearance follows pathway i for which, except for highly persistent materials (Class Y), f_i is assumed to be 1.0; for Class Y substances, only 0.9 is biologically cleared and the remaining fraction, 0.1, is assumed to be permanently retained within L and subject only to radioactive decay.

For dose calculations, Eq. (48a) must include this lymph node clearance and thereby the time integral of activity for material in L is expressed by the following equation:

$$I(t) = \frac{D_P f_h \lambda_h}{\lambda_h + \lambda_r}\left(\frac{f_i}{\lambda_i + \lambda_r} + \frac{(1 - f_i)[1 - \exp(-\lambda_r t)]}{\lambda_r}\right) \tag{49}$$

where t is taken as 18,250 days. For lesser times of integration, the first term of Eq. (49) is replaced by the form in Eq. (48).

Apparently Brain and Valberg [18] viewed the lymphatic portion of the ICRP lung model in a different light. Their equation for the integrated residence time of a material in the lymph nodes after a single acute exposure is

$$I(t) = \lambda_h f_h D_P \sum_s \frac{f_s}{\lambda_i - \lambda_s - \lambda_r}\left(\frac{1 - \exp[-(\lambda_s + \lambda_r)t]}{\lambda_s + \lambda_r} - \frac{1 - \exp(-\lambda_i t)}{\lambda_i}\right) \tag{50}$$

where the subscript s denotes all pathways clearing compartment P, viz., e, f, g, and h. It seems, therefore, that their equation differs from the ICRP concept in which $D_P f_h$ varies only with different depositions, D_P, due to change in particle size and different classifications of material. In other words, Brain and Valberg viewed the lymph node buildup as a function of the total alveolar burden as did Mercer and Thomas.

Additional and improved studies of lymph node kinetics are needed. Of special value will be experiments which reveal the nature of particulate clearance from the lymph nodes where presently, quantitative information is lacking. Attention should also be given the considerable differences in the lymphatic drainage of the lungs among various species and their impact on nodal kinetics.

Acknowledgments

This paper is based in part on work performed under contract with the U.S. Atomic Energy Commission at the University of Rochester Atomic Energy Project and has been assigned Report No. UR-3490-598.

Without the frequent discussions of this fascinating topic with my colleague, Dr. Robert W. Kilpper, and the many helpful suggestions he provided, I doubt that this chapter would have been possible. The author is also extremely grateful to Dr. Thomas T. Mercer for his constructive criticism and the opportunity to utilize some of the new kinetic models under consideration by his ICRP task group. Also, the excellent reviews of the manuscript by Drs. P. A. Valberg, J. D. Brain, D. F. Proctor, F. A. Smith, and L. Leach are gratefully acknowledged with the full understanding that all of the errors remaining in this paper are my own. Finally, but not least, my special appreciation to Ms. Alison Blum for her tireless cooperation through many revisions.

References

1. R. E. Albert and L. C. Arnett, Clearance of radioactive dust from the human lung, *Arch. Ind. Health,* **12**:99-106 (1955)
2. R. E. Albert, M. Lippmann, H. T. Peterson, Jr., J. Berger, and D. Bohning, Bronchial deposition and clearance of aerosols, *Arch. Intern. Med.,* **131**: 115-127 (1973).
3. R. E. Albert, M. Lippmann, J. Spiegelman, A. Luizzi, and N. Nelson, The deposition and clearance of radioactive particles in the human lung, *Arch. Environ. Health,* **14**:10-13 (1967).
4. R. E. Albert, M. Lippmann, J. Spiegelman, C. Strehlow, W. Briscoe, P. Wolfson, and N. Nelson, The clearance of radioactive particles from the human lung. In *Inhaled Particles and Vapours II.* Edited by C. N. Davies. New York, Pergamon, 1966, pp. 361-377.
5. B. Altshuler, N. Nelson, and M. Kuschner, Estimation of lung tissue dose from the inhalation of radon and daughters, *Health Phys.,* **10**:1137-1161 (1964).
6. I. Andersen, G. R. Lundqvist, P. L. Jensen, and D. F. Proctor, Human response to controlled levels of sulfur dioxide, *Arch. Environ. Health,* **28**:31-39 (1974).

7. I. Andersen, G. R. Lundqvist, and D. F. Proctor, Human nasal mucosal function in a controlled climate, *Arch. Environ. Health,* **33**:408-420 (1971).

8. I. Andersen, G. R. Lundqvist, and D. F. Proctor, Human nasal mucosal function under four controlled humidities, *Am. Rev. Respir. Dis.,* **106**: 438-449 (1972).

9. B. G. Bang, A. L. Mukherjee, and F. B. Bang, Human nasal mucus flow rates, *Johns Hopkins Med., J.,* **121**:38-48 (1967).

10. A. D. Barton and R. V. Lourenco, Bronchial secretions and mucociliary clearance, *Arch. Intern. Med.,* **131**:140-144 (1973).

11. D. V. Bates, B. R. Fish, T. F. Hatch, T. T. Mercer, and P. E. Morrow, Deposition and retention models for internal dosimetry of the human respiratory tract, *Health Phys.,* **12**:173-208 (1966).

12. K. G. Bensch and E. A. M. Dominguez, Studies of the pulmonary air-tissue barrier: Part Iv. Cytochemical tracing of macromolecules during absorption, *Yale J. Biol. Med.,* **43**:236-241 (1971).

13. H. Berke and L. M. Roslinski, The roentgenographic determination of tracheal mucociliary transport rate in the rat, *Am. Ind. Hyg. Assoc. J.,* **32**:174-178 (1971).

14. A. Bianco, F. R. Gibb, R. W. Kilpper, S. Landman, and P. E. Morrow, Studies of tantalum dust in the lungs, *Radiology,* **112**:549-556 (1974).

15. A. Black, J. C. Evans, E. H. Hadfield, R. G. Macbeth, A. Morgan, and M. Walsh, Impairment of nasal mucociliary clearance in woodworkers in the furniture industry, *Br. J. Ind. Med.,* **31**:10-17 (1974).

16. D. V. Booker, A. C. Chamberlain, J. Rundo, D. C. F. Muir, and M. L. Thomson, The elimination of five micron particles from the human lung, *Nature,* **215**:30-33 (1967).

17. J. D. Brain, Free cells in the lungs; Symposium on pulmonary responses to inhaled materials, an evaluation of model systems, *Arch. Intern. Med.,* **126**:477-487 (1970).

18. J. D. Brain and P. A. Valberg, Models of lung retention based on ICRP Task Group report, *Arch. Environ. Health,* **28**:1-11 (1974).

19. K. A. Brownlee, *Statistical Theory and Methodology in Science and Engineering.* New York, Wiley, 1965.

20. J. A. Burton, T. H. Gardiner, and L. S. Schanker, Absorption of herbicides from the rat lung, *Arch. Environ. Health,* **29**:31-33 (1974).

21. P. Camner and K. Philipson, Intra-individual studies of tracheobronchial clearance in man using fluorocarbon resin particles tagged with ^{18}F and ^{99m}Tc. In *Inhaled Particles III,* Vol. 1. Edited by W. H. Walton. Old Woking, Surrey, England, Unwin, Gresham Press, 1971, pp. 157-163.

22. P. Camner, K. Philipson, and L. Fribert, Tracheobronchial clearance in twins, *Arch. Environ. Health,* **24**:82-87 (1972).

23. P. Camner, K. Philipson, L. Friberg, B. Holma, B. Larsson, and J. Svedberg, Human tracheobronchial clearance studies with fluorocarbon resin particles tagged with ^{18}F, *Arch. Environ. Health,* **22**:444-449 (1971).

24. N. Cooke and F. B. Holt, The solubility of some uranium compounds in simulated lung fluid, *Health Phys.,* **27**:69-77 (1974).

25. R. G. Cuddihy and J. A. Ozog, Nasal absorption of CsCl, $SrCl_2$, $BaCl_2$ and $CeCl_3$ in Syrian hamsters, *Health Phys.* **25**:219 (1973).
26. M. B. Dolovich, J. Sanchis, C. Rossman, and M. T. Newhouse, Aerosol penetrance (AeP): A sensitive index of peripheral airway obstruction, *Fed. Proc.,* **33**:365 (Abst.) (1974).
27. H. J. Einbrodt, H. Kinny, and H. Kortemme, Quantitative Untersuchungen uber den Lymphtransport von Blei aus der menschlichen Lunge, *Arch. Hyg.,* **153**:105-108 (1969).
28. S. J. Enna and L. S. Schanker, Absorption of drugs from the rat lung, *Am. J. Physiol.,* **223**:1227-1231 (1972).
29. S. J. Enna and L. S. Schanker, Phenol red absorption from the rat lung: Evidence of carrier transport, *Life Sci.,* **12**:231-239 (1973).
30. J. Ferin and L. J. Leach, The effect of SO_2 on lung clearance of TiO_2 particles in rats, *Am. Ind. Hyg. Assoc. J.,* **35**:260-263 (1973).
31. W. Findeisen, Uber das Absetzen kleiner, in der Luft suspendierten Teilchen in der menschlichen Lunge bei der Atmung, *Pflügers Arch.,* **236**: 367-379 (1935).
32. M. V. Fisher, P. E. Morrow, and C. L. Yuile, Effect of Freund's complete adjuvant upon clearance of iron-59 oxide from rat lungs, *J. Reticuloendothel. Soc.,* **13**:536-556 (1973).
33. F. A. Fry and A. Black, Regional deposition and clearance of particles in the human nose, *Aerosol Sci.,* **4**:113-124 (1973).
34. G. Gamsu, R. M. Weintraub, and J. A. Nadel, Clearance of tantalum from airways of different caliber in man evaluated by a roentgenographic method, *Am. Rev. Respir. Dis.,* **107**:124-224 (1973).
35. F. R. Gibb and P. E. Morrow, Alveolar clearance in dogs after inhalation of iron-59 oxide aerosol, *J. Appl. Physiol.,* **17**:429-432 (1962).
36. I. S. Goldberg and R. V. Lourenco, Deposition of aerosols in pulmonary disease, *Arch. Intern. Med.,* **131**:88-91 (1973).
37. G. M. Green, Alveolobronchiolar transport mechanisms, *Arch. Intern. Med.,* **131**:109-114 (1973).
38. E. D. Gupton and P. E. Brown, Chest clearance of inhaled cobalt-60 oxide, *Health Phys.* **23**:767-769 (1972).
39. A. K. M. M. Haque and A. J. L. Collinson, Radiation dose to the respiratory system due to radon and its daughter products, *Health Phys.,* **13**:431-443 (1967).
40. J. Heyder, J. Gebhart, G. Heigwer, C. Roth, and W. Stahlhofen, Experimental studies of the total deposition of aerosol particles in the human respiratory tract, *Aerosol Sci.,* **4**:191-208 (1973).
41. A. C. Hilding, Ciliary activity and course of secretion currents of the nose, *Mayo Clin. Proc.,* **6**:285-287 (1931).
42. A. C. Hilding, Phagocytosis, mucus flow and ciliary action, *Arch. Environ. Health,* **6**:61-73 (1963).
43. H. C. Hodge, H. E. Stokinger, W. F. Neuman, W. F. Bale, and A. E. Brandt, *Pharmacology and Toxicology of Uranium Compounds,* Vol. 1, Part 4. Edited by C. Voegtlin and H. C. Hodge. New York, McGraw-Hill, 1953, Chap. 26.

44. P. B. Hoffer, J. Bernstein, and A. Gottschalk, Fluorescent techniques in thyroid imaging, *Semin. Nucl. Med.,* **1**:379-389 (1971).
45. B. Holma, Short-term lung clearance in rabbits exposed to a radioactive bi-disperse (6 and 3 μ) polystyrene aerosol. In *Inhaled Particles and Vapours II.* Edited by C. N. Davies. New York, Pergamon, 1967, pp. 189-201.
46. K. Horsfield, G. Dart, D. E. Olson, G. F. Filley, and G. Cumming, Models of the human bronchial tree, *J. Appl Physiol.,* **31**:207-217 (1971).
47. R. F. Hounam, A. Black, and M. Walsh, Deposition of aerosol particles in the nasopharyngeal region of the human respiratory tract, *Nature,* **221**: 1254-1255 (1969).
48. ICRP Committee 2 Report, *Limits for Intakes of Radionuclides by Workers.* Personal communication with J. Vennart.
49. Committee IV Report, *Evaluation of Radiation Doses to Body Tissues from Internal Contamination due to the Occupational Exposure.* ICRP Publication 10, New York, Pergamon, 1968.
50. ICRP Publication 19, *The Metabolism of Compounds of Plutonium and Other Actinides.* New York, Pergamon, 1972, pp. 5-9.
51. J. Iravani, Clearance function of the respiratory ciliated epithelium in normal and bronchitic rats. In *Inhaled Particles III,* Vol. I. Edited by W. H. Walton. Old Woking, Surrey, England, Unwin, Gresham Press, 1971, pp. 143-146.
52. J. Iravani, Koordination der Flimmerbewegung im Bronchialepithel der Ratte, *Plügers Arch.,* **305**:199-209 (1969).
53. A. T. Isitman, R. Manoli, G. H. Schmidt, and R. A. Holmes, An assessment of alveolar deposition and pulmonary clearance of radio pharmaceuticals after nebulization, *Am. J. Roentgenol. Radium Ther. Nucl. Med.,* **120**:776-781 (1974).
54. W. Jacobi, The dose to the human respiratory tract by inhalation of short-lived 222-Rn and 220-Rn decay products, *Health Phys.,* **10**:1163-1174 (1964).
55. J. A. Jacques, *Compartmental Analysis in Biology and Medicine.* New York, Elsevier, 1972, Chaps. 1, 4, and 7.
56. L. J. Johnson, P. N. Dean, and H. M. Ide, In vivo determination of the late-phase lung clearance of ^{239}Pu following accidental exposure, *Health Phys.,* **22**:410-412 (1972).
57. G. M. Kanapilly, O. G. Raabe, C. H. T. Goh, and R. A. Chimenti, Measurement of in vitro dissolution of aerosol particles for comparison to in vivo dissolution in the lower respiratory tract after inhalation, *Health Phys.,* **24**:497-507 (1973).
58. K. H. Kilburn, Clearance mechanisms in the respiratory tract, *Handbook of Physiology, Reactions to Environmental Agents,* Section 9. Bethesda, American Physiological Society, 1977.
59. K. H. Kilburn, Functional morphology of the distal lung, *Int. Rev. Cytol.,* **37**:153-270 (1974).
60. R. W. Kilpper, A. Bianco, F. R. Gibb, S. Landman, and P. E. Morrow, The uptake and retention of insufflated tantalum by lymph nodes. In *Radiation*

and the Lymphatic System, Proc. 14th Ann. Hanford Biology Symp. Richland, Washington, 1974, CONF 740930 (1976). pp. 46-53.

61. E. J. King, B. A. Maguire, and G. Nagelschmidt, Further studies of the dust in lungs of coal miners, *Br. J. Ind. Med.*, **13**:9-23 (1956).
62. W. Kosterkötter and G. Bünemann, Animal experiments on the elimination of inhaled dust. In *Inhaled Particles and Vapours.* Edited by C. N. Davies. New York, Pergamon, 1961, pp. 327-337.
63. P. Kotrappa, Calculation of the burden and dose to the respiratory tract from continuous inhalation of a radioactive aerosol, *Health Phys.*, **17**:429-432 (1969).
64. C. LaBelle and H. Brieger, Fate of inhaled particles in early postexposure period: II. Role of pulmonary phagocytosis, *Arch. Environ. Health,* **1**: 423-427 (1960).
65. H. D. Landahl, On the removal of airborne droplets by the human respiratory tract. II. The nasal passages, *Bull. Math. Biophys.*, **12**:161-169 (1950).
66. H. D. Landahl, T. N. Tracewell, and W. H. Lassen, On the retention of airborne particulates in the human lung, *Arch. Ind. Hyg. Occup. Med.*, **3**: 359-366 (1951).
67. J. M Lauweryns and J. H. Baert, The role of the pulmonary lymphatics in the defenses of the distal lung: Morphological and experimental studies of the transport mechanisms of intratracheally instillated particles, *Ann. NY Acad. Sci.*, **221**:244-275 (1974).
68. L. J. Leach, E. A. Maynard, H. C. Hodge, J. K. Scott, C. L. Yuile, G. E. Sylvester, and H. B. Wilson, A five-year inhalation study with natural uranium dioxide (UO_2) dust–I. Retention and biologic effect in the monkey, dog and rat, *Health Phys.*, **18**:599-612 (1970).
69. L. J. Leach, C. L. Yuile, H. C. Hodge, G. E. Sylvester, and H. B. Wilson, A five-year inhalation study with natural uranium dioxide (UO_2) dust–II. Post exposure retention and biologic effects in the monkey, dog and rat, *Health Phys.*, **25**:239-258 (1973).
70. G. P. Lewis and L. Coughlin, Lung "soot" accumulation in man, *Atmos. Environ.*, **7**:1249-1255 (1973).
71. M. Lippmann, Deposition and clearance of inhaled particles in the human nose, *Ann. Otol. Rhinol. Laryngol.*, **79**:519-528 (1970).
72. M. Lippmann and R. E. Albert, The effect of particle size on the regional deposition on inhaled aerosols in the human respiratory tract, *Am. Ind. Hyg. Assoc. J.*, **30**:257-275 (1969).
73. R. V. Lourenco, M. F. Klimek, and C. J. Borowski, Deposition and clearance of 2 μ particles in the tracheobronchial tree of normal subjects–smokers and non-smokers, *J. Clin. Invest.*, **50**:1411-1420 (1971).
74. R. V. Lourenco, R. Loddenkenper, and R. W. Carong, Patterns of distribution and clearance of aerosols in patients with bronchiectasis, *Am. Rev. Respir. Dis.*, **106**:857-866 (1972).
75. P. C. Luchsinger, J. E. Kilfeather, and B. LaGarde, Particle clearance from the human tracheobronchial tree, *Am. Rev. Respir. Dis.*, **97**:1046-1050 (1968).
76. H. Matthys, M. Müller, and N. Konietzko, Quantitative and selective

bronchial clearance studies using ^{99m}Tc-sulfate particles, *Scand. J. Respir. Dis. [Suppl.]*, **85**:33-37 (1974).

77. T. T. Mercer, On the role of particle size in the dissolution of lung burdens, *Health Phys.*, **13**:1211-1221 (1967).
78. T. T. Mercer, A. C. Allison, J. R. Casley-Smith, C. R. Rylander, and C. M. West, Task Group on Respiratory Absorption and Elimination Mechanisms Report to ICRP Committee 2, April 1975. (In preparation.)
79. P. E. Morrow, Alveolar clearance of aerosols, *Arch. Intern. Med.*, **131**:101-108 (1973).
80. P. E. Morrow, Dynamics of dust removal from the lower airways: Measurements and interpretations based upon radioactive aerosols. In *Ariway Dynamics*, Springfield, Ill., Charles C Thomas, 1970, pp. 299-312.
81. P. E. Morrow, Lymphatic drainage of the lung in dust clearance, *Ann. NY Acad. Sci.*, **200**:46-65 (1972).
82. P. E. Morrow, Models for the study of particle retention and elimination in the lung. In *Inhalation Carcinogenesis*, Oak Ridge, Tenn., AEC, 1970, pp. 103-119.
83. P. E. Morrow, Theoretical and experimental models for dust deposition and retention in man, *Rev. Environ. Health*, **1**:186-212 (1974).
84. P. E. Morrow, F. R. Gibb, and H. D. Beiter, Inhalation studies of uranium trioxide, *Health Phys.*, **23**:273-280 (1972).
85. P. E. Morrow, F. R. Gibb, H. Davies, and M. Fisher, Dust removal from the lung parenchyma: An investigation of clearance simulants, *Toxicol. Appl. Pharmacol.*, **12**:372-396 (1968).
86. P. E. Morrow, F. R. Gibb, and K. Gazioglu, The clearance of dust from the lower respiratory tract of man: An experimental study. In *Inhaled Particles and Vapours II*. New York, Pergamon, 1966, pp. 351-359
87. P. E. Morrow, F. R. Gibb, and K. M. Gazioglu, A study of particulate clearance from the human lungs, *Am. Rev. Respir. Dis.*, **96**:1209-1221 (1967).
88. P. E. Morrow, F. R. Gibb, and L. Johnson, Clearance of insoluble dusts from the lower respiratory tract, *Health Phys.*, **10**:543-555 (1964).
89. P. E. Morrow, F. R. Gibb, and L. J. Leach, The clearance of uranium dioxide dust from the lungs following single and multiple inhalation exposures, *Health Phys.*, **12**:1217-1223 (1966).
90. M. T. Newhouse, F. J. Wright, M. Dolovich, and O. L. Hopkins, Clearance of RISA aerosol from the human lung. In *Airway Dynamics Physiology and Pharmacology*. Edited by A. Bouhuys. Springfield, Ill., Charles C Thomas, 1970, pp. 313-317.
91. D. Newton and J. Rundo, Long-term tobacco smoking and mucociliary clearance, *Arch. Environ. Health*, **26**:86-89 (1971).
92. S. J. Normann, Kinetics of phagocytosis. II. Analysis of *in vivo* clearance with demonstration of competitive inhibition between similar and dissimilar foreign particles, *Lab. Invest.*, **31**:161-169 (1974).
93. S. J. Normann, Kinetics of phagocytosis. III. Two colloid reactions,

competitive inhalation and degree of inhibition between similar and dissimilar foreign particles, *Lab. Invest.*, **31**:286-293 (1974).

94. M. Ogata, A. Tanaka, E. Yokomura, K. Kumashiro, S. Yamamoto, and S. Seno, Intake of lead particles through lung alveoli by lead fume inhalation, *Acta Med. Okayama*, **27**:211-219 (1973).

95. D. E. Olson, M. F. Sudlow, K. Horsfield, and G. F. Filley, Convective patterns of flow during inspiration, *Arch. Intern. Med.*, **131**:51-57 (1973).

96. J. F. Park, D. L. Catt, D. K. Craig, R. J. Olson, and V. H. Smith, Solubility changes of ^{238}Pu oxide in water suspension and effect on biological behavior after inhalation by beagle dogs. In *Proc. 3rd Int. Congr. IRPA*. Edited by W. Snyder. Washington, D.C., 1974, pp. 719-724.

97. M. A. Parsont, W. L. Holley, and W. D. Burnett, The effect of particle size on organ distribution of radioactive material deposited in the lungs, *Health Phys.*, **22**:143-148 (1972).

98. T. J. Pedley, R. C. Schroter, and M. F. Sudlow, Flow and pressure drop in systems of repeatedly branching tubes, *J. Fluid Mech.*, **46**:365-383 (1971).

99. R. F. Phalen and P. E. Morrow, Experimental inhalation of metallic silver, *Health Phys.*, **24**:509-518 (1973).

100. D. F. Proctor, I. Anderson, and G. Lundqvist, Clearance of inhaled particles from the human nose, *Arch. Intern. Med.*, **131**:132-139 (1973).

101. D. F. Proctor and H. N. Wagner, Clearance of particles from the human nose, *Arch. Environ. Health*, **11**:366-371 (1965).

102. M. F. Quinlan, S. D. Salman, D. L. Swift, H. N. Wagner, and D. F. Proctor, Measurement of mucociliary function in man, *Am. Rev. Respir. Dis.*, **99**: 13-23 (1969).

103. O. Raabe, Some important considerations in use of power functions to determine clearance data, *Health Phys.*, **13**:293-295 (1967).

104. A. Rescigno and G. Segre, *Drug and Tracer Kinetics*. Waltham, Mass., Blaisdell, 1966, Chaps. 1 and 2.

105. J. Sadé, N. Eliezer, A. Silberberg, and A. C. Nevo, The role of mucus in transport by cilia, *Am. Rev. Respir. Dis.*, **102**:48-52 (1970).

106. J. Sanchis, M. Dolovich, R. Chalmer, and M. T. Newhouse, Regional distribution and lung clearance mechanisms in smokers and non-smokers. In *Inhaled Particles and Vapours III*, Vol. 1. Edited by W. H. Walton. Old Woking, Surrey, England, Unwin, Gresham Press, 1972, pp. 183-188.

107. C. L. Sanders, The distribution of inhaled plutonium-239 dioxide particles within pulmonary macrophages, *Arch. Environ. Health*, **18**:904-912 (1969).

108. R. Santa Cruz, J. Landa, J. Hirsch, and M. A. Sackner, Tracheal mucous velocity in normal man and patients with obstructive lung disease: effects of terbutaline, *Am. Rev. Respir. Dis.*, **109**:458-463 (1974).

109. R. G. Shorter, J. L. Titus, and M. B. Divertis, Cytodynamics in the respiratory tract of the rat, *Thorax*, **21**:32-37 (1966).

110. W. S. Snyder, The use of the lung model for estimation of dose. *Proc. 12th Annual Bio-Assay and Analytical Chemistry Meeting, Gatlinburg, Tennessee, CONF-661018,* 1967, pp. 74-86.

111. A. A. Spritzer, J. A. Watson, J. A. Auld, and M. A. Guetthoff, Pulmonary macrophage clearance, *Arch. Environ. Health,* **17**:726-730 (1968).

112. L. M. Steckel and C. M. West, Characterization of Y-12 uranium process materials correlated with in vivo experience, Union Carbide Nuclear Division–Y-12, Plant Report Y-15 44-A, July 28 (1966).

113. K. L. Swinth, J. F. Park, G. L. Voelz, and J. H. Ewins, In vivo detection of plutonium in the tracheobronchial lymph nodes with a fiber optic coupled scintillator. In *Radiation and the Lymphatic System, Proc. 14th Ann. Hanford Biology Symp.* Richland, Washington, 1974, CONF 740930 (1976). pp. 59-66.

114. G. V. Taplin, N. D. Poe, and A. Greenberg, Lung scanning following radioaerosol inhalation, *J. Nucl. Med.,* **7**:77-87 (1966).

115. G. V. Taplin, N. D. Poe, T. Isawa, and E. K. Dore, Radioaerosol and xenon gas inhalation and lung perfusion scintigraphy, *Scand. J. Respir. Dis. [Suppl.],* **85**:144-158 (1974).

116. M. Taylor, The origin and functions of nasal mucus, *Laryngoscope,* **84**: 612-636 (1974).

117. J. Thomas, A method for calculation of the absorbed dose to epithelium of the respiratory tract after inhalation of daughter products of radon, *Ann. Occup. Hyg.,* **7**:271-284 (1964).

118. R. G. Thomas, An interspecies model for retention of inhaled particles. In *Assessment of Airborne Particles.* Edited by T. Mercer, P. Morrow, and W. Stöber. Springfield, Ill., Charles C Thomas, 1972, pp. 405-418.

119. R. G. Thomas, Transport of relatively insoluble materials from lung to lymph nodes, *Health Phys.,* **14**:111-117 (1968).

120. R. G. Thomas, W. C. Eqing, D. L. Catron, and R. O. McClellan, In vivo solubility of four forms of barium determined by scanning techniques, *Am. Ind. Hyg. Assoc. J.,* **34**:350-359 (1973).

121. M. L. Thomson and P. Pavia, Long-term tobacco smoking and mucociliary clearance, *Arch. Environ. Health,* **26**:86-89 (1973).

122. M. L. Thomson and D. Pavia, Particle penetration and clearance in human lung–Results in healthy subjects and subjects with chronic bronchitis, *Arch. Environ. Health,* **29**:214-219 (1974).

123. M. L. Thomson, D. Pavia, and M. W. McNicol, A preliminary study of the effect of guiaphenesin on mucociliary clearance from the human lung, *Thorax,* **28**:742-747 (1973).

124. M. L. Thomson and M. D. Short, Mucociliary function in health, chronic obstructive airway disease and asbestosis, *J. Appl. Physiol.,* **26**:535-539 (1969).

125. A. Toigo, J. J. Imarisio, H. Murmal, and M. N. Lepper, Clearance of large carbon particles from the human tracheobronchial tree, *Am. Rev. Respir. Dis.,* **87**:487-492 (1963).

126. G. E. Tremble, Clinical observations on the movement of nasal cilia: An experimental study, *Laryngoscope,* **58**:206-224 (1948).

127. A. D. Tucker, J. H. Wyatt, and D. Undery, Clearance of inhaled particles from alveoli by normal interstitial drainage pathways, *J. Appl. Physiol.*, **35**:719-732 (1973).
128. S. A. Tyler, On a modification of the power function description of body burden from measured retention. Argonne National Laboratory, semi-annual report ANL-5841, p. 132 (1958).
129. H. N. Wagner, V. Lopez-Majano, and J. K. Langan, Clearance of particulate matter from the tracheobronchial tree in patients with tuberculosis, *Nature,* **205**:252-254 (1965).
130. J. G. Wagner, *Biopharmaceutics and Relevant Pharmacokinetics.* Hamilton, Ill., Drug Intelligence Publications, 1971, Chaps. 35, 36, 38, and 41.
131. E. R. Weibel, *Morphometry of the Human Lung.* New York, Academic Press, 1963.

15

Cough

DAVID E. LEITH

Harvard University School of Public Health
Boston, Massachusetts

The cough reflex is the watchdog of the lungs.

C. Jackson

I. Introduction

To cough is "to expel air from the lungs suddenly and usually in a series of efforts with an explosive noise made by the opening of the glottis" [134]. Perhaps because the clearance function of coughing is so well-known, it is not made explicit in this dictionary definition nor in the several other definitions of a cough, including "frequent repetition of coughing, being a symptom of disease."

Coughing is one member of a class of respiratory maneuvers in which the respired gas acts as a fluid coupling which transmits energy from the respiratory muscles to other sites in the respiratory system, for purposes outlined in Table 1. Besides transmitting the energy lost in flowing gas and for the many forms of sound production, several such maneuvers are used to move material other than gases, including tissues, secretions, and foreign materials. These are, for the most part, clearance mechanisms. Some are widely effective, but other remarkably localized ones exist for several regions of the upper airways. Many of them include maneuvers to narrow the passages through which gas flows, which increases

TABLE 1 Physiological Acts in Which the Respired Gas Acts as a Hydraulic Fluid to Transmit Energy from the Respiratory Muscles to Other Sites in the Respiratory System

Energy from respiratory muscles is used for:

(A) Ventilation: moving the gas itself

- Breathing: gas exchange
- Panting: thermoregulation
- Sniffing: olfaction

(B) Sound production: psychosocial uses

- Phonation, singing
- Whistling
- Snorting
- Bronx cheer

(C) Moving material: outward or inward

- Coughing: lower airway, larynx
- Forced expiration: lower airway, larynx
- Clearing throat: hypopharynx
- Hawking: oropharynx
- Spitting: mouth
- Sneezing: upper airways
- Nose-blowing: nasopharynx, paranasal sinuses, nose
- Sniffling: retaining secretions in nose
- Snuffling: nasopharynx, nose, paranasal sinuses

(D) Miscellaneous acts

- "Clearing" ears, sinuses

gas velocities and steepens velocity gradients across the stream, and maneuvers to oscillate the tissues and materials along the airway walls. Both presumably increase the effectiveness of the maneuver in clearing the airway. The sounds associated with the oscillations, as well as the nature of the materials moved, are regarded as inelegant, a cultural attitude which probably accounts for the absence of elegant terms by which we may refer to these acts.

There is an interesting interplay of some of these clearance mechanisms associated with the crossover of respiratory and alimentary tracts in the pharynx. There are powerful airway clearance mechanisms for the larynx and lower airway (cough) and for the nose and nasopharynx (sneeze); these have virtually unsuppressible reflex triggers. But reflex expulsion of ingested material from the mouth, oropharynx, and hypopharynx is ordinarily inappropriate. Thus reflexes protect the upper and lower airways during swallowing, and during clearance of the mouth and oropharynx by acts which are themselves usually initiated voluntarily rather than reflexly. Associated senses allow awareness of the location and nature of materials in the mouth and pharynx, much less so in the upper airways and perhaps not at all in lower airways. In each of the two crossing tracts, however, some of these centrally organized maneuvers can be initiated voluntarily (coughing, swallowing), while others (like gagging and sneezing) usually cannot. Further discussion can be found in Proctor's chapter in the *Handbook of Physiology*, [108].

Coughing is rare in complete health. Even persons who cannot cough—for example, those paralyzed by neurological diseases—may get along well for years. This suggests that normally the clearance of the respiratory tract is satisfactorily managed by other mechanisms—for example, macrophages and the mucociliary system. But when those systems fail, or when they are overloaded by foreign materials or by secretions abnormal in kind or amount, coughing is a fast and powerful adjunct. It is of course a universal human experience during common illnesses such as minor respiratory infections.

Coughing has significance other than its obvious function in clearing material already present in the airways. A preventive function is probably provided by the cough receptors in the epipharynx and aditus laryngis; epipharyngeal and laryngeal coughs expel materials which might otherwise be aspirated into the airway [64]. Coughing can be triggered at the extremes of lung volume, apparently by airway stretch and by airway closure at high and low lung volumes (Chap. 16). It can limit inspiration at lung volumes below total lung capacity (TLC) when lung recoil forces are abnormally great, as after a period of oxygen breathing near RV. Perhaps this mechanism plays a role in preventing application of excessive pressure to the lung. No physiological significance is obvious for the cough elicited at low volumes, though it is used clinically for the purpose [129]. Coughing has psychosocial functions. It may be used voluntarily as a discreet sign, or unconsciously with symbolic meaning [42], or as a tic [10,67]. Frequently, coughing occurs without any apparent function in the usual sense; that is, in allergy, in irritant atmospheres, and in other settings where neither clearance nor other useful result is seen.

Finally, the cough is used by physicians and others in several ways. It is an index of disease which finds wide use in epidemiology [130,139,141] and as a tool (or a problem) in differential diagnosis [5,12,15,125,128]. In these contexts its strong association with smoking and chronic bronchitis must be considered one of its most important aspects [141]; its presence is part of the clinical definition of the latter. It is used in guiding, and evaluating the response to, therapy in both clinical settings and drug trials [25,37,72]. It is useful in physical examination of the lungs, of the body wall (for example, hernias and prolapses), and of the nervous system [16]. Reexpansion of a collapsed lung by connecting a chest tube to a one-way valve (e.g., underwater seal) requires that pleural pressure periodically rise above atmospheric; the cough is one act which does this. Some of these are discussed further below.

Neural aspects of the control and organization of coughing are discussed in Chap. 16.

II. Normal Physiology of Coughing

This section draws heavily upon several descriptive papers which are well worth reading [68,104,120,135,143]. In order to set the stage for more detailed consideration of the interlocking mechanics of respiratory, circulatory, and cerebrospinal fluid systems during coughing, I will start with a general account of a "typical" cough sequence, and of some of the variations which can occur.

A. General Description and Normal Variations

Coughing usually starts with a brief rapid inspiration of a volume of air larger than the normal resting tidal volume, as shown in Fig. 1. The glottis is then closed for about 0.2 sec. During that time the pressure in abdominal, pleural, and alveolar spaces is raised to 50-100 mmHg or more by an expiratory effort which includes agonist-antagonist interaction between inspiratory and expiratory muscles, of both rib cage [6] and abdomen-diaphragm [3]. Abdominal pressure thus exceeds intrathoracic pressure. Circulatory and cerebrospinal fluid systems are affected as might be expected during this brief violent Valsalva maneuver [45,91,119,120]. Intraocular pressure also rises.

The glottis is suddenly opened actively [62,132] as subglottic pressure continues to rise [68,143; Fig. 2]. Expiratory flow at the mouth accelerates rapidly; within 30-50 msec, flow reaches a peak which may exceed 12 liters/sec [62]. Oscillations of tissue and gas cause a characteristic explosive sound and may play a role in suspending secretions in the moving gas stream [132]. During this time the lower trachea and other intrathoracic airways collapse, contributing a transient "spike" of flow on top of the more sustained expiratory flow through the airways from lung parenchyma (Figs. 1, 11C).

About a half-second later, after a liter of gas or less has been expired [62, 68], flow is stopped by one of two methods: either the glottis closes with a characteristic "second sound," as shown in the upper panel of Fig. 1, or respiratory muscle agonist-antagonist activity is adjusted so that alveolar pressure falls to zero (lower panel, Fig. 1). The sequence may be repeated rapidly several times, sweeping down through the lung volume toward residual volume and progressively collapsing more and more of the intrathoracic airways [94].

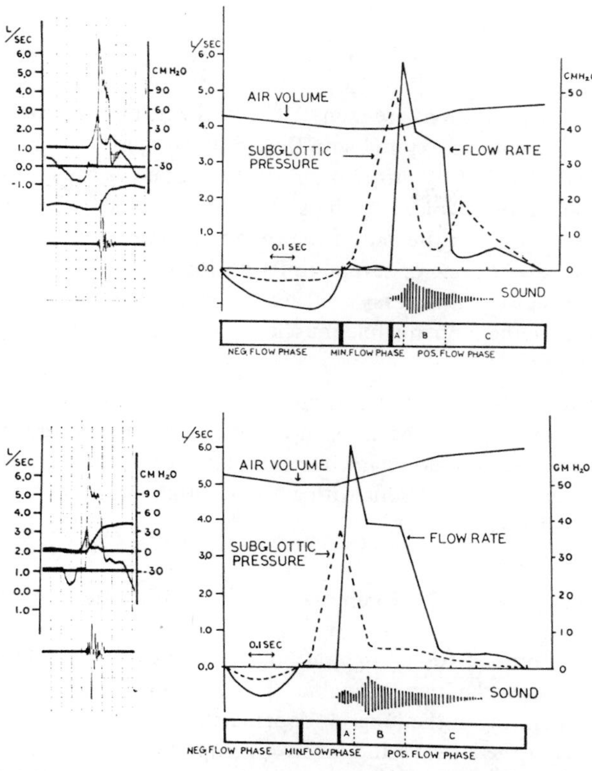

FIGURE 1 Subglottic pressure, air flow, and volume change at the mouth, and sound production during single voluntary coughs; the signals are diagramed on the right. (From Yanagihara et al. [143].)

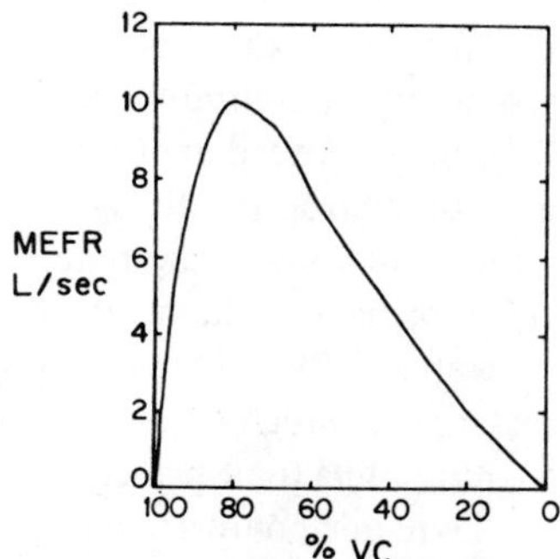

FIGURE 2 Maximum expiratory flow-volume (MEFV) curve. This curve is the mean of tests of five normal men between the ages of 25 and 35 years. Maximum expiratory flow rates (MEFR) in liters per second. (Reprinted from the *Archives of Environmental Health,* **14**:5-9, 1967, copyright 1967, American Medical Association.)

The normal variations are many. The initial inspiration may not occur. Starting volume, volume expired, and flow rates are quite variable, as are the pressures used. Expiratory effort often starts just before the glottis closes [143], causing a characteristic voiced "huh" sound. A similar sound may occur as the glottis closes abruptly at the end of the cough. A series of coughs often occurs; inspiration may occur one or several times during such a series [132]. Involuntary paroxysms of coughing may continue for many seconds, during which time the glottis may remain open while muscle effort and pleural pressure rise and fall several times.

Effective clearance is not entirely dependent on glottis closure. Clearing lower airways by sharp forced expiration without glottis closure is not uncommon [110]. There is no common name for this maneuver, but Negus refers to it as a "bovine" cough [101]. Persons with a tracheostomy or a laryngectomy learn to "cough" effectively.

B. Background: The Expiratory Flow-Limiting Mechanism

Coughing is a form of forced expiration; it utilizes the maximum expiratory flow rates of which the lung is capable. These upper limits to flow are set by a mechanism operating in the lung. It depends upon lung elastic recoil forces and the properties of the airways and involves compression of downstream (mouthward) portions of the airways by dynamic forces associated with flow. An important feature of the mechanism is that maximum flows are reached by relatively gentle expiratory effort; above that easily reached level, changes in expiratory effort do not result in changes in flow.

These effort-independent flow maxima set upper limits to pulmonary ventilation, which are expressed in several common pulmonary function tests (the maximum voluntary ventilation, the forced expired volume, the maximum midexpiratory flow, and others). In obstructive diseases such as asthma, emphysema, and bronchitis, the maximum flows are severely reduced and can become a limit to aerobic metabolism; but in normal individuals the available flows far exceed those needed even in heavy exercise. Thus Mead et al. [94] said: "In healthy individuals the only circumstance in which (these) mechanisms . . . come into play naturally is during coughing; thus their principal pertinence is to expectoration rather than ventilation. Dynamic compression of the intrathoracic airways is undoubtedly an essential part of an effective cough since it makes possible the high kinetic energy of the airstream required to move material at the airway wall."

This section attempts to provide an intuitive grasp of the important parts of the flow-limiting mechanism. A brief introduction is available in an article by Macklem and Mead [86], and more detailed accounts are found in publications by Fry and Hyatt [40], Pride and Permutt et al. [107], Mead and co-workers [94], and Macklem and Mead [85].

Clearly it is not possible to expire at infinite flow rates. What flows are possible? Peak flow, i.e., the highest "instantaneous" expiratory flow near the onset of a forced expiration, is a common pulmonary function measurement; values around 600 liters/min (10 liters/sec) are reasonable for healthy young adults. The peak flows are related to body size, of course; a normal value close to 2 vital capacities/sec is a convenient, though very rough, rule of thumb.

Can those high flows be maintained throughout an entire expiratory vital capacity (VC) maneuver? No; in fact, having accelerated to a peak value, maximum expiratory flows fall in a rough proportion with lung volume; the relationship is conveniently represented as a maximum expiratory flow-volume (MEFV) curve (Fig. 2). Thus maximum expiratory flows are said to be an effort-independent function of lung volume.

In order to understand why maximum flows are lower at low lung volumes, it is convenient to turn to a mechanical analogy, the Starling resistor (Fig. 3). Consider flow through a collapsible tube traversing a chamber in which pressure can be held at specific levels. Such a system can operate in three modes. First, if inlet pressure P_i and outlet pressure, P_o are both greater than chamber pressure, P_c, the tube is everywhere open and its pressure-flow characteristics are the familiar ones of a pipe: raising P_i, or lowering P_o, causes increased flow. Next, if P_i and P_o are both less than P_c, the tube is everywhere collapsed and (ideally) no flow occurs. The last mode is the one of interest. When P_i is greater than P_c, but P_o is lower than P_c, a region of collapse is seen near the outlet, as shown in Fig. 3. Under these conditions lowering P_o does not increase the flow. The downstream constriction simply narrows a bit more. All the extra pressure drop is dissipated in the compressed segment, and no change in upstream flow, geometry, or pressure distribution occurs. However, increasing P_i still does increase flow, and increasing P_c will diminish flow. But if we fix the *difference* between

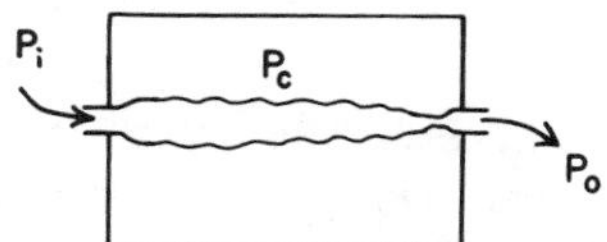

FIGURE 3 Diagram of a Starling resistor, in which a collapsible tube traverses a chamber where the pressure is P_c. Inlet pressure is P_i, outlet pressure is P_o. Fluid flows from inlet to outlet through the tube. When $P_i > P_c > P_o$, a constriction appears at the downstream portion of the tube within the chamber, and flow depends on $(P_i - P_c)$ and the tube's upstream geometry. Flow is independent of changes in P_o or $(P_i - P_o)$.

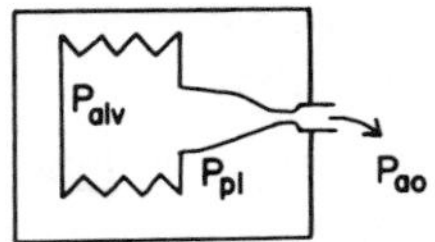

FIGURE 4 During a forced expiration, the respiratory system behaves like a Starling resistor. When $P_{alv} > P_{pl} >> P_{ao}$, flow is related to $(P_{alv} - P_{pl})$, which is the elastic component of transpulmonary pressure, and on the geometry of an upstream portion of the airways.

P_i and P_c, we can change them up and down equally, without changing flow. In sum, flow has become independent of $(P_i - P_o)$ and is now dependent on $(P_i - P_c)$. If $(P_i - P_c)$ is constant, changing either P_i or P_o does not change flow.

When we refer to a Starling resistor, it is understood that it is operating in the mode where the flow depends on $(P_i - P_c)$. During forced expiration, the respiratory system may be viewed as a peculiar Starling resistor system (Fig. 4) in which the difference $(P_i - P_c)$ is a function of lung volume, where alveolar pressure is P_i and pleural pressure is P_c. The difference between them, $(P_{alv} - P_{pl})$, is the elastic or static component of transpulmonary pressure, $P_{st(L)}$ and varies with lung volume.

During a forced expiration, the expiratory muscles are used to raise pleural pressure, P_{pl}, well above pressure at the airway opening, P_{ao}. But the pressure within the trachea exceeds P_{ao} by only a small amount (because of the resistance of extrathoracic airways) so a collapsing pressure is applied to intrathoracic airways. They narrow, and when effort is high enough, the system behaves like a Starling resistor. Since we can regard $P_{st(L)}$ as the effective driving pressure for maximum expiratory flow rates, we now see why MEFR diminishes with lung volume.

Flow of course is influenced by the size and collapsibility of airways, by lung elasticity, and by other interacting factors which we should sidestep here. Several different ways of looking at the underlying mechanics have proven useful [29,40,94,107].

Mead [94] pointed out that when expiratory effort and flow were high enough, a pressure drop equal to $P_{st(L)}$ would occur between alveoli and some point in the airways. At such points the pressure would equal the pleural pressure; these are equal pressure points, EPP, and the airways between alveoli and the EPP are referred to as the upstream segment. By definition, during maximum flow, the resistance of the upstream segment, R_{us}, is equal to $P_{st(L)}$ divided by MEFR. Since the pressure, flow, and resistance of the upstream segment are fixed (at any given lung volume), it can be shown that its geometry is fixed; that is to say, the location of EPP is fixed when flow reaches maximum.

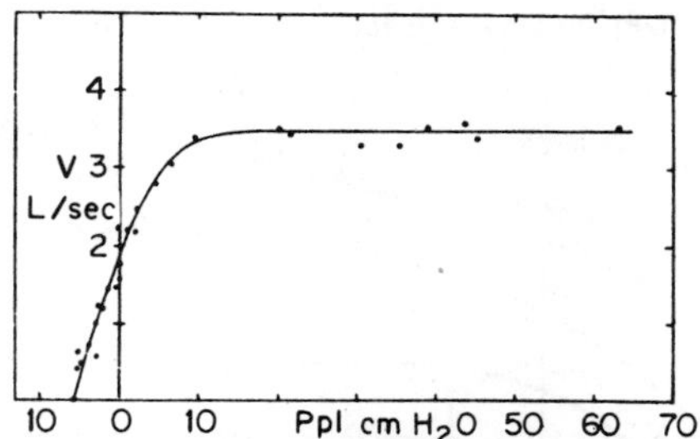

FIGURE 5 An isovolume pressure-flow (IVPF) curve at 33% VC in a normal man. At that volume, in repeated expiratory VC maneuvers ranging from slow to forced, simultaneous values of pleural (esophageal) pressure and expiratory flow are recorded. (From Macklem and Mead [86].)

By definition, the downstream resistance from EPP to mouth equals P_{pl} divided by MEFR; P_{pl}, and therefore R_{ds}, varies with effort.

As a last step in this section, we can consider the relationship between pleural pressure (referred to P_{ao}) and expiratory flow at some selected lung volume. By plotting values of pressure and flow at the instant a subject passes through that volume in each of a series of increasingly rapid expirations, we can draw a curve, referred to as an isovolume pressure-flow (IVPF) curve, which looks like the one shown in Fig. 5. We see that in order to hold volume constant, with flow equal to zero, pleural pressure must be subatmospheric by enough to counterbalance the lung recoil. As pleural pressure rises, so does alveolar pressure (and by the same amount, since volume, and therefore the elastic component of transpulmonary pressure, are constant). The chord slope of the pressure-flow curve is the airway resistance. As pleural pressure rises and becomes positive, the pressure-flow curve levels off; the flat part of the IVPF curve expresses the effort-independent nature of MEF, and the maximum value of flow attained is "unique" to the lung volume being considered for this individual. A family of similar curves can be drawn for different lung volumes in the same individual (Fig. 6). They show that the maximum flow is lower, and is achieved at a lower pleural pressure (P_{max}), at low lung volumes, where lung recoil is lower.

Hyatt and Flath [48] have plotted P_{max} as a function of lung volume, along with the maximum static pressures and the maximum dynamic pressures of which the ventilatory muscles are capable (Fig. 7). Within the cross-hatched area, flow varies with pressure. Within the region bounded by the P_{max} line and the maximum dynamic expiratory effort line, flow is independent of pressure, but the compression of the downstream segment, and its resistance, varies directly with pressure. At any given lung volume, the difference between static and

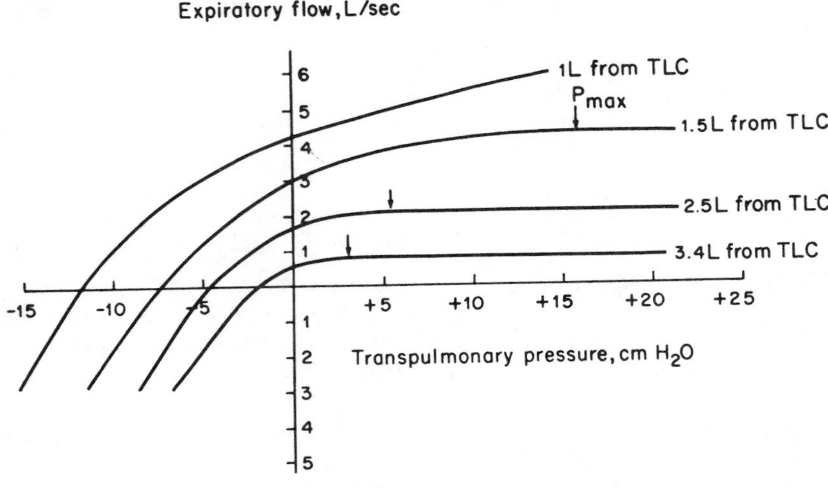

FIGURE 6 A family of IVPF curves at different lung volumes in a normal subject. As lung volume diminishes, so does the static (elastic) component of transpulmonary pressure. Arrows indicate the pressures which just suffice to reach maximum flow (P_{max}) at each lung volume. (From A. Bouhuys (ed.) *Airway Dynamics,* 1970. Courtesy of Charles C Thomas, Publisher, Springfield, Illinois [49].)

dynamic maximum pressures can be attributed to force-velocity relationships of expiratory muscles. At lower volumes the expiratory flows—and therefore the velocity of muscle shortening—is less, and the difference between the static and dynamic pressures is less.

In summary, this section has reviewed some aspects of respiratory mechanics which apply to the cough mechanism. MEFRs are an effort-independent function of lung volume, determined by a mechanism operating in the lung and analogous with a Starling resistor. Flow maxima depend upon lung recoil and airway properties. The transpulmonary pressures which just suffice to reach MEFR (P_{max}) are relatively low and vary with lung volume. Greater pressures do not vary the location of EPP or the geometry of upstream airways, but do cause greater dynamic compression of downstream airways. Maximum muscle pressures vary with lung volume and with expiratory flow rate. Now we will return to a more detailed description of mechanical events in coughing.

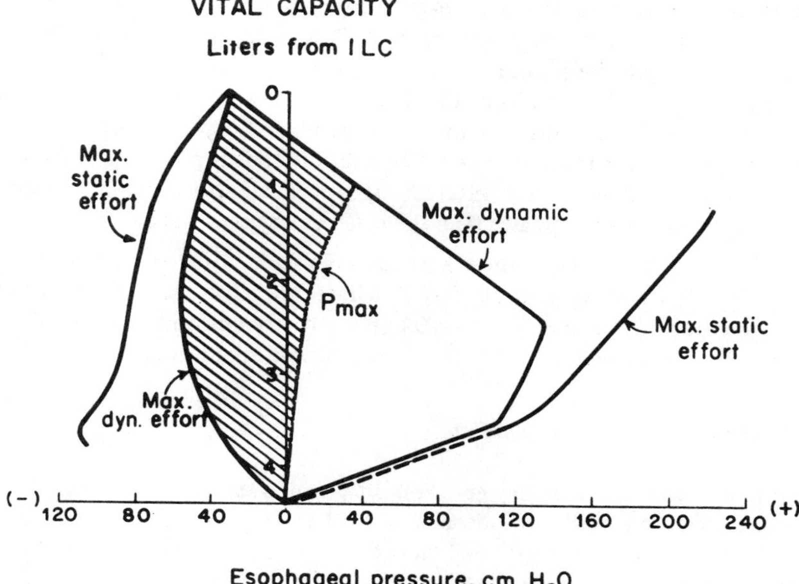

FIGURE 7 Relationship of pleural (esophageal) pressure to lung volume during maximum static efforts and during maximum forced inspiratory and expiratory vital capacity maneuvers. The relationship of P_{max} and lung volume is indicated by the dotted line. See text. (From Hyatt and Flath [48].)

C. The Respiratory System in Coughing

1. Lung Volume

Initial lung volumes are said to be high, usually more than one resting tidal volume above FRC. Like many ventilatory activities, however, spontaneous coughing may be different from voluntary coughing during laboratory studies. When subjects were instructed to give a single cough into a face mask [143], three males inspired about 0.5 liter and two females inspired about 0.2 liter; the single cough resulted in expiration of about 1.1 liters and 0.6 liter respectively. Variability was great. In another study [46], the combined volume of the first three consecutive maximal voluntary coughs in healthy young adults was equivalent to about 85% of their forced vital capacity, FVC. Since the functional residual capacity of upright humans is about 35-45% of the vital capacity, these subjects must have started well above FRC, probably near 90% of TLC. Loudon and

Shaw [80] found the volume of air expelled per cough during 45 coughs in 9 normal subjects was 2258 ml ± 455 ml (SD), about 45% of their mean FRC. Other authors report inspiration and expiration of 1.7 to as much as 2.5 liters in a single cough cycle. Knudson et al. [62] show a series of coughs over the VC range with volume changes of about a liter at high lung volumes, falling progressively to perhaps 0.2 liter near RV (Fig. 11B); their purposes, and instructions to the subjects, were different. It is probable that variability in spontaneous coughing is even greater than these values suggest.

The initial high lung volumes have several effects. Greater expiratory muscle pressures and higher expiratory flow rates are achievable. The effects of gravity on the lung are minimized, so that more nearly uniform inflation of lung regions exists, and the number of closed lung units is minimized.

2. *Pressures: The Role of Muscles*

Pressure and flow events during coughing are so rapid that great care is needed to assure accurate records. Knudson et al. [62] found it necessary to fill their esophageal balloon system with helium and to match carefully the delays between pressure and other signals. Nevertheless, much of what is shown in older papers appears useful.

After, or just before, the glottis closes following inspiration, the expiratory muscles begin to raise pressure throughout the system (Fig. 1). When pleural pressure reaches about 50-100 mmHg the glottis opens; pressure in the trachea falls, but esophageal pressure continues to rise, reaching levels of 100-200 cmH_2O or more in normal people. After about a half-second, pressure falls. When it has fallen below P_{max}, flow also decreases.

Presumably the pressures available during coughing are limited in some way by strength, which varies with age and sex as described by Cook et al. [28]. Ventilatory muscle strength also appears to vary with physical fitness, increasing in some athletes and decreasing with general debility.

Peak pressures are said to be 50-100% greater during cough than during forced expirations [68,80]. If that is true, one would look to explanations of two kinds: first, in control of reflex as compared to voluntary maximum acts, and second, in expiratory muscle geometry and force-length and force-velocity relationships.

Bucher [18] concluded that the larynx plays a double role in the cough mechanism, reinforcing it both by storing and coordinating the expiratory impulse and by reflexly increasing net expiratory muscle activity. Floersheim, cited by von Leden [132], came to the same conclusion, that the glottis "modifies the cough reflex by increasing the intrapleural pressure by 20%." Presumably such a reflex potentiation would involve some combination of increased agonist and decreased antagonist activity. Proctor [108] discusses this aspect of reflex organization of coughing.

But the glottis also introduces differences in the timing of volume and flow events during cough compared with forced expirations, and intrinsic muscle properties might then result in higher pressures. Two different mechanisms are involved [3].

First, the velocity of shortening of expiratory muscles can be regarded as depending on the rate of change of thoracic gas volume ($\dot{V}_{TG}$). Thoracic gas volume changes when there is flow at the airway opening ($\dot{V}_{ao}$) and when thoracic gas is undergoing compression or expansion ($\dot{V}_c$). The latter can be substantial. For example, if alveolar pressure rises by 100 cm H_2O in 0.2 sec in a person coughing at a lung volume of 5 liters, the volume change of about 0.5 liter due to compression results in a $\dot{V}_c$ averaging 2.5 liters/sec. $\dot{V}_c$ values up to 35 liters/sec have been reported in some studies [34,52]. Closing the glottis during the phase of thoracic gas compression dissociates $\dot{V}_c$ and $\dot{V}_{ao}$ in time, decreases $\dot{V}_{TG}$ and the velocity of muscle shortening, and (perhaps) maximizes muscle pressures.

Second, if flow at the mouth is allowed to occur during the phase of rising effort and pressure, they reach their peak after a substantial volume has been expired. The glottis allows peak pressure to be reached, therefore, at higher volumes where muscle force-length relationships and geometry are more advantageous.

The rise of tension in isometric muscle contraction is approximately exponential in time, with a time constant of about 0.1 sec. In the respiratory system it may be longer [96] and in patients with chronic obstructive lung diseases it is greater than in normal people [89]. The duration of glottis closure in the initial phase of coughing is about 0.2-0.3 sec, appropriate timing if high pleural pressures are to be achieved before the start of the expiratory phase. The period of closure must vary with age and disease, but I could not find out whether it is adjusted to optimize coughing in the face of changing mechanics of the respiratory system.

3. *The Glottis*

The importance of the glottis in coughing has been debated [18,101,132,143], and though a case can be made, as above, for its value, the fact remains that effective airway clearance is possible by cough-like maneuvers not utilizing the larynx.

During the inspiratory phase, the glottis actively dilates, as is usual during inspiration [132].

Active closure involves both glottis (ventricular bands or false cords) and supraglottic structures. von Leden and Isshiki [132] review the ample evidence that these, and not epiglottis or the true vocal cords, are used to restrain the very high tracheal pressures encountered in coughing and the somewhat similar events during laughter and glottal strokes.

There is general agreement that the opening of the glottis, at the onset of the expiratory phase of coughing, is an active process. This is supported by animal studies in which airflow was diverted through a tracheostomy by Floersheim, cited by von Leden [132], by electromyographic investigations of laryngeal muscles [35], by cinephotographic observations of rapid and extensive abduction of the arytenoid cartilages [132], and by the timing of the rise of expiratory flow [62].

At the same time, and superimposed upon the active motions of the glottis during abduction, are violent oscillations of the mucous membranes and underlying structures. These are described in von Leden and Isshiki's reports of high-speed cinephotography of the larynx during coughing [132], and are said to "represent the passive response of these structures to the stormy air flow." They describe, for example, an unusual maneuver of the epiglottis, which appears to flap so violently in the breeze that its tip may strike the posterior pharyngeal wall several times. These authors, stressing the potential for laryngeal trauma that lies in repeated coughing, suggest ready use of antitussive medicines.

The quality of the sound produced by coughing is quite variable and can be quite distinctive. It may obviously reflect the nature and quantity of secretions. At other times it appears more dependent upon the properties of the oscillating tissues. Theodos [128] says that pressure on the trachea by aortic aneurysm, tumor, or lymph nodes can produce a "brassy" cough. "Tracheal rattles" are described, and "fluttering" of the expiratory flow in gas and liquid-filled [116] lungs has been ascribed to elastic and inertial forces in the fluid stream and airway walls. Inflammation may change airway properties enough to cause characteristic sounds.

4. *Expiratory Flows and Transients*

Among the most interesting aspects of expiratory flow during cough are those associated with the extremely rapid collapse of intrathoracic airways when the glottis opens. This transient event occurs with a time constant between 3 and 8 msec in normal humans, with the expulsion of 50-150 ml air from intrathoracic airways. As a result, a transient spike of "supramaximal" flow is superimposed on the maximum flows coming from the lung parenchyma [62]. This spike is especially obvious as an initial volume step in spirograms of persons with obstructive lung diseases [30,34], and their flow traces during coughing (Fig. 2). The conflicting interpretations in the older literature are presently best understood in the light of a careful, thorough, recent study by Knudson et al. [62].

The basic relationships have been mentioned already. Just before the glottis opens, intrathoracic airways are distended by a pressure difference equal to the static (elastic component of) transpulmonary pressure; in fact the intrapulmonary airways probably are exposed to even greater transmural pressures because at high lung volumes, peribronchial pressure is more negative than pleural pressure. As the glottis opens, air escapes and pressure within the airways falls. But pleural pressure remains high, or is still rising. Thus transmural pressures diminish everywhere along intrathoracic airways, and the previously distended airways relax toward their undistended cross sections; their volume decreases. This is more pronounced in the downstream (mouthward) airways, since pressure within the airways falls progressively from alveoli to mouth. As the EPP migrates upstream in intrathoracic airways, negative transmural pressures are applied to airways downstream from it. The resulting dynamic compression accounts for most of the airways volume change (Fig. 8).

Simultaneous with the collapse of the downstream airways, flow begins to occur through them from the lung parenchyma. The sum of these two flow components–*from* and *through* collapsing airways–accounts for most of the flow measured at the mouth (gas expansion and any change in volume of extrathoracic airways also influence flow at the mouth). The two flow components, from lung and from collapsing intrathoracic airways, have different time courses because they depend on different mechanical systems. The dynamic compres-

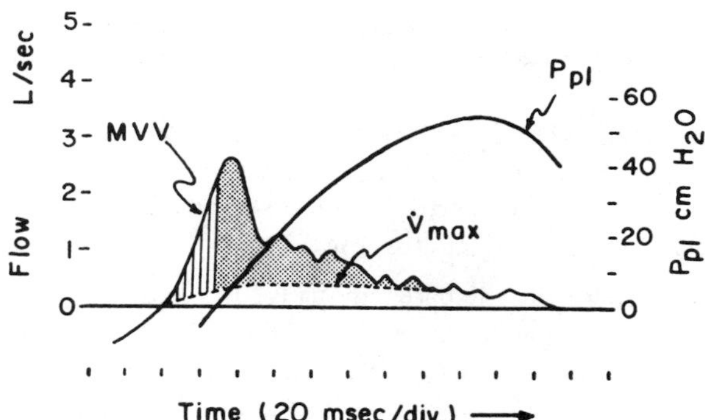

FIGURE 8 Flow and pleural (esophageal) pressure during the expiratory phase of a maximum voluntary ventilation maneuver (MVV), in a patient with obstructive disease. Dashed line labeled $\dot{V}_{max}$ is parenchymal flow. Vertically hatched area represents volume displaced from airways by passive collapse (relaxation); stippled area, the volume displaced by dynamic compression. (From Ref. 62.)

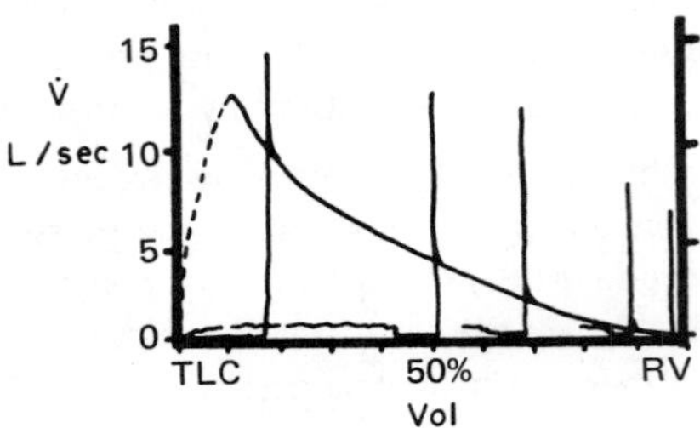

FIGURE 9 Five separate flow transients triggered at P_{pl} of 80 cmH_2O, shown in flow-volume representation superimposed on this normal subject's MEFV curve [62].

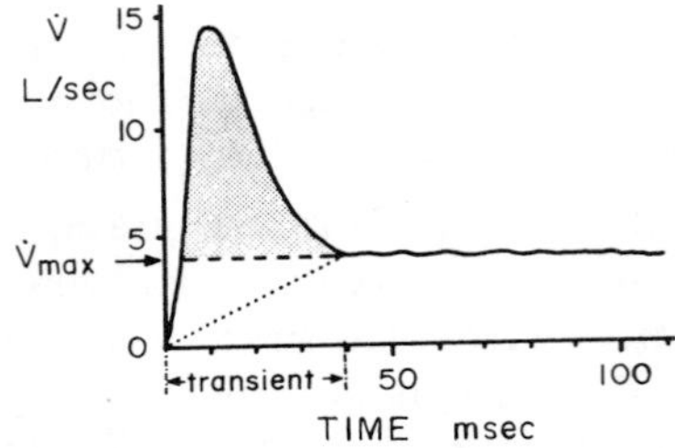

FIGURE 10 A triggered flow transient plotted in time. End of the transient is defined by the point at which flow falls from supramaximal levels to $\dot{V}_{max}$: Dashed line represents parenchymal flow if the migration of EPP was instantaneous. Stippled area represents the ΔVaw used in subsequent analyses. Dotted line represents parenchymal flow if EPP migration was slow. (From Ref. 62.)

sion is complete within about 40-80 msec (depending on the lung volume at the time) so that, while the volume discharge is small, the instantaneous flow attributable to this mechanism can approach 10 liters/sec during "triggered transients" made by opening a valve at the mouth (Fig. 9).

In contrast, flow from the parenchyma is sustained in time, falling relatively slowly as lung volume decreases. The timing of the rise of flow from the parenchyma is uncertain (Fig. 10). It has been suggested [14] that a "finite time" was required for airway collapse, which allowed initially high flows to come from the parenchyma, thus accounting for the initial spike of flow. Knudson and his colleagues examined this possibility in excised dog tracheas [62] and could not demonstrate that the simulated parenchymal flow reached maximum value before dynamic collapse had occurred. They conclude that the EPP migrate rapidly, though not instantaneously, to their "steady-state" location.

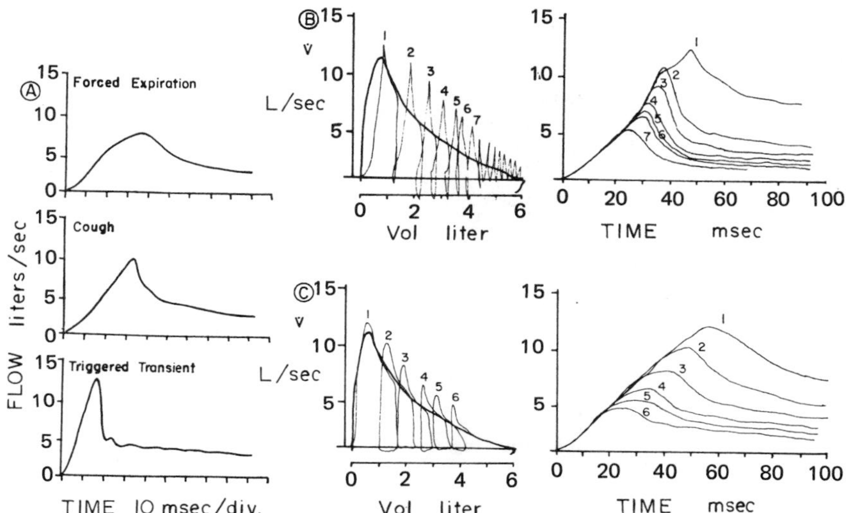

FIGURE 11 (A) Flow-time representations of forced expiration, cough, and triggered transient performed at the same lung volume in a normal subject. (B) On the left is the flow-volume representation of a series of voluntary coughs beginning at TLC and progressing sequentially down the VC, superimposed on the subject's MEFV curve. On the right, the numbered coughs are represented as flow in time. Here the flow "plateau" referred to by Langlands is clearly shown. (C) A series of brief rapid expiratory efforts are shown in the same way as the coughs; the glottis is open throughout. Transient spikes are less "sharp" and deceleration less abrupt. All curves are from the same normal subject. (The figure and most of the legend are from Knudson et al. [62].)

Flow transients are less apparent in records made at high lung volumes (and flows) in young normal persons (Fig. 11), and may be overlooked if measuring devices are used which cannot respond rapidly, for example, some peak flow meters and spirometers. Nevertheless they have been observed for years [14,21, 30,41,46,68,80,143] and their origin clearly described. Loudon and Shaw [80] said "during coughs, the peak flow rate occurs before or during airway narrowing; presumably it is contributed to by the expulsion of dead space air." Gandevia [41] refers to a sudden collapse of airways at the beginning of forced expiration, and Langlands' fine paper [68], which shows the relationship between supramaximal and maximal flow in both normal and bronchitic subjects (Fig. 12), accounts for the former by the transient collapse.

Campbell and Young [21] and other authors correctly perceived that inertia in spirometers could introduce a "bounce" into the spirogram with the abrupt deceleration of the transient to the more sustained flow, and some con-

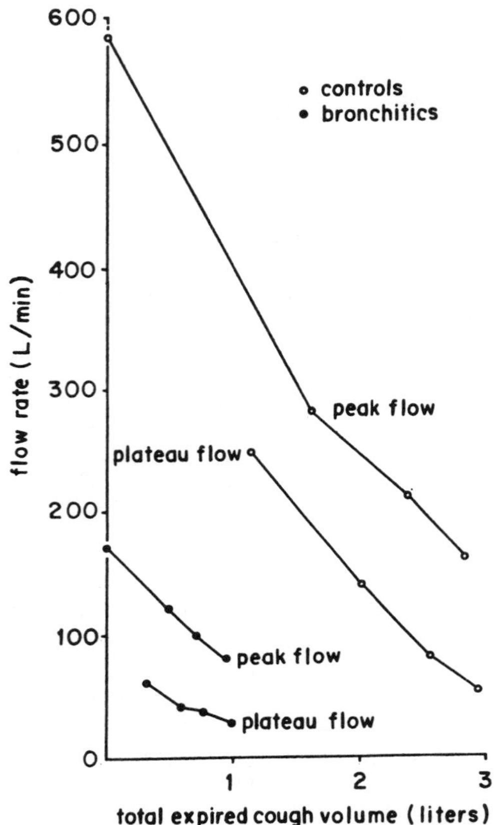

FIGURE 12 Mean peak flow rate and mean plateau flow rate (supramaximal flow and $\dot{V}_{max}$, respectively, in the terminology of Knudson et al.) for each of the first four in a series of voluntary coughs in normal and bronchitic subjects, plotted against volume expired from TLC. (From Langlands [68].)

fusion persists about the interrelations between man and machine in making such spirograms. Mead [92] gives relevant references and also points out the respiratory system's insensitivity to external loads while it is operating on its MEFV curve.

5. Airways in Coughing

Airways narrow during coughing. What are the mechanisms, which airways are involved, how much do they narrow and what are the factors which influence the site and degree of narrowing? What effects does narrowing have on the cough mechanism?

The mechanisms for airway narrowing during coughing are two: the dynamic compression discussed above, and contraction of smooth muscle in airway walls. We are not concerned here with the relationship between airway size and lung volume, and will set aside consideration of airway hysteresis [60]. The complex and active field of airway mechanics cannot be adequately reviewed here [83]. The evidence for reflex bronchoconstriction is discussed in Chap. 16 by Widdicombe.

In 1949 Di Rienzo [32] asserted that during coughing a peristaltic wave of smooth muscle contraction swept up the airways toward the larynx, clearing secretions ahead of it; "one breathes with the thorax," he said, "and one coughs with the bronchi." Nobody agrees with that view. Other radiographers [47] cannot confirm his bronchographic observations of "bronchial vomiting," and physiologists think that dynamic collapse of airways must start at the thoracic inlet and follow the EPP upstream as lung volume diminishes. Thus the airways would tend to be cleared in a sequence which starts in the trachea and moves towards the periphery [94]. This idea is confirmed by more recent bronchographic studies [110], by the use of catheters for measurement of intrabronchial pressure [87], by use of "retrograde catheters" for measurement of pressures in peripheral airways, and by cinephotography of extrapulmonary airways in excised lungs [85].

How far upstream can the region of dynamic compression extend? It varies with lung volume. At high volumes it includes only trachea and other extrapulmonary airways of excised dog lung [85]. It does not extend beyond the segmental airways until lung volume is less than about 25% VC [87], but then goes far out in the lung and at least theoretically could include the entire airway, at least to the sites where closure occurs in 0.5-1.0 mm bronchi [85].

But Cavagna et al. [22] showed that airways can remain open at a static transpulmonary pressure of minus 2 cmH_2O; that is to say, pleural pressure is greater than alveolar pressure. At that volume, therefore, the EPP is upstream of the alveolus! Cavagna also showed that the airways remain open to lower lung volumes during oxygen uptake from the occluded lung than during mass flow out of the airway, lending some support to the idea that dynamic narrowing may influence airway-closing mechanics, in the direction of closing at higher volumes than might otherwise occur.

What happens during coughing at sites of closure is not well-known. If critical closure occurs at dynamically narrowed sites, flow stops at that point and the pressure distal to the point of closure rises to alveolar pressure. Local transmural pressure then may suffice to reopen the airway. Oscillation of this kind may account for the dynamic wheezing of forced expiration.

Even in closed airways filled with secretions, fluids are extruded up into more central airways. This "tussive squeeze" at low lung volumes feeds materials into larger airways, whence they can be cleared by the "bechic blast." These terms, originating with the Jacksons, are reintroduced with relish by Huizinga in his Chevalier Jackson Memorial Lecture [47].

The degree of narrowing is effort-dependent, in the downstream segment. Its resistance—and total transpulmonary resistance—therefore varies with effort, and can reach extremely high values. The calculation of these peak resistances has been popular, but their significance is limited. The effort-dependence of airway compression is clearly shown by the work of Knudson et al. [62], who measured the increasing volumes displaced from airways during flow-transients made at increasing pleural pressures.

The degree to which airways are narrowed in the collapsed region influences the effectiveness of airway clearance. Narrowing of the airway, at any given flow rate, increases linear velocity of the flowing gas. Since kinetic energy of the moving gas varies with the square of its linear velocity, decreasing the cross section to one-fifth, for example, will increase the gas energy by 25 times; it is on this basis that several authors assert that dynamic narrowing is even more important for effective coughing than are high expiratory flows [94,113].

At bronchoscopy and by bronchography, estimates of the degree of narrowing have ranged up to 80% reduction in tracheal cross section, with estimated velocities approaching 25,000 cm/sec, or three-quarters of the speed of sound. Airway cross section varies with the transmural pressure and depends on elastic properties, which may be expressed as curves of cross-sectional area plotted against transmural pressure.

Smooth muscle contraction changes the shape of the pressure-area curve in different ways at different levels in the airway. Tracheal muscle contraction can narrow the trachea at most transmural pressures but can also stiffen it by apposing the ends of its semilunar cartilages [61,103]. It therefore resists collapse more than in the relaxed state, maintaining a greater cross-sectional area at very negative transmural pressures. Bronchoconstriction tends to narrow small airways which do not resist compression. Both of these effects would tend to shift the EPP upstream, lengthening the compressed segment, and perhaps making cough effective in more remote airways.

Peribronchial pressure is difficult to measure and its physiology is complicated. There is evidence that pressure in the connective tissue space of the bronchovascular bundle is lower than pleural pressure, especially at high lung volumes [83]. Currently accepted ideas about the mechanical interdependence between adjacent structures in the lung suggest that when they are nonuniformly inflated, restoring forces are created tending to maintain uniform inflation.

During coughing, the collapse of intrapulmonary airways to very low cross sections at a time when the surrounding parenchyma is still at a high volume would be expected to set up such restoring forces. They would be expressed as a fall in peribronchial pressure, which would tend to minimize the fall in bronchial transmural pressure and the change in area. The potential for disruption of peribronchial alveoli is discussed below in Sec. III.A.

6. *Two-Phase Flow*

Rohrer [112] suggested that air could push plugs of material up the airways. Other authors have seen that high gas velocity makes this process more effective [113], and that dynamic collapse of airways contributes to increased velocities. In this section we examine the relationship between gas velocity and clearance of materials up through tubes, estimate the distribution of velocities in the airways during coughing, and then review some relevant experiments.

Coughing has been regarded as an example of two-phase cocurrent upflow [23,24,73]. In a chemical engineers' handbook [106] we find the following:

> Transference of momentum. Acceleration of one fluid in order to transfer its momentum to a second is a principle commonly used in . . . pumping from inaccessible depths.
>
> For upflow, the following general types of flow pattern have been observed where the values of the superficial velocities given are representative for liquids with viscosities less than about 100 centipoise and gas densities about that of air.
>
> 1. Bubble or aerated flow, in which the gas is dispersed as fine bubbles throughout the liquid, occurs for gas superficial velocities below about 2 ft/sec (60 cm/sec).
> 2. Piston, plug, or slug flow, in which the gas flows as large plugs, occurs for gas superficial velocities from about 2 to about 30 ft/sec (60 to 1000 cm/sec).
> 3. Annular or film flow, in which the liquid flows up the pipe as an annulus and the gas flows as a core, occurs for liquid superficial velocities less than 2 ft/sec and gas superficial velocities over 30 ft/sec (1000 cm/sec).
> 4. Mist flow, in which the liquid is carried as fine drops by the gas phase. Data indicate that this probably occurs for superficial gas velocities over about 70 ft/sec ($>$ 2500 cm/sec).

"Superficial velocity" is the average speed of the gas up the tube, and is simply the flow rate divided by the cross-sectional area of the tube.

The flow regimes are illustrated in Fig. 13.

In order to estimate the superficial velocity at various levels in the airway during cough, Leith [73] divided normal MEFRs by total cross sections derived from measurements of Rohrer for uninflated lung and Weibel for partially inflated lung, recognizing the difficulty of estimating appropriate dynamic cross-sections from these static data. Figure 14 indicates the regions in which mist

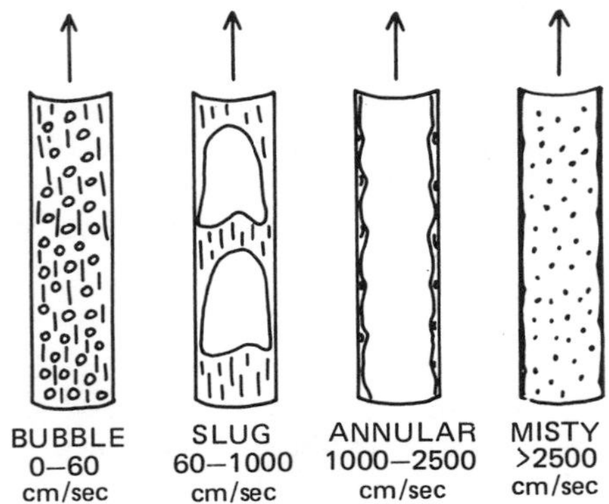

FIGURE 13 Four main types of two-phase cocurrent upflow, with the corresponding superficial velocity of the gas.

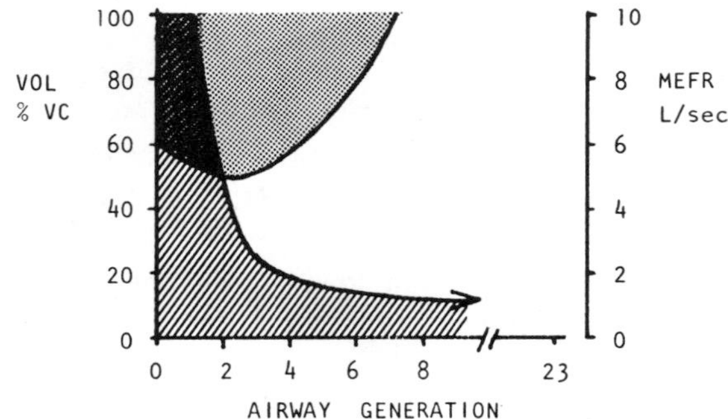

FIGURE 14 Airway regions in which gas superficial velocity exceeds 1500 cm/sec. In the stippled area this is the case even in the absence of dynamic narrowing. Where dynamic narrowing occurs (cross-hatched area) those high superficial velocities may exist far out in the lung even at low flow rates, but that is uncertain. See text.

flow might be expected for ordinary liquids. In the cross-hatched region, velocities over 2500 cm/sec can occur even without dynamic compression. The dashed line shows the airways which can be compressed; high velocities may occur in all such regions.

This rough approach, of course, confirms the idea that cough is most effective at high lung volumes where high flows are available; but it also suggests that cough pumping may be effective in uncompressed airways at high flow rates. That view is not generally held, but if true, would be of interest in some kinds of airway abnormalities, in which the EPP does not progress upstream in the usual way and intrathoracic airways are not compressed [84,94]. It would be interesting to know how effectively the long extrathoracic (therefore uncompressed) trachea of horses and giraffes is cleared by coughing.

In regions where airway compression occurs, gas velocities may be very high. Estimates range up to half or even three-quarters of the speed of sound [113]; that is, in the range of 16,000-24,000 cm/sec. These vastly exceed the minimum velocities necessary for mist pumping of ordinary liquids, but perhaps have some significance in clearing very viscid, tenacious materials, or solids.

A thick annulus of fluid can profoundly influence the pressure-flow behavior of a tube. Clarke and coworkers [24] conclude that significant effects can be expected in human airways. When waves or ripples appear in the liquid annulus, much increased energy losses occur and local resistance increases (Fig. 15). Flow-dependence of resistance should result, most marked where lumens are small and liquid layers are thick. This raises the interesting possibility that EPP may be "called" upstream to such regions, especially during the bronchoconstriction associated with coughing.

7. *Effectiveness of Coughing*

Defining and measuring cough effectiveness has been approached in several ways. Harris and Lawson [46,71] developed an index of "scrubbing action" based on measurements of flow and tracheal cross section during cough. They concluded that about 59, 26, and 15% of the total scrubbing action occurred in the first, second, and third cough in a continuous sequence. They noted that peak velocity came after the time of peak flow, since maximum narrowing had not occurred at the instant of peak flow. This is consistent with the view that the process of airway collapse contributes to peak flow.

Barach, Bickerman, and their colleagues published a series of papers in the early 1950s dealing with cough mechanics and artificial coughing [6,11,13]. They found that Thorotrast in aqueous suspension, thickened with gastric mucin, was suitable for semiquantitative measurement of clearance by cough-like maneu-

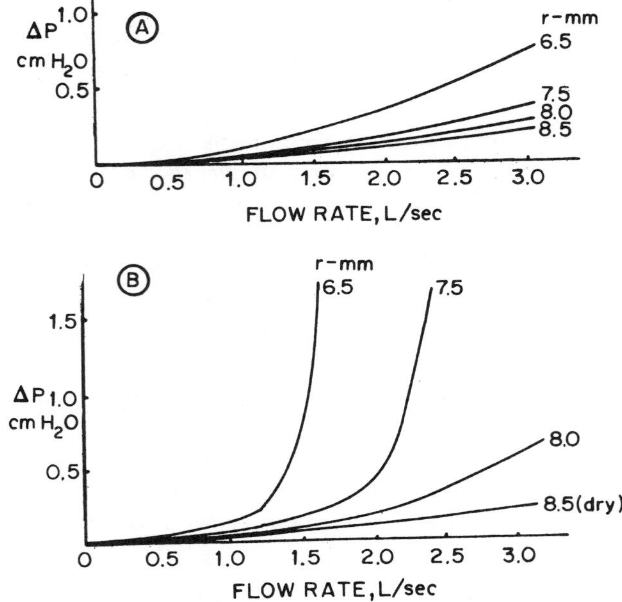

FIGURE 15 (A) Pressure-flow curves in dry tubes with lumen radius 8.5 mm and smaller. (B) Similar curves in dry tube with lumen radius 8.5 mm and with lumen reduced by a liquid annulus to the same radii as those shown in (A). When the gas and liquid begin to interact, energy losses increase abruptly and markedly. (From Clarke et al. [24].)

vers after instillation into the airways of anesthetized dogs. "Virtually all" of the material could be removed by artificial coughing which was probably less effective than spontaneous coughing would be. There was little or no clearance from control animals. In other studies they reported clearance of solid objects (lead shot, paper clips) from dogs' airways. Better methods of measuring cough effectiveness would be very useful.

Maximum expiratory flow rates vary inversely approximately with the square root of gas density. Thus at altitude or at depth, or while breathing gases other than air, changes in cough effectiveness are possible. Since offsetting changes in mass and maximum flows occur, the kinetic energy of the flowing gas may not change except insofar as the force-velocity behavior of expiratory muscles is involved, with resulting changes in effort-dependent downstream compression of airways. This might tend to diminish effectiveness of cough at altitude and perhaps to enhance it when gas density is increased. Several investigators have considered these issues, among them Dr. A. L. Barach who kindly called them to my attention (personal communication).

D. Circulatory and Cerebrospinal Fluid Systems

Coughing is like a brief but strong Valsalva maneuver, with related effects on the circulatory and cerebrospinal fluid systems. A thorough review is not appropriate for this chapter, but because some of the complications of coughing involve these two systems, they will be mentioned briefly. Sharpey-Schafer's chapter in the *Handbook of Physiology* remains a good description [120].

When pressure in the thorax and abdomen rises abruptly at the start of a cough, there is an initial sharp rise in systemic arterial pressure as the left heart maintains its transmural pressures during systole. To the extent that arterial runoff then is to regions not exposed to increased pressure, the load on the left heart is diminished, and it tends to operate at lower volumes. Simultaneously, venous return into the thoracoabdominal cavity decreases, so the blood volume begins to be redistributed to regions outside that cavity. Though venous reservoirs within the abdomen are exposed to pressure greater than pleural pressure, heart filling diminishes and stroke volume decreases. At the same time, the pressure in the cerebrospinal fluid rises, due in part to communication between peridural veins and prevertebral veins, which are exposed to the pressure in thorax and abdomen. A slight shift of volume into the peridural space is enough to equalize CSF and thoracoabdominal pressures. The increases in CSF pressure and arterial pressure initially are nearly equal, so that the vascular transmural pressures within the cranium are nearly constant [45]. But within a few heartbeats, the stroke volume and cardiac output diminish. Though arterial pressure may still be quite high compared with atmospheric pressure, the difference between arterial pressure and CSF pressure is decreasing. That difference is the effective perfusion pressure for the brain, where the critical closing pressure for small vessels depends upon both their smooth muscle tone and upon the surrounding pressure of the CSF [31]. The difference between arterial and CSF pressure can fall below 20 mmHg [45], and cerebral hypoperfusion and anoxia can occur. This is especially likely when hyperventilation and hypocarbia have induced smooth muscle contraction in the cerebral circulation. Thus tussive syncope (see below) is one member of a class of events which includes micturition syncope [44,115], weight-lifter's blackout [27], the "messtrick" [120], and the widely practiced children's trick known as a "fainting lark" in English (translated into the "bird syndrome" in the Spanish literature).

It is worth noting that the same low perfusion pressures then exist for viscera within the thorax and abdomen, too, including the coronary arteries [45].

The normal circulatory responses to Valsalva-like maneuvers include reflex vasodilation; their absence tends to make syncope less likely. The same is true when congestive heart failure exists [120].

The influences of elevated CSF pressure on circulatory dynamics of brain and spinal cord have been studied for decades, but only a few relatively complete investigations deal with the effects of cough and Valsalva maneuvers. The concepts of critical closing pressure [102] and the "vascular waterfall" [105] do not appear to have been widely applied yet in this field, though the pressure-flow relationships have been well-described [36]. While one author explicitly shows the critical closing behavior of the cerebral circulation [31], other recent reviewers make no mention of these concepts [70,90].

III. Pathophysiology of Coughing

A. Maladaptive Features of Coughing

1. Trauma

Lung disruption during forced expiratory maneuvers appears well documented [99,11]. Such maneuvers include coughing, expulsive and Valsalva maneuvers, vomiting, and even nose-blowing. It is puzzling at first that the lung could be disrupted at a time when it is getting smaller, but a plausible mechanism is suggested in one of the Macklins' remarkable papers [88]. They were considering Valsalva maneuvers, during which thoracic blood volume diminishes. If intrapulmonary blood vessel diameters decrease while the surrounding lung remains inflated, the vessel wall tends to pull away from adjacent alveoli. The pressure in the connective tissue space of the bronchovascular bundle must fall, the Macklins reasoned, and a big pressure difference is created which forces air through the walls of perivascular alveoli. It enters the connective tissue space and spreads along the bronchovascular bundle to the hilum and mediastinum. This hypothesis was supported by experiment. It anticipates, and appears to be another statement of, more recent ideas about mechanical interdependence among non-uniformly distended structures in the lung [93].

But the duration of a cough, or a series of coughs, in normal persons is not enough for much redistribution of thoracic blood to occur. Furthermore lung volume diminishes so rapidly that intrathoracic pressures cannot remain high for more than a couple of seconds. So vessel collapse seems unlikely. But airways do collapse, rapidly, and to a marked degree. The same mechanism Macklin applied to intrapulmonary vessels during Valsalva maneuvers can be applied to the intrapulmonary airways during cough. One would expect the effect to be pronounced if lung volume were high at the same time that airway collapse were pronounced—for example, because of much increased resistance in peripheral airways. Pulmonary interstitial emphysema and pneumomediastinum most frequently occur in children with asthma [111]. Air in the bronchovascular bundle allows narrowing of both the airways and the pulmonary vessels, with obvious consequences to resistance and closure, the distribution of gas and blood, and right heart loads. From the mediastinum air spreads to other interstitial spaces and can enter pleural, pericardial, and peritoneal cavities. In lung disruption due to expiratory effort, air embolism of cerebral and coronary arteries apparently never occurs[99], though it is a dominant and lethal part of lung disruption by overdistension [53]. Perhaps only in the latter case are vessels overextended lengthwise and torn across.

It is not clear whether destruction of parenchyma could occur adjacent to airways, though coughing has been suggested as a traumatic cause of pulmonary emphysema [5,38].

Trauma to airways and larynx probably occurs [38,132].

Trauma to the body wall presumably is due to violent muscle forces and to big transmural pressures associated with coughing, which may exceed voluntary maximum pressures. Pulled rectus abdominus muscles occur [4]. Inguinal and other hernias, vaginal prolapses, and other body wall abnormalities are affected and surgeons may delay their repair until chronic cough has been treated. During and after surgery of thorax, abdomen, central nervous system, eye, and other structures, coughing may be troublesome.

Cough fractures of ribs occur in infants [63] and adults [133] and are to be distinguished from stress fractures and fatigue fractures. Most frequently they involve one or several lower ribs in the axillary line, often on the same side as a preexisting lung lesion. They are easily overlooked. Pleuritic pain always is present and pleural effusion, pneumothorax, even hemoptysis may occur. Fractured vertebrae are reported [12]. Cough fractures are more common in males, and when bone strength is abnormally decreased.

2. *Tussive Syncope*

Fainting associated with coughing was described by Charcot in 1876. Since then hundreds of cases have been reported. The two major mechanisms proposed are reflected in two names given to the syndrome: laryngeal epilepsy and modified fainting lark. The literature is large and fascinating, but since the focus of this chapter is supposed to be on clearance mechanisms, only a brief description is given, drawn largely from several good short reviews [91,104,118,123].

Tussive syncope occurs in children [57] as well as adults. The latter are almost always vigorous middle-aged men with a chronic cough. They seldom volunteer the history of syncope on cough; the physician must seek it [91]. Virtually all who suffer tussive syncope have an obstructive airway disease—asthma or chronic bronchitis. The fainting fit is always associated with a paroxysm of coughing; unconsciousness may result within 10 sec. There is no prior aura, and no convulsion or incontinence of urine or feces. Coughing stops with unconsciousness, and recovery occurs within a few more seconds, without post-ictal state. The episodes are so abrupt that death may result if they occur during hazardous activities.

Most authors agree that the usual mechanism is cerebral hypoperfusion and hypoxia attendant upon a fall in cardiac output and a rise in CSF pressure, though the latter is often not considered. Why should this syndrome occur almost exclusively in persons with obstructive diseases? McIntosh and colleagues say that both the magnitude and duration of intrathoracic pressure rise are greater in persons with cough syncope than in those without it. In persons with severe obstructive disease, a cough paroxysm simulates a violent and long-sustained Valsalva maneuver. Though the glottis is open, expiratory flow is low and lung volume stays high, as shown in Fig. 16, panels ii–v. The associated increase in pressure can be accounted for partly on the basis of muscle force-length behavior (Fig. 17). It is also true that the decreased velocity of shortening will contribute to the increased pressures. Thus the expiratory muscles can exert nearly static maximum efforts throughout the cough paroxysm; that is not the case in normal persons who quickly expire to low lung volumes. In addition, it seems certain that the expiratory muscles are stronger, due to a "training effect," in people with chronic cough, probably including smokers. McIntosh and his colleagues [91] say that esophageal and CSF pressures over 300 mmHg are "not uncommon," but that is certainly above the usual range of pressure for normal people [28].

Sharpey-Schafer [118] reports one individual who, during coughing paroxysms, maintained intrathoracic pressures of 450 mmHg "for many seconds"—by far the highest I've heard of. Along with the sex-related incidence of obstructive diseases, sex and age-related differences in strength probably contribute to the apparent vast preponderance of vigorous middle-aged men among those who suffer cough syncope; Kerr and Derbes report only three women in their series of 290 cases [58].

The mechanisms by which the sustained Valsalva-like maneuver leads to cerebral hypoperfusion were discussed above.

Figure 18 shows the relation between pulmonary capillary wedge pressure (as an index of thoracoabdominal pressure) and the pressure measured by a catheter in a femoral artery during coughing leading to syncope. One may suspect that the "femoral artery" catheter was also exposed to thoracoabdominal pressure in this case, for the two pressures track one another closely after the first two heartbeats. But the very absence of a difference between them demonstrates the virtual absence of a perfusion pressure for thoracoabdominal (and

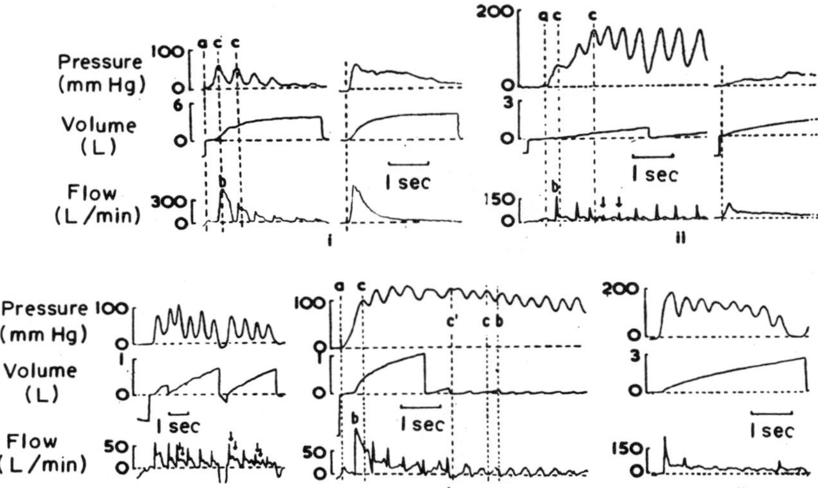

FIGURE 16 Panels i and ii show a series of voluntary coughs and a forced expiration in a normal and in a bronchitic subject. The transpulmonary pressure and pneumotachographic measuring systems had response times of less than 0.05 sec. Panels iii–v are from bronchitic subjects. In iv, as pressure rises flow falls to zero, according to Langlands, from whom the figure is taken [68]. Pressure stays high throughout.

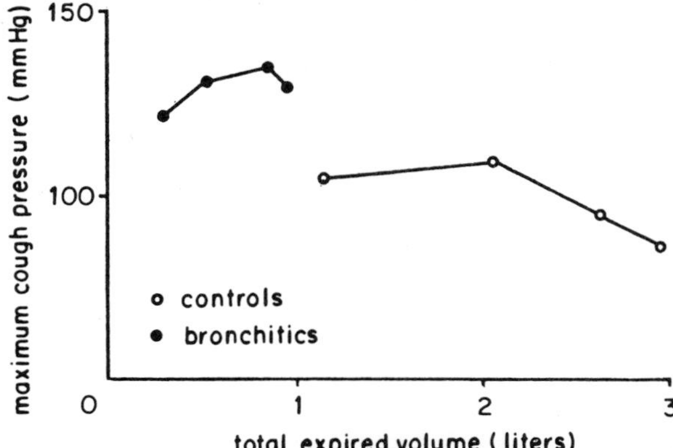

FIGURE 17 Mean maximum transpulmonary pressure of each of the first four in a series of voluntary coughs in normal and bronchitic subjects, plotted against the volume expired from TLC. Pressures are higher in bronchitics but are measured at higher lung volume and lower flows. Values are within normal range of static maxima. (From Langlands [68].)

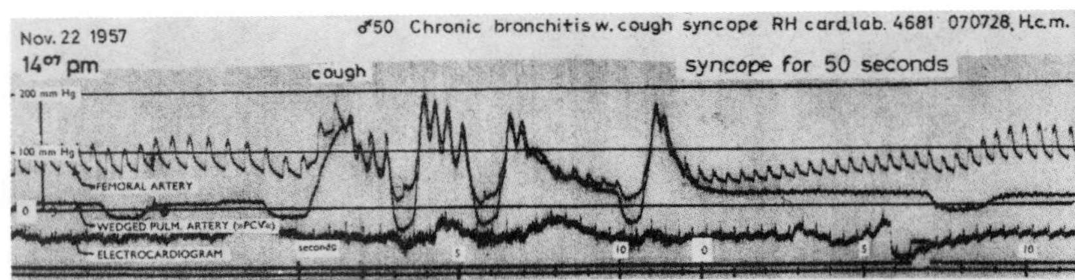

FIGURE 18 Simultaneous measurements of pressures in the femoral artery and a wedged pulmonary artery (PCV) and an electrocardiogram during coughing leading to syncope. During cough the two pressures become identical and their fluctuations appear to represent repetitive cough efforts rather than cardiac systole. (From Pedersen et al. [104.)

cerebral) viscera. A low cardiac output is suggested by the low arterial pressures during the inspirations between coughing episodes, and after the last one.

It is tempting to dismiss the "laryngeal epilepsy" mechanism originally postulated by Charcot, but that appears unwise in view of thoughtful reports like that of Morgan-Hughes [97]. He discusses four patients suffering episodes of unconsciousness precipitated by coughing. Two proved to have cerebral tumors and two had atheromata narrowing the internal carotid arteries. Many questions remain about cause and effect, but other authors also emphasize the need for careful assessment of neurological and circulatory systems of persons with cough syncope [69,127]. Even when the cause is clearly respiratory, the diagnosis and treatment of obstructive disease associated with wheezing and cough syncope is not simple, though some authors have said otherwise [1].

Vagal reflex influences on the heart have been implicated as the basis for cough syncope [39]. Irani and Sanchis [50] describe a patient who developed transient second-degree A-V block on deep inspiration, Valsalva, and coughing.

Other mechanisms for tussive syncope, reviewed (but not subscribed to) by McIntosh et al. [91] seem less useful to me and are omitted here.

3. *Miscellaneous Events*

A miscellaneous group of respiratory and circulatory events associated with coughing is listed here.

Coughing can precipitate wheezing, reduced expiratory flow rates, and asthma attacks [122,126]. Reflex bronchoconstriction as part of the cough reflex, or in response to the same irritants which initiated coughing, is discussed in Chap. 16. A relation exists with exercise-induced asthma [126]. Hypocapnia, and local mechanical irritation of airway due to collapse during coughing, have been suggested as contributing factors.

Sudden reverse pressure and flow transients in the venous system are invoked in several settings. Pulmonary embolism is said to result when venous thrombi are dislodged. Kinking and even knotting of venous catheters have caused failure of ventriculoatrial shunts used to treat hydrocephalus [100].

Paroxysmal cough has been induced by temporary transvenous pacemakers [55], and vagal afferent stimulation can lead to discharges in phrenic and abdominal muscle nerves [142].

Experienced bronchographers report that bronchographic medium can be almost explosively distributed in patterns interpreted as alveolar filling, at the time of coughing. It is not clear whether it results from prior inspiration. This suggests the operation of a mechanism which presumably could distribute other materials in the lung during coughing, for example, septic secretions. The role of coughing in transmission of disease between persons is well-known [79,81].

Urinary incontinence and other more or less severe inconvenience may attend coughing.

B. Failures of the Cough Mechanism

This section deals not only with cough failures but also with the kinds of change which, if severe enough, lead to failure. Examples are given to illustrate the range of possibilities.

It is convenient to list three categories of failure of the cough pump. I will call them drive, feed, and structural failure.

Any pump needs an energy source to drive it. Here we are concerned with the mechanisms by which pleural pressure is raised during coughing. The neural apparatus which controls the expiratory muscles, and the musculoskeletal apparatus itself, must be relatively intact.

Failures of the driving system can result from decreased sensitivity of cough receptors. Examples include topical anesthesia, inflammation or irritation [64], trauma (for example, by endotracheal tubes) or adaptation.

Central processing can allow depression by neurological illness or injury, by drugs, by hyperthermia [65], and in age or debility. Inhibition by voluntary and reflex mechanisms occurs when pain is associated with coughing, for example, in postsurgical patients, and those with rib fractures. Voluntary suppression may be easier than is usually supposed [38].

Muscular and efferent neural abnormalities obviously can interfere with or prevent coughing. Myasthenia, spinal cord injuries, curare-like drugs, and cholinesterase inhibitors are examples.

Pumps must also be fed appropriate materials. This one must have fed into it from below not only the secretions and other materials it clears, but also the high flows of air which constitute the hydraulic coupling between muscles and airway secretions. If it is correct that coughing is effective only in larger airways, then we rely on the mucociliary system to feed secretions into them. Many things can impair mucociliary function. Abnormal kinds or quantities of secretions exist in mucoviscidosis, cholinergic crisis, asthma, and dehydration; the ability of the cilia to sweep them up the airway is diminished. Ciliary function may be abnormal when irritants like SO_2 or tobacco smoke are inhaled, or in diseases such as influenza. These are discussed elsewhere.

The airflows available for coughing are diminished in the obstructive diseases like asthma, emphysema, and chronic bronchitis. The reductions may be extreme, to maximum expiratory flows of a liter per second or less over most of the vital capacity even in ambulatory persons. When expiratory flows are very low, the ability to clear large airways is diminished. The energy available in the moving gas stream is decreased, and abnormal degrees and patterns of airway collapse occur [21,49].

Campbell and Young [21] observed that "in many patients a relaxed exhalation produced a greater expired volume than a forceful exhalation." They ascribed this to excessive tracheobronchial collapse. Anything which decreases expiratory flow throughout a prolonged expiration will decrease the expired volume, because breath-holding ability or other factors set a limit to the duration of such maneuvers. Decreases in flow can result from true "negative effort-dependence", but alveolar gas compression during forced expirations also results in lower flows throughout the maneuver, because true lung volume (as would be measured plethysmographically), and therefore lung recoil and expiratory flows, are less than they would be at all instants during a less vigorous expiration. This is the more likely explanation for the decreased VC during forced as compared with relaxed maneuvers.

Langlands [68] shows striking data which are interpreted as showing that flow at the mouth decreased markedly as a function of expiratory effort in some bronchitics (at a time when expiratory flow is so low that the volume expired during the maneuver is quite small). This too would be attributable to a decrease in lung volume by gas compression, and other usual causes of "negative effort-dependence," except for Langlands' assertion that flow *stops* at high effort (Fig. 17, panel iv). If that is true, one is forced to conclude that all airways were closed and that some reopened when the expiratory effort was relaxed and the thoracic gas reexpanded. Clearly if airways are closed, cough clearance of regions downstream from them is not possible.

Nonuniform behavior of the lung characterizes many lung diseases. The influences of such inhomogeneities on coughing are not well-known. Gravity-dependent differences in regional lung volumes are more marked in persons with decreased lung recoil, and may not disappear even at high lung volumes, if the maximum transpulmonary pressures are low. Closure of dependent regions persists at volumes above the upright FRC even in normal people after the age of 65 [8]. Postural changes appear to be rational as a means of promoting lung clearance in such circumstances. When bronchospasm is present, some lung units may remain closed at all lung volumes, and their clearance by either cough or mucociliary activity is doubtful.

To the extent that the extrathoracic trachea is not subjected to dynamic compression, gas velocities in it may fall too low for effective clearance if expiratory flow rates are low. Postural drainage may assist clearance of secretions brought to that level, but not farther, by cough.

Finally, if we take the narrow view that the airways themselves from the sixth or seventh generation of branching out to the mouth constitute the actual structure of the pump itself, we can consider how structural abnormalities can impede pump function.

Two basic mechanisms often coexist: those which decrease expiratory flows and those which change the effectiveness with which the airstream scrubs the airway walls. These are discussed well in an article by Macklem, Fraser, and Brown [84].

Decreased flows can result from excessively collapsible airway regions, for example in tracheomalacia. Apparently the flow-limiting segment can be held at too easily collapsed regions, instead of moving progressively upstream with decreasing lung volume. Dynamic compression does not occur in regions upstream of such a site until lung volumes and flows are very low, and cough clearance is probably ineffective under those conditions. Flows may be very much decreased by severe narrowing of the airway, for example, in tracheal stenosis or extrinsic compression by tumor or vascular structures. A distinction should be made between intrathoracic and extrathoracic narrowing of this kind, since the former is subjected to dynamic narrowing but the latter may be dynamically widened, during expiration.

Abnormal contours of the airway walls impede cough clearance. In bronchiectasis and bronchomegaly, secretions residing in outpockets along the airway are poorly cleared. During bronchography, one can see fluid radiopaque media raised by coughing become trapped just above the narrowing caused by thyroid enlargement, pooling there until, during the next inspiration, inflowing air and gravity again take it into the thoracic airways. Persons who work in intensive care areas are aware of the tendency for secretions to accumulate at the distal end of endotracheal tubes, where the mucus escalator ends, because the noncollapsible tube does not permit effective cough clearance unless flow is high. Abnormal shapes of collapsing airways might impair cough function [110]. Bronchoscopists describe excessive collapse of widened tracheas, with apposition of inner walls laterally; secretions are trapped there, while air flow is confined to a restricted channel medially.

C. Consequences of Cough Failure

There is general agreement that absence of effective cough is life-threatening, but there is little more to go on than uniform clinical experience. Aspiration of gastric contents or secretions from oral and nasal cavities is more likely when the cough reflex is absent. Obstruction of airways, if not cleared, leads to plugging, atelectasis, and gas exchange abnormalities which may be very severe. Atelectasis and retention of secretions, and failure to clear irritants and bacteria seem to predispose to acute and chronic infection. Bronchomegaly and infection are closely associated [54]. But does the infection occur because of existing airway deformation and inadequate clearance, or does chronic infection cause tissue destruction and airway deformation? And why does one quadriplegic patient do well for months or years, while another paralyzed or comatose patient dies a respiratory death in a few weeks?

IV. Clinical Aspects of Cough

A. Cough as an Index of Disease

Popular knowledge recognizes the association of cough with many kinds of diseases. Infection ranging from acute viral upper respiratory infections and influenza, to pertussis, bronchitis, pneumonia, and tuberculosis, as well as allergy and various occupational exposures, the smoker's cough, and such feared diseases as lung cancer are all familiar examples.

Medical texts and articles furnish long lists, because coughing is an easily noted sign and symptom which is useful in diagnosis and management of adult and pediatric diseases [5,76,82,125]. Bickerman's chapter in the second edition of *Clinical Cardiopulmonary Physiology* [12] is a good example; it includes a table of causes which exemplify the broad range of diseases and suggest the difficulty of the differential diagnosis (Table 2).

The distinction between coughing and throat-clearing is sometimes unclear, the latter frequently associated with sinusitis and postnasal drip [141].

Cough is associated with mechanical irritation of the visceral pleura; thus it is said to occur at the time of rupture of blebs at the lung surface, when rib fractures occur, and during medical procedures like pleural taps.

TABLE 1 Some Causes of Cough (By permission: H. A. Bickerman, Chap. 31 in *Clinical Cardiopulmonary Physiology* 2nd ed. 1960, Grune and Stratton.)

Infectious

Viral: common cold, atypical pneumonia, psittacosis, measles, influenza
Bacterial: the pneumonias, tuberculosis, pertussis
Mycotic: histoplasmosis, coccidioidomycosis, moniliasis, actinomycosis, blastomycosis
Spirochetal: syphilis, Vincent's infection
Rickettsial: typhus, Q fever
Parasitic: ascariosis, distomiasis

Irritative

Chemical: noxious gases and fumes, smoke
Mechanical: retained secretions, foreign bodies, improper use of voice
Thermal: exposure to marked variations in temperature

Allergic

Asthma, vasomotor rhinitis
Loeffler's pneumonia, eosinophilic granuloma

Neoplastic

Intraluminary: benign, malignant
Extraluminary with compression: lymphomas, Hodgkins, etc.

Vascular

Heart failure with pulmonary congestion
Pericarditis
Pulmonary embolism, pulmonary infarction
Compression due to aneurysm

Pneumoconiosis

Silicosis, berylliosis, asbestosis, hemochromatosis

Unknown Etiology

Collagen disorders: disseminated lupus erythematosus, periarteritis nodosa, scleroderma
Sarcoidosis
Pulmonary fibrosis, granulomatosis

Psychogenic

Habit spasm or "tic," tension states

It would be fun to write a chapter about unusual causes of cough. Banyai [5] mentions osteophytes of the cervical spine, aneurysm of the ascending palatine artery, neurilemmoma of the vagus nerve, intralobar sequestration (Rokitansky's syndrome) and others. Wolff [137] cured three cases of chronic cough —some of them socially incapacitating, as severe coughing can be—by removal of hairs touching the tympanic membrane. Mital and Agarwala report a patient who coughed up a bronchogenic carcinoma [95].

The presence or absence of coughing in response to stimulation by tracheal catheter is used as an index of a patient's ability to protect his own airway from aspiration of foreign materials, and is one of the criteria used in decisions about tracheal intubation or extubation [37].

As an index of disease in epidemiology, coughing has special importance [77]; for example, it is used in surveys of smoking [141], air pollution [78], occupational health, and the influence of weather on respiratory diseases [75].

Wynder and coworkers [139] state "Persistent cough, together with the production of phlegm, is common in the American male population . . . the most important factor in persistent cough is cigarette smoking." They assert that "The most effective way to reduce cough is to discontinue cigarette smoking," and cite followup data which show that 77% of smokers with a bronchial cough are freed of their cough when they stop smoking, 54% within 4 weeks [140]. These authors feel that chronic cough is taken too lightly by the public and physicians alike, since "bronchial cough usually indicates that the ciliated bronchial epithelium has been destroyed and/or that the overlying mucus is so viscous that it can no longer be effectively moved upward by ciliary motion." They regard bronchial cough as a precursor of disease including recurrent infection, chronic destructive bronchitis, and possibly cancer.

B. Suppressing Cough

When cough is nonproductive, painful, traumatic, inconvenient, or downright dangerous (as in tussive syncope), its suppression may be desirable. Many drugs are available which have this effect, including alcohol [9,20], codeine, and other agents. Commercial cough medicines are many; the search for new agents is continuous and the reports on their effectiveness abound [25,33,43,138]. I will not review them.

In anesthesia, intensive care, bronchoscopy, radiology, and research laboratories, instrumentation of the airways of humans and animals is frequent. Topical anesthesia, general and intravenous "local" [124] anesthetics, narcotics or other depressants, and curare-like drugs are all used at times in various combinations, to permit safe invasion of the airways. Adaptation of (or damage to) receptors occurs within hours, so that fully conscious people can tolerate endotracheal or tracheostomy tubes without difficulty.

Voluntary suppression of coughing apparently is feasible, and can be assisted by voluntary acts like quick inspiratory maneuvers [38].

C. Facilitating Cough

The same stages of coughing can be considered as in the section above on cough failure.

Facilitating the cough drive can start with its triggering by mechanical, osmotic, or chemical irritation of cough receptors. Tracheal catheters (both laryngeal and percutaneous), instillation of liquids, or inhalation of irritants such as citric acid aerosols [136] and SO_2 are used for clinical and laboratory purposes. This also triggers bronchoconstriction [122].

Withdrawing of inhibitory reflexes, for example due to pain, also permits more effective coughing. The trade-off between analgesia and cough depression is a matter of judgment when narcotics are used for this purpose in the postoperative period. Mechanical support of abdominal or thoracic incisions by binders or by manual compression is useful [7].

Direct stimulation of peripheral nerves apparently can induce coughing but is not applied clinically [55,137,142], nor is central stimulation [56,98].

Attention to musculoskeletal function of the drive mechanism is exemplified by adequate reversal of curariform drugs, management of myasthenia, and maneuvers intended to maintain mobility of the rib cage.

Some quadriparetics are apparently "able to trigger a reflex contraction of the abdominal muscles at the end of a deep inspiration and thus actively assist their own cough" [59].

Does muscle training have a place? Stronger inspiratory muscles may allow cough to start at higher lung volumes where it is presumably more effective. Weak expiratory muscles obviously would tend to diminish cough clearance, but, at least in persons with chronic cough, the expiratory muscles may already be stronger than in normal persons [110,118]. The evidence is slender that such muscle training is feasible.

Feed mechanisms involve both the airflow available and the mucociliary system. Hydration, mucolytics, inhaled mist, expectorants and other modalities are used to try to improve mucus properties and flow.

Expiratory flow rates can be increased by bronchodilators by inflation to high starting volumes voluntarily (including glossopharyngeal breathing) [2] or passively, and when expiration is assisted by manual compression of the body wall [59]. Postural drainage is helpful as are some of the maneuvers of chest physical therapy such as chest vibration and the various forms of percussion.

Rainer [109] and others have advocated surgical procedures to stiffen the extrapulmonary intrathoracic airways, in situations where excessive collapsibility was thought to be responsible for decreased expiratory flows. The results have not been encouraging and some authors consider the procedure useless [84], but it is not clear that no benefit is ever derived.

Glottic rehabilitation with return of cough has been reported [74].

D. Cough Substitutes and Treatment of Failure

The list of things we can do when the cough mechanism fails is disappointingly short. It is found in texts and articles on intensive respiratory care and on chest physical therapy.

Great care in filtering, warming, and humidifying inspired air, the use of mucolytic and bronchodilator agents, intermittent positive pressure breathing, deep breathing and sighing, postural changes, and chest physical therapy all are directed toward optimizing the function of mucociliary clearance mechanisms.

Often endotracheal intubation or tracheostomy is used to facilitate the steps above, to protect the airway from the entrance of foreign materials, and to permit convenient suctioning of the airway by catheter or fiberoptic bronchoscope. The substitution of a suction catheter for a cough is a poor bargain, but often the only one available. It is a dirty technique which is incompletely effective, in a limited distribution in the airways, and which is traumatic to the airway mucosa. Atelectasis [17] and severe acute circulatory disturbances may occur during suctioning, because the interior of the trachea is connected to wall suction by a catheter which itself can nearly occlude the endotracheal tube through which it is passed, or around which the larynx may close reflexly if no endotracheal tube is present. Profound hypoxia [131], vagal stimulation [121], acute right-heart strain and left-heart loading can attend the very low lung volumes and intrathoracic pressures which result.

Lung lavage is a potentially powerful clearance technique whose cautious exploration continues [117]. Since expiration from the liquid-filled lung usually takes place at maximum flow rates, driven by a water column as great as a meter in height, this technique really is not only lavage but liquid-filled artificial coughing in a manner and degree never contemplated in the air-filled lung. The mechanics of liquid-filled coughing are not well worked out. Recoil forces are probably less during deflation in the water-filled than in the air-filled lung, because the air-liquid interface is absent. The density and viscosity of the expired medium are profoundly different; violent flow oscillations are commonly observed during expiration, and maximum expiratory flows are between one-fiftieth and one-hundredth of the corresponding air-filled values [116]. The location of the flow-limiting segment, and linear velocities at the choke point, are not known to me. The mechanics of airway clearance must be changed when the expired medium is a liquid with density comparable with that of mucus. I have no idea about what happens to them when slightly denser fluorocarbons immiscible with water are respired, reintroducing interfacial phenomena. Such liquids are respired in some animal experimental settings, and human use has been proposed [19,114].

E. Artificial Coughing

Barach, Bickerman, and others developed artificial coughing methods and devices, described in a series of articles in the early 1950s [6,11,13]. Starting with passive expiration after inflation of the relaxed respiratory system to static pressures of 40 cmH_2O, they progressed to methods which abruptly opened a valve to expose the airway to a pressure of -60 cmH_2O or more, for a period of seconds. This technique, referred to as exsufflation with negative pressure (EWNP), produced high expiratory flows and was shown effective in clearing viscous radiopaque materials and dense foreign bodies from the airways of anesthetized dogs. The mechanics of forced emptying of lungs by sucking on the airway are comparable with those which apply when pleural pressure is raised (with exceptions having to do with extrathoracic airways and the presence of cannulas in the airways). Therefore EWNP presumably can produce the dynamic narrowing of airways downstream of the flow-limiting segment which is necessary for the highest linear velocities in those regions. Trauma to mucosa at the entrance of airway cannulas appears equally probable in spontaneous and passive coughing, as long as similar pressures are involved. The potential for forced expiration to dangerously low lung volumes exists, so either the duration, the volume change, or the minimum thoracic gas volume should be controlled, though this does not appear to have been done systematically in most cases. Clinical trials with apparently valuable results were reported by several investigators including Colebatch in 1961 [26], but the method has not been widely used and is unknown to most respiratory intensivists in my experience. The equipment was cumbersome and perhaps the idea was ahead of its time by a decade, for widespread interest in respiratory intensive care did not blossom until mechanical ventilators and blood gas analysis became widely available. If so, its reintroduction might now result in wider use of such methods, which, if improved in fairly obvious ways, could become clinically applicable techniques capable of clearing more airways, more completely than current methods, with less danger of trauma, sepsis, and cardiorespiratory complications.

V. Looking Ahead

I come away from this necessarily incomplete review with questions in five categories of basic and applied science.

First, evolutionary, comparative, and developmental aspects of coughing, which have not been covered here. When does the cough reflex appear, in evolution and in the individual? And how is it distributed among species? The tench coughs [144]. What nonmammalian species cough and which don't? Why? Did dinosaurs cough? How could we know? Does life style influence coughing? One supposes that burrowing animals or residents of dusty desert, plain, and barn would have different clearance demands from eagle, bat, or seal. Irving and Scholander saw a porpoise close its blowhole, never to breathe again, after a few drops of fresh water were splashed into it [51].

Does size influence the need for cough, or its effectiveness? I've never heard a mouse cough, and Korpas [66], cited by Widdicombe in Chap. 16, says rats do not cough. Reynolds numbers go down as airway diameter diminishes at any given gas velocity; simple calculations indicate Reynolds numbers of 100 or less in the trachea of mice at rest, and what about the capacity to suspend and clear droplets of mucus from a trachea less than a millimeter in diameter? Should those who use small animals in studies of airway physiology and inhaled particles take account of such scale factors?

Shapes vary widely among animals. I see no mechanism for dynamic compression of most of the trachea in geese, horses, and giraffes. Is dynamic compression really important? Can an elephant blow his nose effectively or must he sniffle?

Second, physiological aspects of coughing. During cough and Valsalva maneuvers the intracranial and thoracoabdominal viscera form a complex interlocking system of Starling resistors, whose functioning is not fully understood. Coughing in the liquid-filled lung looks interesting. Are expiratory muscles really stronger in persons with chronic cough? How is liquid radiopaque medium suddenly spread widely through alveoli during the expulsive phase of coughing, if the bronchographers are correct? How far out in the lung does cough really work? Is collateral ventilation significant in the cough clearance of airway obstructions (Proctor, personal communication)? How can the effectiveness of coughing best be measured?

Third, maladaptive effects of coughing. Plausible suggestions have been made that coughing is traumatic to the mucous membranes lining airways, and to the alveoli surrounding them. If so, it seems very important to find out about it.

Fourth, mechanisms of cough failure. Until these are better understood, prevention and intervention are difficult to explore thoroughly.

Fifth, and most important, therapies are needed to optimize cough and other clearance mechanisms, to slow or prevent the deterioration of those mechanisms in disease, and to treat the consequences of their loss. Artificial coughing merits reexamination, not only in paralyzed patients with normal lungs as in the past, but also in forms which might be helpful for those with other kinds of cough failure.

Acknowledgment

We thank the authors, editors, and journals for their permission to use materials from the works cited in the figure legends.

References

1. D. W. Aaronson, R. N. Rovner, and R. Patterson, Cough syncope—Case presentation and review, *J. Allergy,* **46**:359-363 (1970).
2. J. E. Affeldt, Neuromotor paralysis. In *Handbook of Physiology,* Section 3: *Respiration,* Vol. II. Edited by W. O. Fenn and H. Rahn. Washington, D.C., American Physiological Society, 1965, Chap. 46.
3. E. Agostoni, Action of respiratory muscles. In *Handbook of Physiology,* Section 3: *Respiration,* Vol. I. Edited by W. O. Fenn and H. Rahn. Washington, D.C., American Physiological Society, 1964, Chap. 12, pp. 380-381.
4. R. L. Anderton, Rectus abdominal muscles pulled by coughing, *JAMA,* **222**: 486 (1972).
5. A. L. Banyai, A symptom connoting many causes and sequels, *Chest,* **60**(4): 335 (1971).
6. A. L. Barach, G. J. Beck, H. A. Bickerman, and H. E. Seanor, Physical methods simulating mechanisms of the human cough, *J. Appl. Physiol.,* **5**:85-91 (1952).
7. D. Barlow, A cough-belt to prevent and treat postoperative pulmonary complications, *Lancet,* **2**:736 (1964).
8. R. Begin, A. D. Renzetti, A. H. Bigler, and S. Watanabe, Flow and age dependence of airway closure and dynamic compliance, *J. Appl. Physiol.,* **38**:199-207 (1975).
9. H. Berkowitz, The effect of ethanol on the cough reflex, *Clin. Sci. Mol. Med.,* **45**:527-531 (1973).
10. B. A. Berman, Habit cough in adolescent children, *Ann. Allergy,* **24**:43-46 (1966).
11. H. A. Bickerman, Exsufflation with negative pressure (E.W.N. P.): Elimination of radiopaque and foreign bodies from bronchi of anesthetised dogs, *Arch. Intern. Med.,* **93**:698-704 (1954).
12. H. A. Bickerman, Bronchial drainage and phenomena of cough. In *Clinical Cardiopulmonary Physiology,* 2nd ed. Edited by B. L. Gordon. New York, Grune and Stratton, 1960, Chap. 31.

13. H. A. Bickerman, G. J. Beck, C. Gordon, and A. L. Barach, Physical methods simulating mechanisms of the human cough: Elimination of radiopaque material from the bronchi of dogs, *J. Appl. Physiol.*, **5**:92-98 (1952).
14. W. S. Blumenthal, F. J. DeMaio, and L. Cander, The relationship between air flow transients, intrathoracic pressure, and airway geometry during cough, *Clin. Res.*, **10**:404 (Abstr.) (1962).
15. R. Bookman, Cough in allergic respiratory disease, *Ann. Allergy*, **29**:367-371 (1971).
16. E. Bors, Simple methods of examination in paraplegia. II. The cough response of the external anal sphincter, *Med. Serv. J. Can.*, **22**:662-667 (1966).
17. B. Brandstater and M. Muallem, Atelectasis following tracheal suction in infants, *Anesthesiology*, **31**:468-473 (1969).
18. K. Bucher, Pathophysiology and pharmacology of cough, *Pharmacol. Rev.*, **10**:43-58 (1958).
19. H. W. Calderwood, J. H. Modell, B. C. Ruiz, J. E. Brogdon, and C. I. Hood, Pulmonary lavage with liquid fluorocarbon in a model of pulmonary edema, *Anesthesiology*, **38**:141-144 (1973).
20. B. Calesnick and H. Vernick, Antitussive activity of ethanol, *Q. J. Stud. Alcohol*, **32**:434-441 (1971).
21. A. H. Campbell and I. F. Young, Tracheobronchial collapse, a variant of obstructive respiratory disease, *Br. J. Dis. Chest*, **57**:174-181 (1963).
22. G. A. Cavagna, E. A. Stemmler, and A. B. DuBois, Alveolar resistance to atelectasis, *J. Appl. Physiol.*, **22**:441-452 (1967).
23. S. W. Clarke, The role of two-phase flow in bronchial clearance, *Bull. Physiopathol. Respir. (Nancy)*, **9**:359-372 (1973).
24. S. W. Clarke, J. G. Jones, and D. R. Oliver, Resistance to two-phase gas-liquid flow in airways, *J. Appl. Physiol.*, **29**(4):464-471 (1970).
25. B. M. Cohen, Respiratory and cough mechanics in antitussive trials. Responsivity of objective indices to the treatment of acute upper respiratory tract infections, *Respiration*, **32**(1):32-45 (1975).
26. J. Colebatch, Artificial coughing for patients with respiratory paralysis, *Aust. N. Z. J. Med.*, **10**:201-212 (1961).
27. D. Compton, P. McN. Hill, and J. D. Sinclair, Weight-lifter's blackout, *Lancet*, **2**:1234-1237 (1973).
28. C. D. Cook, J. Mead, and M. M. Orzalesi, Static volume-pressure characteristics of the respiratory system during maximal efforts, *J. Appl. Physiol.*, **19**:1016-1022 (1964).
29. S. V. Dawson and E. A. Elliott, Expiratory flow limitation at wave speed, *Fed. Proc.*, **33**:324 (Abstr.) (1974).
30. H. Dayman, Mechanics of airflow in health and in emphysema, *J. Clin. Invest.*, **30**:1175-1190 (1951).
31. R. C. Dewey, H. P. Pieper, and W. E. Hunt, Experimental cerebral hemodynamics. Vasomotor tone, critical closing pressure, and vascular bed resistance, *J. Neurosurg.*, **41**:597-606 (1974).

32. S. Di Rienzo, Bronchial dynamism, *Radiology,* **53**:168-186 (1949).
33. N. B. Eddy, Codeine and its alternates for pain and cough relief, *Ann. Intern. Med.,* **71**:1209-1212 (1969).
34. J. N. Evans and M. Jaeger, Rates of volume displacement at the mouth and thorax during various respiratory maneuvers, *Fed. Proc.,* **32**:445 (Abstr.) (1973).
35. K. Faaborg-Anderson, Electromyographic investigation of intrinsic laryngeal muscles in humans, *Acta Physiol. Scand. [Suppl. 140],* **41**:77-83 (1957).
36. J. K. Farrar, Jr. and M. R. Roach, The effects of increased intracranial pressure on flow through major cerebral arteries in vitro, *Stroke,* **4**:795-806 (1973).
37. T. W. Feeley and J. Hedley-Whyte, Weaning from controlled ventilation and supplemental oxygen, *N. Engl. J. Med.,* **292**(17):903-906 (1975).
38. C. M. Fisher, The possible role of coughing in the pathogenesis of pulmonary emphysema, *Can. Med. Assoc. J.,* **91**:351-352 (1964).
39. C. K. Francis, J. B. Singh, and B. J. Polansky, Interruption of aberrant conduction of atrioventricular junctional tachycardia by cough, *N. Engl. J. Med.,* **286**:357-358 (1972).
40. D. L. Fry and R. E. Hyatt, Pulmonary mechanics: a unified analysis of the relationship between pressure, volume, and gas flow in the lungs of normal and diseased human subjects, *Am. J. Med.,* **29**:672-689 (1960).
41. B. Gandevia, The spirogram of gross expiratory tracheobronchial collapse in emphysema, *Q. J. Med.,* **32**:23-31 (1962).
42. M. Grotjahn, Smoking, coughing, laughing, and applause—a comparative study of respiratory symbolism, *Int. J. Psychoanal.,* **53**:345-349 (1972).
43. S. Grzybowski, Cough medicines, *Can. Med. Assoc. J.,* **92**:619-620 (1965).
44. J. H. Haldane, Micturition syncope, *Can. Med. Assoc. J.,* **101**:712-713 (1969).
45. W. F. Hamilton, R. A. Woodbury, and H. T. Harper, Jr., Arterial, cerebrospinal, and venous pressures in man during cough and strain, *Am. J. Physiol.,* **141**:42-50 (1944).
46. R. S. Harris and T. V. Lawson, The relative mechanical effectiveness and efficiency of successive voluntary coughs in healthy young adults, *Clin. Sci.,* **34**:569-577 (1968).
47. E. Huizinga, The "tussive squeeze" and the "bechic blast" of the Jacksons, *Ann. Otol. Rhinol. Laryngol.,* **76**:923-934 (1967).
48. R. E. Hyatt and R. E. Flath, Relationship of air flow to pressure during maximal respiratory effort in man, *J. Appl. Physiol.,* **21**:477-482 (1966).
49. R. E. Hyatt, R. Sittipong, S. Olafsson, and W. A. Potter, Some factors determining pulmonary pressure-flow behavior at high rates of airflow. In *Airway Dynamics.* Edited by Bouhuys. Springfield, Ill., C. C Thomas, 1970, pp. 43-60.
50. F. Irani and J. Sanchis, Inspiration- and cough-induced atrioventricular block, *Can. Med. Assoc. J.,* **105**:735-736 (1971).

51. L. P. Irving, P. Scholander, and S. W. Grinnell, The respiration of the porpoise, *Tursiops truncatus, J. Cell. Comp. Physiol.,* **17**:145-168 (1941).
52. Marc J. Jaeger, Coughing and forced expiration at reduced barometric pressure, *Fed. Proc.,* **31**:322 (Abstr.) (1972).
53. R. E. James, Extra-alveolar air resulting from submarine escape training: A post-training roentgenographic survey of 170 submariners. Naval Submarine Medical Center Report 550. Bureau of Medicine and Surgery U.S. Navy, 1968.
54. R. F. Johnston and R. A. Green, Tracheobronchiomegaly, *Am. Rev. Respir. Dis.,* **91**:35-50 (1965).
55. J. Kang, M. Gupta, P. A. Catangay, and F. Raia, Paroxysmal cough induced by transvenous pacemaker, *Am. Heart J.,* **81**(5):719-720 (1971).
56. Y. Kase, Y. Wakita, G. Kito, T. Miyata, T. Yuizono, and M. Kataoka, Centrally-induced coughs in the cat, *Life Sci.,* **9**:49-59 (1970).
57. R. M. Katz, Cough syncope in children with asthma, *J. Pediatr.,* **77**:48-51 (1970).
58. A. Kerr, V. J. Derbes, The syndrome of cough syncope, *Ann. Intern. Med.,* **39**:1240-1253 (1953).
59. Nell A. Kirby, M. J. Barnerias, and A. A. Siebens, An evaluation of assisted cough in quadriparetic patients, *Arch. Phys. Med. Rehabil.,* **47**:705-710 (1966).
60. R. J. Knudson and D. E. Knudson, Pressure-flow relationships in the isolated canine trachea, *J. Appl. Physiol.,* **35**:804-812 (1973).
61. R. J. Knudson and D. E. Knudson, Effect of muscle constriction of flow-limiting collapse of isolated canine trachea, *J. Appl. Physiol.,* **38**:125-131 (1975).
62. R. J. Knudson, J. Mead, and D. E. Knudson, Contribution of airway collapse to supramaximal expiratory flows, *J. Appl. Physiol.,* **36**(6):653-667 (1974).
63. I. Kopcsányi, A. Laczay, and L. Nagy, Cough fracture of ribs in infants with dyspnea, *Acta Paediatr. Acad. Sci. Hung.,* **10**(2):93-98 (1969).
64. J. Korpás, P. Bilcik, and E. Fraenkel, Changes in coughing in cats with experimental or spontaneous inflammation of the respiratory tract, *Physiol. Bohemoslov.,* **14**(5):488-494 (1965).
65. J. Korpás and Z. Tomori, The effect of hyperthermia on cough and respiration, *Physiol. Bohemoslov.,* **7**:527-531 (1958).
66. J. Korpás and Z. Tomori, *Cough and Other Respiratory Reflexes.* Bratislava, Czechoslovakian Academy of Science, 1975.
67. H. Kravitz, R. M. Gomberg, R. C. Burnstine, S. Hagler, and A. Korach, Psychogenic cough tic in children and adolescents. Nine case histories illustrate the need for re-evaluation of this common but frequently unrecognized problem, *Clin. Pediatr.,* **8**:580-583 (1969).
68. Jean Langlands, The dynamics of cough in health and in chronic bronchitis, *Thorax,* **22**:88-96 (1967).
69. S. J. Larson, Herniated cerebellar tonsils and cough syncope, *J. Neurosurg.,* **40**:524-528 (1974).

70. N. A. Lassen, Control of cerebral circulation in health and disease, *Circ. Res.*, **34**:749-760 (1974).
71. T. V. Lawson and R. S. Harris, Assessment of the mechanical efficiency of coughing in healthy young adults, *Clin. Sci.*, **33**:209-224 (1967).
72. George C. Leiner, S. Abramowitz, M. J. Small, and V. B. Stenby, Cough peak flow rate, *Am. J. Med. Sci.*, **251**:211-214 (1966).
73. D. E. Leith, Cough, *J. Am. Phys. Ther. Assoc.*, **48**(5):439-447 (1968).
74. R. B. Lewy, Glottic rehabilitation with Teflon injection—the return of voice, cough and laughter, *Acta Otolaryngol. (Stockh.)*, **58**:214-220 (1964).
75. R. G. Loudon, Weather and cough, *Am. Rev. Respir. Dis.*, **89**:352-359 (1964).
76. R. G. Loudon, Cough in health and disease, *Aspen Emphysema Conf.*, **10**:41-53 (1967).
77. R. G. Loudon and L. C. Brown, Cough frequency in patients with respiratory disease, *Am. Rev. Respir. Dis.*, **96**:1137-1143 (1967).
78. R. G. Loudon and J. F. Kilpatrick, Air pollution, weather and cough, *Arch. Environ. Health*, **18**:641-645 (1969).
79. R. G. Loudon and R. M. Roberts, Droplet expulsion from the respiratory tract, *Am. Rev. Respir. Dis.*, **95**:435-442 (1967).
80. R. G. Loudon and G. B. Shaw, Mechanics of cough in normal subjects and in patients with obstructive respiratory disease, *Am. Rev. Respir. Dis.*, **96**:666-677 (1967).
81. R. G. Loudon and S. K. Spohn, Cough frequency and infectivity in patients with pulmonary tuberculosis, *Am. Rev. Respir. Dis.*, **99**:109-111 (1969).
82. P. MacArthur, Coughs and colds in childhood, *Practitioner*, **208**:191-197 (1972).
83. P. T. Macklem, Airway obstruction and collateral ventilation, *Physiol. Rev.*, **51**:368-436 (1971).
84. P. T. Macklem, R. G. Fraser, and W. G. Brown, Bronchial pressure measurements in emphysema and bronchitis, *J. Clin. Invest.*, **44** 6):897-905 (1965).
85. P. T. Macklem and J. Mead, Factors determining maximum expiratory flow in dogs, *J. Appl. Physiol.*, **25**:159-169 (1968).
86. P. T. Macklem and J. Mead, The physiological basis of common pulmonary function tests, *Arch. Environ. Health*, **14**:5-9 (1967).
87. P. T. Macklem and N. J. Wilson, Measurement of intrabronchial pressure in man, *J. Appl. Physiol.*, **20**:653-663 (1965).
88. M. T. Macklin and C. C. Macklin, Malignant interstitial emphysema of the lungs and mediastinum as an important occult complication in many respiratory diseases and other conditions: Interpretation of clinical literature in light of laboratory experiment, *Medicine*, **23**:281-357 (1944).
89. L. Marazzini, F. Vezzoli, and G. Rizzato, Intrathoracic pressure development in chronic airways obstruction, *J. Appl. Physiol.*, **37**:575-578 (1974).
90. G. I. Mchedlishvili, N. P. Mitagvaria, and L. G. Ormotsadze, Vascular mechanisms controlling a constant blood supply to the brain ("autoregulation"), *Stroke*, **4**:742-750 (1973).

91. H. D. McIntosh, E. H. Estes, and J. V. Warren, The mechanism of cough syncope, *Am. Heart J.,* **52**:70-82 (1956).
92. J. Mead, Theory and methodology in respiratory mechanics with glossary of symbols. In *Handbook of Physiology,* Section 3: *Respiration,* Vol. I. Edited by W. O. Fenn and H. Rahn. Washington, D. C., American Physiological Society, 1964, Chap. 11, p. 370.
93. J. Mead, T. Takishima, and D. Leith, Stress distribution in lungs: A model of pulmonary elasticity, *J. Appl. Physiol.,* **28**:596-608 (1970).
94. J. Mead, J. M. Turner, P. T. Macklem, and J. B. Little, Significance of the relationship between lung recoil and maximum expiratory flow, *J. Appl. Physiol.,* **22**:95-108 (1967).
95. O. P. Mital and M. C. Agarwala, Expectoration of a bronchogenic carcinoma, *Br. J. Dis. Chest,* **62**:52-53 (1968).
96. P. Mognoni, F. Saibene, G. Sant'Ambrogio, and E. Agostoni, Dynamics of the maximal contraction of the respiratory muscles, *Respir. Physiol.,* **4**:193-202 (1968).
97. J. A. Morgan-Hughes, Cough seizures in patients with cerebral lesions, *Br. J. Med.,* **2**:494-496 (1966).
98. M. Mori and Y. Sakai, Re-examination of centrally-induced cough in cats using a microstimulation technique, *Jpn, J. Pharmacol.,* **22**:635-643 (1972).
99. W. P. Munsell, Pneumomediastinum, *JAMA,* **202**:689-693 (1967).
100. S. E. Natelson and W. Molnar, Malfunction of ventriculoatrial shunts caused by the circulatory dynamics of coughing, *J. Neurosurg.,* **36**:283-286 (1972).
101. V. E. Negus, *The Comparative Anatomy and Physiology of the Larynx.* New York, Hafner, 1949.
102. J. Nichol, F. Girling, E. B. Claxton, and A. C. Burton, Fundamental instability of small blood vessels and critical closing pressure in vascular beds, *Am. J. Physiol.,* **146**:330-344 (1961).
103. C. R. Olsen, A. E. Stevens, N. B. Pride, and N. C. Staub, Structural basis for decreased compressibility of constricted tracheae and bronchi, *J. Appl. Physiol.,* **23**:35-39 (1967).
104. A. Pedersen, E. Sandoe, E. Hvidberg, and M. Schwartz, Studies on the mechanism of tussive syncope, *Acta Med. Scand.,* **179**:653-661 (1966).
105. S. Permutt and R. L. Riley, Hemodynamics of collapsible vessels with tone: The vascular waterfall, *J. Appl. Physiol.,* **18**:924-932 (1963).
106. R. H. Perry, C. H. Chilton, and S. D. Kirkpatrick (eds.), *Chemical Engineers' Handbook,* New York, McGraw-Hill, 1963.
107. N. B. Pride, B. S. Permutt, R. L. Riley, and B. Bromberger-Barnea, Determinants of maximal expiratory flow from the lungs, *J. Appl. Physiol.,* **23**:646-662 (1967).
108. D. F. Proctor, Physiology of the upper airway. In *Handbook of Physiology,* Section 3: *Respiration,* Vol. I. Edited by W. O. Fenn and H. Rahn. Washington, D.C., American Physiological Society, 1964, Chap. 8.

109. W. G. Rainer, R. S. Mitchell, G. F. Filley, and B. Eiseman, Significance of tracheal collapse in pulmonary emphysema—cinefluorographic observations, *Surg. Forum,* **12**:70-72 (1961).
110. J. E. Rayl, Tracheobronchial collapse during cough, *Radiology,* **85**:87-92 (1965).
111. P. F. Roe and B. N. Kulkarni, Pneumomediastinum in children with cough, *Br. J. Dis. Chest,* **61**:147-150 (1967).
112. F. Rohrer, Die Mechanik des Hustens, *Schweiz. Med. Wochenschr.,* **2**: 765-767 (1921).
113. B. B. Ross, R. Gramiak, and H. Rahn, Physical dynamics of the cough mechanism, *J. Appl. Physiol.,* **8**:264-268 (1955).
114. D. J. Sass, E. L. Ritman, P. E. Caskey, N. Banchero, and E. H. Wood, Liquid breathing: Prevention of pulmonary arterial-venous shunting during acceleration, *J. Appl. Physiol.,* **32**:451-455 (1972).
115. B. S. Schoenberg, Micturition syncope—not a single entity, *JAMA,* **229**: 1631-1633 (1974).
116. W. H. Schoenfisch and J. A. Kylstra, Maximum expiratory flow and estimation CO_2 elimination in liquid-ventilated dogs' lungs, *J. Appl. Physiol.,* **35**:117-121 (1973).
117. J. M. Seidman and A. A. Sasahara, Bronchopulmonary lavage (Editorial), *N. Engl. J. Med.,* **286**:1262-1263 (1972).
118. E. P. Sharpey-Schafer, The mechanism of syncope after coughing, *Br. Med. J.,* **2**:860-863 (1953).
119. E. P. Sharpey-Schafer, Effects of coughing on intrathoracic pressure, arterial pressure, and peripheral blood flow, *J. Physiol. (Lond.),* **122**:351-357 (1953).
120. E. P. Sharpey-Schafer, Effect of respiratory acts on the circulation. In *Handbook of Physiology,* Section 2: *Circulation,* Vol. III. Edited by W. F. Hamilton. Washington, D.C., American Physiological Society, 1965, Chap. 52.
121. C. Shim, N. Fine, R. Fernandez, and M. H. Williams, Cardiac arrhythmias resulting from tracheal suctioning, *Ann. Intern. Med.,* **71**:1149-1153 (1969).
122. B. G. Simonsson, F. M. Jacobs, and J. A. Nadel, Role of autonomic nervous system and the cough reflex in the increased responsiveness of airways in patients with obstructive airway disease, *J. Clin. Invest.,* **46**: 1812-1818 (1967).
123. J. L. Skolnick and D. E. Dines, Tussive syncope, *Minn. Med.,* **52**:1609-1613 (1969).
124. F. R. Smith and P. C. Kundahl, Intravenously administered lidocaine as cough depressant during general anesthesia for bronchography, *Chest,* **63**:427-429 (1973).
125. M. J. Sokoloff, Cause and treatment of chronic cough, *JAMA,* **218**: 1711-1712 (1971).
126. D. C. Stanescu, and D. B. Teculescu, Exercise- and cough-induced asthma, *Respiration,* **27**:377-383 (1970).

127. J. M. Sutherland and J. H. Tyrer, "Cough syndrome" with suggestions as to the possible role played by cerebral atherosclerosis, *Med. J. Aust.*, **1**: 39-42 (1965).
128. P. A. Theodos, History and physical examination. In *Clinical Cardiopulmonary Physiology*, 3rd ed. Edited by B. L. Gordon, R. A. Carleton, and L. P. Faber. New York, Grune and Stratton, 1969, Chap. 8, pp. 418-419.
129. P. Ungvarski, Mechanical stimulation of coughing, *Am. J. Nurs.*, **71**:2358-2361 (1971).
130. United States Department of Health, Education and Welfare. Smoking and health. Report of the Advisory Committee to the Surgeon General of the Public Health Service. Public Health Service Publication No. 1103. U.S. Government Printing Office. Washington, D.C., 1964.
131. B. J. Urban and S. W. Weitzner, Avoidance of hypoxemia during endotracheal suction, *Anesthesiology*, **31**:473-475 (1969).
132. H. von Leden and N. Isshiki, An analysis of cough at the level of the larynx, *Arch. Otolaryngol.*, **81**:616-625 (1965).
133. W. T. Warmington, Four cases of cough fracture, *Ulster Med. J.*, **35**:72-74 (1966).
134. *Webster's New International Dictionary*, 2nd ed. Edited by W. A. Neilson. Springfield, Mass., Merriam, 1960.
135. J. L. Whittenberger and J. Mead, Research in tuberculosis and related subjects. Respiratory dynamics during cough, *Trans. 48th Meeting Natl. Tuberc. Assoc., New York, 1952*, pp. 414-418.
136. F. O. Winther, Experimentally induced cough in man by citric acid aerosol. An evaluation of a method, *Acta Pharmacol. Toxicol. (Kbh.)*, **28**:108-112 (1970).
137. A. P. Wolff, M. May, and D. Nuelle, The tympanic membrane. A source of the cough reflex, *JAMA*, **223**:1269 (1973).
138. World Health Organization. Opiates and their alternates for pain and cough relief. Report of a WHO scientific group. *WHO Tech. Rep. Serv.*, **495**:1-19 (1972).
139. E. L. Wynder and E. P. Fairchild, Jr., The role of a history of persistent cough in the epidemiology of lung cancer, *Am. Rev. Respir. Dis.*, **94**:709-720 (1966).
140. E. L. Wynder, P. L. Kaufman, and R. L. Lesser, A short-term followup study on ex-cigarette smokers, with special emphasis on persistent cough and weight gain, *Am. Rev. Respir. Dis.*, **96**:645-655 (1967).
141. E. L. Wynder, F. R. Lemon, and N. Mantel, Epidemiology of persistent cough, *Am. Rev. Respir. Dis.*, **91**:679-700 (1965).
142. S. Yamamoto, Reflex discharges in phrenic and abdominal muscle nerves to vagal afferent nerve stimulation, *Exp. Neurol.*, **13**:402-417 (1965).
143. N. Yanagihara, H. von Leden, and E. Werner-Kukuk, The physical parameters of cough: The larynx in a normal single cough, *Acta Otolaryngol. (Stockh.)*, **61**:495-510 (1966).
144. S. Young, Electromyographic activity during respiration and coughing in the tench *(Tinca tinca L.)*, *J. Physiol. (Lond.)*, **227**:18P-19P (1972).

16

Respiratory Reflexes and Defense

J. G. WIDDICOMBE

St. George's Hospital Medical School
London, England

I. Introduction

The particular advantages which nervous reflexes contribute to the defense of the respiratory system (and thereby to the body as a whole) are two: first, the promptness of the response in situations where delay could be fatal; and secondly, the fact that a reflex can quickly and powerfully link up sensors and effectors, and recruit into the defensive response most of the physiological activities of the body. These are general characteristics of the nervous system. Without their involvement in respiratory defense we would have to rely on slow local changes, possibly poorly coordinated and depending for intercommunication on humoral or bloodborne information systems. Given this quick and powerful means of reacting to invasion, the body need not restrict its use to emergencies; the same defensive forces can be called into action in less urgent situations, including those of whose existence we may be unaware.

The respiratory tract reflexes can be set up by a variety of stimuli: by inhaled "foreign bodies," by smokes and particles, and by irritant and noxious gases and aerosols. Each of these stimuli invades the respiratory system from outside and needs to be dealt with. The invading agent may be dealt with by means other than defensive reflexes, for example, by mucociliary clearance or conditioning processes in the nose; reflex and nonreflex clearance mechanisms may coexist. The respiratory system may also be attacked from within. Excess mucus in the airways can be a hazard to health and require removal. In various diseases of the respiratory tract and lungs the defensive reflexes are evoked and, even if there is no intruder to be expelled, the motor responses may be beneficial.

A respiratory defensive reflex is one where the motor responses tend to eliminate the cause of disease or disorder, or to counteract or lessen the structural or physiological damage which may be caused. As such the reflexes are essentially "pathophysiological" rather than physiological, but the underlying components of the defensive mechanism may also play a role in healthy conditions. A distinction between "protective" and "defensive" respiratory reflexes has been drawn [62]. This classification may provide a convenient subdivision of a long list of mechanisms, but it is doubtful if it is semantically justified or conceptually useful. "Expulsive" and "nonexpulsive" are other possible labels, but their application to individual defensive reflexes might be controversial and confusing.

It is usually not difficult to define a *primary* defensive reflex. For example, inhalation of cigarette smoke can cause coughing. However, this is the first brush stroke on the picture. For completion we must delineate, inter alia: (a) where the smoke is acting, since the cough reflex can arise from the larynx, trachea, and bronchi, and each response has different characteristics; (b) whether there are local changes, for example, in mucus secretion or release of bioactive substances, which may modify the excitatory processes of the reflex; (c) whether there are important primary reflex actions other than coughing, for example, bronchoconstriction, hypertension, mucus secretion, etc.; (d) whether the primary reflex responses lead directly to *secondary* reflex actions, say via blood gas or hemodynamic changes; and (e) to what extent the responses are affected by conditioning or are influenced by voluntary control. Even when these factors have been studied there will remain unanswered many questions about the neurophysiology of the reflexes and their interactions.

This chapter will deal chiefly with defensive reflexes in the subhuman mammal, in particular the cat, so loved by neurophysiologists. Less work has been done with man, because the methods for studying reflexes are essentially analytical and the surgical invasions required are often inappropriate for human investigations. There has been some research on submammalian species, and this will be discussed briefly later.

First, structure of receptors in the respiratory tract will be considered, since these are believed to be the first cellular links in the defensive reflex chain; the evidence, largely indirect, for this belief will be discussed. It will become apparent at this stage that the nomenclature of respiratory receptors is controversial and unsatisfactory, so a brief section dealing with this problem will be interposed. Next the physiological behavior of the various receptors will be described based mainly on evidence from "single-fiber" recording of action potential traffic. Little is known of the way in which the chemical or mechanical environment of the receptors stimulates or inhibits them, but the emphasis in this book is probably more on the defensive responses than on receptor physiology. Therefore, these reflex motor responses are next discussed in detail, classified in order of the motor systems–respiratory, laryngeal, bronchomotor, cardiovascular, and secretomotor; a short section on respiratory sensation, although not a reflex, is appropriate here. Having dealt with these motor systems, the chapter then concerns the responses from each anatomical site, nose, larynx, etc.; this approach involves some repetition, which is justified, since it brings the pathophysiological mechanisms into a logical framework of the respiratory defenses. Finally, there are short discussions on two topics of more general interest; the comparative physiology of defensive reflexes, and the interaction of primary defensive reflexes with secondary effects. These last two discussions are important when we consider the defensive reflexes in man, because much of our knowledge is based on experiments with animals lower than man, and on experiments with conditions designed to isolate primary components of the total responses. In intact man this artificial situation does not exist, and it is the integrated response of primary and secondary effects which is of chief importance.

II. Histological Structure of Respiratory Tract Receptors

The nervous receptors for the defensive reflexes lie in and under the epithelium of the airways, where they are well situated to respond to mechanical and chemical stimuli, even if weak. Strong stimuli may change the discharge of endings lying deeper in the airway walls [104] and even outside the airways [86], but it is unlikely that this effect is an important component of the defensive reflexes. The epithelial nerve endings are often referred to generically as "irritant" receptors (but see below).

The histological research on respiratory irritant receptors is surprisingly thin [32]. Many early light-microscopic studies showed that there were receptors in the epithelium, but gave little information about the relationship between receptor terminals and their tissue environment. More recent electron-microscopic work is helping to clarify the picture, but at present there is no comprehensive survey of the structure of receptors at any anatomical site in the respiratory tract. Even when receptor structure has been worked out, it is not always possible to say which receptors are responsible for which reflex.

As might be expected, the configuration of the receptors depends on the cellular nature of the epithelium in which they lie: namely, columnar cell in the nose, trachea, and bronchi, squamous cell in the pharynx and vocal folds, and thin cell in the alveolar wall.

A. Nasal Receptors

These endings have been little studied histologically, and most of the studies have been related more to the sense of smell than to defensive reflexes (see review by Graziadei [38]). The trigeminal nerves carry most of the afferent fibers which respond to chemical odors and irritants, both myelinated [17] and nonmyelinated fibers being concerned [19]. We know that end-organs in the nasal epithelium can give rise to various forms of smell sensation, sometimes associated with sniffing, to pain, and, as will be described later, to defensive reflexes such as sneeze, apnea, and the diving reflex, and also to many nonrespiratory reflexes [4,104]. Which receptors are responsible for which response is not known.

B. Pharyngeal Receptors

The afferent innervation of the pharynx is mainly involved in the swallowing reflex, which is not relevant to this chapter, since it is only defensive in the sense that a pharyngeal foreign body should not be allowed to remain in place. However, irritation of the epithelium of the epipharynx (or nasopharynx, the posterior wall above and behind the soft palate) sets up a powerful defensive reflex, the "aspiration reflex" [48,62,99] or "sniff reflex" [11]. This mucosa contains fine afferent nerve terminals connected to myelinated fibers which run in the glossopharyngeal nerve (Fig. 1) [32]. The terminals seem to lie under the squamous cell layer, and therefore might be mechanically protected by it. Neither three-dimensional delineation nor electron-microscopic studies seem to have been done. Receptors with nonmyelinated fibers do not seem to have been described, but it is unlikely that they are absent, since pain (presumably from nociceptors) can be evoked from the epipharynx.

C. Laryngeal Receptors

The larynx and its associated structures, especially the epiglottis and the vocal folds, are an extremely sensitive source of origin of defensive reflexes. Therefore, it is not surprising to find that the epithelium is the site of many afferent end-organs. In general three types of receptor have been described on the basis of light microscopy. Electron microscopy does not seem to have been done.

First, there are myelinated afferent nerve fibers under the epithelium which split into fine nerve branches which spread among the epithelial cells of the mucosa [82,101]. By analogy with receptors in the lower respiratory tract, these endings are most probably responsible for the cough and other defensive reflexes. They are found especially in the vocal folds and the dorsal supraglottis area, and the fibers from them travel in the superior laryngeal nerves, which contain the main afferent supply of the larynx.

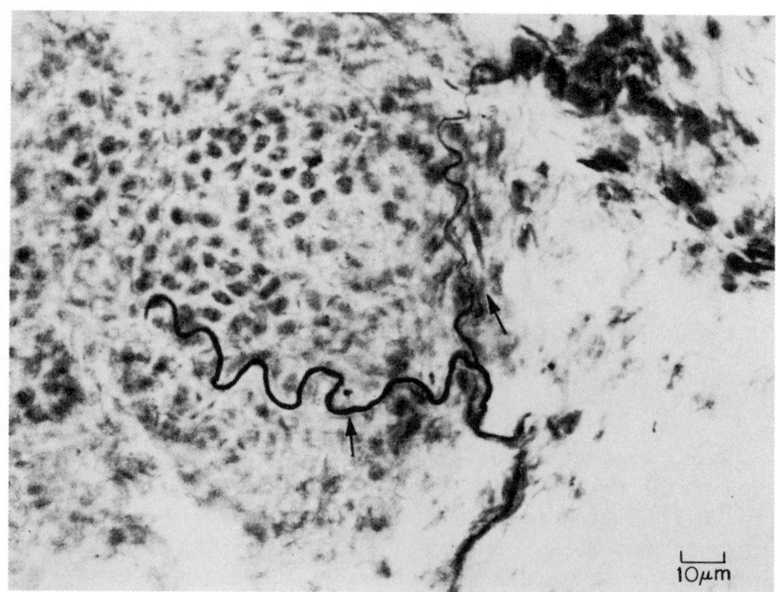

FIGURE 1 Frozen section of cat epipharyngeal region showing nerve fibers ramifying among epithelial cells. X550. Schofield's silver stain. Photograph by Mrs. A. M. S. White. (From Fillenz and Widdicombe [32].)

Second, there are specialized nervous structures, such as large hederiform endings, corpuscles, and taste buds [30,40,56,57]. The last receptors are especially copious in the epiglottis of ungulates, such as the lamb, and are presumably related to reflex swallowing from the larynx, as well as to taste. To this group may possibly be added the subepithelial cells of Langhans with rosettes of nonmyelinated nerve terminals [7] (the function of which, and whether they are afferent or efferent, is unknown).

Third, there are fine ("free") nerve endings with nonmyelinated afferent fibers, found in all parts of the laryngeal mucosa. These receptors are probably pain or nociceptive endings, since they resemble those found in nearly all viscera. However, there is also some evidence that they may play a part in defensive reflexes from the larynx.

Thus there are many types of afferent end-organ in the laryngeal epithelium, and, even in the absence of more definitive histological studies, they provide the structural basis for the several different patterns of defensive reflex which can be elicited from this region.

D. Tracheobronchial Receptors

Light microscopy shows nerve fibers entering and ramifying in the epithelium of the airways, from trachea to the respiratory bronchioles [32]. Histochemical studies suggest that they are afferent rather than motor. There are no major differences in appearance at different levels of the airways. Although no careful histological counts have been done, some microscopic studies indicate that the concentration of receptors is lower in the smaller airways [29], and other investigations indicate the opposite [46]. Physiological evidence indicates that the receptors are in a higher concentration in the trachea and large bronchi [6,73, 104]. Electron microscopy shows afferent fibers on the luminal side of the tracheobronchial basement membrane [50,75]. Both light and electron microscopy show the receptor terminals reaching almost to the ciliary layer (Figs. 2 and 3), a picture consistent with a high receptor sensitivity to intraluminal irritants. The receptors branch prolifically, both beneath the epithelium and within its base; the network sends vertical twigs between the columnar cells toward the surface. P. Jeffery (personal communication) has found nerve fibers, afferent in appearance, in cross section 1-2 μm from the luminal surface of the epithelium of cat and rat (Fig. 3), usually with structures resembling desmosomes and tight junctions just outside. The site and appearance of the receptors, and the fact that they have myelinated nerve fibers, are indirect but good evidence that they are the irritant receptors responsible for defensive reflexes.

A further nervous ending in the airways is that associated with clusters of myoepithelial or neurosecretory cells [45,63], although the functions of these clusters is controversial, and it is not even clear if the nerves are afferent or efferent. Free, presumably nociceptive, endings have also been described in the airway wall [29,106], but their precise structure has not been worked out.

Recently von During et al. [102] have drawn the three-dimensional structure of a receptor in a small bronchus of the rat (Fig. 4). Although they concluded that it was a "pulmonary stretch receptor," and as such would be unlikely to be involved in defensive reflexes, it had terminals which paraded under the epithelium; this appearance suggested that it might respond to intraluminal irritants. A similar structure has been described by Jabonero and Sabadell [49]. The pictures are an important advance in our visualization of the complex structure of airway receptors.

E. Alveolar Receptors

Receptor activity and reflexes from the alveoli have been extensively studied by Paintal [78,80]. The endings have nonmyelinated fibers and their histological appearance has recently been determined [47,69]. Since they are stimulated

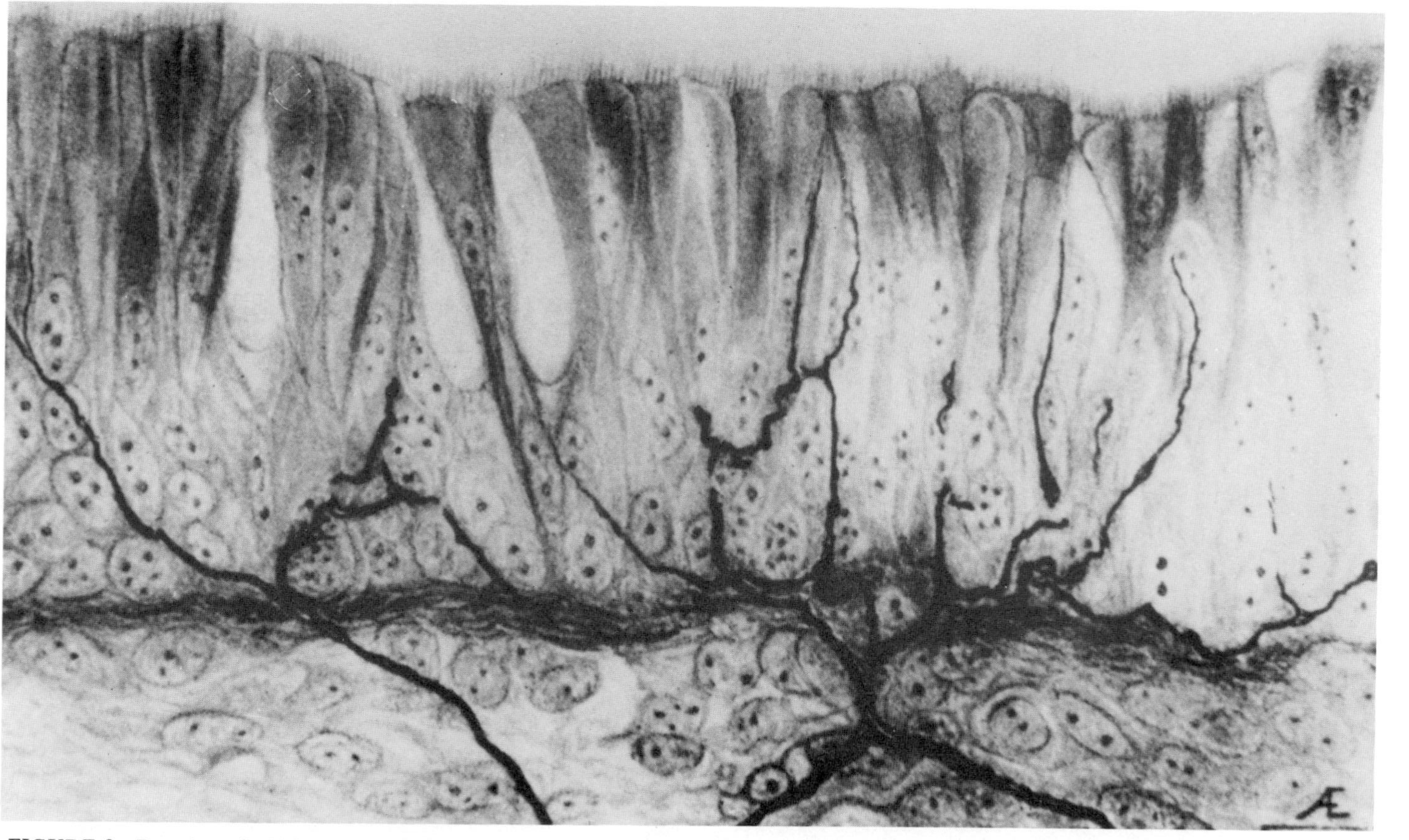

FIGURE 2 Drawing of a light microscopic picture of an epithelial irritant receptor. Note the ramification of nerve terminals between the columnar and mucous cells of the epithelium.

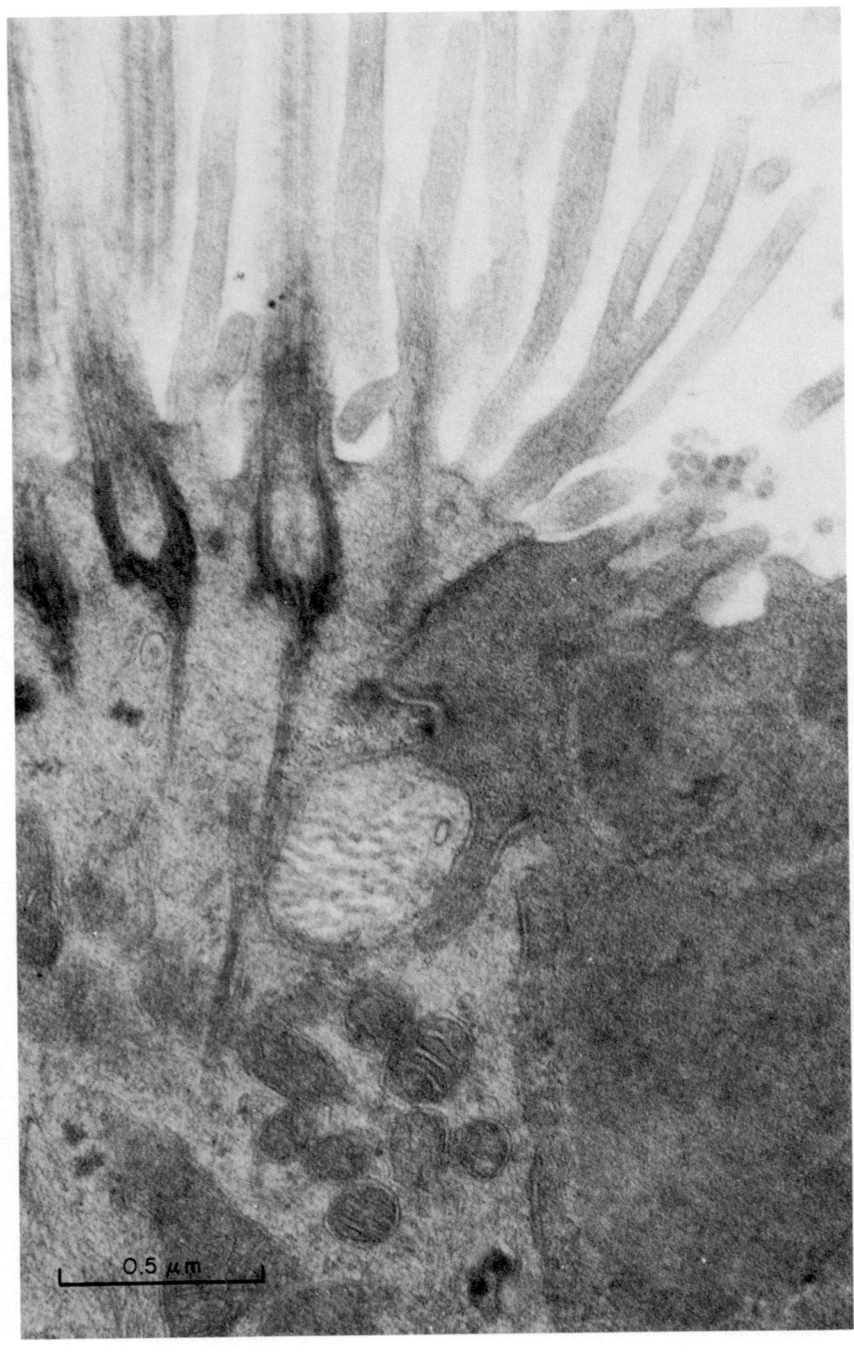
0.5 μm

by alveolar interstitial edema and may give rise to unpleasant sensation [80], they may be nociceptors; Paintal [80] has christened them J-receptors, short for "juxtapulmonary capillary receptors." In the context of this chapter, although the alveolar endings are not in the respiratory tract, it is important that they are stimulated by inhaled irritant gases such as chlorine, ammonia, ethyl ether, and halothane.

III. A Note on Nomenclature of Respiratory Tract Receptors

This is a confused subject and an important one, for we need to define what we are talking about; histologists and physiologists have intra- and interdisciplinary disagreements. In this chapter we will give a physiological terminology, based partly on the belief that receptors should be named after the stimulus they usually "receive," and partly on what seems to be developing as the nomenclature accepted by neurophysiologists active in the field.

All the receptors to be described in detail lie in the epithelium. All respond to mechanical stimulation. Most of those receptors with myelinated fibers are very sensitive to inhaled dusts, irritant gases, and aerosols; these will be called "irritant receptors," a name used in 1963 [75], and generally accepted since. Those with myelinated fibers, but relatively insensitive to inhaled irritants, will be called "mechanoreceptors." Those receptors with nonmyelinated fibers are more difficult to name. The endings in the alveolar wall have been termed J-receptors by Paintal [80], as described above. Similar receptors exist in the laryngeal [13], and bronchial epithelium [21,22]. Endings in each of the three sites have many properties in common. Since they are stimulated by inhaled irritant gases and tissue damage, and probably cause pain or unpleasant sensation, it is likely that they are "nociceptive endings" in the sense that Sherrington [92] applied this term to similar receptors in visceral and somatic tissues. If a generic term is needed for groups of nerve endings with nonmyelinated fibers in all three (and other) sites, nociceptors or C-fiber receptors [34], might be appropriate; J-receptor is clearly unsuitable as a general term. More specialized receptors (taste buds, smell receptors, etc.) will be given their conventional names.

FIGURE 3 Electron micrograph of cat trachea showing a "sensory" terminal axon within surface epithelium between a ciliated cell (on the left) and a goblet cell (on the right), and within 1 μm of the airway lumen. Note the neurotubules in the axon. Glutaraldehyde and osmium tetroxide: uranyl acetate and lead citrate ×54,000. (Photomicrograph by courtesy of Dr. P. Jeffery.)

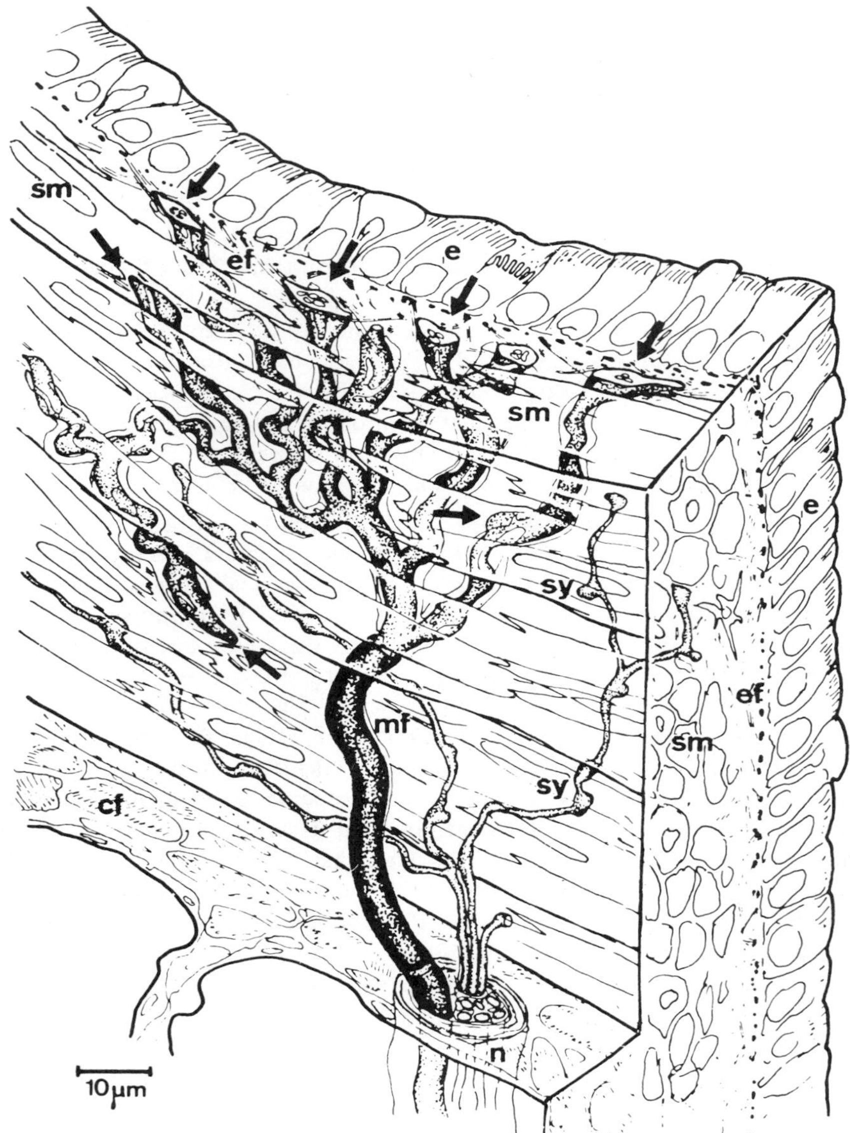

FIGURE 4 Three-dimensional reconstruction of a receptor in the wall of a bronchiole of a rat. Note the receptor terminations under the basement membrane and in the smooth muscle layer (arrows). e, epithelium; sm, smooth muscle; n, nerve bundle; mf, myelinated nerve fiber; ef, elastic network; sy, efferent nerve terminals; cf, collagen fibers. (From von During et al. [102].)

Where relevant, mention will be made of dissenting views, of which there will be many. A good review of the problems of nomenclature is given by Armstrong and Luck [6].

Having discussed the histological structure and naming of the respiratory tract receptors, we will now consider the stimuli that excite them.

IV. Physiological Stimuli to Respiratory Tract Receptors

The method used most extensively for studying respiratory tract receptor physiology is the electrical recording of action potentials from single nerve fibers from the endings. This method has several advantages. It allows anatomical localization of the receptor [86]. It gives a fairly precise quantitative assessment of the activation or inhibition of the receptor, showing what agents or conditions can change the discharge or sensitivity of the receptor. By "tapping the telephone wires" we know the signals being transmitted to the central nervous system and, if given other information about the reflex responses to those signals, we can draw conclusions about the relative strength of the motor effects of the different stimuli. Thus the method allows conclusions to be drawn both about the functions of the receptors in health and disease and about the defensive reflexes which may be elicited. The technique also has limitations, however. It is selective, since it is easier to record from myelinated afferent fibers, and therefore receptors with these fibers have mainly been studied. Receptors with nonmyelinated nerves have been infrequently studied, although there is no reason to doubt their importance. The method analyzes only one part of a complex system, and accurate extension of the information provided depends on the valid analysis of the other components; for example, single-fiber technique may involve cutting the afferent nerve and abolishing the reflex of the whole defensive system; studies of the intact reflexes are an essential supplement to the single-fiber work. Even the information obtained about receptors is limited, since the method tells very little about the ways in which the receptor terminals are influenced by their tissue and cellular environment: for example, how a receptor potential is set up or modified by the physical and chemical changes around the nerve endings. In this respect we lack knowledge of receptor physiology obtained for endings such as the Pacinian corpuscle and the primary endings in the muscle spindle. Yet this information is important if we are to understand the basic mechanisms of the defensive reflexes.

A. Irritant Receptors

These have been studied, by single fiber recording, for receptors in the larynx [3,13,85,94], trachea and bronchi [6,31,58,66,70,71,73,86,88,90,104]. In the lower airways they have the highest concentration in the trachea and the large bronchi near the hilum of the lung [6,73,104]. They have small-diameter myelinated afferent fibers, in the Aδ group, in the vagus nerves. All the receptors are stimulated by mechanical deformation of the epithelium with, for example, a thread or catheter. The discharge is characteristically irregular, possibly suggesting a near-random process in the receptor terminals during the development of action potentials. Since the irritant receptors are mechanosensitive, it is not surprising that they are excited by large inflations and deflations of the appropriate part of the respiratory tract (Fig. 5), and play a physiological role during such deformations [58,59]. Such stimulation, even when maintained, gives a rapidly adapting discharge, and often an off-response when the stimulus is removed. Because of their activation by lung collapse or deflation, Buff and Koller [16] prefer to call these receptors "collapse" or "deflation" endings. In quiet breathing in the anesthetized animal, the endings are usually silent, or show a weak discharge with respiratory modulation.

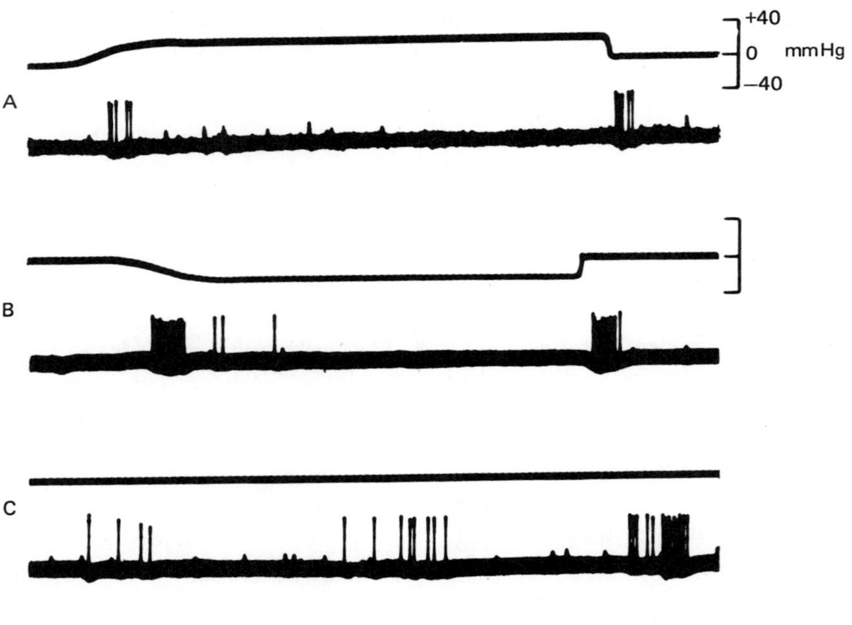

FIGURE 5 Action potentials (lower traces) from a rapidly adapting receptor in the trachea of a cat. Upper traces, intratracheal pressure. Inflation (A) and deflation (B) of the trachea causes rapidly adapting discharges from the receptor. In (C), the tracheal epithelium was gently touched with a catheter, causing further activity. (From Widdicombe [104].)

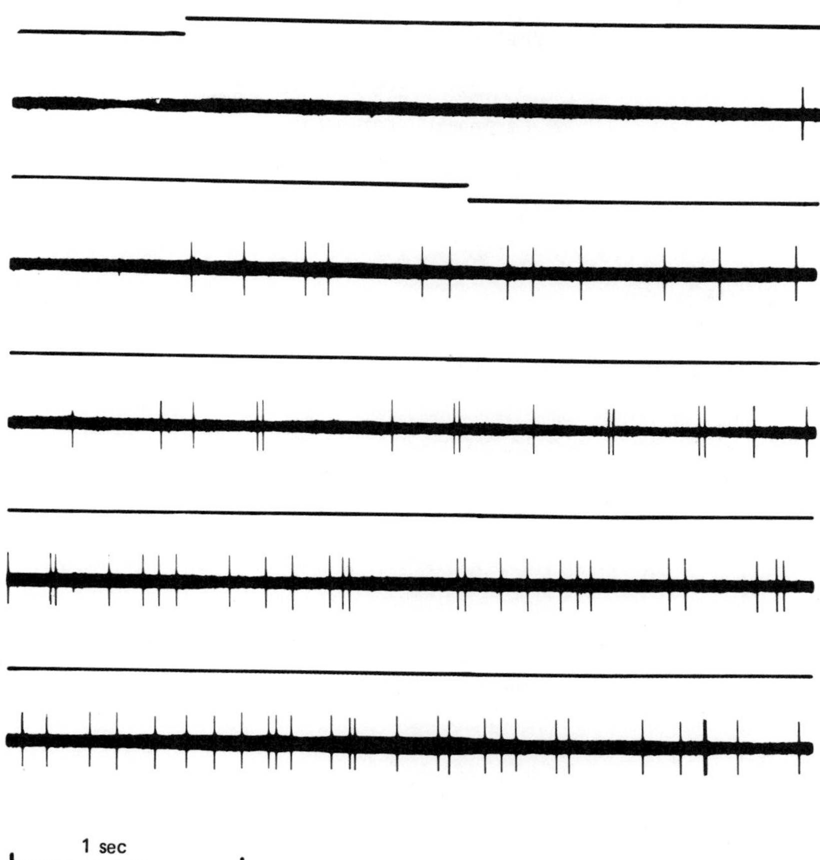

FIGURE 6 Response of a laryngeal epithelial receptor (type 1) to insufflation of cigarette smoke into the larynx of a cat. Single-fiber recording from the superior laryngeal nerve. Upper trace signal, smoke administered during upward deflection. Note irregular discharge of action potentials after a latency, and after discharge. (From Boushey et al. [13].)

The receptors are stimulated by intraluminal irritants, gases, or aerosols, acting chemically or mechanically. These include "inert" carbon dust, cigarette smoke (Fig. 6), and a range of chemicals (Table 1). The susceptibility of the receptors varies greatly, between sites, between irritants, and between receptors. For example, those in the larynx are little affected by carbon dust, possibly because the squamous cell layer over the vocal folds protects them. Some of the negative results may be explained by a protective action, mechanical or chemical buffering, of a mucus layer, although this is speculative. Obviously, too, the

TABLE 1 Responses of Respiratory Tract Receptors to Various Irritants

Irritant stimulus	Receptor[a]				
	Epipharyngeal	Laryngeal (Type 1)	Laryngeal (Type 2)	Lung irritant	Alveolar (Type J)
Catheter	+	+	+	+	
Carbon dust		0	0	+	
Cigarette smoke		+	–	+	
Ammonia	0	+	+	+	+
Sulfur dioxide		+	0	(+)	
Ethyl ether				+	+
Halothane				0	+
Histamine	0	0	0	+	(+)
Carbon dioxide	0	+	–	0	0

[a]+, strong stimulation; (+), weak stimulation; 0, no effect; –, inhibition; blank, not tested.

response will depend on the strength of the stimulus; in terms of gaseous chemicals the concentration at the receptor is crucial, and irritant gases such as sulfur dioxide may be largely absorbed in the nose and upper respiratory tract [14]. Interaction of more than one chemical stimulus on the receptors has not been studied, but investigation of the reflex actions indicates that synergistic effects may be expected.

Irritant receptors are also stimulated or sensitized by changes in the mechanical properties of the airway wall underlying the receptor site. Thus those in the lungs and trachea are stimulated by contraction of airway smooth muscle [70] (Fig. 7), and sensitized by decreases in lung compliance which lead to greater mechanical pull on the airways during the respiratory cycle [89]. This behavior may be especially important in acute experimental lung diseases, such as bronchoconstriction, microembolism, anaphylaxis, congestion, and edema, each of which stimulates lung irritant receptors; presumably the stimulation contributes to or causes reflex changes in breathing and other variables seen in these conditions. In this respect it is important that tracheobronchial irritant receptors are stimulated by anaphylactic reactions in the lungs, and by inhalation of histamine aerosols [70,86,90].

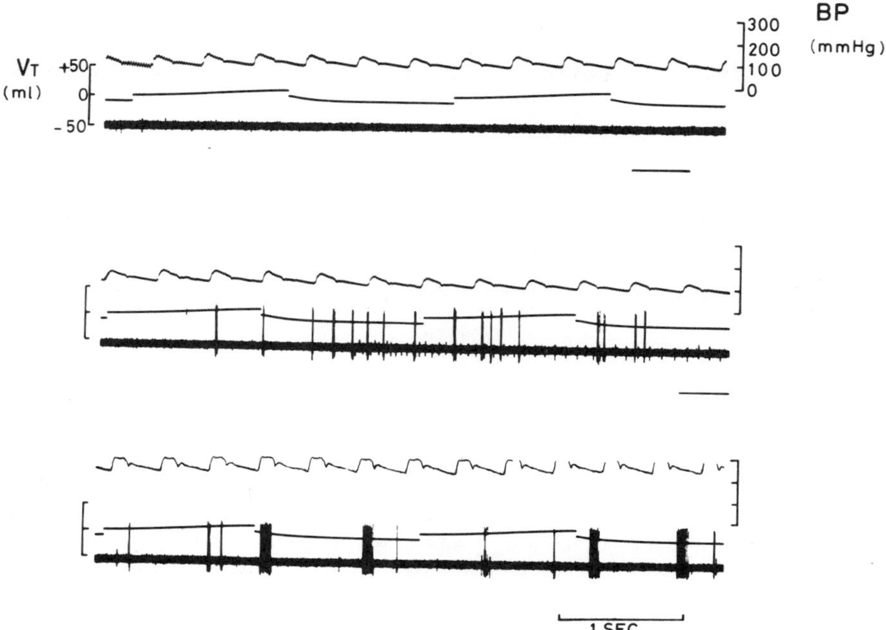

FIGURE 7 Response of a pulmonary irritant receptor to intra-right atrial injection of histamine acid phosphate, 100 μg/kg (at signal in uppermost record) in a vagotomized, paralyzed, artificially ventilated rabbit. 5.5 sec between upper two traces, 20.5 sec between lower two. Histamine caused an increase in blood pressure and a receptor discharge without clear relation to respiratory phase. (From Mills et al. [70].)

B. Receptors with Nonmyelinated Fibers

Primarily, those receptors in the alveolar wall have been studied. They are activated by strong concentrations of irritant gases, by microembolism and by alveolar edema [6,20,78,79]. Paintal has concluded that the main pathophysiological stimulus to the alveolar J-receptors is an increase in alveolar interstitial fluid volume. Similar receptors occur in the laryngeal mucosa [13] and in the walls of the bronchial tree [21,22] and these are stimulated by intraluminal irritants or histamine aerosol. The relative importance of receptors with nonmyelinated fibers in the three sites in defensive reflexes has yet to be determined.

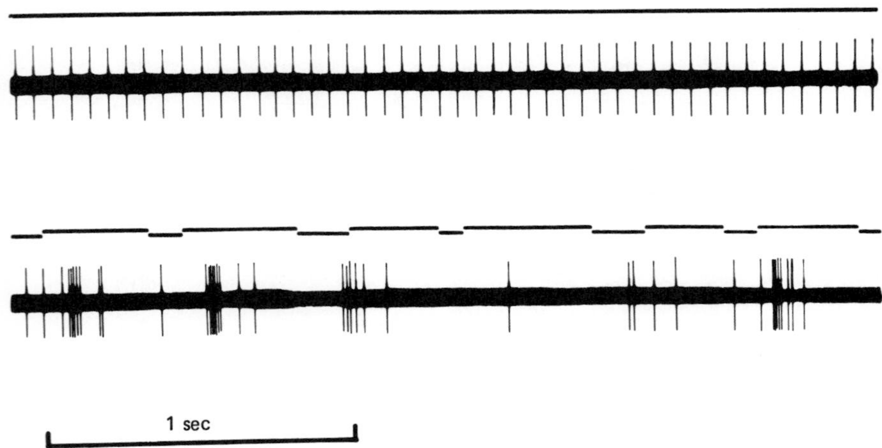

FIGURE 8 This record shows firing in a type 2 laryngeal fiber and its response to a gentle mechanical stimulus. In the upper record the fiber was not stimulated. In the lower record a linen thread was drawn across the receptive field of the fiber with each signal (upward deflection of the trace). This alternately excited and inhibited fiber activity. Records continuous. Upper trace, signal; lower trace, action potentials. (From Boushey et al. [13].)

C. Other Respiratory Tract Receptors

Receptors in the epipharynx, presumably responsible for the aspiration reflex, are rapidly adapting with an irregular discharge on mechanical stimulation, but are not here called irritant receptors, since they seem insensitive to chemical stimuli, at least from the limited studies which have been published [76]. As in the case of the vocal folds, the squamous cell nature of the epithelium may have a protective role.

In the laryngeal epithelium are endings ("type 2") which have a spontaneous regular discharge and are mechanosensitive, but are little affected by most chemical irritants [13] (Fig. 8). They are stimulated by ammonia vapor, and inhibited by carbon dioxide. Pulmonary stretch receptors are in the tracheobronchial tree, with highest concentration in the trachea and large bronchi [72]. They can be localized in the airway smooth muscle, both on indirect [106] and direct evidence [8]. They are stimulated by inhaled ammonia and some volatile anesthetics [106], inhibited by carbon dioxide [10,74], and influenced by the degree of smooth muscle tone [8].

D. Receptor Behavior in Disease

Repeated chemical or mechanical stimulation of irritant receptors may result in a decreasing response over a time span of a few minutes [104]. However, the receptors are not totally inhibited, and the depression of activity could be due to changes in the immediate environment of the receptor or its surrounding tissues [89].

Repeated acute stimulations over several hours lead to reduced threshold and increased activity of the receptor [70], and there is also indirect evidence that animals chronically exposed to irritant gases have a sensitized lung irritant receptor response [28]. Sensitization of irritant receptors in humans with chronic lung disease has also been suggested [93]. These phenomena have not been put on a quantitative basis, and have only been studied for irritant endings in the lungs of rabbits, but they clearly are potentially important in considerations of reflex activity in chronic lung disease or chronic exposure to irritant gases or aerosols.

V. Reflex Patterns of Response

Now that we have considered the structure of airway receptors and the various stimuli which activate them, the next stage is to discuss the reflex results of this activation. Excitation of a defensive afferent pathway to the central nervous system results in motor responses in most or all of the outputs from the brainstem (Table 2). Those affecting breathing have been studied most extensively, but the others can be powerful and important.

Most of the experimental studies of defensive reflexes have features which make their application to man limited. They are nearly all with anesthetized animals, and the nature and depth of the anesthetic will determine the size or even the presence of the reflex being studied. A good example is the sneeze reflex, which is very readily blocked by anesthesia, and therefore has been little investigated; by contrast the "aspiration reflex" can withstand anesthesia deep enough to suppress completely spontaneous breathing [62]. In addition, the reflex stimulus is usually given through a tracheal cannula, so that the reflexogenic areas of the upper respiratory tract are bypassed. Finally, there may be striking species differences; for example, the rat has virtually no cough reflex.

A. Respiratory Reflexes

The pattern of respiratory response to stimulation of airway epithelial receptors varies with the site of stimulation and the nature and strength of the stimulant

TABLE 2 Summary of Reflex Responses to Stimulation of Respiratory Tract Receptors

Receptor	Respiration	Bronchi	Larynx	Blood pressure	Airway mucus
Nasal	Apnea, or sneeze	Dilation	Constriction	Increase	Secretion
Epipharyngeal	Inspirations	Dilation	? Dilation	Increase	Secretion
Laryngeal	Apnea, expirations or cough	Constriction	Constriction	Increase	Secretion
Tracheal irritant	Cough	Constriction	Constriction	Increase	Secretion
Lung irritant	Hyperpnea	Constriction	Constriction	Unknown	Unknown
Alveolar type J	Tachypnea	? Constriction	Constriction	Decrease	Unknown

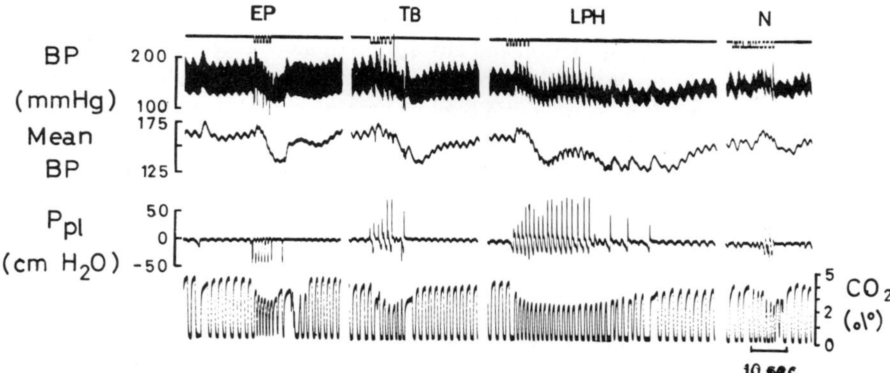

FIGURE 9 Changes in systemic arterial blood pressure (BP), mean blood pressure (mean BP), intrapleural pressure (P_{pl}), and tidal CO_2% caused by mechanical stimulation of the epipharyngeal (EP), tracheobronchial (TB), laryngopharyngeal (LPH), and nasal (N) mucosae, in an anesthetized spontaneously breathing cat. Signals for stimulation are at the top of the record. (From Tomori and Widdicombe [99].)

(Fig. 9) [32,106]. From the nose, sneezing, from the epipharynx, sniffing, and from the larynx and the trachea, coughing, may tend to remove the irritant stimulus and defend the organism from invasion [62,87]. The mechanical events of these reflexes are considered elsewhere in this volume (Chapter 15), and here only two comments are made. First, the cough and sneeze are, almost by definition, preceded by a deep inspiration; at least on theoretical grounds, this may have the adverse effect of increasing the inhalation of the irritant substance. Presumably this is compensated for by the added mechanical efficiency of the subsequent expulsive effort. Second, all experimental work shows that stronger concentrations of chemical irritants are needed to provide expulsive coughing and sneezing than are required to elicit other defensive reflexes from the respiratory tract, at least in the anesthetized animal [13,62]; we do not know whether this difference in reflex sensitivity depends on receptor thresholds or on the number of receptors recruited and their discharge frequencies. The nonexpulsive reflexes include an apneic response from the nose, possibly related in mechanism to the diving reflex of aquatic animals [4,5] and inhibition of breathing from the larynx [13]. The latter reflex merits further comment. Weak irritation of the laryngeal mucosa causes inhibition of breathing, whether the irritation is mechanical or chemical, and this is probably true also for man. Stronger stimulation is required to produce either an expiratory reflex [60,60a] or the cough reflex. It is not known whether the same receptors, but with different discharge frequencies, are involved in all three reflex patterns of response.

Stimulation of irritant receptors in the lungs does not seem to cause coughing [71], unless perhaps the stimulus is very strong. On mechanical grounds it is unlikely that coughing would protect the lungs from a foreign body deep in the airways, or prevent the action and absorption of a chemical irritant diffusely distributed deep in the lungs. The chemical and mechanical stimuli which excite lung irritant receptors all cause rapid shallow breathing, and there may be hyperventilation [16,53,54,70]. It must be emphasized, however, that the evidence concerning the action of lung irritant receptors on breathing is inferential, and we lack direct and convincing experimental data.

B. Laryngeal Reflexes

Changes in laryngeal caliber play a conspicuous part in all the defensive reflexes. For coughing and sneezing, the sudden opening of a previously closed larynx during the expulsive phase may be mechanically important in aerodynamic terms in removing a solid body in the airways; it must be said that this conventional view is based on little experimental evidence, and tracheostomized patients do not seem to be at a severe disadvantage through the lack of a laryngeal component in coughing.

Weaker irritant stimuli to the airways also cause reflex changes in laryngeal caliber, in the absence of coughing or sneezing [97]. During apneic responses from the nose, the larynx closes during the apnea and subsequent expiratory phases, and the same is true with the inhibition of breathing seen on weak irritation of the larynx (Fig. 10). Indeed, for the larynx, the reflex with the lowest minimum adequate stimulus is constriction of the larynx in the expiratory phase, without significant change in the pattern of breathing. This is not peculiar to the anesthetized experimental mammal, since the same phenomenon is seen in healthy unanesthetized man [42].

Irritation of the lungs also causes expiratory constrictions of the larynx, together with hyperpnea (Fig. 11) [95]. The functional significance of this laryngeal reflex has not been established, but it might increase the duration of expiration and functional residual capacity, and thereby promote gas exchange in the lungs. The importance of expiratory resistance to airflow in the larynx has recently been emphasized in relation to its effect on the pattern of breathing [9,36], and extension of this research to irritative conditions of the respiratory tract is urgently required. Changes in laryngeal calibre are one of the reflex changes seen in a variety of acute experimental lung conditions, including pneumothorax, anaphylaxis, and bronchoconstrictions [27,95,96].

C. Bronchomotor Reflexes

Reflex bronchoconstriction has been known for many years to occur on inhalation of dust and irritant gases, in experimental animals and man (see Refs. 105

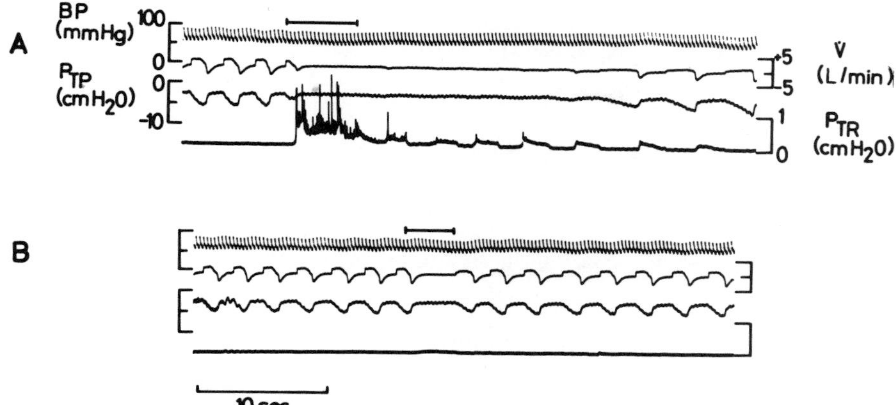

FIGURE 10 Effect of insufflation of 1:10[4] ammonia vapor into the larynx when the superior laryngeal nerves are intact (A) and cut (B). Note the apnea, absence of expiratory efforts, and increase in laryngeal resistance. From above down: signal, blood pressure, lower tracheal flow, transpulmonary pressure, and upper tracheal pressure (translaryngeal pressure). The signal above the blood pressure is the timing of insufflation. The rapid changes in translaryngeal pressure may be due to mucus in the larynx or to vibration of the vocal cords. (From Szereda-Przestaszewska and Widdicombe [97].)

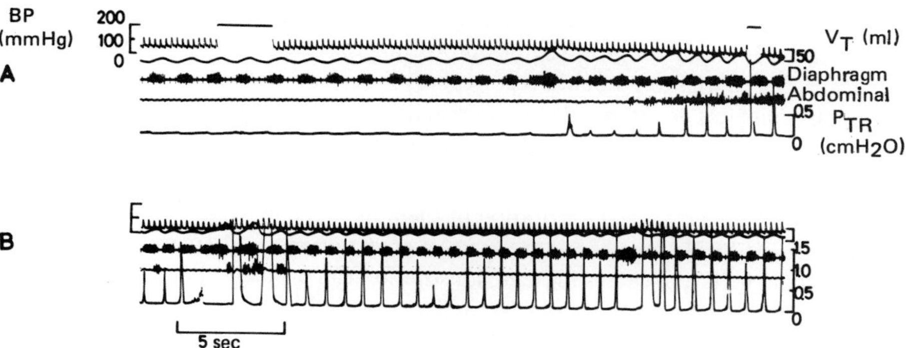

FIGURE 11 Effect of histamine aerosol on (from above downward) blood pressure, tidal volume, diaphragm electromyogram, abdominal electromyogram, and translaryngeal pressure at constant airflow. Histamine caused an increase in laryngeal resistance in the expiratory phase and rapid breathing.

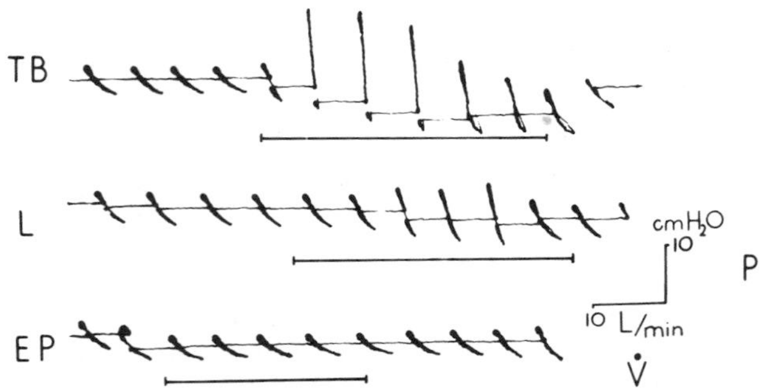

FIGURE 12 Oscilloscope records of total lung resistance changes during mechanical stimulation of tracheobronchial (TB), laryngeal (L) and epipharyngeal (EP) mucosae in an anesthetized, paralyzed, and artificially ventilated cat. Calibrations are in pressure (P) and flow ($\dot{V}$), and periods of mechanical stimulation are indicated by bars. Each sloping line corresponds to one pump cycle (pump frequency, 30 cycles/min; photographic paper moved horizontally in each expiratory pause), and its slope is proportional to total lung resistance. Thus an increase in slope indicates an increase in resistance, and a decrease in slope a decrease in resistance. (From Tomori and Widdicombe [99].)

and 107). In analytical experiments it can be produced by irritation of the mucosa of the larynx, trachea, and bronchi (Fig. 12). The physiological advantage of this constriction is not very clear. In timing, it is slow and long-lasting relative to events like coughing and apnea; it lacks respiratory phase, as would be expected from the time constants of the bronchial neuromuscular system. Bronchoconstriction increases the rigidity of the airways, and may render them less liable to collapse in the vigorous movements of coughing and hyperpnea [81]. The constriction may increase the impaction and absorption of aerosols and gases in the larger airways, thus protecting the alveoli [98]. In theory deadspace ventilation should decrease, but this effect is offset by the increase in physiological deadspace due to uneven distribution of inspired air [16]. Any advantages of bronchoconstriction should outweigh the disadvantage of an increased airways resistance and work of breathing.

Perhaps surprisingly, irritation of the nose and epipharynx causes bronchodilatation [2,99], together with laryngeal constriction. Early work indicating that nasal irritation causes bronchoconstriction can probably be explained by diffusion of the irritating gases to the larynx, the bronchoconstrictor reflex from the latter site being dominant. Any physiological function of this bronchodilator reflex is obscure, as is its relation to the diving reflex.

D. Cardiovascular Reflexes

Mechanical or chemical irritation of most parts of the respiratory tract causes reflex hypertension (Fig. 13). This is true for the epipharynx, nose, larynx, and

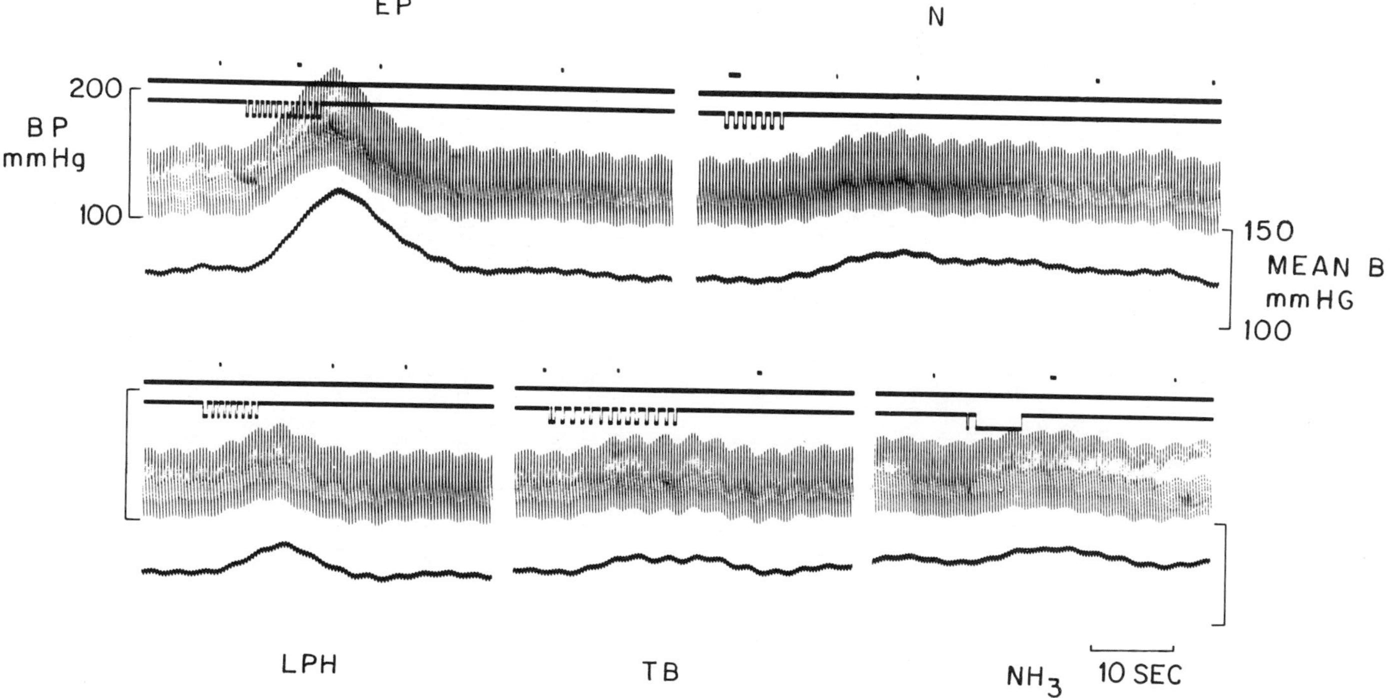

FIGURE 13 Representative changes in systolic, diastolic, and mean blood pressures on epipharyngeal (EP), nasal (N), laryngeal (LPH), and tracheobronchial (TB) stimulation and on intranasal insufflation of ammonia (NH_3) in a paralyzed cat. (From Tomori and Widdicombe [99].)

tracheobronchial tree [99]; this is the order for decreasing size of response for the anesthetized cat. In paralyzed man, mechanical stimulation of the epipharynx and tracheobronchial tree also causes hypertension, presumably reflex [23]. The response from the nose has been extensively studied in experimental animals, since it is an important part of the diving reflex, and includes vasoconstriction in various vascular beds, release of catecholamines from the adrenal medulla, and sympathetic stimulation of the heart [4,24,67,103].

The primary reflex changes in blood pressure may be masked by the hemodynamic effects of acts such as coughing (Fig. 9), and the hypotensive response in "cough syncope" [91] is a good example of this. A vasomotor action from lung irritant receptors has yet to be established.

It is more difficult to be definite about any primary reflex changes in heart rate due to irritation of the respiratory tract. Although strong stimulation of the nose and larynx can cause bradycardia [4,24,67,106] related to the diving reflex from the former site, the stimuli have usually been strong, and the involvement of secondary reflexes from arterial baroreceptors due to blood pressure changes has to be considered. Cardiac arrhythmias due to stimulation of the unanesthetized laryngeal mucosa have been described [51], and may be mediated by changes in vagal and sympathetic motor controls of the heart.

E. Reflex Secretion of Mucus

Chemical irritation of the respiratory tract causes secretion of mucus. This is partly a direct action of the irritant on the secretory cells, but, in addition, irritation of the larynx and trachea causes reflex secretion of mucus from the trachea of the cat [33] (see Chap. 10). Recent studies have shown that this is due to motor secretory activity in both the parasympathetic (vagal) and sympathetic systems, and is especially prominent on stimulation of the larynx [35]. Irritation of the nasal mucosa has a similar reflex action on tracheal mucus output, but no response has been seen on chemical irritation of the lungs. Teleologically one would expect reflex mucus secretion at a site peripheral rather than central to the irritant focus, so that the mucus might travel centrally to counteract the deleterious effects of the irritant. In the cat it is not established whether the reflexly stimulated mucus output comes from mucus glands or goblet cells. However, a similar reflex secretion has been demonstrated in the goose [84], which has goblet cells in the trachea but no mucus glands, so presumably both secretory systems may be involved in mammals.

F. Respiratory Sensation

For obvious reasons, this can easily be studied only in unanesthetized man. Mechanical irritation of the respiratory tract, for example with a catheter, causes unpleasant sensation or even pain, with a quality and timing which suggest strongly that it is due to stimulation of irritant or epithelial receptors [83]. The other methods of exciting irritant receptors in the experimental animal, for example inhalation of irritant gases and aerosols, also cause unpleasant sensation in man, and the same is seen in lung diseases and conditions known to activate lung irritant receptors [71,108]. At least in some instances in man, this unpleasant sensation can be prevented by local anesthetization of the vagus and glossopharyngeal nerves, or by inhalation of a local anesthetic aerosol which would paralyze surface receptors [39].

Thus it is certain that irritant and epithelial receptors can cause pain or unpleasant sensation when adequately stimulated. Presumably the wide diversity of qualities of this sensation are due to the various patterns of involvement of the different types of epithelial receptor as is also true for somatic unpleasant sensation, for example, in the skin. The role of "nociceptive" endings in the respiratory tract with nonmyelinated afferent fibers deserves special study in this regard.

VI. Defensive Reflexes from Individual Sites

So far in this chapter the defensive reflexes have been considered in rather general terms. This is because, for most conditions, the activation of reflexes does not occur at one particular site. Inhalation of gaseous irritants or aerosols will usually lead to deposition and reflex activation at many areas, and it is difficult to define the relative importance of the various zones of excitation. Respiratory diseases such as infections are seldom localized to one part of the airways. Thus the total defensive reflex responses will be the resultant of many different afferent stimulations. However, there are situations in man where the involvement is localized to one part of the respiratory tract, and this is the usual condition in analytical studies in the experimental animal. For this reason, and also to bring together the experimental evidence on the primary defensive reflexes, this section will summarize the effects of local irritant stimulation of the respiratory system, at the cost of some repetition.

A. The Nose

In man, irritation of the nasal mucosa is customarily considered to cause sneezing. In the experimental animal, nasal irritation seldom causes sneezing, possibly because the latter reflex is readily susceptible to general anesthesia, but more likely because weak stimuli produce not sneezing but the "diving reflex," of which apnea or inhibition of breathing is the most conspicuous respiratory component. Concurrently there is hypertension due to vasoconstriction in many vascular beds and release of catecholamines from the adrenal medulla, bradycardia, constriction of the larynx, especially in expiration and during the apnea, bronchodilation, and mucus secretion in the trachea [4,24,67,84]. The overall similarity between the diving reflex and the response to nasal mucosal irritation is striking, both in the pattern of motor response and also in our ignorance about the receptors and afferent mechanisms involved. For the diving reflex it is not clear whether the main physiological stimulus is external "wetness" or the entry of water into the nares; for the irritant reflex response we do not know which mucosal receptors are stimulated—"smell," "irritant," or "nociceptive"—largely because we know little about the physiology of these receptors. "Non-irritant odors" can elicit respiratory reflexes from the nose [1]. "Irritant gases" cause qualitatively similar reflex changes. For man, the sensation due to nasal stimulation or irritation varies greatly in quality and intensity. Further research is needed to show whether different chemical and mechanical stimuli work through different afferent pathways, or whether the same pathways are involved in different patterns and degrees.

With regard to the motor responses to nasal stimulation, the diving reflex has a clear teleological advantage in causing apnea, laryngeal closure, and "centralization" of circulating blood. The respiratory and laryngeal changes on nasal irritation may also be advantageous, but it is more difficult to envisage the advantage of bronchodilation, tracheal mucus secretion, and the hemodynamic effects. The nose, of such visual prominence and sensitivity, has been relatively neglected by physiologists.

B. The Epipharynx

This area was for long regarded as the "no-man's-land" of the upper respiratory tract, until Ivanco et al. [48] in an extensive series of investigations [62,100] established the properties of the "aspiration reflex." This is the rapid and repetitive series of vigorous inspiratory efforts caused by mechanical stimulation of the epipharyngeal mucosa [77]. The reflex is "sniff-like" [11], without alternating expiratory efforts, and is one of the most powerful reflex drives to inspiration yet studied. Unlike some other respiratory reflexes, it is very resistant to anesthesia and hypothermia, and causes a powerful arousal reaction. It is associated with reflex hypertension, tachycardia, and bronchodilatation. Single-fiber recordings from the afferent nerves of the receptors show that the endings are mechanosensitive and rapidly adapting, but are not sensitive to those chemical irritants tested [76]. Thus the reflex is not strictly an irritant reflex, but presumably acts to remove a foreign body in the back of the nose by pulling it into the pharynx where it is either swallowed or coughed up. The aspiration reflex could be important in the newborn, when the nasal passages have to be cleared at the start of breathing. In adult man the cardiovascular response, including hypertension and venoconstriction, may be more powerful than the respiratory effects [23]. The reflex has been activated in man to treat chronic hiccough.

C. The Larynx

The weakest effective mechanical or chemical stimulation of laryngeal irritant receptors causes laryngeal closure, in man and experimental animals [42,96]. Stronger stimulations also lead to inhibition of breathing, hypertension, bradycardia, bronchoconstriction, and tracheal mucus secretion [4,24,67,84]. The analogy with the diving reflex is clear; protection is provided by the reflex changes, until asphyxial blood gas alterations become dangerous to the organism.

With stronger stimuli, in particular discrete mechanical stimulation with a catheter to the vocal folds, the "expiration reflex" (a short expiratory effort without preceding inspiration) is elicited [60a,61]. This has been extensively studied by Korpas and his colleagues, who describe the function of the reflex as the vigorous expulsion of a potential laryngeal obstruction. The expiration reflex, unlike the cough reflex, is resistant to general anesthesia, and is especially powerful in the newborn. It is especially interesting that Korpas has shown that this reflex is active in man, and is enhanced in inflammatory conditions of the laryngeal mucosa [62]. Reflex laryngeal constriction also occurs.

Even stronger stimuli to the larynx cause coughing, characterized by an initial inspiratory effort before the expulsive expiration [12].

Recording action potentials in single afferent fibers from laryngeal mucosal receptors shows that there are at least three types: type 1, rapidly adapting irritant receptors; type 2, spontaneously firing mechanosensitive endings less responsive to irritants; and "nociceptive" endings with nonmyelinated fibers [13]. There are probably also "taste-receptors" in the larynx of some species. The role of the different receptors in the various laryngeal reflexes has yet to be worked out, but presumably in most forms of laryngeal stimulation the total reflex and sensory responses are due to the interaction of all the receptor systems.

D. The Trachea

Stimulation of irritant receptors in the tracheal epithelium ("cough receptors") causes coughing, hypertension, laryngeal constriction and bronchoconstriction. The respiratory pattern of the cough produced by tracheal stimulation differs from that seen when the larynx is irritated [62]. There seems to be no investigation of whether weaker stimulation of tracheal irritant receptors causes inhibition of breathing rather than coughing, as is true for the larynx.

Cough receptors in the trachea are sensitized in experimental inflammation of the respiratory tract [62] and are stimulated by drugs which contract the underlying smooth muscle [71]. They are paralyzed by local anesthetic aerosols, and the reflex is rather susceptible to general anesthesia. The sensitivity of tracheal cough receptors in human respiratory diseases merits study, since the animal experiments of Korpas and Tomori [62] indicate that great variations in threshold may occur; severe epithelial damage may abolish the cough reflex. The action of mucus either in stimulating cough receptors, or in protecting them from inhaled irritants, also requires investigation. Furthermore, although the primary reflex effects of stimulation of cough receptors have been frequently studied, the secondary responses—blood gas and hemodynamic changes—have received less attention, although they can be conspicuous.

E. The Bronchi

Irritant receptors within the lungs do not seem to cause coughing, since those conditions which stimulate them vigorously cause hyperpnea rather than coughing [71]. However, the "pure" respiratory response to activation of lung irritant receptors is still controversial. Reflex laryngeal constriction in expiration and bronchoconstriction are established.

Although in general irritation of the trachea causes coughing, whereas irritation of the interpulmonary bronchi causes hyperpnea, the distinction is probably not hard and fast. Mechanical stimulation of the bifurcations of the larger bronchi can produce a cough, and the conditions in which excitation of bronchial irritant receptors leads to either coughing or hyperpnea or both in sequence have not been defined.

The lung irritant receptors have a nonpathological role, since they seem to be responsible for the deep sighing, augmented breaths which open up collapsed lung, especially in the newborn [89]. The hyperpnea, as distinct from coughing, due to inhaled irritant gases and aerosols is probably due to stimulation of lung irritant receptors. In acute lung diseases such as pneumothorax, bronchoconstriction, microembolism, anaphylaxis, and pulmonary congestion and edema, lung irritant receptors provide or contribute to the reflex hyperventilation [53,54], and they are probably involved in the associated unpleasant respiratory sensation in man [108]. In this respect, the reinflation of collapsed lung is a powerful stimulus to lung irritant receptors [89] and causes pain or distressing sensation in man [15].

Lung irritant receptors are exquisitely sensitive to intraluminal mechanical and chemical irritants, and yet are paradoxically tough in that repeated stimulation over hours does not diminish their sensitivity but may instead lead to a reduction in threshold [28,70]. By analogy between experimental animals and man, they are probably important in acute and chronic human lung disease, in providing respiratory drive and sensation.

F. The Alveoli

J-receptors in the alveolar wall are stimulated by strong concentrations of irritant gases, and cause reflex apnea followed by tachypnea, hypotension, and bradycardia [80]. Their most usual stimulus seems to be the volume of interstitial fluid in the alveolar wall, and in experimental lung disease they are activated in pulmonary microembolism, congestion, and edema. An important reflex from them is the inhibition of spinal reflexes via a pathway ascending to the subcortical areas of the brain [26,52]. The reflex role of alveolar J-receptors on the inhalation of irritant gases has yet to be established, but Paintal's important studies of their physiology raise two general problems. First, do similar receptors, with similar reflex actions, also exist in the tracheal and bronchial wall? They have been identified in the laryngeal mucosa [13] and the bronchial wall [21,22] and might be expected to occur throughout the respiratory tract if they are visceral nociceptors. Second, can other respiratory tract receptors also have an action on spinal reflexes and skeletal muscular tone?

VII. General Considerations

In this last section are discussed some aspects of the defensive reflexes which seem worth comment because of their relevance either to general neurobiology, or to the human condition in health and disease.

A. Comparative Physiology

Fishes have a well-developed cough mechanism, in one respect more complicated than for mammals, since they can cough either forward or backward [43,44,87, 109]. This is possible because their ventilatory system is unidirectional, water passing through the buccal cavity to the opercular or parabranchial cavities and out over the gills. Ventilation is achieved by a double pump system, the buccal pump rostrally and the opercular or parabranchial pumps caudally; the system is very similar to the double series pump on each side of the heart. Introduction of irritant chemicals into the buccal cavity causes forward coughing, with reversal of the pump action, while irritation of the gills or in the caudal chambers causes backward coughing. Details of the muscular-sphincteric processes and of the water pressures and flows at different sites in the ventilatory system have been worked out by Hughes [43] and Young [109]. Some fish, such as mackerel, have lost the power of active irrigation of the gills and rely for ventilation on a ram action in swimming; presumably they cannot cough.

Amphibia, and some reptiles, seem unable to cough, since they cannot significantly increase intrapulmonary pressure by active muscle contraction [87]. Ventilation consists of filling the lungs by a positive pressure buccal pump, followed by laryngeal closure. Expiration is passive due to the elastic forces derived from the lungs. The larynx has primarily a sphincteric role. Whether it is reflexly closed in response to irritation does not seem to have been established. Amphibia also exhibit tidal ventilation, with the larynx closed, and gas exchange in the pharynx. Here the muscular arrangements should allow forced expulsive reflexes, equivalent to coughing.

The development, in reptilia, of a rib cage and inspiratory and expiratory muscles in the trunk, and the loss of the buccal pump, should provide the first situation in evolution for the occurrence of full-scale defensive reflexes, including from the lungs, such as coughing or sneezing seen in the mammal. Again, however, there is no report in the literature of such reflexes.

With birds, the general impression is that the defensive reflexes, especially the expulsive ones, are weak compared with those in mammals [55]. However, there are descriptions of coughing [110], expiratory efforts [18], and apneas [41] provoked either by mechanical stimulation of the larynx or trachea, or by inhalation of irritant gases. Hypertension and transient laryngeal closure also occur [64]. Interestingly, there is a reflex decrease in total airways resistance [18], the opposite of that seen in mammals. If this airway dilation occurs in the bronchi which bypass the lungs, then the result could be to divert the irritating gas into the air sacs and away from the gas-exchanging areas, thereby protecting the lungs at the expense of diminished lung ventilation. Birds, as would be expected, have a powerful diving reflex on immersion of the bill or beak into water [24,64]. This includes apnea, laryngeal closure, and profound circulatory adjustments. Even if the diving reflex is not strictly a "defensive reflex," its existence in sophisticated form must depend on very similar integrative mechanisms.

Finally, it should be pointed out that the defensive reflexes differ considerably in strength between different mammalian species. Three examples among common laboratory animals are the powerful cough reflex of the cat, the strong nasal apneic and hemodynamic reflexes of the rabbit, and the virtual absence of a true cough reflex in the rat [62].

B. Reflex Interactions

A reflex such as the cough may have an illusory simplicity: it appears as an accentuated tidal breath with transient interruption of the expiratory phase by glottis closure. Yet there are a number of reasons for challenging the illusion.

1. The multiple outputs of the defensive reflexes—respiratory, laryngeal, cardiovascular, bronchomotor, secretomotor and possibly spinal—point to a highly complex integrating system in the brain, about which little is known and which is, thankfully, outside the scope of this chapter.
2. Many of these resultant changes—e.g., in blood pressure, or blood gas tensions—could cause secondary effects which become as important to the organism as the primary reflexes, for example, cough syncope.
3. A particular example of a secondary action is the fact that the vigorous movements of coughing will themselves stimulate irritant receptors in the respiratory tract, and this could lead to self-augmenting or -perpetuating patterns. An example of such a positive feedback is that stimulation of lung irritant receptors causes bronchoconstriction, and bronchoconstriction stimulates lung irritant receptors. The importance of such mechanisms, especially in disease, needs to be studied [107].
4. Some degree of voluntary control of our defensive reflexes is possible, and we can voluntarily mimic the cough reflex, but probably not accurately the other defensive reflexes [25]. There are clinical indications that central nervous conditioning may be important in determining the occurrence and strength of the defensive reflexes.
5. For somatic afferent pathways, the phenomenon of "gating" is important; activity in one afferent pathway can open or close a gate to permit or prevent the effectiveness of a second afferent pathway, for example, in reflexes from the skin [68]. Does a similar mechanism exist for respiratory tract reflexes?
6. In relation to the last point, it seems highly unlikely that any naturally occurring stimulus in the respiratory tract influences only one group of receptors. Even with a stimulus localized, for example, to the larynx, animal experiments show that two or three groups of receptors will be activated. With inhaled irritants or aerosols, or in respiratory disease, the resultant

reflex changes must nearly always be due to the interaction of activities in more than one afferent pathway [37]. This consideration must apply especially to "provocation tests," where the pattern of involvements of the different afferent systems will depend on the chemical nature of the irritant, its particle size and solubility, the flow pattern of inhalation, etc.

VIII. Conclusions

This chapter has reviewed some aspects of the defensive reflexes from the respiratory tract. Their strength and importance in healthy man is common experience. Their complexity as physiological integrating mechanisms is formidable and little understood. Their significance in respiratory and nervous disease must be considerable, but the manner and extent of their modification in disease processes have been neglected, except for acute pathological conditions in experimental animals. They provide an example where the collation of information from analytical studies in animals and integrative studies in man should, in the future, lead to important advances in our understanding of pathophysiological processes.

References

1. W. R. Allen, Effect on respiration, blood pressure and carotid pulse of various inhaled and insufflated vapors when stimulating one cranial nerve and various combinations of cranial nerves. III. Olfactory and trigeminals stimulated, *Am. J. Physiol.,* **88**:117-129 (1929).
2. J. V. Allison and D. A. Powis, Adrenal catecholamine secretion during stimulation of the nasal mucous membrane in the rabbit, *J. Physiol. (Lond.),* **217**:327-336 (1971).
3. B. L. Andrew, A functional analysis of the myelinated fibres of superior laryngeal nerve of the rat, *J. Physiol. (Lond.),* **133**:420-432 (1956).
4. J. Angell James and M. de B. Daly, Nasal reflexes, *Proc. R. Soc. Med.,* **62**:1287-1293 (1969).
5. J. E. Angell James and M. de B. Daly, Some mechanisms included in the cardiovascular adaptations to diving, *Symp. Soc. Exp. Biol.,* **26**:313-341 (1972).
6. D. J. Armstrong and J. C. Luck, A comparative study of irritant and type J receptors in the cat, *Respir. Physiol.,* **21**:47-60 (1974).
7. P. Ardonin and M. Maillet, Etude des fibres nerveuses amyeliniques de la corde vocale, *Acta Otolaryngol. (Stockh.),* **59**:225-233 (1965).
8. D. Bartlett, Jr., P. Jeffery, G. Sant'Ambrogio, and J. C. M. Wise, Location of stretch receptors in the trachea and bronchi of the dog, *J. Physiol. (Lond.),* **258**:409-420 (1976).

9. D. Bartlett, Jr., J. E. Remmers, and H. Gautier, Laryngeal regulation of respiratory airflow, *Respir. Physiol.*, **18**:194-204 (1973).
10. D. Bartlett, Jr. and G. Sant'Ambrogio, Effects of local and systemic hypercapnia on the discharge of stretch receptors in the airways of the dog, *Respir. Physiol.*, **26**:91-99 (1976).
11. H. L. Batsel and J. Lines, Bulbar respiratory neurons participating in the sniff reflex in the cat, *Exp. Neurol.*, **39**:469-481 (1973).
12. H. A. Boushey, P. S. Richardson, and J. G. Widdicombe, Reflex effects of laryngeal irritation on the pattern of breathing and total lung resistance, *J. Physiol. (Lond.)*, **224**:501-513 (1972).
13. H. A. Boushey, P. S. Richardson, J. G. Widdicombe, and J. C. M. Wise, The response of laryngeal afferent fibres to mechanical and chemical stimuli, *J. Physiol. (Lond.)*, **240**:153-175 (1974).
14. J. D. Brain, Uptake of inhaled gases by the nose, *Ann. Otol. Rhinol. Laryngol.*, **79**:529-539 (1970).
15. E. J. Burger and P. Macklem, Airway closure: Demonstration by breathing 100% O_2 at low lung volumes and by N_2 washout, *J. Appl. Physiol.*, **25**: 139-148 (1968).
16. R. Buff and E. A. Koller, Studies on mechanisms underlying the reflex hyperpnoea induced by inhalation of chemical irritants, *Respir. Physiol.*, **21**:271-383 (1974).
17. V. I. But and V. I. Klimova-Cherkasova, Afferentation from upper respiratory tract, *Bull. Exp. Biol. Med.*, **64**:13-16 (1967).
18. D. Callanan, M. Dixon, J. G. Widdicombe, and J. C. M. Wise, Responses of geese to inhalation of irritant gases and injections of phenyl diguanide, *Respir. Physiol.*, **22**:157-166 (1974).
19. N. Cauna, K. H. Hinderer, and R. T. Wentges, Sensory receptor organs of the human nasal respiratory mucosa, *Am. J. Anat.*, **14**:295-300 (1969).
20. H. M. Coleridge, J. C. G. Coleridge, and J. G. Luck, Pulmonary afferent fibres of small diameter stimulated by capsaicin and by hyperinflation of the lungs, *J. Physiol. (Lond.)*, **179**:248-263 (1965).
21. H. M. Coleridge and J. C. G. Coleridge, Two types of afferent vagal C-fiber in the dog lung: Their stimulation by pulmonary congestion, *Fed. Proc.*, **34**:372 (abstract) (1975).
22. H. M. Coleridge and J. C. G. Coleridge, Afferent vagal C-fibres in the dog lung: Their discharge during spontaneous breathing, and their stimulation by alloxan and pulmonary congestion. In *Krogh Centenary Symposium on Capillary Exchange, Pulmonary Oedema and Respiratory Adaptations.* Edited by A. S. Paintal, Delhi, University of Delhi, 1976.
23. J. L. Corbett, J. A. Kerr, C. Prys-Roberts, A. Crampton-Smith, and J. M. K. Spalding, Cardiovascular disturbances in severe tetanus due to overactivity of the sympathetic nervous system, *Anaesthesia*, **24**:198-212 (1969).
24. M. de Burgh Daly, Interaction of cardiovascular reflexes, *Sci. Basis Med.*, 307-332 (1972).
25. J. N. Davis, Autonomous breathing, *Arch. Neurol.*, **30**:480-484 (1974).
26. S. S. Deshpande and M. S. Devanandan, Reflex inhibition of monosynap-

tic reflexes by stimulation of type-J pulmonary endings, *J. Physiol. (Lond.)*, **206**:345-358 (1976).

27. M. Dixon, M. Szereda-Przestaszewska, J. G. Widdicombe, and J. C. M. Wise, Studies on laryngeal calibre during stimulation of peripheral and central chemoreceptors, pneumothorax and increased respiratory loads, *J. Physiol. (Lond.)*, **239**:325-345 (1974).
28. M. Dixon, D. Callanan, R. Penman, and J. G. Widdicombe, Unpublished results (1975).
29. A. F. Elftman, The afferent and parasympathetic innervation of the lungs and trachea of the dog, *Am. J. Anat.*, **72**:2-28 (1943).
30. W. H. Feindel, The neural pattern of the epiglottis, *J. Comp. Neurol.*, **105**: 269-280 (1956).
31. P. Ferrer and E. A. Koller, Uber die Vagus afferenzen des Meerschweinchens und ihre Bedeutung dur die Spontanatmung, *Helv. Physiol. Pharmacol. Acta*, **26**:365-387 (1968).
32. M. Fillenz and J. G. Widdicombe, Receptors of the lungs and airways. In *Handbook of Sensory Physiology*, Vol. 3. Edited by E. Neil. Heidelberg, Springer-Verlag, 1971, pp. 81-112.
33. H. Florey, H. M. Carleton, and A. Q. Wells, Mucus secretion in the trachea, *Q. J. Exp. Pathol.*, **13**:269-284 (1932).
34. S. I. Frankstein and Z. N. Sergeeva, Tonic activity of lung receptors in normal and pathological states, *Nature*, **210**:1054-1055 (1966).
35. J. T. Gallagher, P. W. Kent, M. Passatore, R. J. Phipps, and P. S. Richardson, The composition of tracheal mucus and the nervous control of its secretion in the cat, *Proc. R. Soc. Lond. [Biol.]*, **192**:69-76 (1975).
36. H. Gautier, J. E. Remmers, and D. Bartlett, Control of the duration of expiration, *Respir. Physiol.*, **18**:205-221 (1973).
37. M. Glogowska and J. G. Widdicombe, The role of vagal reflexes in experimental lung oedema, bronchoconstriction and inhalation of halothane, *Respir. Physiol.*, **18**:116-128 (1973).
38. P. P. C. Graziadei, The olfactory mucosa of vertebrates. In *Handbook of Sensory Physiology*, Vol. IV: *Chemical Senses*, Part 1. Edited by L. M. Beidler. Heidelberg, Springer-Verlag, 1971, pp. 27-58.
39. A. Guz, M. I. M. Noble, J. H. Eisele, and D. Trenchard, Experimental results of vagal block in cardiopulmonary disease. In *Breathing: Hering-Breuer Centenary Symposium*. Edited by R. Porter. London, Churchill, 1970, pp. 315-328
40. S. Hatakeyama, Histological study on the nerve distribution in the larynx in the cat, *Arch. Jpn. Histol.*, **19**:369-389 (1960).
41. W. A. Hiestand and W. C. Randall, Species differentiation in the respiration of birds following CO_2 administration and location of inhibitory receptors in the upper respiratory tract, *J. Cell Physiol.*, **17**:333-340 (1941).
42. J. E. Hinkle and K. R. Tantum, A technique for measuring reactivity of the glottis, *Anesthesiology*, **35**:634-641 (1971).
43. G. M. Hughes, *Comparative Physiology of Vertebrate Respiration*. London, Heinemann, 1963.

44. G. M. Hughes and G. Shelton, Respiratory mechanisms and their nervous control in fish, *Adv. Comp. Physiol. Biochem.*, **1**:275-364 (1962).
45. K. S. Hung and C. G. Loosli, Bronchiolar neuro epithelial bodies in the neo natal mouse lungs, *Am. J. Anat.*, **140**:191-199 (1974).
46. K. S. Hung, M. S. Hertweck, J. D. Hardy, and C. G. Loosli, Ultrastructure of nerves and associated cells in bronchiolar epithelium of the mouse lung, *J. Ultrastruct. Res.*, **43**:426-437 (1973).
47. K. S. Hung, M. S. Hertweck, J. D. Hardy, and C. G. Loosli, Electron microscopic observation of nerve endings in the alveolar walls of mouse lungs, *Am. Rev. Respir. Dis.*, **108**:328-333 (1973).
48. I. Ivanco, J. Korpas, and Z. Tomori, Ein Beitrag zur Interozeption der Luftwege, *Physiol. Bohemoslov.*, **5**:84-90 (1956).
49. V. Jabonero and J. Sabadell, The sensory innervation of the smooth musculature of the respiratory tract, *A. Mikrosk. Anat. Forsch.*, **86**:213-243, (1972).
50. P. Jeffery and L. Reid, Intra-epithelial nerves in normal rat airways: A quantitative electron microscopic study, *J. Anat.*, **114**:35-45 (1973).
51. M. Johnstone, Respiratory and cardiac control during endotracheal intubation, *Br. J. Anaesth.*, **24**:36-50 (1952).
52. M. Kalia, Effects of certain cerebral lesions on the J reflex, *Pflügers Arch.*, **343**:297-308 (1973).
53. W. Karczewski and J. G. Widdicombe, The role of the vagus nerves in the respiratory and circulatory responses to intravenous histamine and phenyl diguanide in rabbits, *J. Physiol. (Lond.)*, **201**:271-292 (1969).
54. W. Karezewski and J. G. Widdicombe, The role of the vagus nerves in the respiratory and circulatory reactions to anaphylaxis in rabbits, *J. Physiol. (Lond.)*, **201**:293-304 (1969).
55. A. S. King and V. Moloney, The anatomy of respiration. In *Physiology and Biochemistry of the Domestic Fowl*, Vol. 1. Edited by D. J. Bell and B. M. Freeman. London, Academic Press, 1971, pp. 93-169.
56. H. Koizumi, On sensory innervation of larynx in dog, *Tohoku J. Exp. Med.*, **58**:199-210 (1953).
57. H. Koizumi, On innervation of taste buds in larynx in dog, *Tohuku J. Exp. Med.*, **58**:211-215 (1953).
58. E. A. Koller, Afferent vagal impulses in anaphylactic bronchial asthma, *Acta Neurobiol. Exp.*, **33**:51-56 (1973).
59. E. A. Koller and P. Ferrer, Studies on the role of the lung deflation reflex, *Respir. Physiol.*, **10**:172-183 (1970).
60. J. Korpas, Expiration reflex from the vocal folds, *Physiol. Bohemoslov.*, **21**:671-675 (1972).
60a. J. Korpas, Differentiation of the expiration and the cough reflex, *Physiol. Bohemoslov.*, **21**:677-682 (1972).
61. J. Korpas and G. Kalocsayova, The expiration reflex from the vocal folds of the rabbit, *Physiol. Bohemoslov.*, **23**:333-340 (1974).
62. J. Korpas and Z. Tomori, *Cough and Other Respiratory Reflexes.* Bratislava, Czechoslovakian Academy of Science, 1975.

63. J. M. Lauweryns, M. Cokelaere, and P. Theunynck, Neuro-epithelial bodies in the respiratory mucosa of various mammals, *Z. Zellforsch.*, **135**:569-592 (1972).
64. L. M. Leitner, M. Roumy, and M. J. Miller, Motor responses triggered by diving and by mechanical stimulation of the nostrils and of the glottis of the duck, *Respir. Physiol.*, **21**:385-392 (1974).
65. L. Luciano, E. Reale, and H. Ruska, Uber eine "chemorezeptive" Sinneszelle in der Trachea der Ratte, *Z. Zellforsch. Mikrosk. Anat.*, **85**:350-375, (1968).
66. J. C. Luck, Afferent vagal fibres with an expiratory discharge in rabbit, *J. Physiol. (Lond.)*, **211**:63-71 (1970).
67. R. J. McRitchie and S. W. White, Role of trigeminal, olfactory, carotid sinus and aortic nerves in the respiratory and circulatory response to nasal inhalation of cigarette smoke and other irritants in the rabbit, *Aust. J. Exp. Biol. Med. Sci.*, **52**:127-141 (1974).
68. R. Melzack and P. D. Wall, Pain mechanisms: A new theory, *Science,* **150**: 971-976 (1965).
69. B. Meyrick and L. Reid, Nerves in rat intra-acinar alveoli: An electron microscopic study, *Respir. Physiol.*, **11**:367-377 (1971).
70. J. Mills, H. Sellick, and J. G. Widdicombe, The role of lung irritant receptors in respiratory responses to multiple pulmonary embolism, anaphylaxis and histamine-induced bronchoconstriction, *J. Physiol. (Lond.)*, **203**: 337-357 (1969).
71. J. Mills, H. Sellick, and J. G. Widdicombe, Epithelial irritant receptors in the lungs. In *Breathing: Hering-Breuer Centenary Symposium.* Edited by R. Porter. London, Churchill, 1970, pp. 77-92.
72. G. Miserocchi, J. Mortola, and G. Sant'Ambrogio, Localisation of pulmonary stretch receptors in the airways of the dog, *J. Physiol. (Lond.)*, **235**: 775-782 (1973).
73. J. Mortola, G. Sant'Ambrogio, and R. Clement, Localization of irritant receptors in the airways of the dog, *Respir. Physiol.*, **24**:107-114 (1975).
74. M. E. K. Y. Mustafa and M. J. Purves, The effect of CO_2 upon discharge from slowly adapting stretch receptors in the lungs of rabbits, *Respir. Physiol.*, **16**:197-212 (1972).
75. J. A. Nadel and J. G. Widdicombe, Reflex control of airway size, *Ann. N.Y. Acad. Sci.*, **109**:712-722 (1963).
76. B. S. Nail, G. M. Sterling, and J. G. Widdicombe, Epipharyngeal receptors responding to mechanical stimulation, *J. Physiol. (Lond.)*, **204**:91-98 (1969).
77. B. S. Nail, G. M. Sterling, and J. G. Widdicombe, Patterns of spontaneous and reflexly-induced activity in phrenic and intercostal motoneurones, *Exp. Brain Res.*, **15**:318-332 (1972).
78. A. S. Paintal, Mechanism of stimulation of type J pulmonary receptors, *J. Physiol. (Lond.)*, **203**:511-532 (1969).
79. A. S. Paintal, The mechanism of excitation of type J receptors, and the J reflex. In *Breathing: Hering-Breuer Centenary Symposium.* Edited by R. Porter. London, Churchill, 1970, pp. 59-71.

80. A. S. Paintal, Vagal sensory receptors and their reflex effects, *Physiol. Rev.*, **53**:159-227 (1973).
81. B. Palombini and R. F. Coburn, Control of the compressibility of the canine trachea, *Respir. Physiol.*, **15**:365-383 (1972).
82. A. Plaschko, Die Nervenendigungen und Ganglien der Respirationsorgane, *Anat. Anz.*, **13**:12-22 (1897).
83. C. Prys-Roberts. In *Breathing: Hering-Breuer Centenary Symposium.* Edited by R. Porter. London, Churchill, 1970, p. 249.
84. P. S. Richardson, M. Passatore, and R. Phipps, Unpublished results (1975).
85. S. R. Sampson and C. Eyzaguirre, Some functional characteristics of the mechanoreceptors in the larynx of the cat, *J. Neurophysiol.*, **27**:464-480, (1964).
86. S. R. Sampson and E. H. Vidruk, Properties of "irritant" receptors in canine lung, *Respir. Physiol.*, **25**:9-22 (1975).
87. G. Satchell, *Comparative Physiology of the Cough.* London, Academic Press, 1975.
88. H. Sellick and J. G. Widdicombe, The activity of lung irritant receptors during pneumothorax, hyperpnoea and pulmonary vascular congestion, *J. Physiol. (Lond.)*, **203**:359-382 (1969).
89. H. Sellick and J. G. Widdicombe, Vagal deflation and inflation reflexes mediated by lung irritant receptors, *Q. J. Exp. Physiol.*, **55**:153-163 (1970).
90. H. Sellick and J. G. Widdicombe, Stimulation of lung irritant receptors by cigarette smoke, carbon dust and histamine aerosol, *J. Appl. Physiol.*, **31**:15-19 (1971).
91. E. P. Sharpey-Schafer, The mechanism of syncope after coughing, *Br. Med. J.*, **ii**:860-863 (1953).
92. C. S. Sherrington, *The Integrative Action of the Nervous System,* 1st ed. New York, Scribner, 1906.
93. B. G. Simonsson, F. M. Jacobs, and J. A. Nadel, Role of autonomic nervous system and the cough reflex in the increased responsiveness of airways in patients with obstructive airways disease, *J. Clin. Invest.*, **46**: 1812-1818 (1967).
94. A. T. Storey, A functional analysis of sensory units innervating epiglottis and larynx, *Exp. Neurol.*, **20**:366-383 (1968).
95. A. Stransky, M. Szereda-Przestaszewska, and J. G. Widdicombe, The effect of lung reflexes on laryngeal resistance and motoneurone discharge, *J. Physiol. (Lond.)*, **231**:417-438 (1973).
96. M. Szereda-Przestaszewska, Changes in laryngeal calibre in anaphylactic shock in rabbits, *J. Physiol. (Lond.)*, **241**:21P (1974).
97. M. Szereda-Przestaszewska and J. G. Widdicombe, Reflex effects of chemical irritation on the upper airways on the laryngeal lumen in cats, *Respir. Physiol.*, **18**:107-115 (1973).
98. M. L. Thomson and M. D. Short, Mucociliary function in health, chronic obstructive airway disease, and asbestosis, *J. Appl. Physiol.*, **26**:535-539 (1969).

99. Z. Tomori and J. G. Widdicombe, Muscular, bronchomotor and cardiovascular reflexes elicited by mechanical stimulation of the respiratory tract, *J. Physiol. (Lond.)*, **200**:25-50 (1969).
100. A. Tomori, K. Javorka, and A. Stransky, Reflex responses to stimulation of the upper respiratory tract, *Acta Neurobiol. Exp.*, **33**:57-70 (1973).
101. C. van Michel, Considerations morphologiques sur les appareils sensoriels de la muqueuse vocale humaire, *Acta Anat.*, **52**:188-192 (1963).
102. M. von During, K. H. Andres, and J. Iravani, The fine structure of the pulmonary stretch receptor in the rat, *Z. Anat. Entwicklungsgesch.*, **143**: 215-222 (1974).
103. S. W. White, R. J. McRitchie, and D. L. Franklin, Autonomic cardiovascular effects of nasal inhalation of cigarette smoke in the rabbit, *Aust. J. Exp. Biol. Med. Sci.*, **52**:111-126 (1974).
104. J. G. Widdicombe, Receptors in the trachea and bronchi of the cat, *J. Physiol. (Lond.)*, **123**:71-104 (1954).
105. J. G. Widdicombe, Regulation of tracheobronchial smooth muscle, *Physiol. Rev.*, **43**:1-37 (1963).
106. J. G. Widdicombe, Respiratory reflexes. In *Handbook of Physiology*, Section 3: *Respiration*, Vol. 1. Washington, D.C., American Physiological Society, 1964, pp. 585-630.
107. J. G. Widdicombe, Reflex mechanisms in bronchial obstruction. In *Bronchitis III*. Royal Van Gorcum: Assem., 1970, pp. 288-294.
108. J. G. Widdicombe, Breathing and breathlessness in lung disease, *Sci. Basis Med.*, 148-160 (1971).
109. S. Young, Coughing in fish, a study of the expulsion reflexes. Ph.D. Thesis, University of London, 1974.
110. E. Zeuthen, The ventilation of the respiratory tract in birds, *Biol. Meddr.*, **17**:1-51 (1942).

17

Pulmonary Lymphatics and Their Role in the Removal of Interstitial Fluids and Particulate Matter

LEE V. LEAK

Howard University College of Medicine
Washington, D.C.

I. Introduction

Although Hippocrates spoke of thin channels containing "White Blood," it was not until 1622 that Aselli [3] recognized a system of lymphatic vessels within the mesentery of a well fed dog. This system of vessels was distinct from the blood vascular system in that a nonpigmented or whitish fluid was observed within their lumina. Following the studies of Aselli, the gross anatomical structure and distribution of the large abdominal lymphatics occupied the attention of many of the leading anatomists of the seventeenth and eighteenth centuries who described the organization of lymphatics in several organs including the lung [4,94]. Rudbeck [105] described a system of irregularly shaped vessels in the pulmonary pleura of the dog and Willis [122] observed a superficial plexus of lymphatics in the lungs of the calf. Others were able to identify a plexus of lymphatics which were closely associated with the walls of bronchi and blood vessels and which communicated with each other [18,49,78,108, 124]; and the pleural cavity by means of stomata within the mesothelium of the pleural surface [58]. The belief that the lymphatic vessels formed an open system was very popular in the 19th century [104]. But, later in the century, small, delicate lymphatic vessels were described [22,27] and the concept that the lymphatics are a system of closed vessels [14,50,74,106] was generally accepted.

The vasculature comprising the lymphatic system is similar to the blood vessels in that it forms a system of endothelial-lined tubes of varying diameters which transport cellular and noncellular components in a liquid (i.e., the lymph). There is no "lymphatic circulation" as is true of the blood vascular system, but rather a unidirectional drainage system whose major vessels (thoracic duct and right lymphatic duct) empty at the junction of the jugular and subclavian veins and whose main branches (collecting lymphatic vessels), for the most part, follow the overall distribution of the arteries and the veins. The final arborization of these collecting vessels extend into the connective tissue spaces where they anastomose with a rich plexus of lymphatic capillaries which drains the interstitial areas of the body (except the central nervous system, bone, cartilage, and teeth). The lymphatic system, therefore, serves a major function in the recovery of connective tissue fluids and proteins that have escaped from blood capillaries and are not returned by the venous limb of the blood vascular system [79]. If the escaped plasma proteins were not removed by the lymphatic vessels, protein molecules would accumulate within the interstitial fluids. This would not only deplete the circulation of plasma colloids, but would also disrupt the balance of forces between the interstitial milieu and lumina of blood vessels which control the exchange of fluids across the wall of blood capillaries and venules [13,36,43,79]. Therefore, the constant removal of fluids from the connective tissue spaces by this one-way drainage system serves an important role in the normal maintenance of fluid homeostasis throughout the body tissues. In addition to returning escaped serum protein to the bloodstream [125], the lymphatics are also important in the response of the organism to infection and in the spread of disease to various tissues of the body [82].

Intimately associated with the lymphatic vessels is a complex system of lymph nodes through which lymph passes on its journey to the central veins. Lymph nodes selectively remove antigens and other foreign substances from lymph, thus playing an integral role in the overall host defense system [26,41,44].

In common with the lymphatic vessels in other regions of the body, the pulmonary lymphatics not only function to maintain fluid homeostasis for this organ but also play a significant role in pulmonary defense mechanisms (Fig. 1a,b). They are also involved in the genesis and development of various respiratory disease processes (e.g., tuberculosis; see Ref. 83) and the metastasis of lung cancer [116,118]. With the advent of improved injection techniques and methods of tissue preparation at the end of the 19th century and the early part of the 20th century, detailed anatomical studies were made on the adult mammalian pulmonary lymphatics [75,84,85] and on embryonic and fetal lymphatics [16,19,37,47,55,91a].

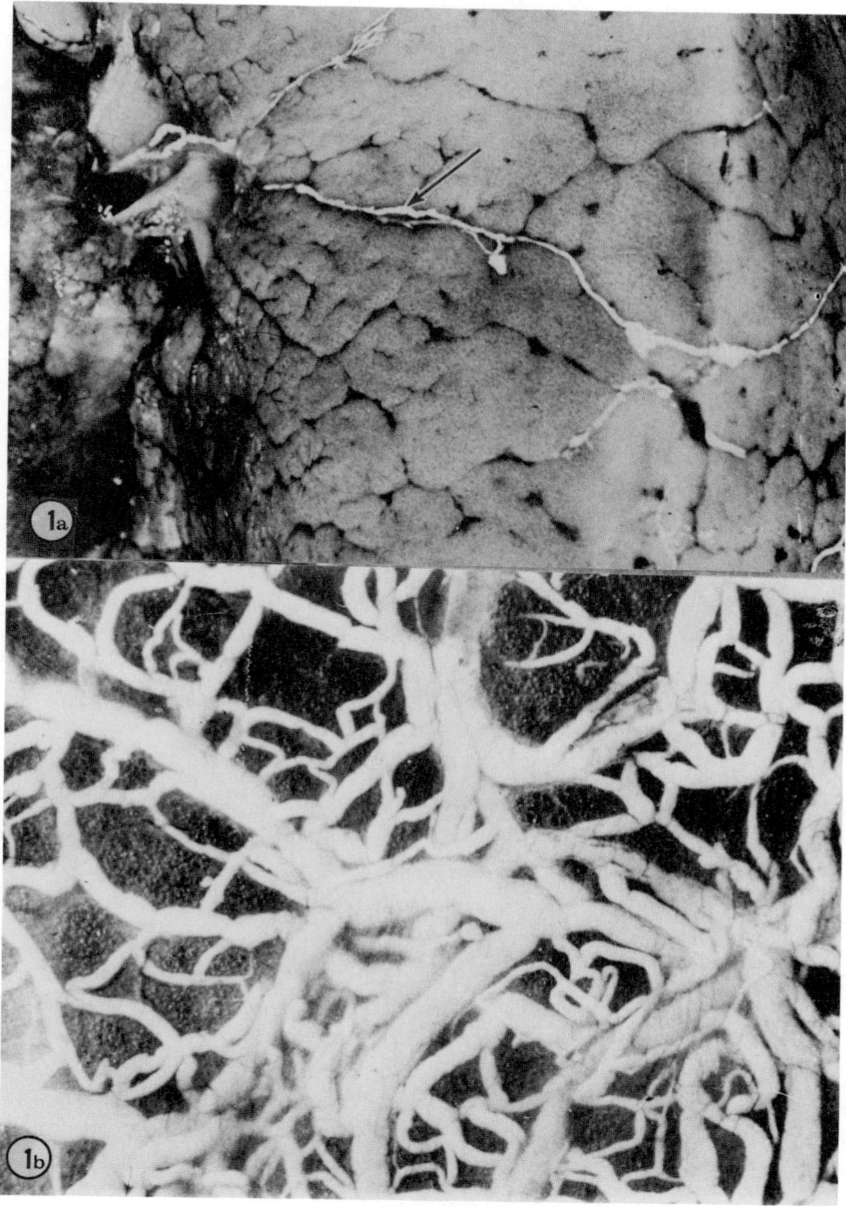

FIGURE 1 (a) Corrosion cast showing pulmonary lymphatic vessels and the location of collecting lymphatics along the interlobular septum (arrow). (b) The rich supply of pulmonary lymphatic is illustrated in this micrograph which is a corrosion cast showing network of lymphatic vessel. (From Ref. 61a.)

The earlier investigators [18,78] divided the pulmonary lymph vessels into two categories: a superficial system, which is distributed within the pulmonary pleura, and a system of deep lymph vessels located in the intrapulmonary tissues. Many of the latter investigators, including Miller, further classified pulmonary lymphatics according to their regional distribution (i.e., pleural, peribronchial, perivascular, or septal). Although significant information regarding pulmonary lymphatics was presented during the early part of the 20th century, many of the findings disagreed as to whether the normal direction of lymph flow in the interlobular septum was outward toward the pleura, from the pleura to the hilum or whether the lymph traveled over the surfaces of the lung, within the pleural lymphatics, directly to the hilum. There was also disagreement regarding the existence, number, and distribution of valves within lymph vessels of the deeper portions of the lung. During the past decade, a number of techniques have been used which provide more information on the organization of pulmonary lymphatics. The radiopaque injection technique [20,119] has provided a method for delineating boundaries of the larger vessels for topographic studies of pulmonary lymphatics for individual lobes, as well as information on the direction of pulmonary lymph flow. The techniques of electron microscopy have also been brought to bear on delineating the ultrastructure of pulmonary lymphatic vessels [57,61,62,64]. The following intrinsic properties of the pulmonary lymphatic system merit consideration:

1. The precise topography and ultrastructure of pulmonary lymphatics and the structural basis of interstitial fluid removal by lymphatics in the lung
2. The ability of pulmonary lymphatic capillaries to propel or drain lymph in a unidirectional stream toward lymphatic collecting vessels
3. The ability of lymphatics to participate in pulmonary defense mechanisms
4. The involvement of lymphatics in the genesis, development, and dissemination of various respiratory disease processes, including the metastasis of lung cancer

In this review, the first of these properties will be dealt with in some detail. In particular, some of the available data on the organization and topography of pulmonary lymphatics will be evaluated. Consideration will be given to those ultrastructural features which enable pulmonary lymphatics to remove large molecules and cells from the interstitial areas of the lung. We will also discuss evidence for the rapid movement of fluid and particulate material across the air interstitial lymph interface and the blood interstitial lymph interface.

II. General Organization of the Lymphatic System

In describing the organization of lymphatic vessels in various tissues of the body, many studies have demonstrated that the uptake of interstitial fluids, proteins, particulate material, and cells by this one-way drainage system is accomplished by extremely thin-walled permeable vessels, the lymphatic capillaries [11,38, 51,70]. These vessels occur at the site of extracellular exchange within the interstitium and provide portals for the return of interstitial plasma protein and fluids which have leaked from blood capillaries. Foreign substances and particulate matter are also removed from the interstitium by this method. Once accumulated in these thin-walled channels, lymph is propelled in a unidirectional flow into vessels which follow the overall distribution of arteries and veins.

The continuity of collecting vessels is interrupted by lymph nodes which provide a filtering, or screening, system for lymph and its content. Lymph from collecting vessels is propelled into the main lymphatic vessels of the body represented by the lumbar vessels, the cisterna chyli, and the thoracic duct which terminates at the junction of the left subclavian and jugular veins, and a number of vessels on the right side of the body which communicate at the union of the jugular and subclavian veins. The components of the lymphatic system are classified as follows.

A. Lymphatic Trunks

These consist of the larger, thick-walled lymphatic vessels which communicate with the central venous system at the base of the neck. The right and left thoracic ducts, the cisterna chyli, and cervical lymphatic vessels make up the major lymphatic trunks. These vessels have a large diameter (4-6 mm) and a thick vascular wall which is organized into three separate tunics: an intima, a media, and an adventitia. The tunica intima consist of a single, continuous layer of endothelial cells which rest on a basement lamina [67]. At selected regions along the length of the vessels, endothelial cells reduplicate and extend into the lumen to form valves. Collagen and elastic fiber provide a filamentous network between the basement lamina and the adjoining smooth muscle cells of the tunica media which comprises the second layer. It is composed of several layers of smooth muscle cells, collagen, and elastic fibers. The smooth muscle cells are circumferentially arranged and are connected to each other by gap junctions (nexus). The outermost layer, the tunica adventitia consists of connective tissue components (i.e., collagen and elastic fibers, fibroblasts, occasional macrophages, and mast cells). In addition, this layer contains blood vessels (vasa vasorum) and nerve bundles which supply the wall of the lymphatic trunks.

B. Lymphatic Collecting Vessels

Like the distributing arteries and medium-sized veins, the collecting lymphatics constitute the main branches of the lymphatic vascular system. They serve as the major channels for the egress of lymph. The diameter of the lymphatic collecting vessels is extremely variable, and there are numerous valves along the length of these vessels. The regular occurrence of valves imparts a beaded pattern which becomes marked when the vessels are dilated. The three tunics (i.e., intima, media, and adventitia) which are characteristic for thick-walled vessels, are also present in the walls of collecting lymphatics. Although a tunica media is present, the smooth muscle cells are not always observed as a continuous layer of cells. Instead, individual smooth muscle cells may be arranged in a spiral or coiled fashion along the length of the collecting vessels.

C. Lymphatic Capillaries

These delicate vessels begin as blind-end tubules or vessels within the interstitium and comprise the extremely thin-walled and permeable vessels located at the sites of exchange between the blood vascular and interstitial areas. Here the lymphatic capillaries act as the primary drainage system to provide a return mechanism for the excess escaped plasma protein, fluids, and cells. Notwithstanding an attenuated wall, the diameter of these vessels is extremely variable, ranging from 20 μm to $\sim$80 μm, and may often appear bulbous or as saccules when fully dilated. The walls of these delicate lymphatics consist of a tunica intima which is formed by a continuous lining of endothelial cells. There are many intercellular junctions which overlap extensively with apposing endothelial cell membranes which are loosely adherent with only few punctate membrane specialization for attachment.

D. Lymphatic Sinusoids

The lymphatic sinusoids constitute the more spacious, endothelial-lined, intercommunicating cavities which are tubular but highly pleomorphic and labyrinthine in shape. The attenuated wall conforms to the contours of the spaces they occupy and the structures they surround [33-35]. In common with lymphatic capillaries, the lymphatic sinusoids serve as drainage sites for interstitial fluids as well as other substances, e.g., hormones secreted in such regions as the interstitial area of the testis [73].

E. Lymphatic Spaces

Recently Fawcett et al. [35] described large, intercommunicating cavities which are filled with protein-rich lymph but whose walls are partially lined by an endothelium. The lumen of these cavities is continuous with the extracellular fluid phase of the surrounding connective tissue matrix. The limiting boundary of these lymphatic spaces is ill-defined in some areas, while in others the endothelial lining is discontinuous but may gradually become continuous in areas where the spaces become confluent with the lumen of a typical lymphatic vessel. The name suggested for these particular structures is discontinuous sinusoids [35].

III. Classification, Topography, and Distribution of Pulmonary Lymphatics

Like other areas of the body, the pulmonary lymphatics are well developed in regions with abundant connective tissue [85]. Therefore, within the interstitial areas of the lung rich in connective tissue components (such as the pleura, interlobular septum, peribronchial, and perivascular regions), an extensively developed plexus of lymphatic vessels can be demonstrated.

The literature on the organization and distribution of pulmonary lymphatics is somewhat contradictory. It is generally agreed that a rich plexus of pulmonary lymphatics abound within the pleura and interlobular septa of large mammals, including the lungs of man. The bronchi, pulmonary arteries, and veins are also surrounded by an interconnecting plexus of lymphatic vessels [47, 55,83,118]. There is no unanimity, however, regarding the existence of alveolar lymphatic vessels or their presence at the air-blood barrier. Although a number of investigators have reported the presence of a system of lymphatics near alveoli [116,117] or surrounding the walls of alveoli [29], others have not been successful in finding lymphatic capillaries beyond the respiratory tree [60,84,99].

A. Pleural Lymphatics

Pulmonary lymphatics were first observed in the pleura of the lung by Rudbeck in 1653 [105] and Willis in 1676 [122]. In 1874 Sappy [107] depicted a superficial or subpleural lymphatic system arranged in an elaborate plexus composed of meshes of irregular polyhedral rings that communicated freely with the lymphatics located in the deeper regions of the lungs. The thickness and complexity of the pleura varies with the size of the animal; for example, in man [85, 89,103] and in cattle [57,122] the pleura is relatively thick, extending into the deeper portions of the lung as interlobular septa (connective tissue septa) to form secondary lobules. However, in smaller animals (such as the rat, rabbit, cat, and dog [85]) the lungs are covered with a thin pleura which does not extend into the deeper portions of the lung.

Miller [85] classified the pleura into a mesothelial layer, an elastic layer, and an areolar layer. Within the areolar layer Miller [84,85] described a single plexus of lymphatics. Because of their location within the subserous connective tissue, the pleural lymphatics are also called subpleural, peripheral, subserous, or superficial lymphatic vessels. Since the lymphatics, along with blood vessels, nerves, and connective tissue components, comprise one of the layers of the visceral covering of the lung, the term "pleural lymphatic" will be used for the superficial lymphatics of the lung.

In 1786 Cruikshank [18] noted that the pleural lymphatics readily fill with an injected dye and that the vessels communicated freely with each other. Subsequent investigators have used this trait to determine the organization and distribution of lymphatic vessels within the pleura. By using injection techniques combined with serial sections, Miller illustrated a rich plexus of lymphatics in the pleura of the dog [83] and in man [84] confirming the earlier observations of Sappy [108].

With the introduction of radiopaque substances, lymphatic vessels and nodes could be visualized in the intact lung [20]. Recently, in vivo radiologic methods have provided additional information on the three-dimensional topography as well as the organization and distribution of pleural lymphatics over the surface of the lung [20]. Although this procedure reveals mainly those vessels which are visible with the unaided eye (0.5-1 mm), the size and distribution of the larger collecting lymphatics within the various lobes of the lung can be illustrated (Fig. 2a). Numerous valves which point in all directions (Fig. 2b) were observed in these large vessels [119] and the distance between them was found to be relatively constant in all parts of a particular lung. Miller [84] had previously observed a similar arrangement; he states that the valves pointed or opened in all directions, thus, permitting "free circulation" of the lymph within the confines of the pleural region.

Since Miller [84] observed valves only in the septal lymphatics which pointed (opened) toward the pleura, he considered that this arrangement precluded the flow of pleural lymph from draining into the deeper lymphatics of the lung.

However, more recent radiologic studies of Trapnell [119] have shown that all valves observed in the interlobular lymphatics pointed away from the pleura and toward the hilum. It is of special interest that a similar arrangement of the valves was observed in cases of lymphangitis carcinomatosis [120]. There were several cases in which the flow of the injection medium drained from the pleura into the deeper lymphatics and then back to the pleura, thus

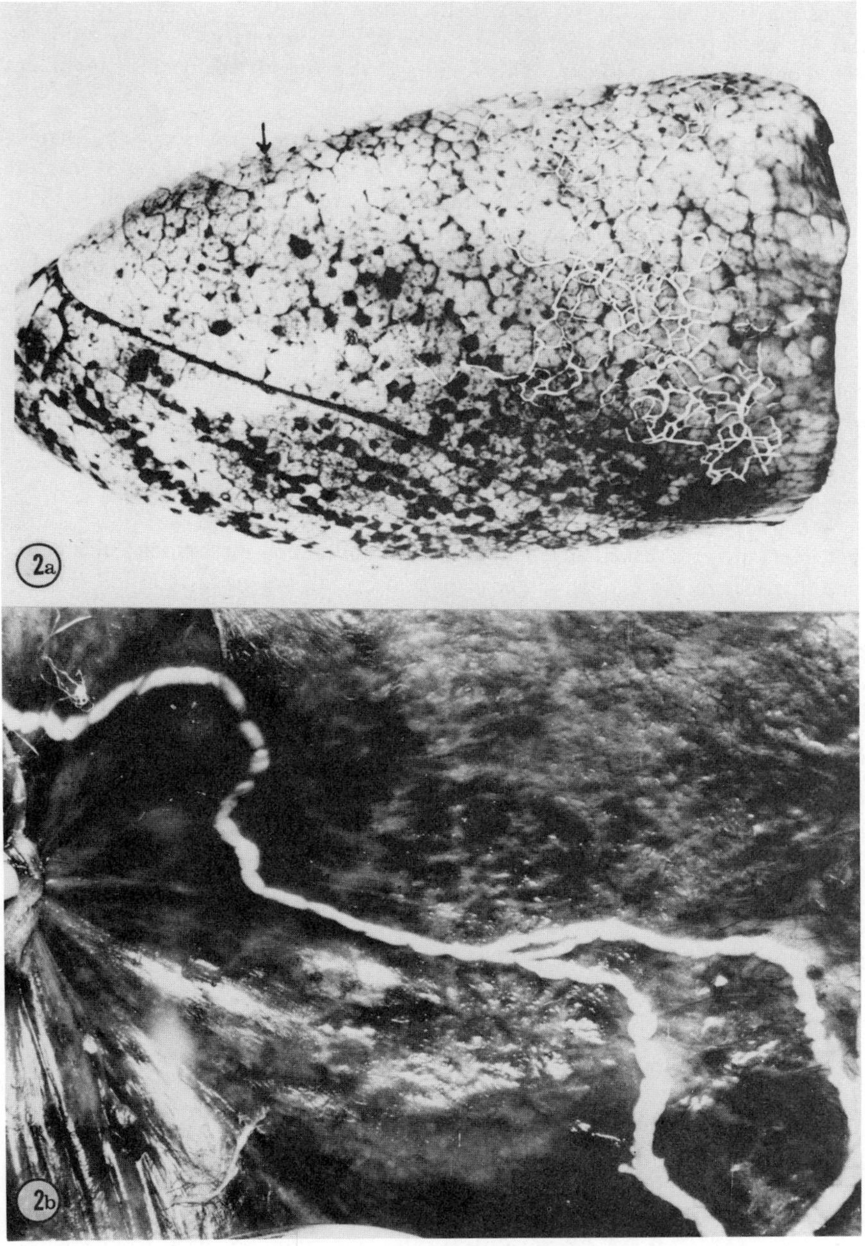

FIGURE 2 (a) Radiograph showing the distribution of pleural lymphatics over the lower lobe. (b) Pleural lymphatics showing valves, the positions of which are indicated by the constrictions in the vessel. (From Ref. 119.)

suggesting an occasional flow toward the pleura. However, the evidence showed that the usual direction of flow in the interlobular lymphatics is away from the pleura and toward the hilum. This finding is also supported by the experiments of other investigators [39,47,55,95,110].

Earlier studies on the distribution of pleural lymphatics suggested that they were located evenly over the entire pulmonary surface [18]. But in more recent studies in which radiographic methods were employed, Trapnell [119] observed an uneven distribution of pleural lymphatics in that many more were found over the left lower lobe than over the upper or middle lobes (Fig. 2a). An uneven distribution of pleural lymphatics in man was also observed by Nagaishi [89], who showed that they were most abundant on the mediastinal surface and very sparse over the costal surfaces of the lung. It should be pointed out that the above studies were carried out on postmortem lung which may account for the uneven labeling of lymphatics.

B. Interlobular Lymphatics

It is generally established that loose collagen containing interstitial fluids and lymph spaces forms a much larger proportion of all organs in fetal life than at later age levels. In the fetal lung, the connective tissue areas forming the pleura, the interlobular septa, and the peribronchial and perivascular regions are extremely extensive. Elaborate lymphatic channels observed in the interlobular septum are closely associated with the interlobular pulmonary veins [19,28,37,91a,110,126]. They form a network of vessels in the interlobular connective tissue surrounding each secondary lobule, which is demarcated by the connective tissue septum. After injecting colloidal carbon into the pleural lymphatics of the fetal lung, Simer [110] observed that the interlobular septa are spaced at intervals of ~1 mm and that each contains lymphatic vessels which drained the carbon from the pleural plexus into the lymphatic channels surrounding the blood vessels and the bronchial tree. The topographical relationship between the interlobular lymphatics and pulmonary veins is also maintained in the adult lung [89,107,118].

C. Intrapulmonary (Deep) Lymphatics

The deep or parenchymatous lymphatics form a network of vessels which are closely associated with the bronchi, arteries, and veins. During the early period of fetal development, an interconnecting lymph plexus is shared by the bronchi and arteries [19]. Later this plexus differentiates into two separate parts; one follows and is closely associated with the bronchi, while the other plexus maintains close association with the arteries. Although differentiated, a connection between the two groups of vessels is maintained, especially at points where the division of bronchi occurs [85].

1. Peribronchial Lymphatics

Miller [85] described two sets of lymphatics in the large bronchial wall. One layer is situated between the muscular and epithelial layer and the second layer is located in the adventitia enclosing the cartilaginous plates of the bronchus (Fig. 3a). The two layers of lymphatics are connected by anastomosing vessels which pass between the plates of cartilage comprising the bronchial wall. In the walls of the smaller bronchi and bronchioles there is only a single plexus of lymphatics (Figs. 3b, 4a,b). As the bronchioles continue to branch and become smaller, the lymphatics are reduced in size and distribution. Earlier, Miller [84, 85] was of the opinion that the bronchial lymphatics terminated at the distal end of the alveolar ducts, while other workers suggested that the lymphatics extended to the region between the terminal and respiratory bronchioles [12,48, 59,64,89,126]. Tobin [116] described lymphatics which accompany branches of pulmonary arterioles and venules to the alveolar walls (alveolar lymphatics). Our studies show lymphatics within the peribronchial connective tissue sheath adjacent to alveoli (Fig. 4a,b), confirming the recent studies of Lauweryns and Baert [62].

2. Perivascular Lymphatics

The abundance of lymphatics within the connective tissue surrounding the pulmonary artery is easily demonstrated in cross and longitudinal sections of the pulmonary artery (Fig. 5a,b). Toward the peripheral region of the lung, both the bronchioles and arterioles are surrounded by a single layer of lymphatics which communicate by anastomosing vessels located between the two. Similarly, a rich plexus of lymphatics surrounds the pulmonary veins. They accompany the smaller veins, originating from the bronchial tree and pleura [85]. In the larger pulmonary vein, the accompanying lymphatic vessels are larger and form an extensive network which surrounds the vein. The scanning electron microscope reveals the topographical relationship between the lymphatics, bronchial tree, and blood vessels (Figs. 6a,b; 7a,b; 8a,b).

IV. Structural Components of Pulmonary Lymphatics

Before electron microscopy was applied to studies of the lymphatic vascular system, it was difficult to distinguish the smaller and thin-walled vessels that terminate within the connective tissue area from those of the collecting vessels.

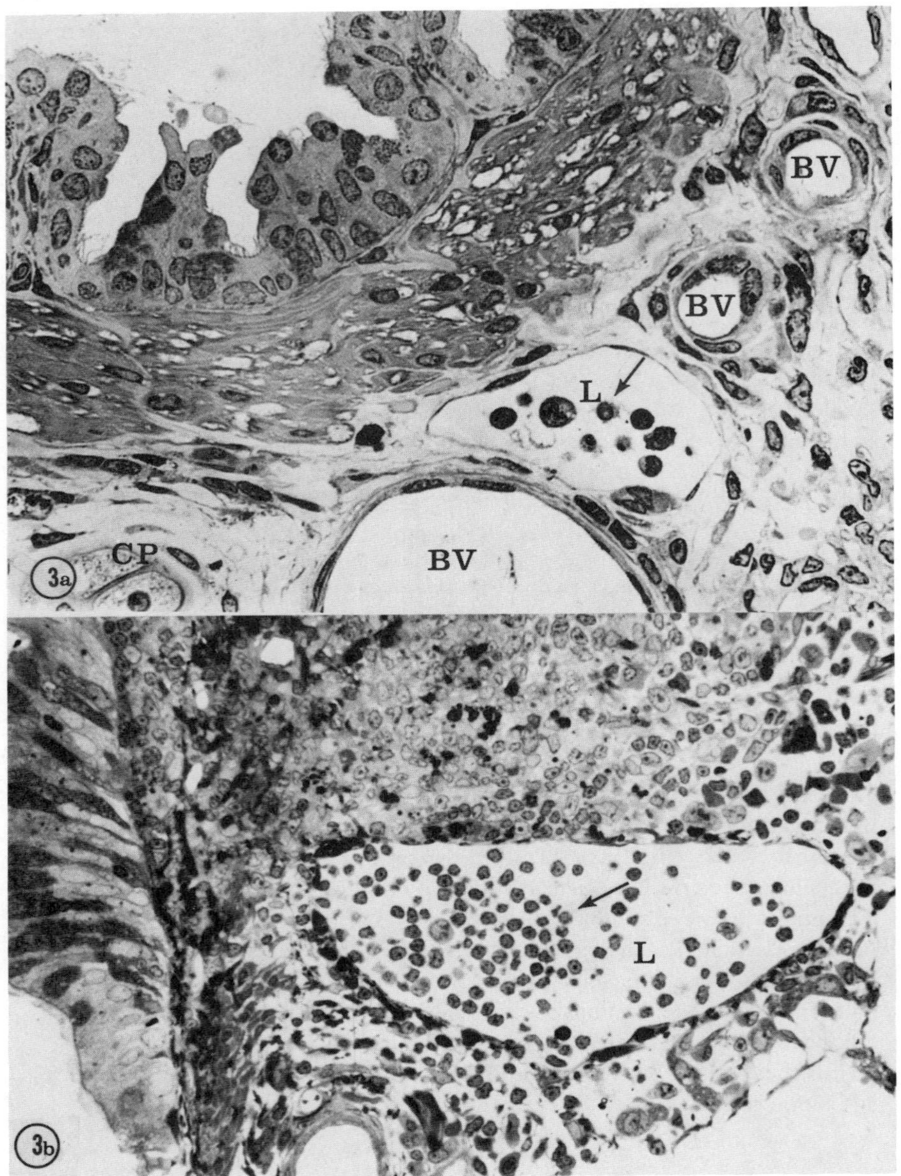

FIGURE 3 (a) Light micrograph showing lymphatic vessel (L) in the adventitia of bronchus. Note large and small lymphocytes in the lymphatic lumen (arrow). Blood vessels (BV) are free of cells and plasma as a result of perfusion fixation. A cartilage plate (CP) is seen in lower left of micrograph. ×1400. (b) Lymphatic collecting vessel (L) whose lumen contains large and small lymphocytes (arrow). ×1400.

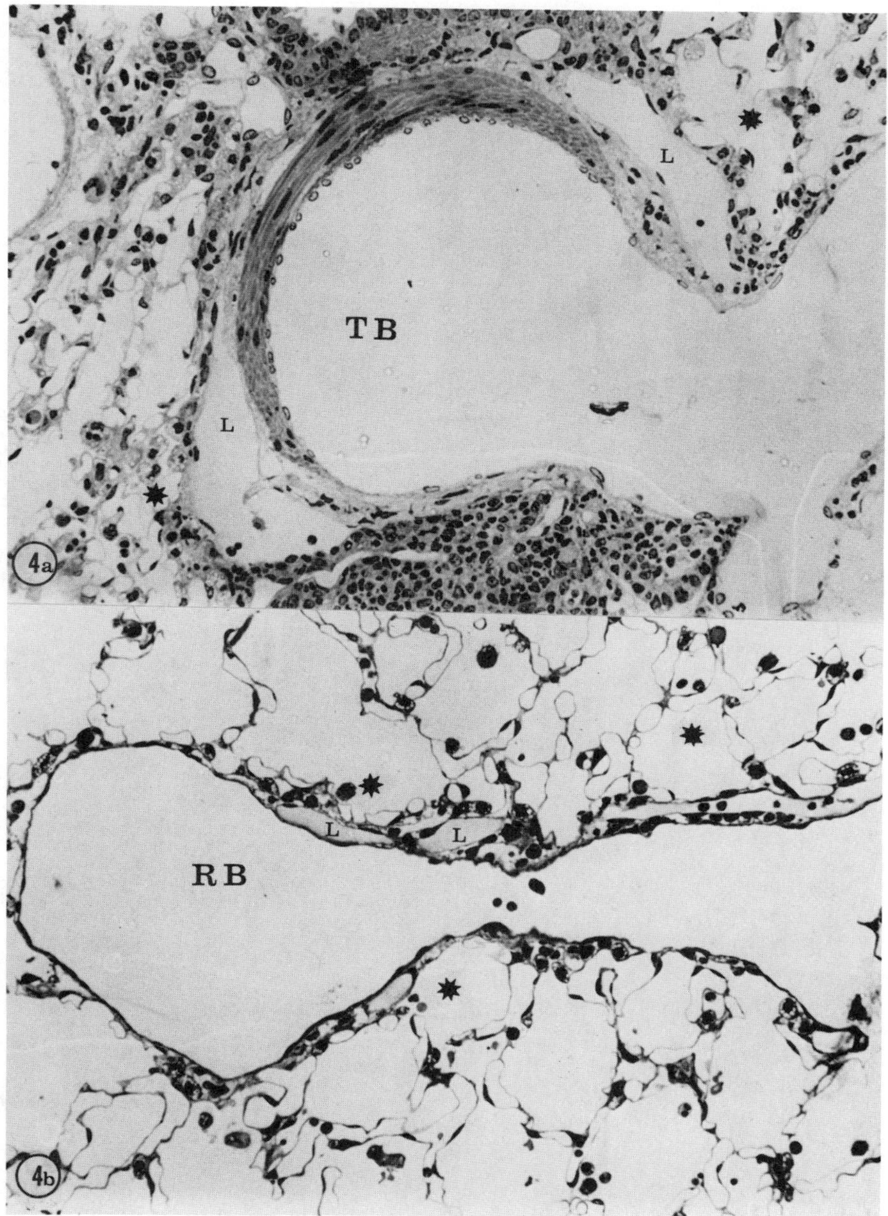

FIGURE 4 (a) Position of lymphatic (L) in relation to a terminal bronchiole (TB) and the adjacent alveoli. ×900. (b) Lymphatics (L) within the connective tissue sheath of a respiratory bronchiole (RB) that are also in close apposition to alveoli (*). ×600.

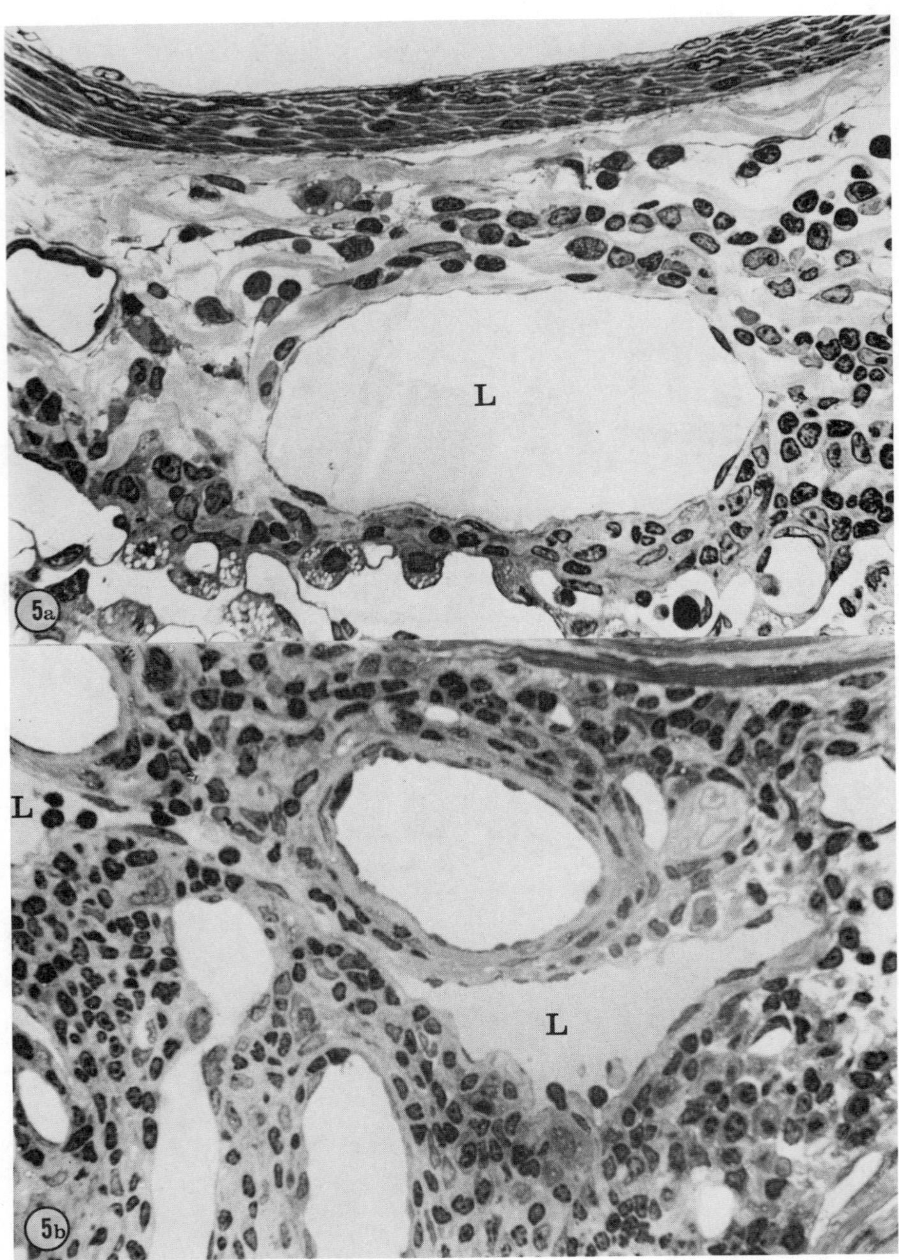

FIGURE 5 (a) and (b) The location of lymphatics (L) within the periarterial connective tissue sheath. (a) ×1400; (b) ×1400.

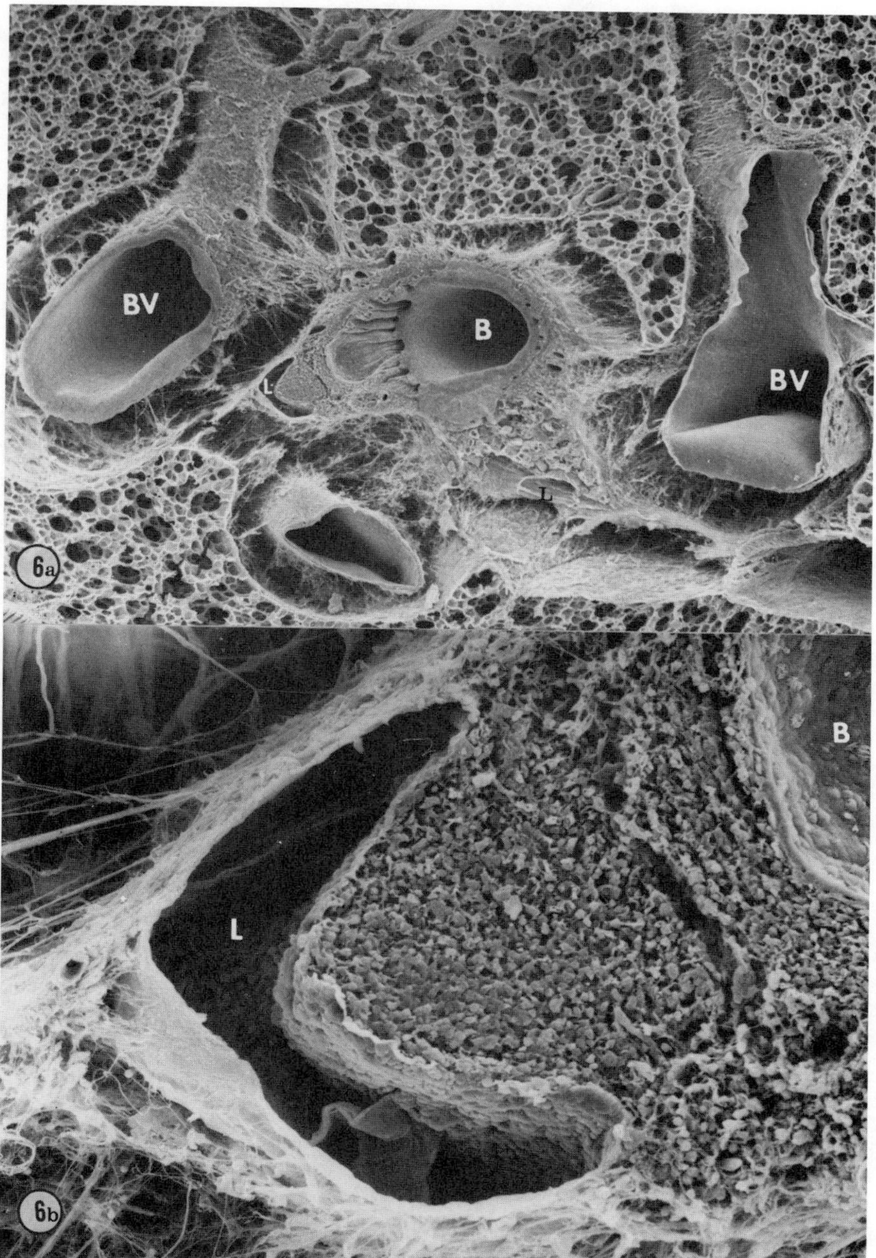

FIGURE 6 (a) The topographical relationship between the bronchial (B), vascular (BV) and lymphatic (L) is shown in this scanning electron micrograph. ×39. An enlargement of the lymphatic vessel which contains valves within its lumen. ×360.

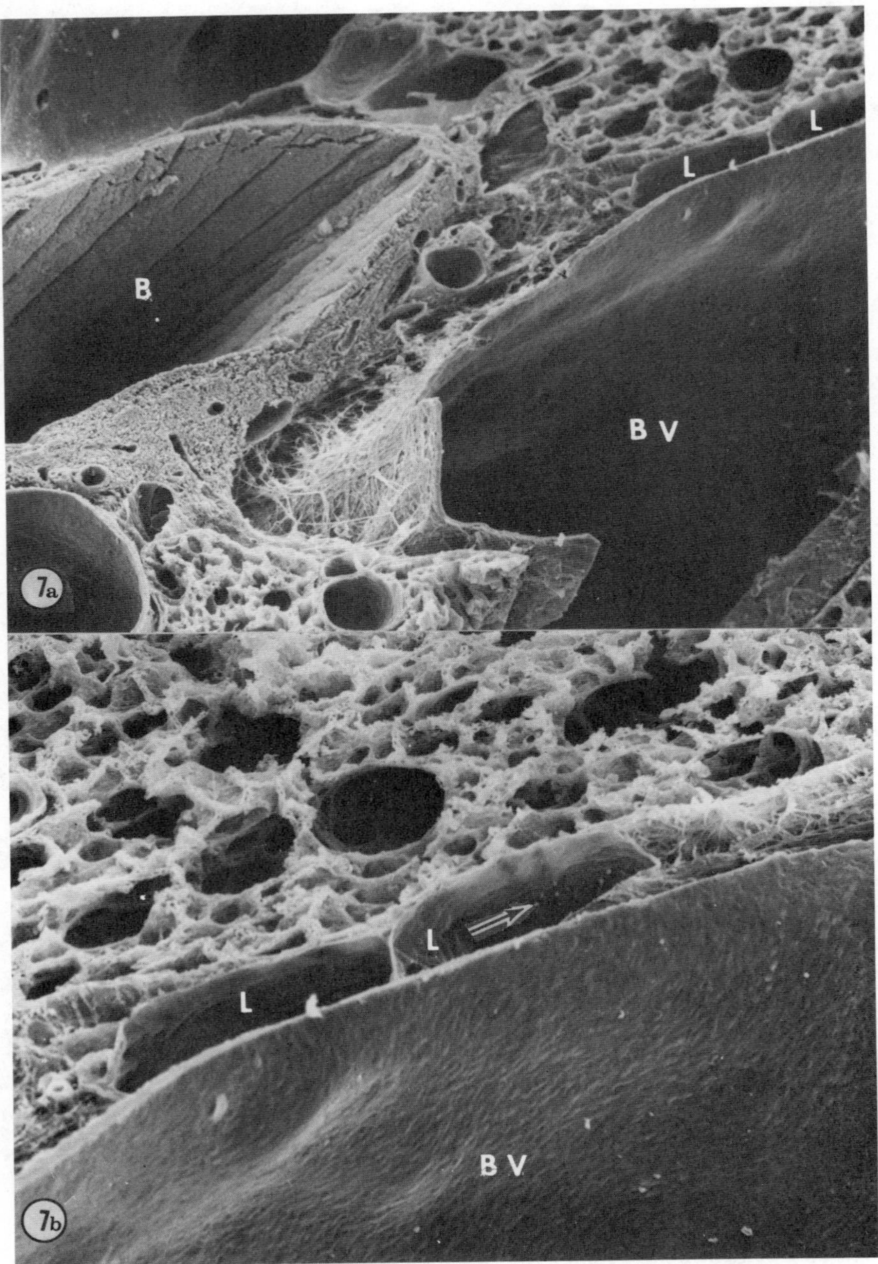

FIGURE 7 Scanning electron micrographs which show branching lymphatics (L) in the periarterial connective tissue sheath. (b) An enlargement which illustrates cells (arrows) within the lymphatic lumen in (a). (a) ×100; (b) ×170.

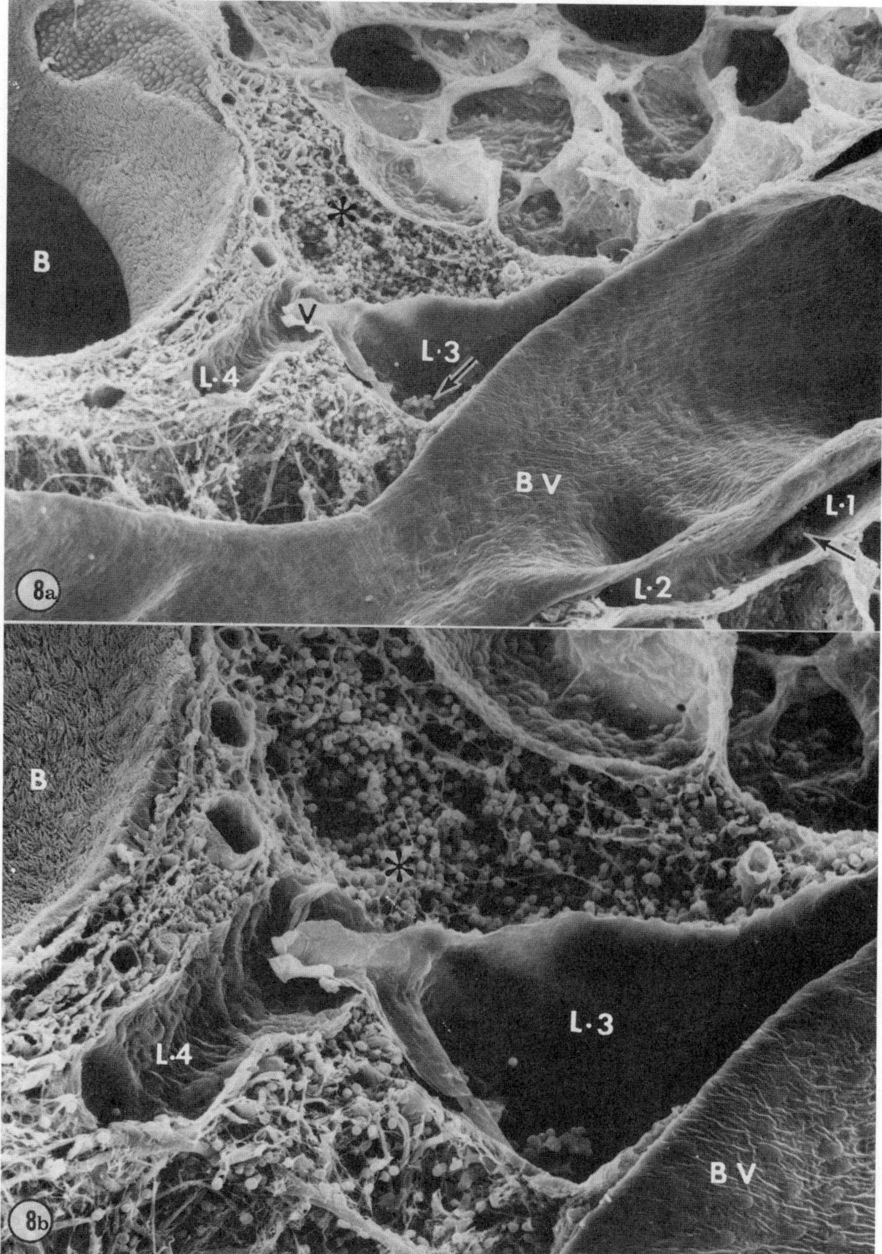

FIGURE 8 The branching of peribronchial and periarterial vessels is demonstrated in the scanning electron micrographs. In (a) parts of lymphatic vessels are seen at L1 and L2 which contain a clump of cells (arrow). L3 also contains a clump of cells (arrow) and forms an anastomosis with L4 by way of a valve (V). Lymphoid tissue (*), similar to that observed in scanning images of lymph nodes surround the lymphatic vessels. Bronchial (B) and blood vessel (BV) are as marked. (a) ×250; (b) ×500.

Embryologically, pulmonary lymphatics enter the hilar region (second month of fetal life) as large vessels. As development continues, they ramify to produce plexiform channels which extend peripherally along bronchi, pulmonary arteries, veins, and the pleura within the connective tissue areas [47,55]. However, from a functional standpoint, uptake into this one-way drainage system commences with the blind end saccules or tubes located at the site of extracellular exchange within the interstitium. Connective tissue fluids and proteins are readily transported across the walls of these lymphatic vessels. The interstitial fluid removed by these vessels (lymph) is concentrated and then propelled into vessels of increasing diameter. Generally referred to as collecting lymphatics, they contain valves and are interrupted at various intervals along their routes by lymph nodes before communicating with the much larger lymphatic trunks. The pulmonary lymphatics located along the bronchial and vascular tree within the connective tissue septa of the interstitium and within the visceral pleura are able to drain continuously the pulmonary connective tissue areas of excess fluids and particulate matter under normal physiological conditions. Therefore, the unidirectional flow process begins at the interstitial lymph interface with uptake by smaller and more permeable vessels, the lymphatic capillaries. As in other regions of the body, the structural arrangement and drainage sequence (i.e., capillary collecting vessels) are also maintained for the pulmonary lymphatic vessels.

A. Ultrastructural Organization of Pulmonary Lymphatic Capillaries

When the techniques of electron microscopy were first applied to the lymphatics [57,64], the fine structure of these vessels was described as being similar to that of lymphatics in other regions of the body. To gain more precise information, we have utilized improved techniques of tissue preservation. By simultaneously applying intravascular and intratracheal perfusion fixation, the lung tissue is allowed to harden in situ, therefore, maintaining the lymphatics in their distended state while preserving their relationship to other structural components of the pulmonary interstitium. With this method, tissue preservation is generally excellent throughout. The blood vessels are cleared of blood cell and plasma content, but the plasma protein within the lymphatic vessels is retained and appears as a dense precipitate. This procedure provides a means by which pulmonary lymphatics can be recognized in routine thick epon sections (light microscopy) as well as ultrathin sections (electron microscopy). Therefore, the precise organization and ultrastructure of lymphatics in the pleura, interlobular septum, peribronchial, and perivascular regions can be routinely observed and identified with some degree of certainty.

Light-microscopic observations of thick epon sections of perfused lung tissue reveal many aspects of pulmonary lymphatics that usually escape detection in routine paraffin sections. The topographical relationship between the lymphatic vessels and the surrounding connective tissue is maintained, providing a more reliable picture of the structural relationship between components of pulmonary tissue. Traditionally, histologists have identified lymphatics by (a) their variable or irregular caliber, (b) a large lumen relative to the thickness in the endothelial wall, (c) an extremely thin endothelial lining which lacks pericytes or a recognizable adventitia as is characterized in cross sectional outlines of blood capillaries, and (d) the lack of blood cells in the lumen. In sections fixed by vascular perfusion, the presence of a uniform gray precipitate within the lymphatic lumen provides an additional criterion because the small blood vessels have been cleared or washed free of blood cells and blood plasma proteins. Therefore, the luminal content within lymphatics remains while blood vessels appear entirely empty (Figs. 3a, 5b).

1. Endothelium

The electron microscope has made it possible to identify additional ultrastructural features which serve as specific criteria for differentiating the lymphatics from blood capillaries [38,70,71]. The lymphatic capillary is lined by a continuous endothelium which is extremely attenuated over major aspects of its diameter (except in the perinuclear region). The basement lamina is lacking, the endothelial cell junctions are often extensively overlapping, and the apposing plasma membranes are loosely adherent with only occasional plasma membrane specializations for attachment. A close topographical relationship is maintained with the adjoining interstitium by way of anchoring filaments which are closely applied to the outer leaflet of the plasmalemma. Cellular projections extend into the connective tissue in close association with anchoring filaments and provide irregular contours along the endothelial surface.

Notwithstanding the extreme attenuations achieved over greater distances of the cytoplasmic area, the pulmonary lymphatic capillary conforms to the lymphatics in other tissues in that it is lined by a continuous endothelium (Fig. 9), the tunica intima.

A continuous basement lamina is lacking, and there are no smooth muscle cells or pericytes that are regularly interposed between the endothelium and the adjacent interstitium. There are, however, numerous anchoring filaments, closely associated elastic fibers and collagen fibrils in intimate contact with the endothelial surface (Figs. 10, 12a,b). The endothelial cytoplasm is very thin over large areas of its circumference, measuring 700-1000 Å in thickness, except where the cytoplasm is thickened to accommodate an elongated nucleus protruding into the vessel lumen (Figs. 9, 11).

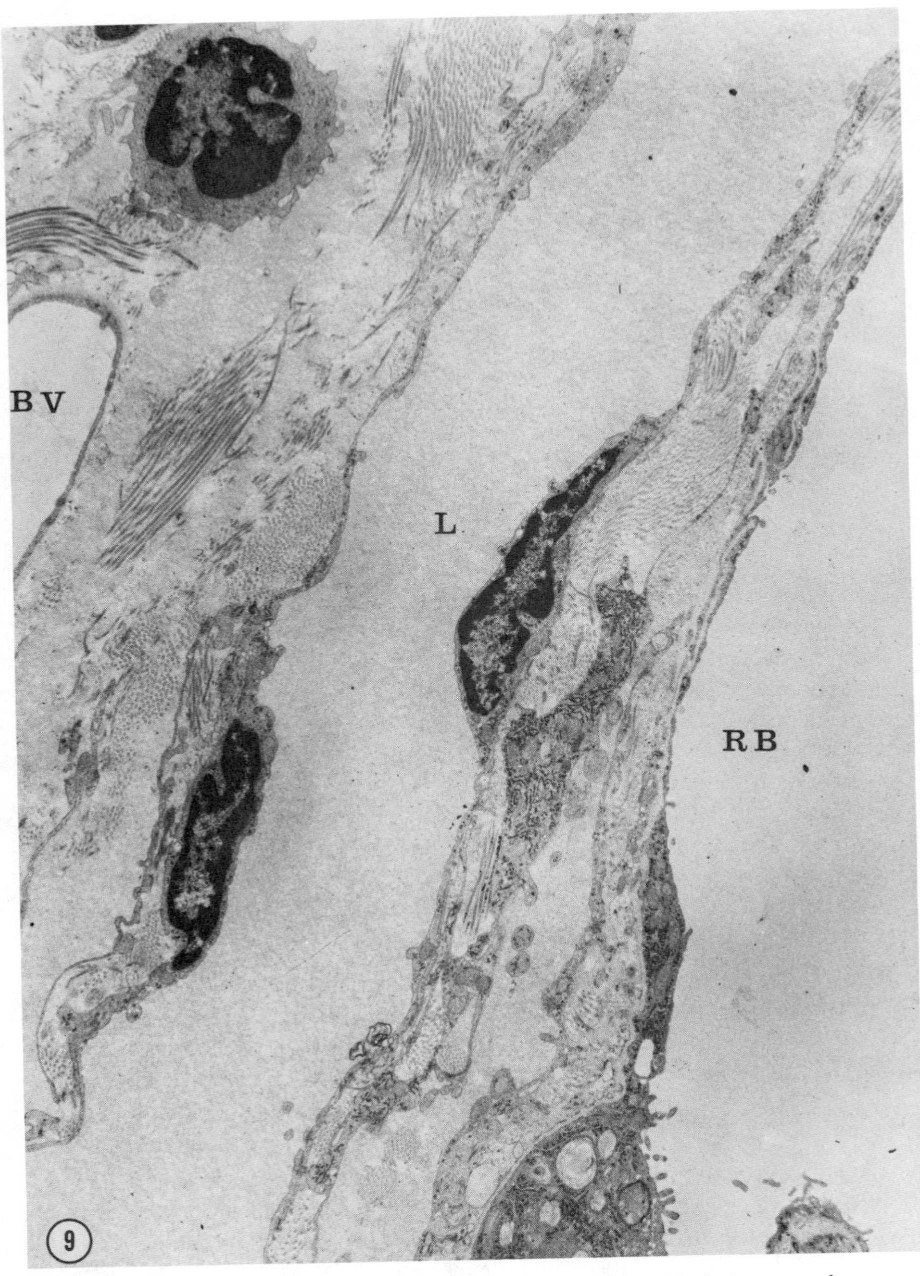

FIGURE 9 A low power micrograph showing the relationship between pulmonary lymphatic (L) and a respiratory bronchiole (RB). A grey flocculant precipitate fills the lymphatic lumen. The lymphatic capillary is lined by a continuous endothelium which is extremely attenuated except in the perinuclear regions. Part of blood vessel (BV) is shown at left of micrograph. ×8000.

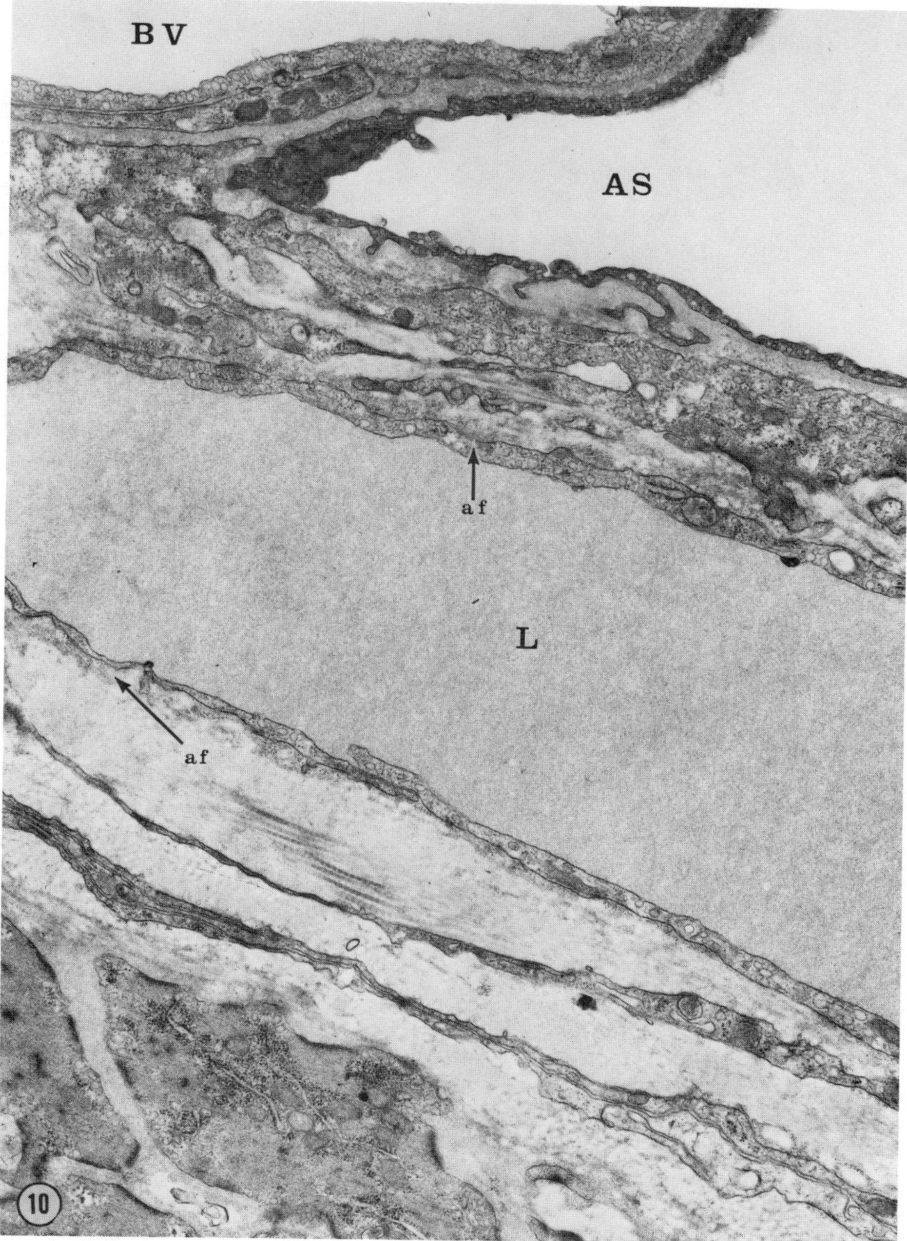

FIGURE 10 Numerous anchoring filaments (af) which are intimately associated with elastic and collagen fibrils extend from the lymphatic (L) wall into the surrounding interstitium. ×20,000.

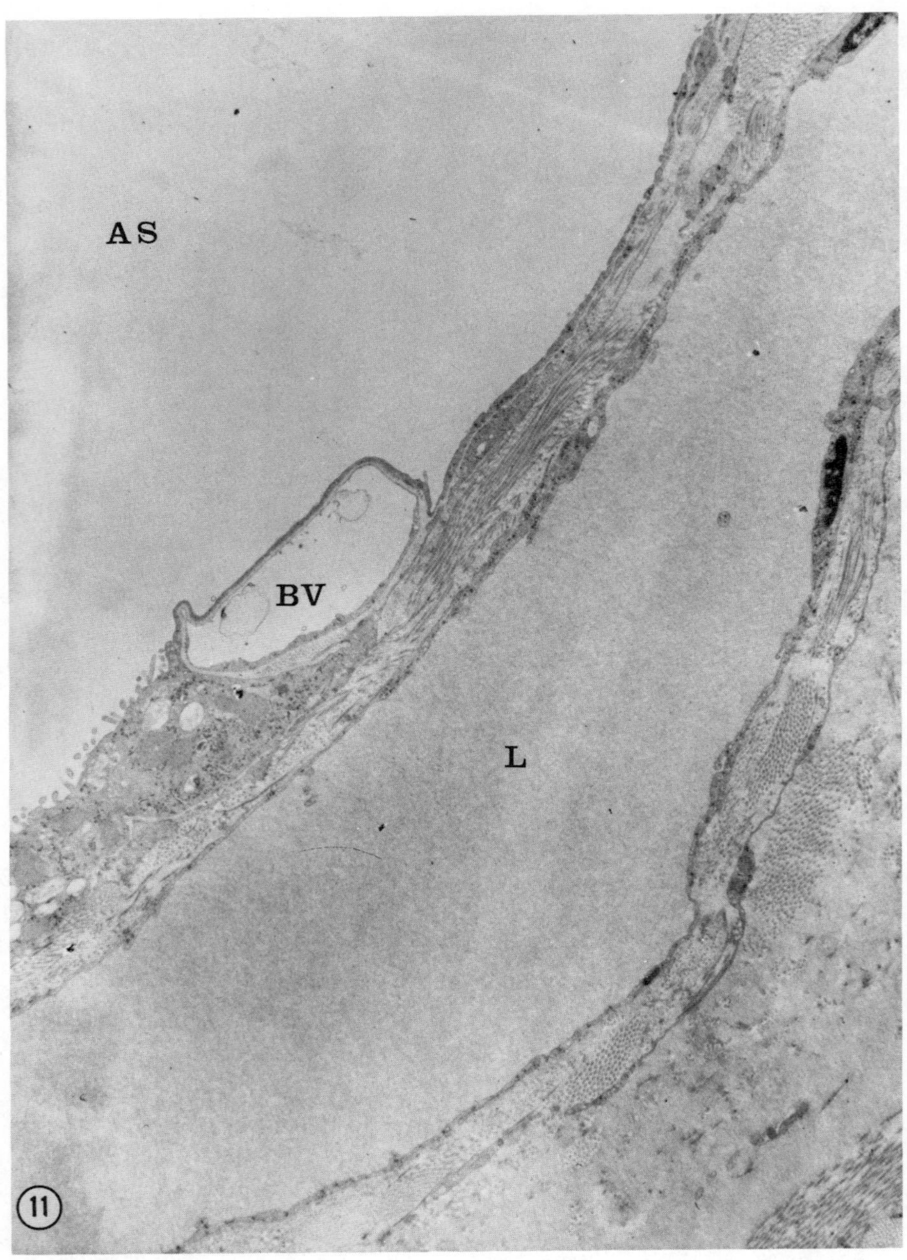

FIGURE 11 Survey electron micrograph which illustrates a lymphatic capillary (L) in juxtaposition to the alveolar space (AS). The blood vessel (BV) is free of its plasma while the lymphatic (L) lumen is filled with a grey precipitate. ×7000.

2. *Cytoplasmic Organelles*

The perinuclear cysterna which surrounds the nucleus is punctated with nuclear pores. The nucleoplasm consists of dense chromatic formations at the periphery, while a network of fine filamentous strands occupy the central region of the nucleus. The nucleolus is observed in the center of the nucleus, or it may be eccentrically located (Fig. 13b).

The extreme attenuations achieved by the cytoplasm over most of the capillary wall is also maintained as a thin rim of cytoplasm between the nucleus and the plasma membrane of both the connective tissue and luminal fronts (Fig. 9). However, much thicker regions of cytoplasm occur in the perinuclear region in which may also be found the cytocentrum which includes a pair of centrioles and a Golgi complex (Fig. 13a,b). Two centrioles are located in the central portion of the Golgi apparatus, one of which is oriented perpendicular to the other. This arrangement is similar to that in collecting lymphatic endothelial cells in the rabbit lung [63], dermal lymphatic capillaries [65,67,68], and a variety of other tissues in various organisms [31].

The Golgi complex consists of crescent-shaped cisterna with closely associated vesicles. Complex multivesicular bodies of various sizes also occur in or around the perinuclear region (Figs. 12b, 13a,b). Some of the vesicles contain an electron dense substance, while others contain dense membranous components. Acid phosphatase has been demonstrated in vesicles and vacuoles near the Golgi complex in dermal lymphatic endothelial cells. The positive reaction for acid phosphatase in a number of vesicles suggests that primary lysosomes are produced in the vicinity of the Golgi complex in collaboration with components of the endoplasmic reticulum [2,21,40,90,91].

The endothelial cells of the pulmonary lymphatic capillary are distinguished by their paucity of either smooth or rough endoplasmic reticulum (Fig. 13a,b). The few randomly dispersed cisterna with attached ribosomes are located mainly within the perinuclear area and occasionally within the thin rim of the cytoplasm. Not all ribosomes are associated with membranes and many are free throughout the cytoplasm as clusters of polyribosomes (Fig. 12b). Since an abundance of endoplasmic reticulum of the rough variety is characteristic of cells in a high rate of protein synthesis for extracellular discharge [9,54,93], the lack of an extensive endoplasmic reticulum within the cytoplasm of the lymphatic endothelial cells seems to indicate that the cells are engaged in only a moderate production of synthetic activity for their own internal use.

Mitochondria are found disposed throughout the perinuclear area, and are also randomly distributed in the attenuated rim of cytoplasm (Figs. 13b, 14). They display the usual form and internal configurations exhibited by

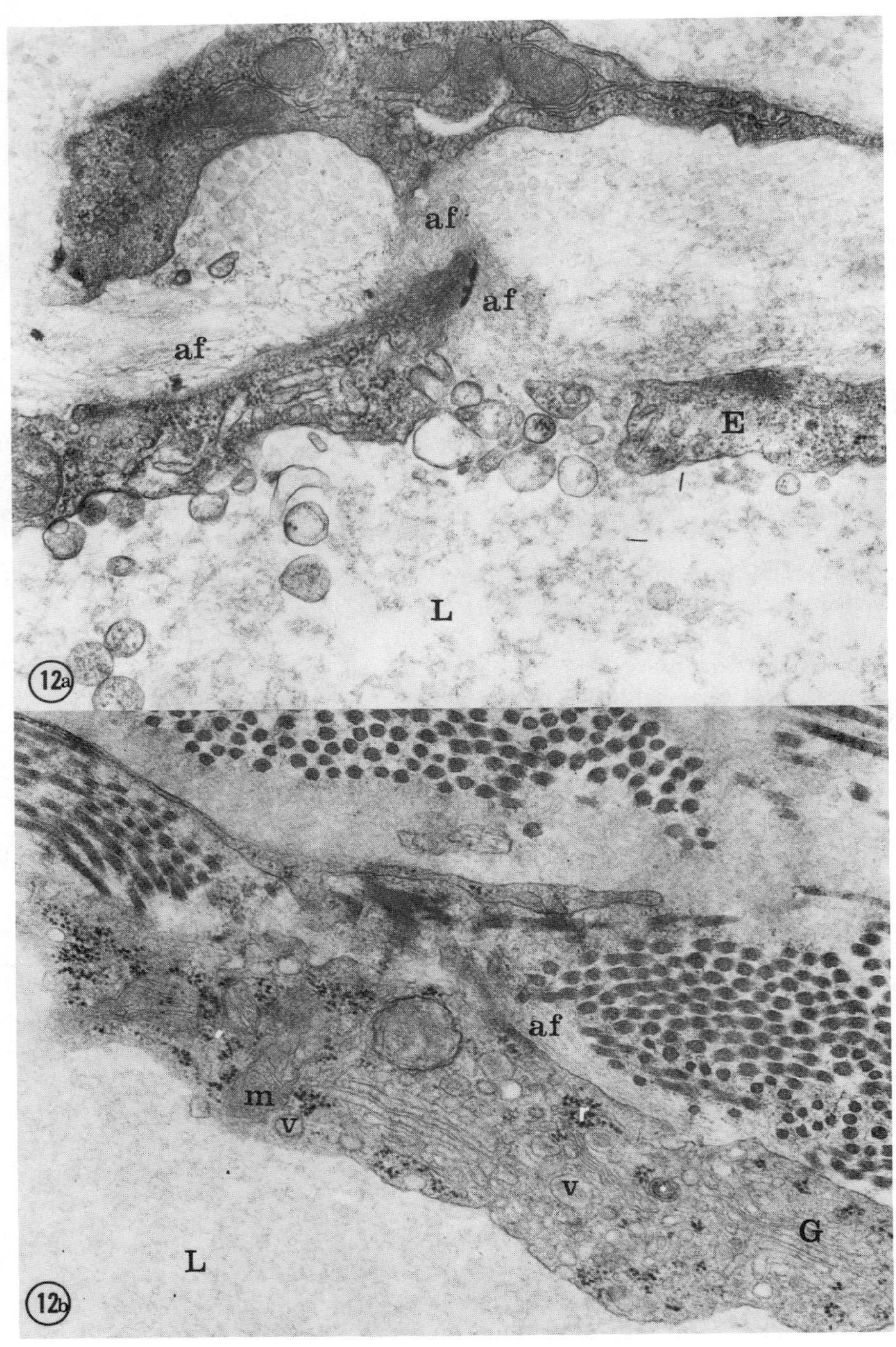
af
af
af
E
L
12a
af
m
v
v
G
L
12b

mitochondria of other cell types, i.e., numerous cristae are formed by enfoldings of the inner membrane (Fig. 14). Microtubules are found in the vicinity of centrioles and in relatively small numbers throughout the cytoplasm. Their form, size, and distribution resemble that observed in the endothelial cells of dermal lymphatic capillaries.

3. Cytoplasmic Filaments

Microfilaments measuring ~60 Å diam are routinely observed within the endothelial cells of pulmonary lymphatic capillaries (Fig. 15). Often they appear in the peripheral cytoplasm subjacent to the plasma membrane, aggregated into small bundles or dispersed throughout the cytoplasm. Although not as numerous as the cytoplasmic filaments seen in dermal capillaries [65,67,68], they are sufficiently organized and distributed throughout the pulmonary lymphatic endothelium to warrant attention as a possible mechanism responsible for the intrinsic contraction of the lymphatic capillary wall [62,72]. Recently much attention has been focused on cytoplasmic filaments in an extremely wide variety of cell types [7,30,45,46,52,96,100,101,121,127]. Majno and Leventhal [76,77] reported in the presence of cytoplasmic filaments in endothelial cells of blood capillaries and suggested a contractile function for these filaments. Biochemical and morphological evidence supports the presence of actin in a wide range of nonmuscle cells [5,53,87,88,97,123]. The regulation of blood flow through capillaries and sinusoids in the liver is believed to be controlled by contractile filaments within the endothelial cells which respond to vasoactive substances [80]. On the basis of rhythmic contraction of dermal lymphatic capillaries observed by cinephotographic methods, a similar contractile function can also be attributed to the numerous cytoplasmic filaments observed in the dermal lymphatic endothelial cells [69]. It is further presumed that a similar condition also exists for the endothelium of the pulmonary lymphatic capillary.

4. Plasmalemmal Vesicles

The endothelial plasma membrane contains numerous specializations along both luminal and connective tissue fronts which range from slight depressions

---

FIGURE 12 (a) Anchoring filaments (af) extend from the lymphatic endothelium (E) into the surrounding interstitium. ×39,000. (b) Anchoring filaments (af), portion of Golgi complex (G) with vesicles (v) of various densities are shown in this electron micrograph. Several of the vesicles (v) contain an electron dense substance (*). Clusters of ribosomes (r) as well as mitochondria (m) are also seen. ×41,000.

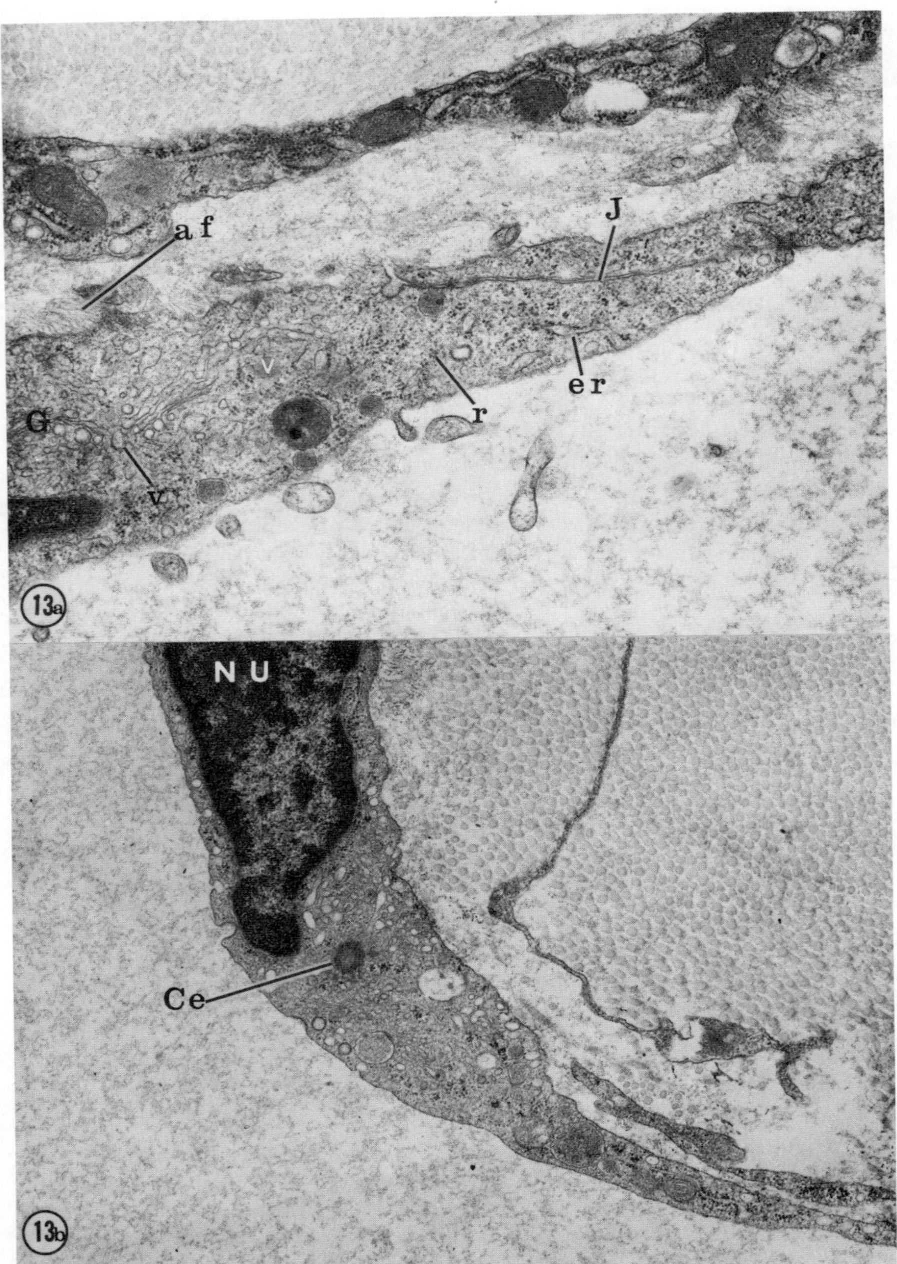

FIGURE 13 These electron micrographs (a and b) depict the perinuclear portion of lymphatic vessels which contain the Golgi (G) and associated vesicles (v) several of which contain an electron dense substance. Part of a nucleolus (NU) and centriole (Ce) are shown in (b). Intercellular junction (J) and anchoring filaments (af) are as marked. Scant cisternae of endoplasmic reticulum (er) as well as free ribosomes (r), are also shown. (a) ×35,000; (b) ×21,000.

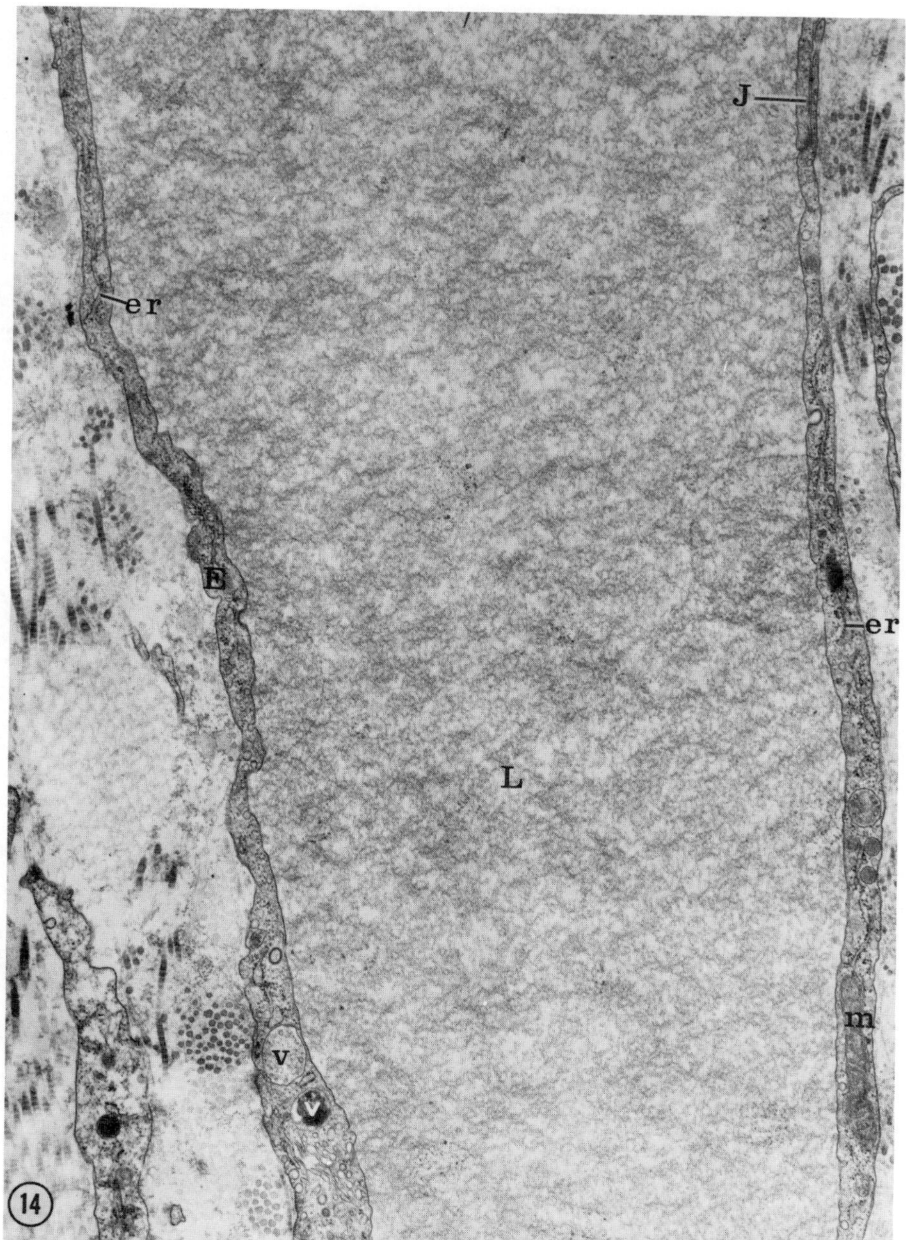

FIGURE 14 Portion of pulmonary lymphatic capillary showing attenuated endothelial cells containing mitochondria (m) endoplasmic reticulum (er) vesicles (v) of varying sizes and content and intercellular junction (J). The lumen (L) contains an electron dense precipitate. ×18,000.

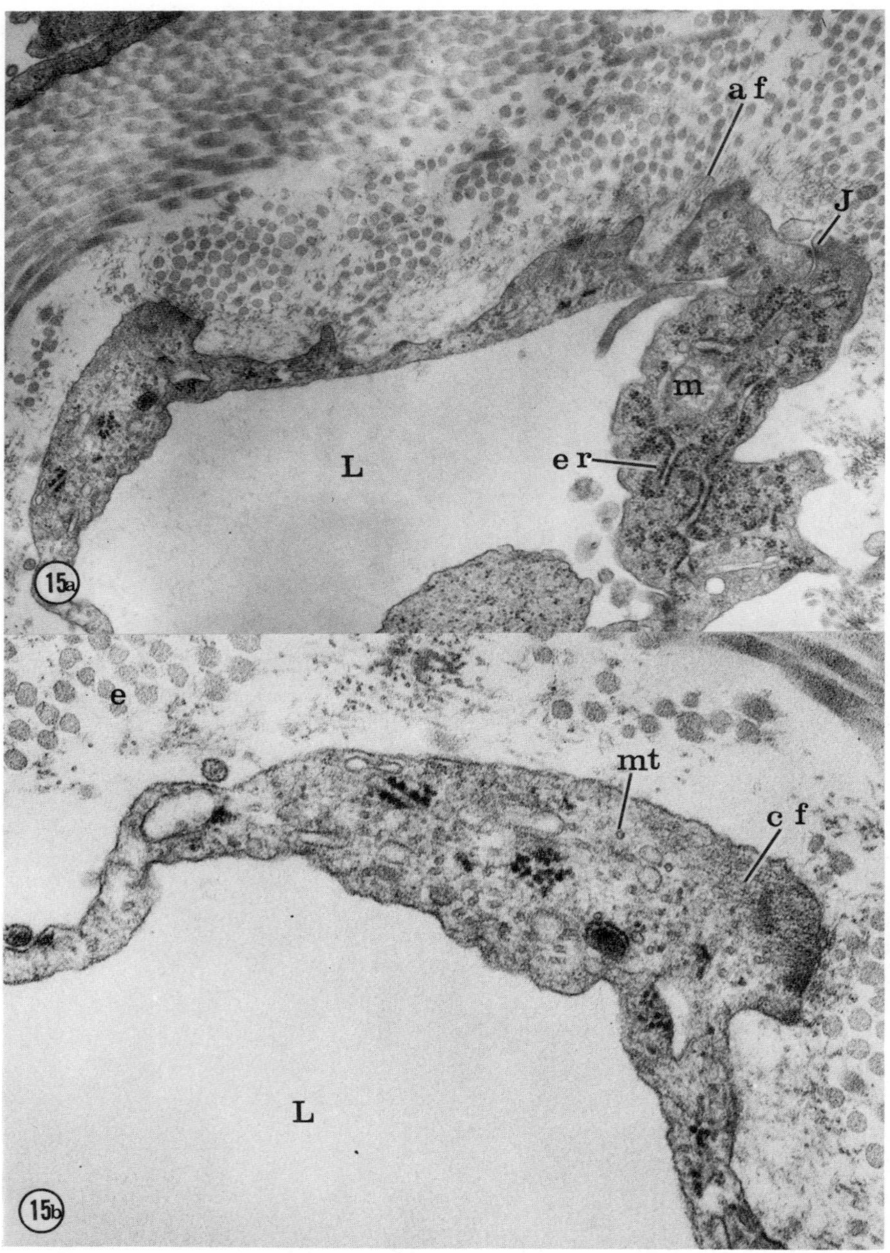

FIGURE 15 Electron micrograph of a portion of lymphatic capillary (L) showing anchoring filaments (af). Cytoplasmic filaments (cf) microtubules (mt) in cross and longitudinal arrangements, mitochondria (m) and endoplasmic reticulum (er) an intercellular junction (J) appears at right of micrograph. (b) shows enlargement of part of (a) which contains cytoplasmic filaments and microtubules. (a) ×30,000; (b) ×63,000.

within the surface of the plasmalemma to vesicles which measure ~750 Å in diameter (Fig. 16a). They occupy positions within the peripheral and midcytoplasmic regions of the endothelial cells. In many regions of the cytoplasm, they are aligned in a chainlike fashion seemingly to form continuous channels (transendothelial channels) throughout the thickness of the endothelium (Fig. 16a,b). Such structures also occur in the thinner regions of the endothelial wall. Studies with lanthanum tracer show that many of the vesicles which appear to lie free in the cytoplasm are in fact open to either the connective tissue or the luminal front since the tracer is located within their lumina. Yet many vesicles lack the tracer and presumably represent those which are completely surrounded by cytoplasm. Much larger vesicles with oval to irregular profiles are also observed in the cytoplasm; these usually contain an electron-dense substance (Fig. 16a).

The role of plasmalemmal vesicles (micropinocytotic vesicles) in the transport of substances across the endothelial cells was proposed earlier by Palade [92]. He described these vesicles in endothelial cells of the blood capillaries and suggested that materials passed from one side of the cell to the other within such structures. Bennett [6] advanced the hypothesis that membrane flow and vesiculation may be important transport mechanisms in carrying particles, molecules, and ions within, into, and out of the cell by way of vesicles. Since these studies, a number of investigators have provided both morphological and experimental evidence which suggest that extracellular materials may in fact be internalized by endothelial cells, as well as a variety of cell types after the formation of inpocketing of the plasma membrane to form vesicles [1,15,32,56,102,112, 114]. Similar observations have also been reported for the lymphatic endothelial cells [10,65,69,71].

5. *Intercellular Junctions*

The pulmonary lymphatic capillary is distinguished by the presence of numerous, extensively overlapping, intercellular junctions which may lack specialization for attachment (Figs. 17a,b, 18a). The intercellular clefts of these junctions are also variable in width. There are focal areas of close approximation (100-250 Å), while widths of 0.5-1 μm may extend for varying lengths of the cleft, presumably to provide an unrestricted passageway (patent junction) to the surrounding interstitium (Figs. 17a, 18b). High magnification of closely apposed areas demonstrate the presence of macula adhaerens (Fig. 18a). Occasionally areas of close apposition are observed in which the intercellular clefts appear to be obliterated by macula occludens. The occurrence of punctate specialization for attachment provides a "spot weld" effect which maintains a close continuity between endothelial cells, along the total length of the vessel, while at the same time permitting specific sites along the intercellular cleft to become easily widened by a separation of apposing endothelial cells. Therefore, patent channels become

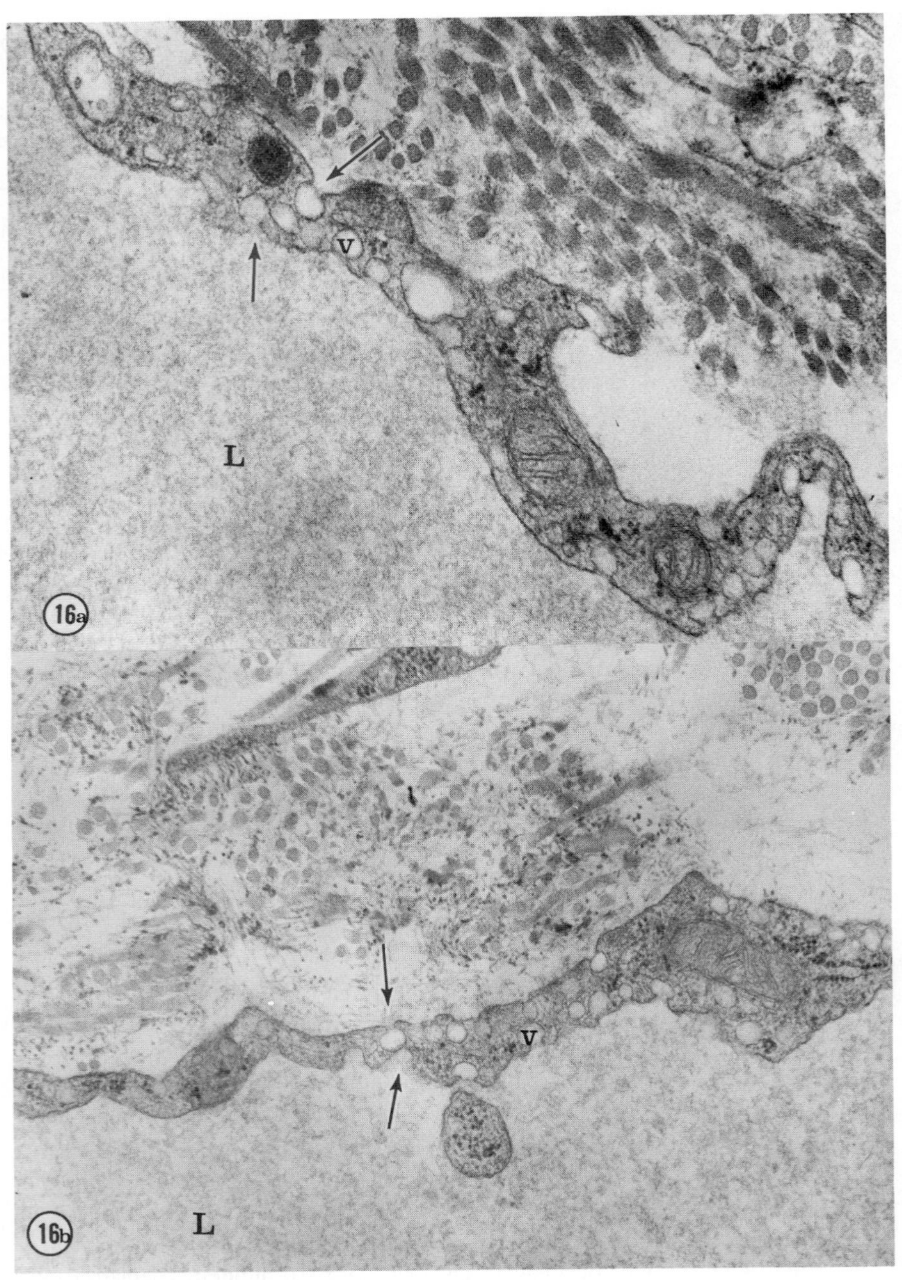

FIGURE 16 The arrangement of plasmalemmal vessels (v) is demonstrated in these electron micrographs. In some areas several vessels are aligned to form transendothelial chains (arrow). (a) ×56,000; (b) ×40,000.

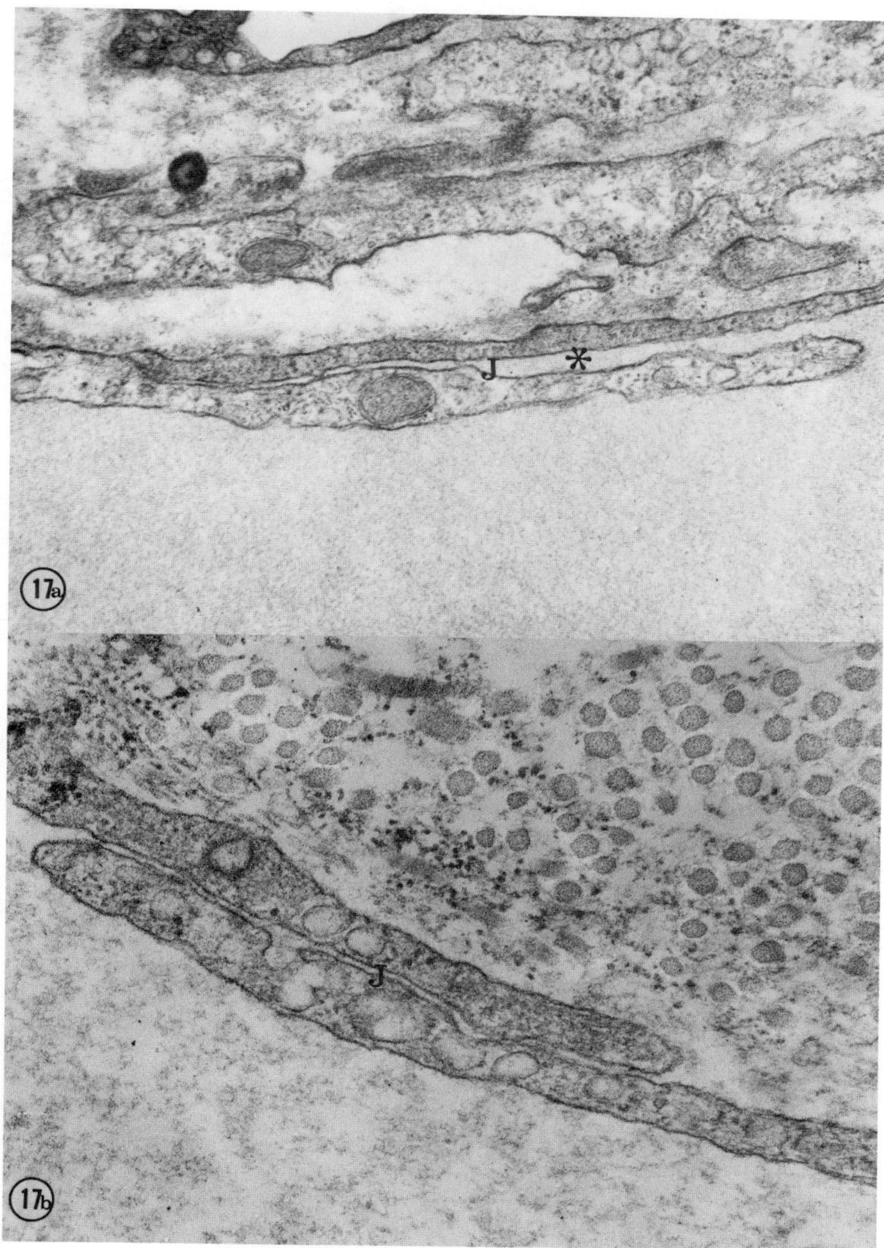

FIGURE 17 Adjacent cells are extensively overlapping to form intercellular junctions (J) with variable distances along the intercellular cleft (*). (a) ×56,000; (b) ×73,000.

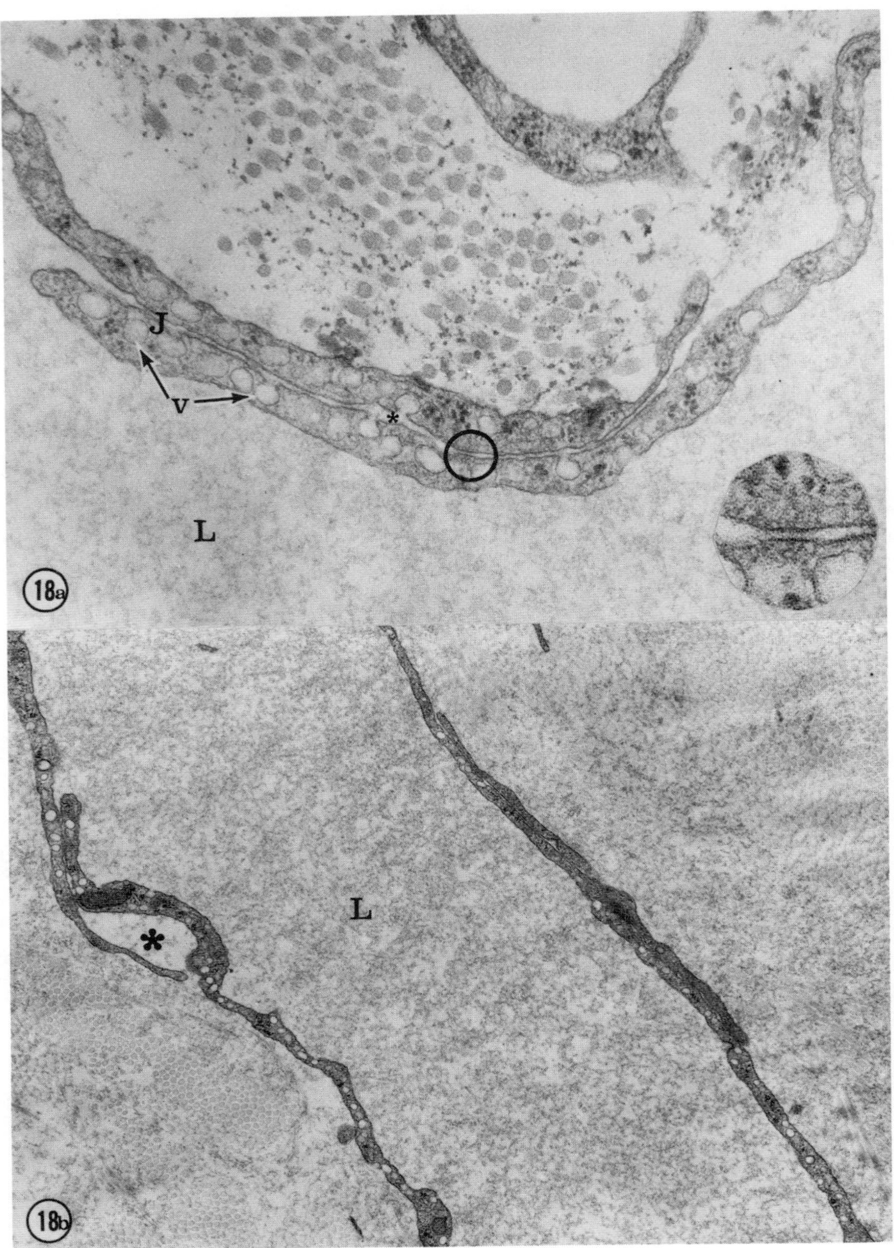

FIGURE 18 Numerous vesicles (v) appear in portions of endothelial cell which overlap (J). Segments of the intercellular cleft (*) in 18b are very wide and contain a dense precipitate similar to that in the lumen (L). Inset in (a) shows enlargement of macula adherens. (a) ×49,000, Inset ×125,000; (b) ×16,000.

readily available to accommodate the rapid passage of excess interstitial fluids and plasma proteins as well as cells into the lymphatic lumen. Some of the terminal cell margins interdigitate so that adjacent cells are closely imbricated with each other, while at other areas, adjacent cells simply abut to form intercellular junctions. Similar junctions were observed in the pulmonary lymphatic capillaries of rabbit and in human infants by Lauweryns and Boussaw [64], as well as the lymphatics in the dermis [8,66].

B. Pulmonary Collecting Lymphatic Vessels

The diameter of the collecting lymphatic vessels varies. The wall is distinguished by the presence of valves and smooth muscle cells (Figs. 19, 20a, 21a,b). The endothelial cells, although attenuated beyond the perinuclear region, form a continuous lining and the opposing cells are held in close apposition by maculae adhaerens. Plasmalemmal vesicles occur along both the connective tissue and luminal fronts of the endothelium. The usual complement of organelles, i.e., mitochondria, Golgi complex, endoplasmic reticulum, are also observed. In addition, microtubules and cytoplasmic filaments are distributed throughout the cytoplasm. The collecting vessels contain valves that are regularly spaced along its length. The periodic constrictions occurring at the base of each valve have the beaded appearance characteristic of the distended vessel (Figs. 1a, 2b). Lymphatic valves consist of leaflets of endothelial cells which originate by a reduplication of the endothelial cells that project into the lumen as folds.

The two layers of endothelial cells are separated by a band of connective tissue containing collagen, elastic fibers, and occasional fibroblasts (Fig. 21a,b). The valvular endothelial cells are also held in close apposition with maculae adhaerens. In common with the valves of veins, the lymphatic valves project into the lumen in the direction of fluid (lymph) flow, which permits a free and rapid movement of lymph toward the larger vessels and lymph trunks. The arrangement of the valves and their unidirectional projection prevents regurgitation.

Lauweryns [61] described the lymphatic valves as "a simple cone or funnel-like formation which is axially or longitudinally suspended in the lymphatic vessel lumen and whose distal or small opening is localized at the deepest point of the funnel." Lauweryns further suggests that this funnel-like architectural arrangement of the valve maintains the one-way flow of lymph and that it would probably be occluded by a flow against the normal direction. Our observations with the scanning electron microscope also reveal a funnel-like arrangement for valves in lymphatic collecting vessels (Fig. 20a,b).

The smooth muscle cells which make up the tunica media of the collecting vessels may vary from single cells which coil around the vessel to several layers of smooth muscle cells (cf. Figs. 19 and 22). The cells are fusiformed cylinders

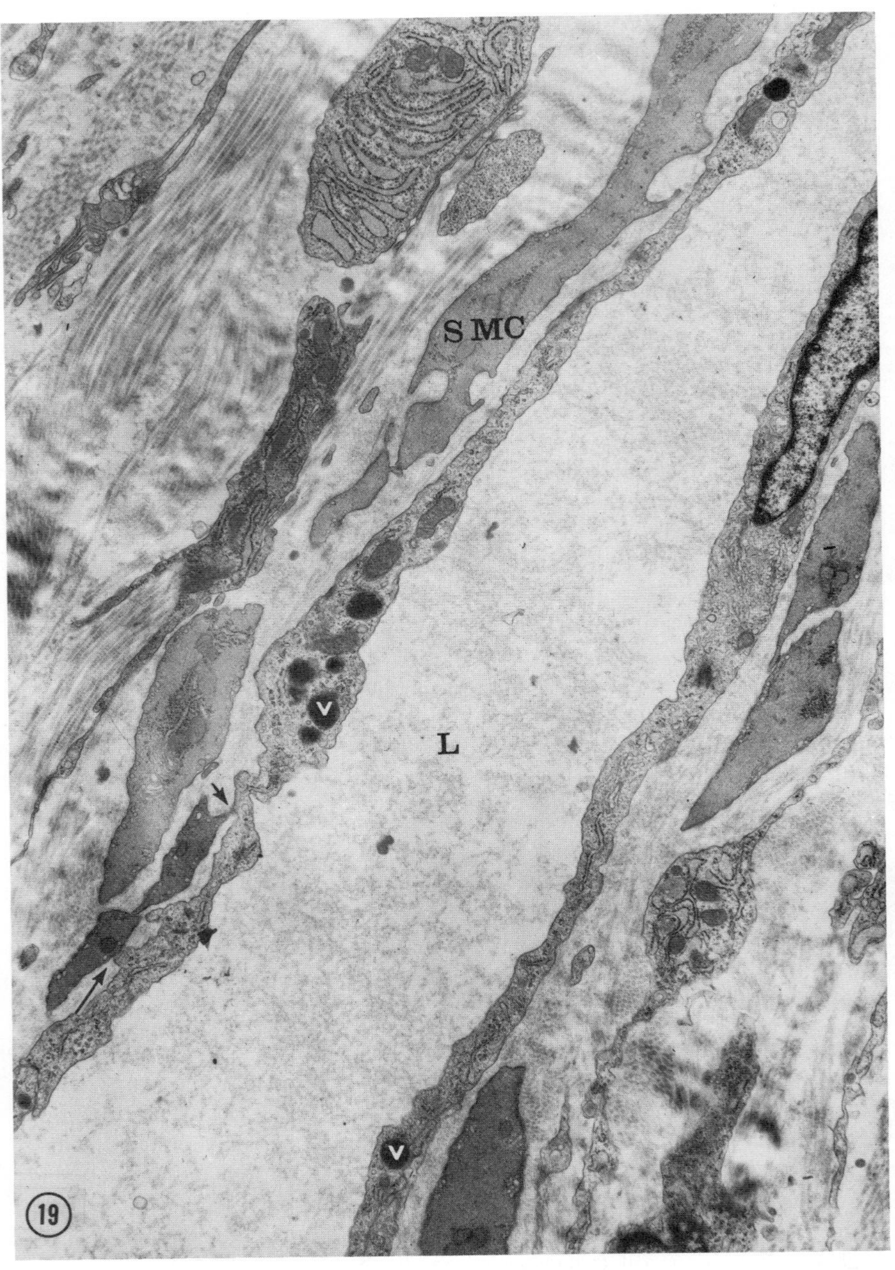

FIGURE 19 Portion of collecting lymphatic with closely associated smooth muscle cells (SMC), some of which make contact with the endothelial cells (arrows). The lumen (L) of collecting vessel also contains a dense precipitate. The endothelial cells contain the usual complement of organelles including large vesicles (v) with an electron dense substance. ×11,000.

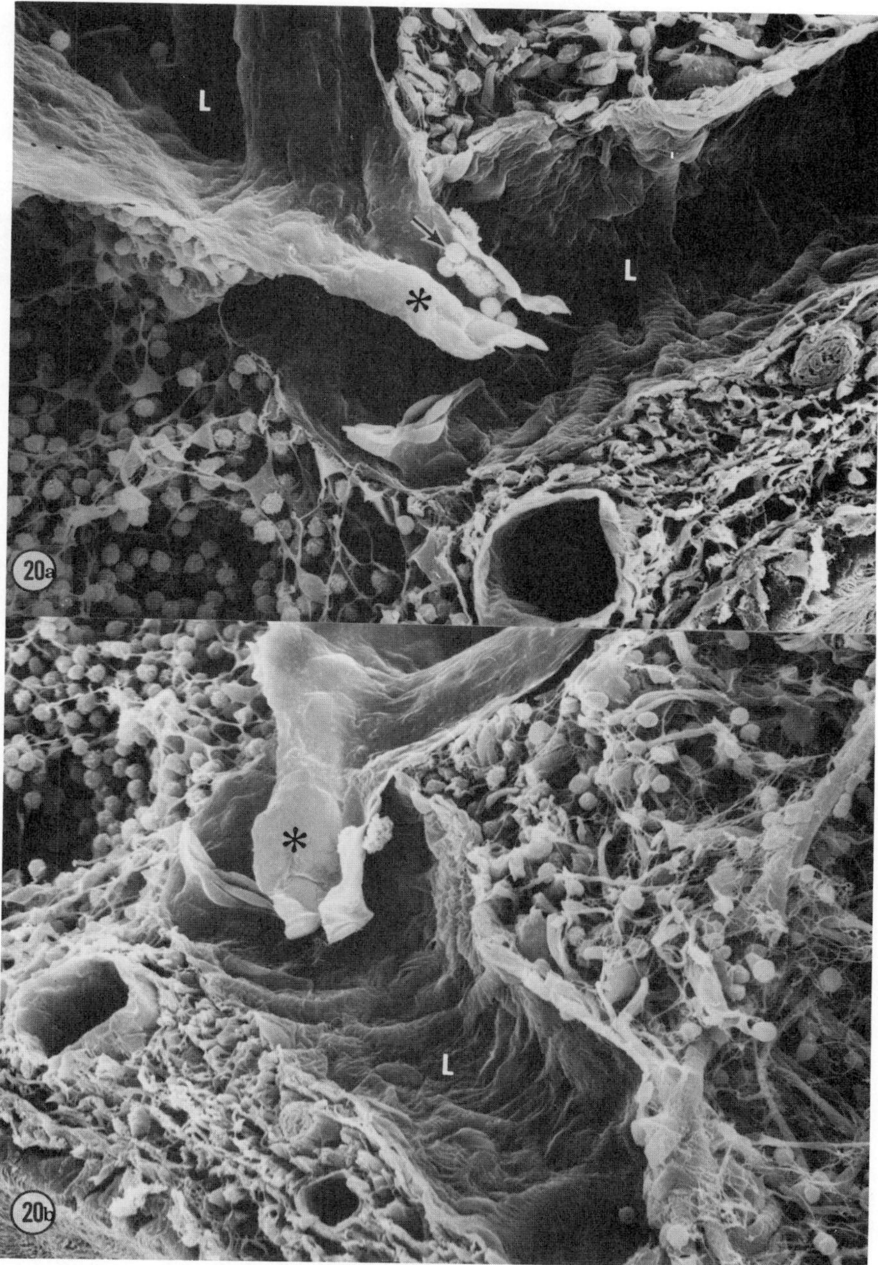

FIGURE 20 Scanning electron micrographs depicting the arrangement of valves (*) in collecting lymphatic vessels (L). Lymphocytes are trapped in the funnel portion of the valve (arrow). In (b) the image has been tilted about 40 degrees to reveal details of the inner aspects of the valve. (a) ×850; (b) ×800.

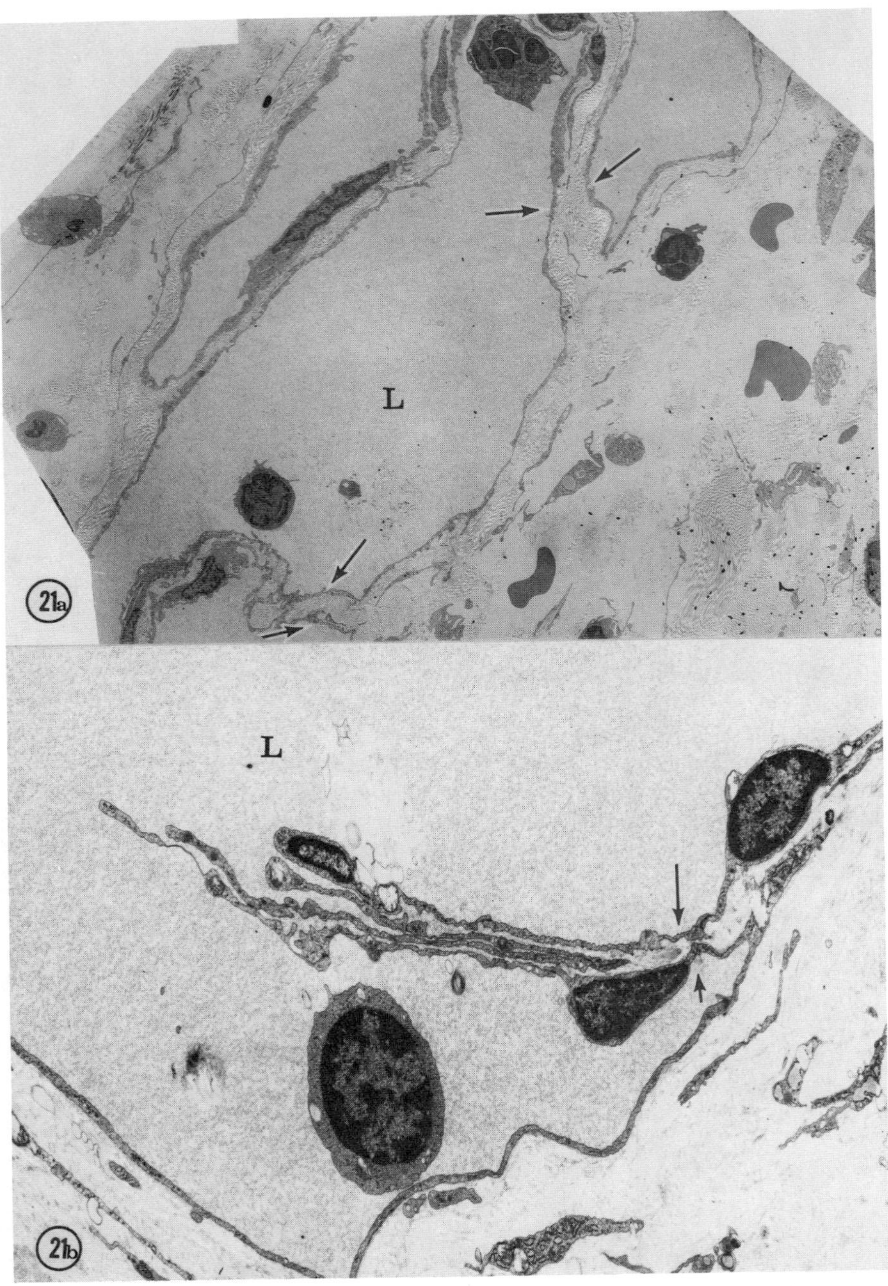

FIGURE 21 Electron micrograph of collecting vessels illustrating the appearance of valves (arrows) which arise as a reduplication of the endothelium which folds into the lymphatic lumen (L). (a) ×3000; (b) ×8000.

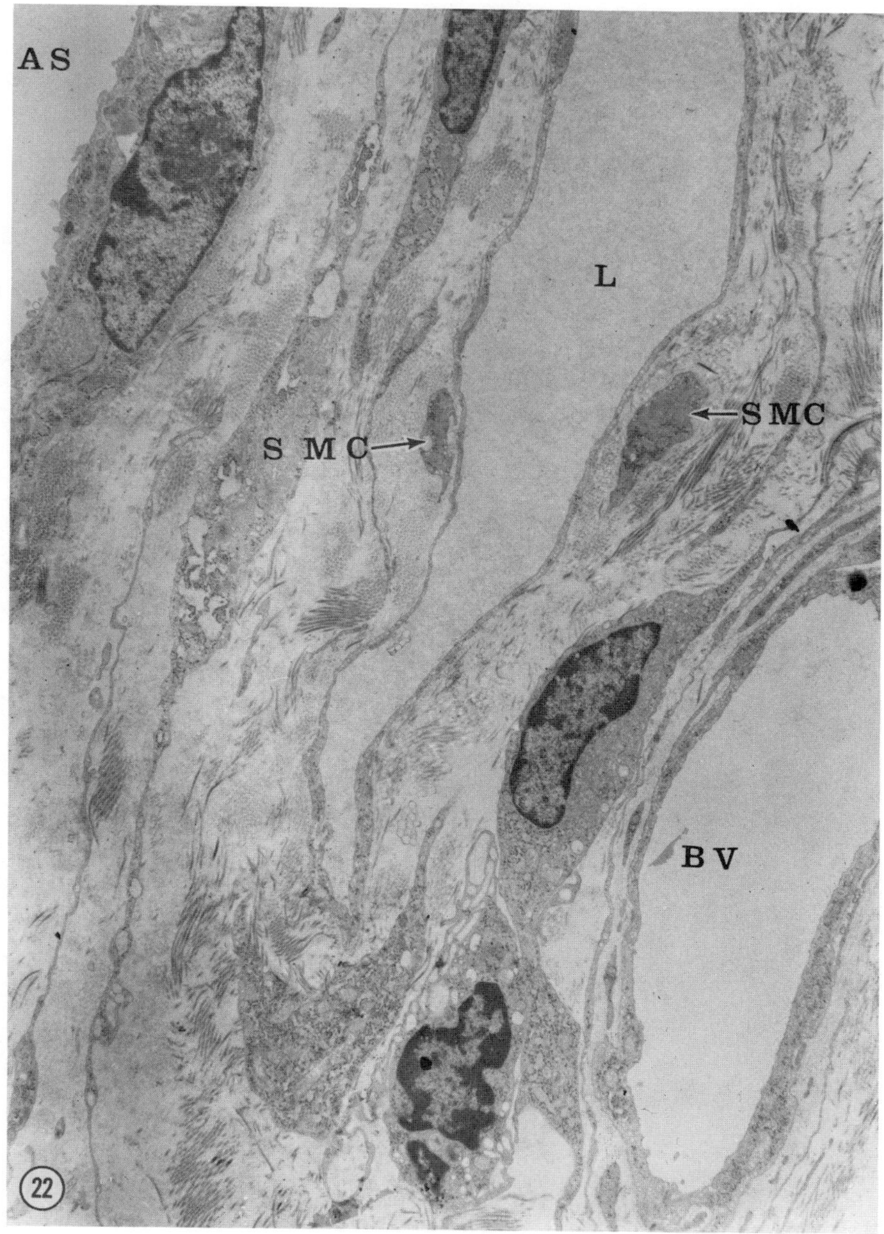

FIGURE 22 The arrangement of an incomplete tunica media where individual smooth muscle cells (SMC) coil along the length of the vessel. Note the relationship of the lymphatic vessel (L) to the adjacent air space (AS) and blood vessel (BV). ×8000.

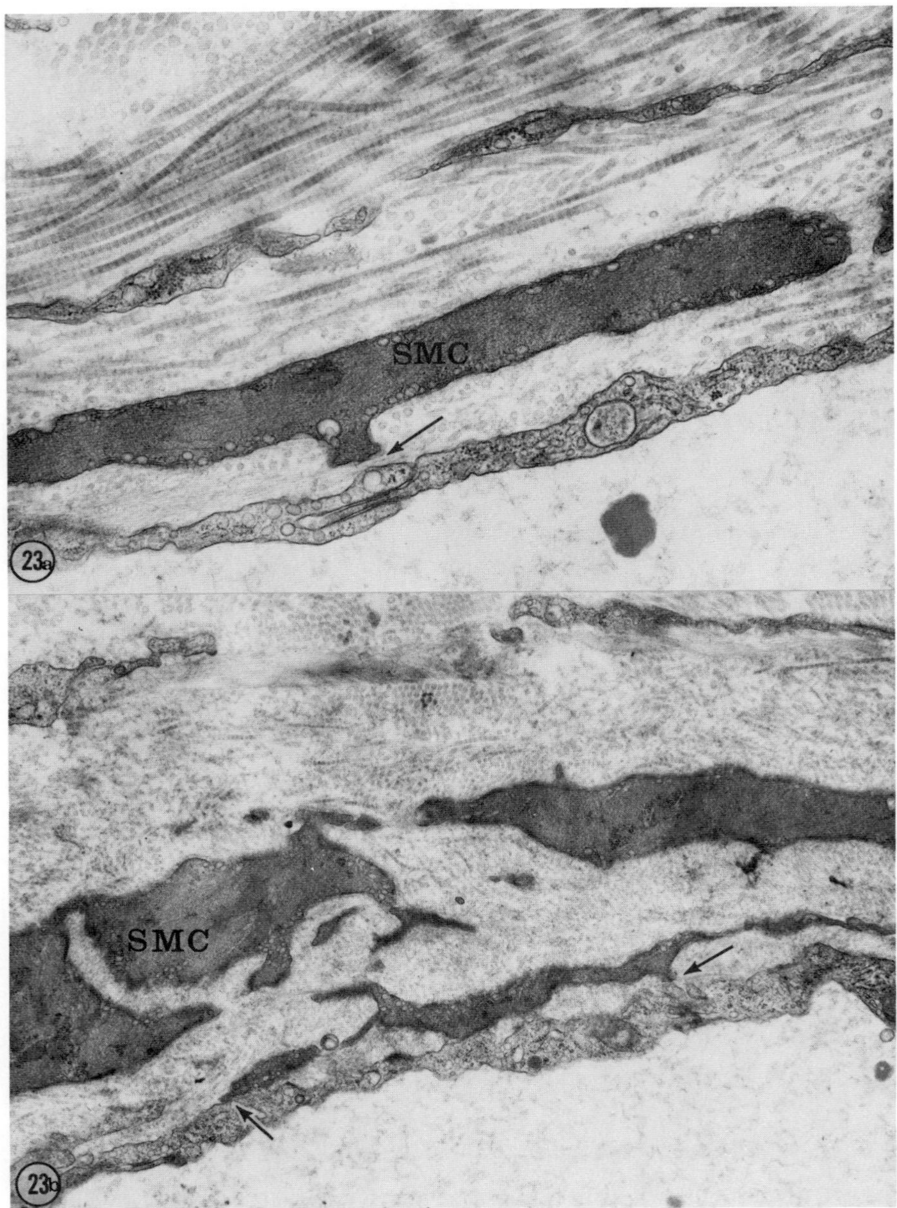

FIGURE 23 The close relationship of the smooth muscle cells (SMC) to the lymphatic endothelium (arrow) is shown in these electron micrographs. (a) ×26,000; (b) ×14,000.

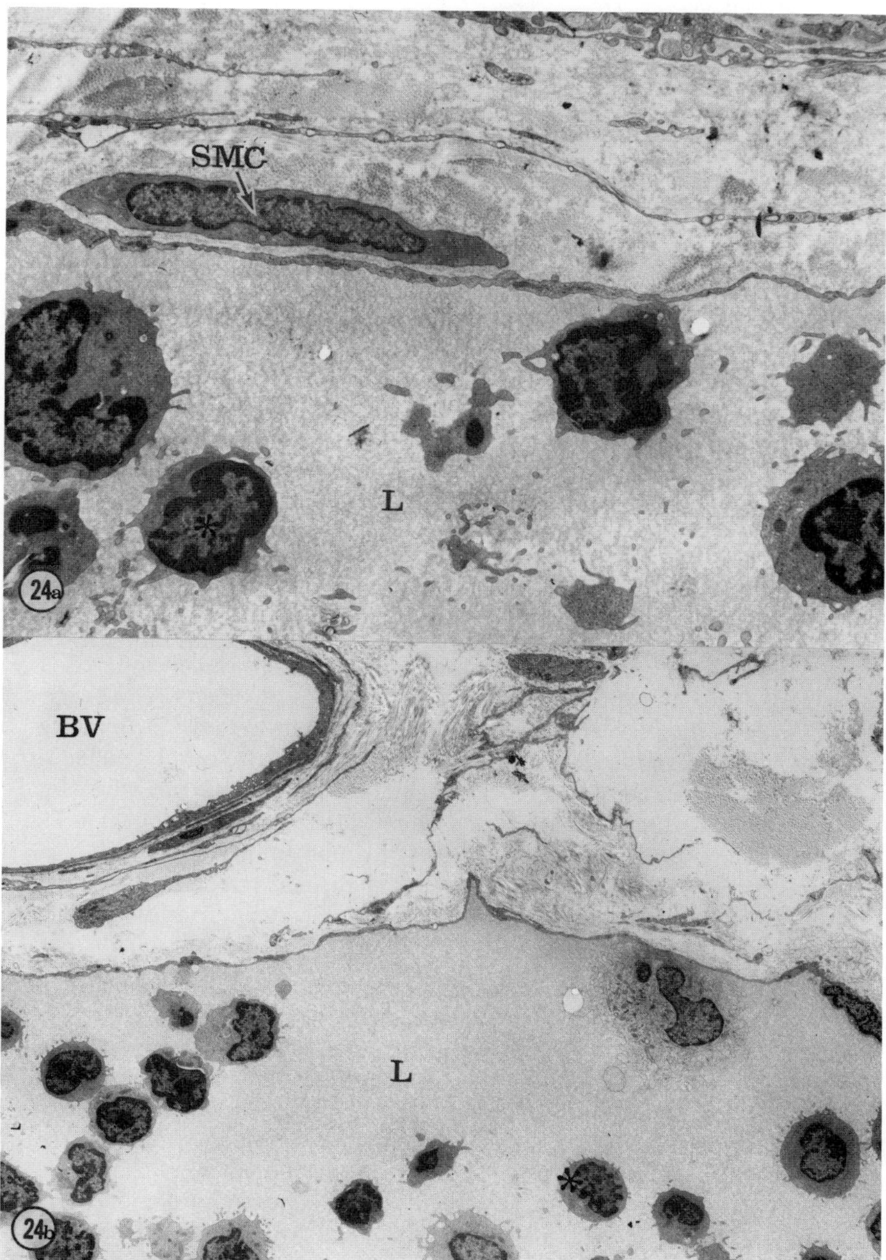

FIGURE 24 Portions of the same lymphatic collecting vessel which contains lymphocytes (*). Part of a smooth muscle cell (SMC) is shown in (a), while (b) represents the opposite side of the same vessel which lacks smooth muscle cells in this portion of its wall. (a) ×5000; (b) ×2000.

with tapering ends. The thickest part of the cell is occupied by an elongated nucleus. Cytoplasmic projections extend from the smooth muscle cell to make contact with the lymphatic wall as suggested in Fig 23a,b. Lymphocytes are often observed within the lumen of collecting vessels (Fig. 24a,b).

V. Interstitial Lymphatic Capillary Interface

Intimate association of the lymphatic capillary wall to the adjacent interstitium is provided by numerous anchoring filaments (Figs. 10, 12a). These filaments appear within a densely staining substance on the external surface of the endothelial cell membrane and extend for varying distances into the surrounding connective tissue between collagen and elastic fibers and connective tissue cells. The anchoring filaments observed around the pulmonary lymphatics are similar in structure and arrangement to those observed in dermal lymphatics [8,67,68,70, 71]. Insertion of the anchoring filaments on the endothelial surface and the extension of the filaments into the surrounding interstitium provides a mechanism for binding the lymphatic wall to the adjoining interstitium.

It is of some historic interest to call attention to the earlier studies of Drinker and Field [24] who suggested that "a further possibility for which no proof exists is that the delicate lymph capillaries are fixed to the surrounding tissues by fine strands of reticulum and that muscular movement by pulling on the strands may induce distortion and temporary openings through which fluid enters eventually to reach a valve trunk from which escape does not occur." Later, Pullinger and Florey [98] investigated lymphatics in both normal and edematous tissues and demonstrated that the lymphatics are intimately associated with the interstitium, notwithstanding increased dilatation of the lymphatics during edema formation.

The presence of anchoring filaments in pulmonary lymphatics confirms our earlier observations for dermal lymphatics and other tissues [72]. They provide a structural basis for "fixing" the lymphatic capillary wall to the adjacent interstitium. With such a mechanism, an increase of fluids and plasma proteins within the interstitium would presumably exert equal pressures around the circumference of the lymphatic vessel, thereby increasing fluid pressure within the interstitial space. There would also be an accompanying movement of collagen bundles, elastic fibers, and other connective tissue components in order to accommodate the increased fluid volume. This would expand the interstitial space and thus produce tension on the collagen bundles and elastic fibrils in which the anchoring filaments are firmly embedded. Therefore, as collagen and elastic fibers are separated by the increased interstitial fluids during both normal and inflammatory conditions, areas of the lymphatic wall would also be pulled along with the collagen and other connective tissue fibers. This would result in a widening of the lymphatic capillary lumen as the extensively and loosely overlapping adjacent endothelial cell junctions could become separated to provide patent intercellular junctions. These patent intercellular junctions permit a rapid movement of fluids as well as particulate materials and cells into the lymphatic capillary lumen. The extent of lymphatic vascular dilatation would vary with the fluid volume and duration of tissue exudate which accumulates within the surrounding connective tissue.

VI. Pulmonary Lymphatic Capillary Permeability

If diffusible substances as well as plasma protein which are constantly lost from the blood capillaries were allowed to accumulate within the interstitium, the blood circulatory system would not only become depleted of its plasma colloids, but this loss would also disrupt the balance of forces responsible for the control of fluid movement and metabolic exchange across the blood vascular wall. Thus, the pulmonary lymphatic vessels, as those in other tissues of the body, subserve the constant removal of pulmonary interstitial fluids and plasma proteins which are not removed at the venular limb of the blood vascular system. This lymph drainage, therefore, prevents a buildup of these components within the pulmonary interstitium and fluid homeostasis is maintained.

Although the overall structural components of the lymphatic system have been described for the lung and various other tissues of the body, two areas of concern remain: (a) the dynamics of fluid movement in the interstitial area, and (b) the mechanisms responsible for the concentration of lymph within the lymphatic capillary and subsequently propel this fluid in a unidirectional drainage pattern to the much larger collecting vessels for return to the systemic circulation. The ultrastructural plan of the lymphatic capillary has been established and, as described above, some answers have been provided for elucidating the topographical relationship of this one-way drainage system to the surrounding interstitium.

VII. Tracer Experiments

The pulmonary lymphatic endothelial cells engulf large molecules and particulate matter from the adjoining interstitial area [57,62]. A number of investigators have taken advantage of this property not only to label pulmonary lymphatics but to ascertain the mechanisms involved in the movement of fluids and large particulate substances from the connective tissue into pulmonary lymphatic vessels. Recent advances in morphological techniques have made it possible to monitor proteins, particulate materials, and cells on their journey from the blood vascular system into the interstitium and their subsequent removal by the lymphatic vascular system [68]. Likewise, substances instilled into the trachea have also been followed across the bronchial and alveolar walls into the pulmonary interstitium for subsequent removal by lymphatic vessels [62].

A. Experiments with Intratracheally Instilled Particulate Tracers

Lauweryns and Baert [62] instilled ferritin and carbon intratracheally into neonatal rabbits and followed the movement and fate of these particles from the pulmonary alveoli. Using electron microscopic methods, these particles were observed within the lymphatic capillary lumen as early as 30 min after their instillation into the trachea.

In an attempt to follow the movement of intratracheally instilled particles in the adult mammalian lung, we have used a suspension of electron-opaque particulate materials of varying sizes (ferritin, ~80 Å, and colloidal carbon ~350 Å diam). These tracer substances were instilled intratracheally into adult mice and rats. After fixation by perfusion, the progress of tracer from the bronchial tree into the interstitium and lymphatic vessels was monitored with the electron microscope at various time intervals (ranging from 15 min up to 1 month). When suspensions of colloidal ferritin were instilled into the trachea, subsequent observation (15-30 min) of perfused, fixed lung tissue showed that the bulk of ferritin appeared within the lumen of the bronchial tree. Ferritin particles also appeared within alveolar macrophages and squamous cells of the alveolar epithelium (Fig. 25a); a few particles were seen within the basal lamina of the alveolar interstitium. No particles were observed within the lymphatics at this early time period. At 2 hr and after, ferritin particles were seen within the alveoli, the interstitial areas around lymphatic vessels, and in vesicles of various sizes within the lymphatic endothelial cells (Fig. 26a,b).

Colloidal carbon is much larger (250-350 Å diam) and is easy to recognize at relatively low magnifications. Its distribution is similar to that of ferritin at 15-30 min after instillation into the trachea (Fig. 25b).

At time intervals greater than 2 hr, the size and number of vesicles in which tracer particles can be observed was greatly increased. In animals observed more than 24-hr after the colloidal carbon instillation, sites of lymphoid tissue and nodes were clearly demarcated by the entrapment of carbon in these areas. In addition to its presence in vesicles within endothelial cells along the bronchial tree and in the pulmonary interstitial macrophages, the tracer appeared in vesicles within the lymphatic endothelial cells (Fig. 27a). The size of the vesicles containing carbon particles were much smaller than the ferritin-containing vesicles of a similar time period. A similar observation was also noted in the studies of Lauweryns and Baert [62]. However, at 3 months (Fig. 28) and later, carbon particles are seen in large vessels within the lymphatic endothelium.

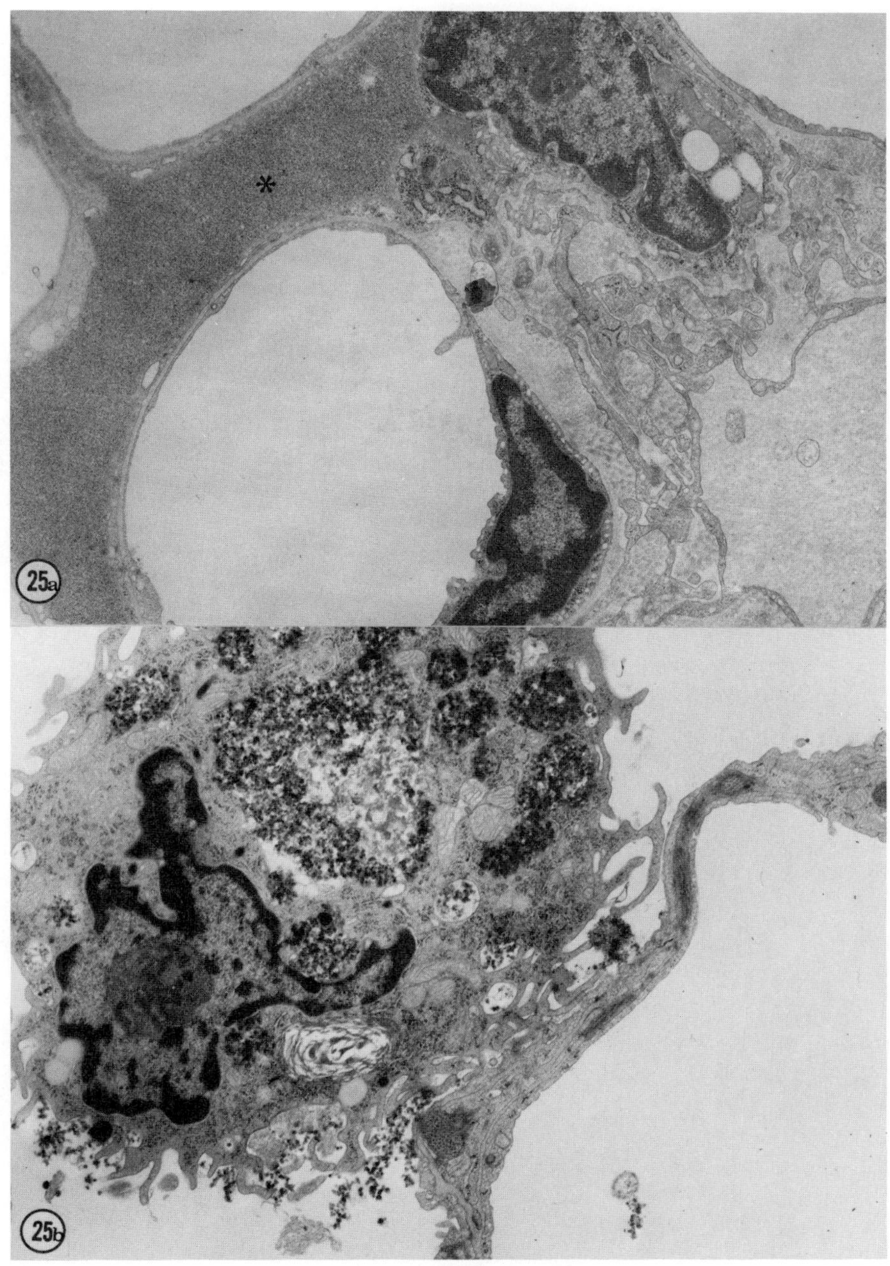

FIGURE 25 (a) This electron micrograph depicts the occurrence of ferritin particles (*) within alveoli. ×20,000. (b) Intratracheally injected carbon is shown within alveolar macrophages. ×13,000.

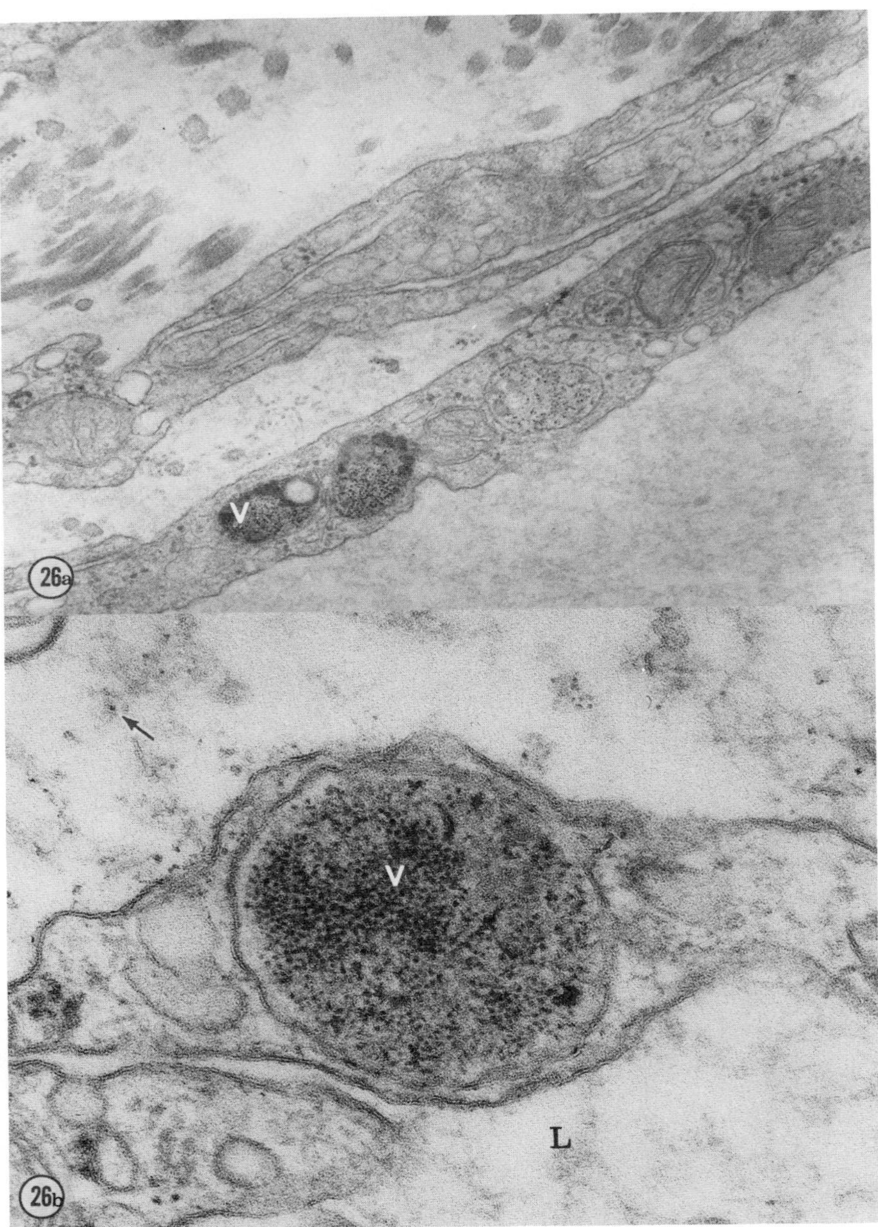

FIGURE 26 The appearance of ferritin within large vesicles (v) and within the interstitium (arrow) at 24 hr after injection into the trachea. (a) ×65,000; (b) ×139,000.

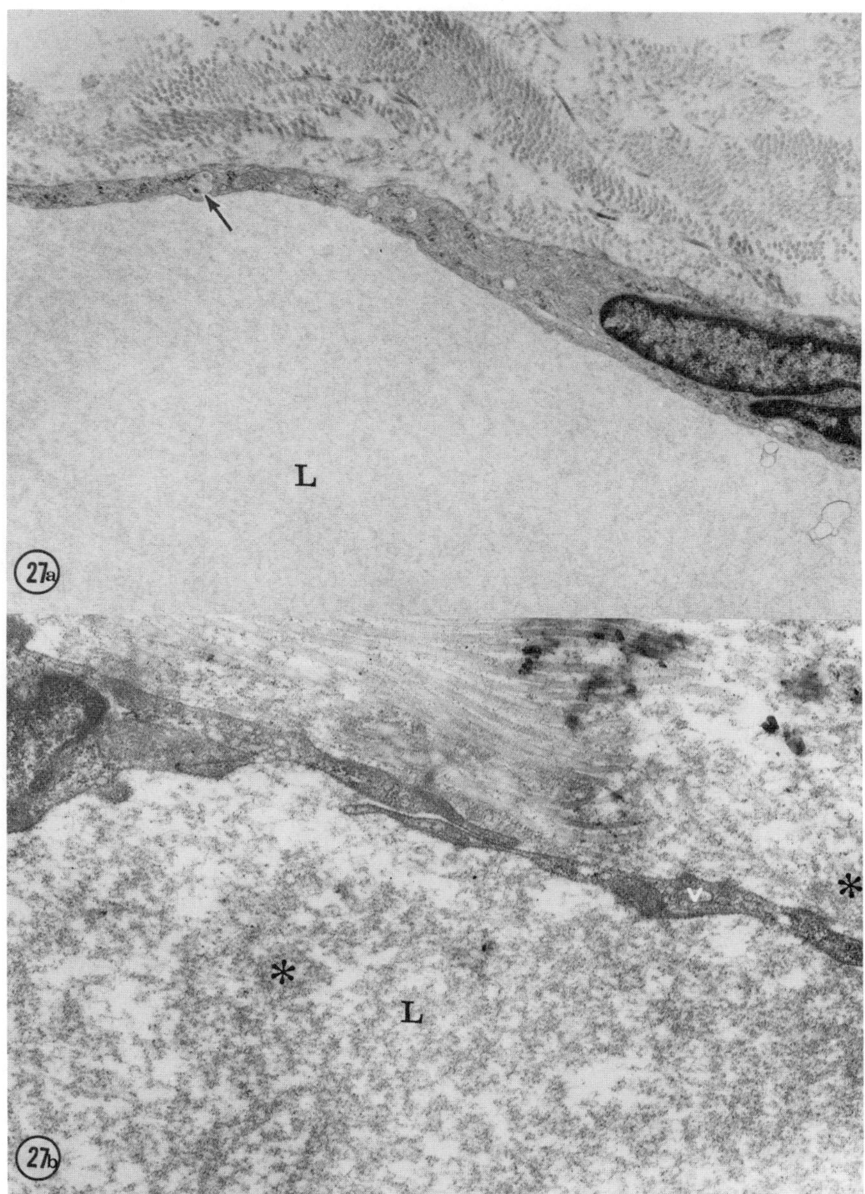

FIGURE 27 (a) The presence of carbon particles (arrow) within vesicle of lymphatic endothelium at 24 hr after an intratracheal injection of colloidal carbon. ×13,000. (b) Part of lymphatic vessel from animal injected with dextran which appears as a very electron dense precipitate (*) in the connective tissue, within vesicles (v) and within the lymphatic lumen (L) at 15 min after an injection of a 10% solution of dextran via the saphenous vein. ×23,000.

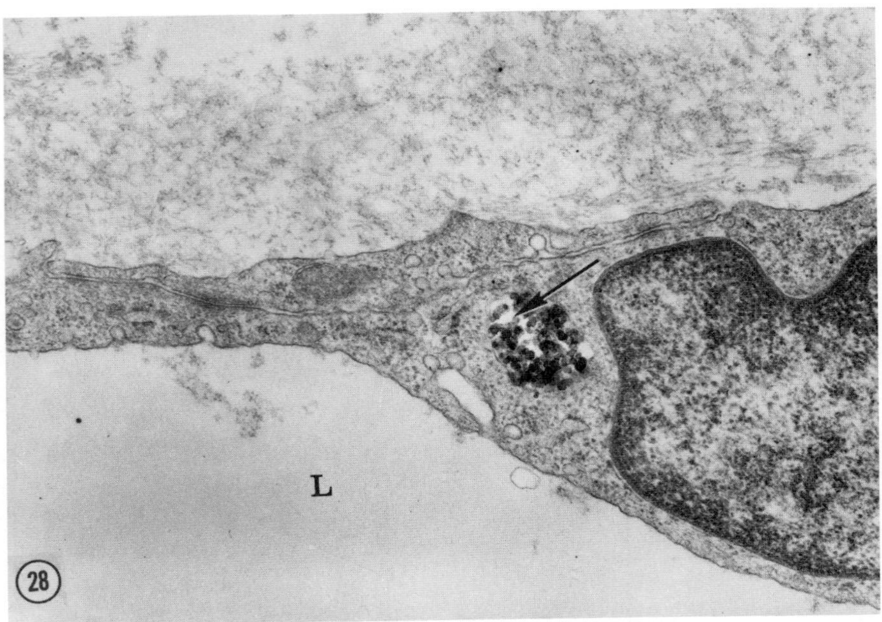

FIGURE 28 Carbon particles (arrow) are in a large vacuole at 3 months after an intratracheal injection of colloidal carbon. ×31,000.

B. Intravascular Injection of Tracer Substances

Interstitial injections of tracer substances permit the tracer to be removed by the lymphatics before their appearance is observed or detected in the blood vascular system. Unfortunately, there is still the possibility of trauma due to unphysiological pressure in the vicinity of the injection site or the production of a mild inflammatory response as indicated by the immigration of macrophages and neutrophils to sites of irritation. This possibility is overcome by using intravenous injections of tracer particles or of substances which can be rendered electron dense by chemical means once the tissue has been fixed and processed. Simionescu and Palade [111] intravenously injected dextran at some distance from the site of tissue to be examined; therefore we injected dextrans of varying molecular weights (60,000 to 300,000) via the saphenous vein of young adult rats. It is well documented that intravascularly injected dextran passes the blood capillary wall and is removed from the interstitium by lymphatic vessels for return to the systemic circulation [42]. In order to observe dextran selectively in the interstitium and the lymphatic vessels, we perfused lungs with saline to free the blood vessels of injected dextran. After fixation with a glutaraldehyde formaldehyde mixture in phosphate buffer at a pH

7.4 at 0°C [111] dextran particles are retained in a homogeneous distribution in the plasma and interstitium, presumably as a result of fixation of the surrounding proteins. This procedure produces an electron-dense product whose density is considerably enhanced by postfixation in osmic acid in a phosphate buffer solution. Examination of pulmonary tissue within 15 min after dextran injections shows the presence of dextran throughout the interstitium and within the pulmonary lymphatic vessels (Fig. 27b). The staining is very intense within 30 min after injection. Dextran gains access to the lymphatic capillary lumen via vesicles and within the intercellular clefts of loosely adherent, overlapping intercellular junctions. It is of special interest to note that the uptake of dextran from the surrounding interstitium by pulmonary lymphatics is very similar to the pattern of movement of peroxidase across the blood-tissue-lymph interface in other tissues of the body [68].

Our studies of pulmonary lymphatics after the instillation of ferritin and colloidal carbon particles into the trachea of young adult rats and mice confirm the findings of Lauweryns and Baert [62] in that the tracer particles are observed within pulmonary lymphatics at various time periods postinjection. The presence of tracer particles within alveolar macrophages and in vesicles within squamous cells of the alveolar epithelium (type I pneumocyte) at short intervals (15-30 min) and their subsequent appearance in pulmonary lymphatic vessels provide morphological evidence to suggest that large particles are able to cross squamous alveolar epithelial cells within vesicles. Once in the connective tissue compartment (which has a negative interstitial fluid pressure [81]) the particles move toward the lymphatics and are subsequently removed in a fashion similar to that in other lymphatic regions of the body. Sorokin and Brain [113] recently demonstrated that iron oxide particles were also taken up by squamous alveolar epithelial cells and that these particles also penetrated the alveolar interstitium. These authors suggest that some of the iron oxide could well find its way passively into juxtaalveolar lymphatics.

Drinker [23] believed that the absorption of microscopically visible particles from the alveoli was mainly a problem of the lymphatic drainage of the lungs. However, the total amount of lymph which is drained from the lung is very slight when compared with that drained from the abdominal viscera [17]. The fact that the normal lung is relatively dry is probably due to the excess of colloid osmotic pressure in the lung capillaries over that of the capillary blood pressure [17,23]. This condition permits very little protein to escape while simultaneously allowing nonprotein fluids to be reabsorbed. Therefore, the small amount of lymph that is drained from the lung under normal circumstances would have a very high level of protein [17]. Drinker [23] was able to increase the flow of pulmonary lymph in the dog by using forced inspiration. Pulmonary lymph drainage is also increased in pulmonary edema [17].

In addition to the tracer studies cited above, other investigators have studied the clearance of proteins [25], inert particles [23,86] iron oxide [113] as well as cultures of virulent type III pneumococci [109] by pulmonary lymphatics. Our studies as well as the work of other investigators show that the size and type of particles (inert, organic, or toxic) affect the speed with which the particles are cleared by pulmonary lymphatics. In the case of toxic substances such as quartz [115], which cause structural damage to the lining alveolar epithelial cells, discontinuities are produced. These expose the injected particles to the underlying connective tissue compartment facilitating their movement toward the pulmonary lymphatics for subsequent removal from the lung.

Notwithstanding a relatively low rate of lymph drainage from pulmonary tissue under normal conditions, there is an extensively elaborate plexus of lymphatic vessels in the lung. These vessels provide a one-way drainage system for the removal of excess interstitial fluids, proteins, particulate matter (i.e., particles removed from the air spaces) and cells (i.e., inflammatory and cancerous) when the pulmonary interstitium is challenged. This constant lymph drainage maintains a condition which facilitates a rapid exchange of gases across the blood-interstitial-air interfaces.

Acknowledgments

The author is indebted to the Allergy and Infectious Disease Institute (A110639) and the Heart and Lung Institute (HL13901) of the National Institutes of Health for support of the personal research cited in this chapter. The technical assistance of Messrs. Henry I. Covington and C. P. Chou is gratefully acknowledged. Gratitude is expressed to Ms. L. Jenkins and Mrs. A. Gill for typing the manuscript.

References

1. E. Anderson, Oocyte differentiation and vitellogenesis in the roach *Periplaneta America, J. Cell Biol.*, **20**:131-155 (1964).
2. E. Anderson, In *Oogenesis.* Edited by J. D. Biggers and A. W. Schultz. Baltimore, Md., University Park Press, 1972, pp. 87-117.
3. G. Aselli, DeLactibus sive lacteis venis, quarto vasorum mesaraicorum genere novo invento Gasp. Aselli. Cremonensis. Anatomici ticinensis Dissertatio qua sententiae convelluntur nel parum perciptae illustrantur. Mediolani, Apud Jo. Baptisam Bidellium (In part in Mangeti Bibl. Anat. II, 636), 1627.
4. T. Bartholin, *Dubia Anatomica de Lacteis Thoracicis publici proposita.* Copenhagen Melch Martzan, 1653, p. 42.

5. O. Behnke, B. I. Kristensen, L. Nillsen, Electron microscopical observations on actinoid and myosinoid filaments in blood platelets, *J. Ultrastruct. Res.*, **37**:351-369 (1971).
6. H. S. Bennett, The concepts of membrane flow and membrane vesiculation as mechanisms for active transport and ion pumping, *J. Biophys. Biochem. Cytol.*, **2**:99 (1956).
7. K. G. Bensch, G. B. Gordon, and L. Miller, Fibrillar structures resembling leiomyofibrils in endothelial cells of mammalian pulmonary blood vessels, *Z. Zellforsch. Mikrosk. Anat.*, **63**:759-766 (1964).
8. J. F. Burke and Lee V. Leak, Lymphatic capillary function in normal and inflamed states. In *Progress in Lymphology*, Vol. II. Edited by M. Viamonte, P. R. Koehler, M. Witte, and C. Witte. Stuttgart, Georg Thieme, 1970, p. 81.
9. L. G. Caro and G. E. Palade, Protein synthesis, storage, and discharge in the pancreatic exocrine cell. An autoradiographic study, *J. Cell Biol.*, **20**: 473-495 (1964).
10. J. R. Casley-Smith, An electron microscopic study of injured and abnormally permeable lymphatics, *Ann. NY Acad. Sci.*, **116**:803-830 (1964).
11. J. R. Casley-Smith and H. W. Florey, The structure of normal small lymphatics, *Q. J. Exp. Physiol.*, **46**:101-106 (1961).
12. A. Celis and J. Porter, Lymphatics of the thorax, *Acta Radiol.*, **38**:461 (1952).
13. F. P. Chinard, G. J. Vosburgh, and T. Enns, Transcapillary exchange of water and of other substances in certain organs of dogs, *Am. J. Physiol.*, **183**:221-234 (1966).
14. E. R. Clark, Observations on living growing lymphatics in the tail of the frog larvae, *Anat. Rec.*, **3**:183-198 (1909).
15. F. Clementi and G. E. Palade, Intestinal capillaries. I. Permeability to peroxidase and ferritin, *J. Cell Biol.*, **41**:33-58 (1969).
16. W. T. Councilman, The lobule of the lung and its relation to the lymphatics, *J. Bost. Med., Sci.*, **4**:165-168 (1900).
17. F. C. Courtice, Hamilton Russell Memorial Lecture. Pulmonary Oedema clinical implications of laboratory experiments, *Aust. N. Z. J. Surg.*, **22**: 177-191 (1953).
18. W. Cruikshank, The anatomy of the absorbing vessels of the human body. London, 1786. Geschichte und Beschreibung der Einsaugenden Gefasse oder Saugardern des menschlichen Körpers (Trans. by Christian F. Ludwig) Leipzig, 1789.
19. R. S. Cunningham, On the development of the lymphatics in the lungs of the pig, *Contrib. Embryol.*, **4**:47-68 (1916).
20. R. J. R. Cureton and D. H. Trapnell, Post-mortem radiography and gaseous fixation of lung, *Thorax*, **16**:138-143 (1961).
21. C. de Duve and R. Wattiaux, Function of lysosomes, *Annu. Rev. Physiol.*, **28**:435-492 (1966).
22. A. Dogiel, Ueber die Beziehungen zwischen Blut und Lymphgefassen, *Arch. Mikrosk. Anat.*, **22**:608-615 (1883).

23. C. K. Drinker, The absorption of toxic and infectious material from the respiratory tract. In *Virus and Rickettsial Diseases,* Symposium Harvard School of Public Health, Cambridge, Mass., Harvard University Press, 1940, p. 381.
24. C. K. Drinker and M. E. Field, *Lymphatics, Lymph, and Tissue Fluid.* Baltimore, Md., Williams and Wilkins, 1933.
25. C. K. Drinker and E. Hardenberg, Absorption from the pulmonary alveoli, *J. Exp. Med.,* **86**:7-17 (1947).
26. C. K. Drinker, M. E. Field, and H. K. Ward, The filtering capacity of lymph nodes, *J. Exp. Med.,* **59**:393-405 (1934).
27. C. J. Eberth and A. Belajeff, Uber die Lymphgefasse des Herzens. *Virchows Arch.,* **37**:124-131 (1866).
28. J. Emery, Connective tissue and lymphatic. In *The Anatomy of the Developing Lung.* Edited by J. Emery. London, Heinemann, Lavenham Press, 1969, Chap. IV, p. 49.
29. S. Engel, The bronchial glands. In *Lung Structure.* Springfield, Ill., Charles C Thomas, 1962, Chap. 9, p. 85.
30. D. W. Fawcett, The fine structure of capillaries, arterioles, and small arteries. In *The Microcirculation.* Edited by S. R. M. Reynolds and B. Zweifach. Urbana, Ill., University of Illinois Press, 1959, p. 1.
31. D. W. Fawcett, Intercellular bridges, *Exp. Cell Res. [Suppl.],* **8**:174-187 (1961).
32. D. W. Fawcett, Physiologically significant specializations of the cell surface, *Circulation,* **26**:1105-1132 (1962).
33. D. W. Fawcett, P. M. Heidger, and Lee V. Leak, Lymph vascular system of the interstitial tissue of the testis as revealed by electron microscopy, *J. Reprod. Fertil.,* **19**:109-114 (1969).
34. D. W. Fawcett, Lee V. Leak, and P. M. Heidger, Electron microscopic observations on the structural components of the blood testis barrier, *J. Reprod. Fertil. [Suppl.],* **10**:105-122 (1970).
35. D. W. Fawcett, W. B. Neaves, and M. N. Flores, Comparative observation on intertubular lymphatics and the organization of the interstitial tissue of the mammalian testis, *Biol. Reprod.,* **9**:500-532 (1973).
36. L. B. Flexner, A. Gelhorn, and M. Merrell, Studies on rates of exchange of substances between blood and extravascular fluids; exchange of water in guinea pig, *J. Biol. Chem.,* **144**:35-40 (1942).
37. G. J. Glint, The development of the lungs, *Am. J. Anat.,* **6**:1 (1906).
38. E. E. Fraley and L. Weiss, An electron microscopic study of the lymphatic vessel in the penile skin of the rat, *Am. J. Anat.,* **109**:85-101 (1961).
39. F. Franke, Uber die Lymphgefasse der Lunge. Zugleich ein Beitrag zur Erklarung der Baucherscheinung bei Pneumonie, *Dtsch. Z.,* **119**:107 (1912).
40. D. Friend and M. G. Farquhar, Functions of coated vesicles during protein absorption in the rat vas deferens, *J. Cell Biol.,* **35**:357-376 (1967).
41. R. A. Good, Immunodeficiency in developmental perspective, *Harvey Lect.,* **67**:1 (1971-1972).

42. G. Grotte, Passage of dextran molecules across the blood-lymph barrier, *Acta Chir. Scand. [Suppl.]*, **211**:8 (1956).
43. A. Guyton, In *Function of the Human Body*, 4th ed., Philadelphia, Pa., Saunders, 1974.
44. J. G. Hall, The response of a node to stimulation with foreign tissue, *Congies. Colloq. Univ. Liege*, **45**:1-8 (1967).
45. K. Hama, On the existence of filamentous structure in endothelial cells of the amphibian capillary, *Anat. Rec.*, **139**:437 (1961).
46. S. S. Han and J. K. Avery, The ultrastructure of capillaries and arterioles of the hamster dental pulp, *Anat. Rec.*, **145**:549 (1963).
47. D. F. Harvey and H. M. Zimmerman, Studies on the development of human lung. I. The pulmonary lymphatics, *Anat. Rec.*, **61**:203 (1935).
48. H. von Hayek, Periarterielle lymphraume, *Anat. Anz.*, **89**:209 (1940).
49. W. Hewson, A description of the lymphatic system in the human subject and in other animals. In *The Works of William Hewson*, 1774. Edited by G. Gulliver. London, Sydenham Society, 1846.
50. W. His, Ueber das Epithel Lymphgefasswurzeln und uber v. Recklinhausen Saftkanalchen, *Z. Wiss. Zool.*, **13**:455-473 (1863).
51. S. Hudock and P. D. McMaster, The lymphatic participation in human cutaneous phenomena. A study of the minute lymphatics of the living skin, *J. Exp. Med.*, **57**:751-774 (1933).
52. H. Ishikawa, R. Bischoff, and H. Holtzer, Mitosis and intermediate-sized filaments in developing skeletal muscle, *J. Cell Biol.*, **38**:538-555 (1968).
53. H. Ishidawa, R. Bischoff, and H. Holtzer, Formation of arrowhead complexes with heavy meromyosin in a variety of cell types, *J. Cell Biol.*, **43**:312-328 (1969).
54. J. E. Jamieson and G. E. Palade, Condensing vacuole conversion and zymogen granule discharge in pancreatic exocrine cells: Metabolic studies, *J. Cell Biol.*, **48**:503-521 (1971).
55. O. F. Kampmeier, The distribution of valves and the first appearance of definite direction in the drainage of lymph in the human lung, *Tuber. Pulm. Dis.*, **18**:360-372 (1928).
56. M. J. Karnovsky, The ultrastructural basis of capillary permeability studied with peroxidase as a tracer, *J. Cell Biol.*, **35**:213-236 (1967).
57. F. Kato, The fine structure of the lymphatics and the passage of China ink particles through their walls, *Nagoya Med. J.*, **12**:221-246 (1966).
58. E. Klein, *The Anatomy of the Lymphatic System*. Vol. II. London, 1875.
59. J. M. Lauweryns, The lymphatic vessels of the neonatal rabbit lung, *Acta Anat. (Basel)*, **63**:427-433 (1966).
60. J. M. Lauweryns, The juxta-alveolar lymphatics in the human lung, *Am. Rev. Respir. Dis.*, **102**:877-885 (1970).
61. J. M. Lauweryns, Stereomicroscopic funnel-like architecture of pulmonary lymphatic valves, *Lymphology*, **4**:125-132 (1971).
61a. J. M. Lauweryns, The blood and lymphatic microcirculation of the lung, *Path. Ann.*, **6**:365-415 (1971).
62. J. M. Lauweryns and J. H. Baert, The role of the pulmonary lymphatics in the defenses of the diseased lung: Morphological and experimental

studies of the transport mechanisms of intratracheally instilled particles, *Ann. NY Acad. Sci.*, **221**:244-275 (1974).

63. J. M. Lauweryns and L. Boussauw, Centrioles and associated striated filamentous bundles in rabbit pulmonary lymphatic endothelial cells, *Z. Zellforsch.*, **131**:417-427 (1972).
64. J. M. Lauweryns and L. Boussauw, The ultrastructure of pulmonary lymphatic capillaries of newborn rabbits of human infants, *Lymphology*, **2**:108-129 (1969).
65. L. V. Leak, Electron microscopic observations on lymphatic capillaries and the structural components of the connective tissue-lymph interface, *Microvasc. Res.*, **2**:361-391 (1970).
66. L. V. Leak, Studies on the permeability of lymphatic capillaries, *J. Cell Biol.*, **50**:300-323 (1971).
67. L. V. Leak, The fine structures and function of the lymphatic system. In *Handbuch der Allgemeinen Pathologie*, Vol. 3, Part 6. Berlin, Springer Verlag, 1972, p. 149.
68. L. V. Leak, The transport of exogenous peroxidase across the blood-tissue lymph interface, *J. Ultrastruc. Res.*, **39**:24-42 (1972).
69. L. V. Leak and J. F. Burke, Studies on the permeability of lymphatic capillaries during inflammation, *Anat. Rec.*, **151**:489 (1965). (Abstr).
70. L. V. Leak and J. F. Burke, Fine structure of the lymphatic capillary and the adjoining connective tissue area, *Am. J. Anat.*, **118**:785-810 (1966).
71. L. V. Leak and J. F. Burke, Ultrastructural studies on the lymphatic anchoring filaments, *J. Cell Biol.*, **36**:129-149 (1968).
72. L. V. Leak and J. F. Burke, Early events of tissue injury and the role of the lymphatic system in early inflammation. In *The Inflammatory Process*, Vol. III. New York, Academic Press, 1974, Chap. 4, p. 163.
73. H. R. Lindner, Partition of androgen between lymph and venous blood of the testis in the ram, *J. Endocrinol.*, **25**:483-494 (1963).
74. W. G. McCallum, The relations between the lymphatics and the connective tissue, *Bull. Johns Hopkins Hosp.*, **14**:1-9 (1903).
75. W. G. McCallum, The pathology of the pneumonia in the USA during the winter of 1917-1918, R.I.M.R. Monograph No. 10, 1919.
76. G. Majno and M. Leventhal, Pathogenesis of histamine type vascular leakage, *Lancet*, **2**:99 (1967).
77. G. Majno, S. M. Shea, and M. Leventhal, Endothelial contraction induced by histamine type mediators, an electron microscopic study, *J. Cell Biol.*, **42**:647 (1969).
78. P. Mascagni, Vasorum lyphaticorum. Corporis human descriptio et iconographia. Siene, 1787.
79. H. S. Mayerson, The physiologic importance of lymph. In *Handbook of Physiology*, Section 2, *Circulation*. Edited by W. F. Hamilton and P. Dow. Washington, D.C., American Society of Physiology, 1963, p. 1035.
80. R. S. McCuskey, Sphincters in the microvascular system, *Fed. Proc.*, **30**: 713 (1971). (Abstr.).
81. B. J. Meyer, A. Meyer, and A. C. Guyton, Interstitial fluid pressure. V. Negative pressure in the lung, *Circ. Res.*, **22**:263 (1968).

82. A. A. Miles and E. M. Miles, The state of lymphatic capillaries in acute inflammatory lesions, *J. Pathol.*, **73**:21-35 (1958).
83. W. S. Miller, The structure of the lung, *J. Morphol.*, **8**:165 (1893).
84. W. S. Miller, Studies on tuberculous infection II. The lymphatics and lymph flow in the human lung, *Am. Rev. Tuberc.*, **3**:193 (1919).
85. W. S. Miller, *The Lung*, 2nd ed. Springfield, Ill., Thomas, 1947.
86. P. E. Morrow, Lymphatic drainage of the lung in dust clearance, *Ann. NY Acad. Sci.*, **200**:46-65 (1972).
87. R. L. Murray and M. W. Dubin, The occurrence of actinlike filaments in association with migrating pibment granules in frog retinal pigment epithelium, *J. Cell Biol.*, **64**:705 (1975).
88. V. T. Nachmias, H. E. Huxley, and D. Kessler, Electron microscope observations on actomyosin and actin preparations from physarum polycephalum, and their interaction with heavy meromyosin subfragment 1 from muscle myosin, *J. Mol. Biol.*, **50**:83 (1970).
89. C. Nagaishi, Pulmonary lymph vessels. In *Functional Anatomy and Histology of the Lung*, Baltimore, Md., University Park Press, 1972, p. 102.
90. A. B. Novikoff, E. Essner, and N. Quintana, Golgi apparatus and lysosomes, *Fed. Proc.*, **23**:1010-1022 (1964).
91. A. B. Novikoff and E. Essner, Pathological changes in cytoplasmic organelles, *Fed. Proc.*, **21**:1130-1142 (1962).
91a. G. Ottaviano, Ricerche. Anast. sui vasi linfatici del pulmone umano, *Morphol. Jb.*, **82**:453 (1938).
92. G. E. Palade, Fine structure of blood capillaries, *J. Appl. Phys.*, **24**:1424 (1953).
93. G. E. Palade, P. Siekevitz, L. G. Caro, Structure, chemistry and function of the pancreatic exocrine cell, *Ciba Found. Symp.*, 23 (1962).
94. J. Pecquet, Experiments nova anatomica in quibus incognitum chyli receptaeulum et ob eo per thoracem usque in ramos usque subclavius vasa lactea deleguntur. Paris, 1651 (In Magel'. Biol. Anat. II:652, and Hemsterhuy's messis aurea; Amsterdam).
95. T. C. Pennell, Anatomical study of the peripheral pulmonary lymphatics, *J. Thorac. Cardiovasc. Surg.*, **52**:629-634 (1966).
96. T. D. Pollard and R. R. Weihing, Cytoplasmic actin and myosin and cell motility, *Crit. Rev. Biochem.*, p. 1 (Jan. 1974).
97. T. D. Pollard, E. Shelton, R. Weihing, and E. D. Korn, Ultrastructural characterization of F. actin isolated from *Acanthamoeba castellanii* and identification of cytoplasmic filaments as F. Actin by reaction with heavy meromyosin, *J. Mol. Biol.*, **50**:91-97 (1970).
98. B. D. Pullinger and H. W. Florey, Some observations on the structure and function of lymphatics: Their behavior in local edema, *Br. J. Exp. Pathol.*, **16**:49-61 (1935).
99. F. Renyi-Vamos, *Das innere Lymphgefass System der Organe.* Verlag der Ungarischen Akademie der Wissenschaften, 1960, Chap. 5, p. 121.
100. J. A. G. Rhodin, Fine structure of vascular walls in mammals, *Physiol. Rev.*, **42** (Suppl. 5):48 (1962).

101. P. Rohlieh and I. Olah, Cross-striated fibrils in the endothelium of the rat myometral arterioles, *J. Ultrastruct. Rev.*, **18**:667-676 (1967).
102. T. F. Roth and K. R. Porter, Yolk protein uptake into the oocyte of the mosquito *Aedes aegypti L.*, *J. Cell Biol.*, **20**:313-332 (1964).
103. H. Rouviere, The terminal collecting trunks of the lymphatic system. In *Anatomy of the Human Lymphatic System,* Ann Arbor, Mich., Edward Bros., 1938, p. 240.
104. F. T. von Recklinghausen, Zur Fellesorption, *Arch. Pathol. Anat.*, **26**:172-208 (1862).
105. O. Rudbeck, Nova exercitatid anatomica exhibens Ductus Hepaticos Aquosos et vasa Glandulorum Serosa, Arosiae, Uppsala, 1653.
106. F. R. Sabin, The origin and development of the lymphatic system, *Bull. Johns Hopkins Hosp.*, **17**:347-440 (1916).
107. P. C. Sappy, Anatomie, physiologic, pathologie de Vaisseaux lymphatiques consideres chez l'homme et les vertebres. Paris, 1874.
108. P. C. Sappy, Description iconographique des vaisseaux lymphatiques chez l'homme et les vertebres. Paris, 1885.
109. R. Z. Schulz, M. F. Warren, and C. K. Drinker, The passage of rabbit virulent type III pneumococci from the respiratory tract of rabbits into the lymphatics and blood, *J. Exp. Med.*, **68**:251 (1938).
110. P. H. Simer, Drainage of pleural lymphatics, *Anat. Rec.*, **113**:269-283 (1952).
111. N. Simionescu and G. Palade, Dextrans and glycogens as particulate tracers for studying capillary permeability, *J. Cell Biol.*, **50**:616 (1971).
112. N. Simionescu, M. Simionescu, and G. E. Palade, Permeability of muscle capillaries to small heme-peptides. Evidence for the existence of patent transendothelial channels, *J. Cell Biol.*, **64**:586-607 (1975).
113. S. P. Sorokin and J. D. Brain, Pathways of clearance in mouse lungs exposed to iron oxide aerosols, *Anat. Rec.*, **181**:581 (1975).
114. B. Stay, Protein uptake in the oocytes of the cecropia moth, *J. Cell Biol.*, **26**:49-62 (1965).
115. F. J. Strecker, Tissue reaction in rat lungs after dust inhalation with special regard to bronchial dust elimination and to the penetration of dust into the lung inerestices and lymphatic nodes. In *Inhaled Particles and Vapours II.* Edited by N. Davis. Oxford, Pergamon, 1967, p. 141.
116. C. E. Tobin, Lymphatic of the pulmonary alveoli, *Anat. Rec.*, **120**:625-635 (1954).
117. C. E. Tobin, Human pulmonic lymphatics, an anatomic study, *Anat. Rec.*, **127**:611-633 (1957).
118. C. E. Tobin, Pulmonary lymphatics, *Am. Rev. Respir. Dis.*, **80**:50-57 (1959).
119. D. H. Trapnell, The peripheral lymphatics of the lung, *Br. J. Radiol.*, **36**:660-672 (1963).
120. D. H. Trapnell, Radiological appearances of lymphangitis carcinomatosis of the lung, *Thorax*, **19**:251-260 (1964).

121. L. Weiss, The structure of fine splenic arterial vessels in relation to hemoconcentration and red cell destruction, *Am. J. Anat.*, **111**:131 (1962).
122. T. Willis, "Pharmaceutice Rationalis," pp. 17, 18, in Opera Omnia 1681, Translated into English in *The Operation of Medicines in Human Bodies,* 1684, part II, p. 13, London, 1675.
123. K. E. Wohlfarth-Bottermann, In *Primitive Motile Systems in Cell Biology.* Edited by R. D. Allen and N. Kamiya. New York, Academic Press, 1964, p. 79.
124. D. W. Wywodzoff, Die Lymphwege der Lung, *Wiener Med. Jahrb.*, **11**:3 (1866).
125. J. M. Yoffey and F. C. Courtice, In *Lymphatics, Lymph and the Lymphomyeloid Complex.* London, New York, Academic Press, 1970.
126. S. K. Zurich, Lung lymphatics. In *Progress in Lymphology,* Vol. II. Edited by M. Viamonte, P. R. Koehler, M. Witte, and C. Witte. Stuttgart, Thieme, 1970.
127. L. O. Zwillenberg and H. H. L. Zwillenberg, Zur Struktur und Funktion der Hülsencapillaren in der Milz, *Z. Zellforsch. Mikrosk. Anat.*, **59**:908-921 (1963).

18

The Integrity of the Air-Blood Barrier

EVELINE E. SCHNEEBERGER

Harvard Medical School and
Children's Hospital Medical Center
Boston, Massachusetts

I. Introduction

Although the delicate structure of the alveolar-capillary barrier is uniquely adapted to the rapid and efficient exchange of oxygen and carbon dioxide, it has a second very important function. It is a barrier which resists the penetration of harmful airborne material. Except for the phagocytic function of alveolar macrophages, relatively little is known of the mechanisms by which the alveolar-capillary membrane acts as a defense of the lung. However, there are at least three attributes of the alveolar epithelium which merit consideration:

1. The *selective permeability* of this epithelium to the diffusion of lipid-insoluble macromolecules is of importance not only in protecting the organism from inhaled noxious material, but it also ensures that the air spaces are not overwhelmed by the small amount of protein and fluid which normally leak from alveolar capillaries [1].
2. *Pinocytotic transport* by type I pneumocytes, from the capillary side of the epithelium to the alveolar surface, provides a mechanism for the delivery of bacteriostatic and other

salutary agents to the alveolar space [2]. Conversely, pinocytotic transport of materials from the alveolus to the interstitial space appears to aid not only in the absorption of lung fluid protein in the newborn period [3,4] but affords a mechanism for the absorption of edema fluid in pathological states.

3. Finally, *phagocytosis* by type I epithelial cells provides an additional, albeit limited, means for the removal of inhaled particulate material [5-7]. Thus the alveolar epithelium functions not only as a selective barrier against inhaled material and material leaked from alveolar capillaries, but its vesicular transport system may serve to protect the organism from harmful intraalveolar substances.

In addition to the barrier functions of the alveolar epithelium, the enormous capillary bed of the lung also plays a defensive role: it removes cells and emboli from the circulation. Situated between the right and left ventricles, this capillary network retains particles which are larger than the diameter of the pulmonary capillaries [8], with the trapped material being subsequently removed. This trapping phenomenon also permits the lung to act as a physiological sieve, by temporarily sequestering circulating leukocytes and megakaryocytes [10-12]. These cells are either released into the circulation again, or they leave the lung possibly by migrating into lymphatic channels or alveolar spaces.

To understand the morphology and function of the alveolar-capillary membrane a brief survey of its ultrastructure and cytochemistry is presented.

II. Ultrastructure and Cytochemistry of the Alveolar-Capillary Barrier

In the mammalian lung, the alveolar-capillary barrier consists of three distinct anatomic layers (Fig. 1). These include the capillary endothelium, the alveolar interstitial space which contains the basement membranes of both endothelial and epithelial cells and a continuous layer of epithelium composed of membranous (type I), and granular (type II) pneumocytes as well as a few brush cells [13]. With appropriate methods of fixation, the alveolar epithelial surface can be shown to be covered by a layer of osmiophilic material which has been interpreted as being surfactant [14]. In its most tenuous portions, the thickness of the human air-blood barrier may range from 0.6 μm to several micrometers, and has an arithmetic mean of about 1.5 μm [15]. In thicker portions of the alveolar wall, amorphous mucopolysaccharide material, elastic and collagen fibers, interstitial macrophages, and a few myofibroblasts are present. It has been estimated that the latter make up about 50% of the alveolar

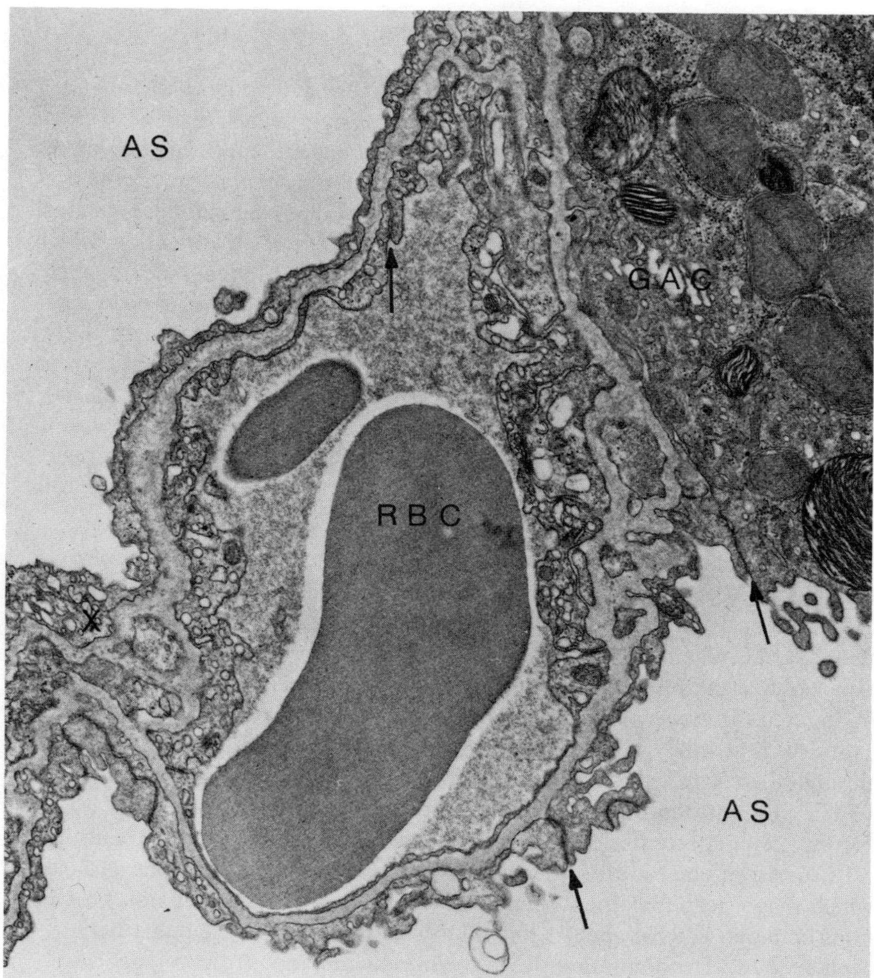

FIGURE 1 Adult mouse lung showing a red blood cell (RBC) in the pulmonary capillary lumen. The alveolar space (AS) is lined by membranous (type I) pneumocytes. Junctions between these cells are indicated (arrows). Pinocytotic vesicles (X) are present in some flat alveolar cells. Fused basement membranes separate epithelial from endothelial cells. The pulmonary endothelium is continuous, nonfenestrated, and contains many pinocytotic vesicles. An endothelial cell junction (arrow is shown between adjacent cells. ×17,000.

interstitial cells. The presence of bundles of intracellular fibrils and the binding of antiactin antibodies strongly suggests that myofibroblasts are contractile and that they may play an important role in the autoregulation of the ventilation/perfusion ratio [16].

A. The Pulmonary Capillary Endothelium

The pulmonary capillary endothelium is continuous, and nonfenestrated and contains large numbers of pinocytotic vesicles, many of which open onto either the luminal or abluminal surface. On the basis of experiments using enzymatic tracers [3,17], it appears that pulmonary capillary vesicles transport protein molecules in a bidirectional manner, similar to that observed in nonfenestrated capillaries of other organs [18]. Recently a further interesting function, which appears to be unique to the lung, has been attributed to the pinocytotic vesicles of pulmonary endothelial cells. Biochemical studies have shown that adenine nucleotides, bradykinin, and angiotensin I are metabolized almost quantitively during their passage through the lungs with virtually no retention of the parent compound nor of their metabolites (see references in Ref. 19). On the basis of cytochemical experiments with adenosine 5′-monophosphate and autoradiographic studies using analogs of angiotensin I and bradykinin, it has been suggested that the requisite hydrolase enzymes may be present in these pinocytotic vesicles [19].

In contrast to the larger arterial vessels of the bronchial and pulmonary circulation [20], pulmonary capillary endothelial cells contain few myofibrils [19]. Other organelles present in these cells are similar to those seen in nonfenestrated capillaries elsewhere [18]. The pulmonary endothelial cells are attached to each other by junctions in which the intercellular space is generally obliterated. However, these areas of adhesion alternate with sites in which a gap, ~40 Å in width, separates adjacent endothelial cells [17] (Fig. 2). It is through these gaps that small water-soluble molecules are thought to diffuse [3,17]. Recent observations made on freeze-fractured alveolar capillary membranes [28] indicate that the junctions between pulmonary capillary endothelial cells consist of one to three interconnected rows of intramembranous particles which show occasional discontinuities (See Fig. 8a, b). The latter are somewhat more common in what appears to be the venular portion of the pulmonary capillary bed. The discontinuities in the intramembranous rows of particles could represent patent areas in the intercellular portions of the junction. However, it remains to be proven whether the intramembranous rows of particles correspond in fact to sites of close apposition of the adjacent unit membranes.

B. The Alveolar Interstitial Space

The alveolar interstitial space, in the thinnest portions of the alveolar-capillary barrier, contains only the fused endothelial and epithelial basement membranes. These, after heavy metal staining, appear as a uniform, dense meshwork of fine filaments which are separated from endothelial and epithelial cells, respectively,

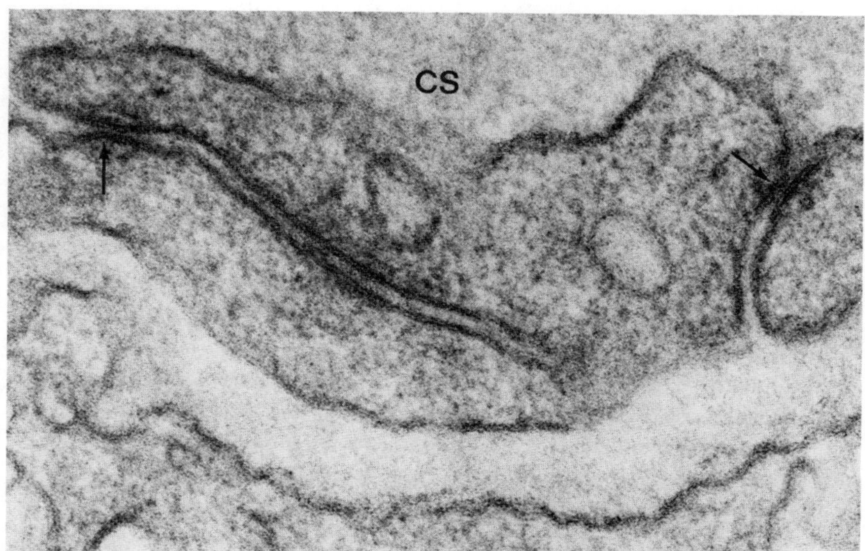

FIGURE 2 Two pulmonary endothelial junctions showing close apposition of the adjacent unit membranes. However, even in the narrowest regions (arrows), a 40 Å wide gap is evident. The capillary space (CS) is at the upper edge. ×140,000. (Reprinted from Ref. 17 by courtesy of the Rockefeller University Press.)

by a narrow, more electron-lucent layer. Chemically the composition of this basement membrane is similar to that of the basement membrane of other organs (see references in Ref. 21) in that it is largely a glycoprotein containing a collagen-like component. Antigenically it is closely related to the glomerular basement membrane [22].

C. The Alveolar Epithelium

The alveolar epithelium is composed of a continuous layer of membranous (type I) pneumocytes interspersed with granular (type II) pneumocytes (Fig. 1). The former are flattened cells which cover a large expanse of alveolar surface with a thin, smooth layer of cytoplasm. With the exception of relatively numerous pinocytotic vesicles, their cellular organelles are inconspicuous. The cuboidal granular pneumocytes, by contrast, contain multivesicular bodies, multilamellar bodies, [23], mitochondria, peroxisomes [24-26], rough endoplasmic reticulum, a prominent Golgi apparatus, and they have blunt microvilli projecting from the surface. Evidence obtained from a number of studies suggests that it is the granular pneumocytes which synthesize and secrete surfactant (see references in

Ref. 27). This surface-active material, present at the interface between alveolar air and alveolar wall, serves to stabilize the alveolar volume. Unlike endothelial cell clefts, those between alveolar epithelial cells are obliterated toward the alveolar lumen by fusion of the outer leaflets of the bounding unit membranes, forming continuous, gasket-like tight junctions or zonulae occludentes (Fig. 3). Following freeze fracture, these pulmonary epithelial zonulae occludentes show the typical network of ridges on the protoplasmic face (PF) and complementary grooves on the exoplasmic face (EF) (see Fig. 9) [28] which have been described in zonulae occludentes of other epithelia [29].

Glycocalyx, rich in acid mucopolysaccharides, covers the epithelial cell membrane facing the alveolus. In the human lung this extracellular coat of type I pneumocytes measures only about 100 Å thickness, while it is much thicker in type II pneumocytes, where it measures 400 Å in thickness [30]. Alkaline phosphatase has been localized to the surface membrane of type II pneumocytes, but it appears to be absent in type I pneumocytes [30]. The presence of both acid phosphatase [30] and esterases [31] in multivesicular and multilamellar bodies of granular pneumocytes raises the question of whether these organelles belong to the lysosomal system. However, the lack of glycocalyx on the limiting membranes of these structures, suggests that they are secretory vacuoles rather than part of the phagocytic system. Indeed by autoradiography it has been shown that radioactive palmitate is incorporated into these organelles, lending support to the contention that they are storage sites for surfactant [27]. Numerous catalase containing peroxisomes are present in granular pneumocytes, [24-26]. The function of peroxisomes in mammalian cells has been variously linked to gluconeogenesis, carbohydrate oxidation, lipid metabolism, and cellular respiration [32,33]. In the latter regard, since the rate of peroxisome respiration is almost directly proportional to ambient oxygen tension, it has been suggested that peroxisomes may play a role in protecting the cell against oxygen toxicity [32,33]. Although this is an intriguing hypothesis, the function of peroxisomes in the lung remains to be established.

D. The Extracellular Alveolar Layer

The extracellular alveolar layer may be best visualized by vascular perfusion fixation [14] or with freeze-substitution techniques [34]. When well preserved, it is a flocculent or granular material with an electron-dense line, measuring ~40 Å in thickness, at its surface. This lining layer may contain small collections of lamellar material similar to that seen in the inclusions of granular pneumocytes, and it completely covers and surrounds alveolar macrophages as they range over the alveolar surface. Physiological and biochemical data [35-37] indicate that this alveolar lining layer consists of two functionally different components:

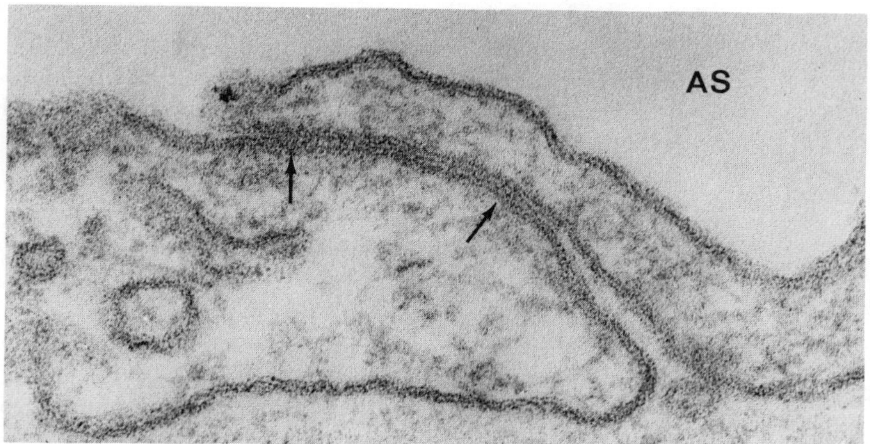

FIGURE 3 A pulmonary epithelial junction showing fusion of the inner leaflets of the adjacent unit membranes in the distal portion of the junction (arrows). The alveolar space (AS) is at the upper edge. ×140,000. (Reprinted from Ref. 17 by courtesy of the Rockefeller University Press.)

a film facing the alveolar space composed of highly surface-active phospholipids, and beneath it a layer (the hypophase) containing surface-active phospholipids in a different physicochemical configuration, as well as proteins and carbohydrates. It is thought that components of the lining layer are recruited from the hypophase during lung expansion, and that they may reenter the hypophase at low lung volumes. Of the materials in the extracellular alveolar lining layer, the saturated phospholipid dipalmitoyl phosphatidyl choline is the major surface active component.

III. Integrity of the Alveolar-Capillary Barrier to Circulating Macromolecules

To maintain its gas exchange function, a number of complex structural and functional adaptations exist in the lung which prevent the accumulation of excess fluid in alveolar septa.

1. In contrast to the systemic capillary pressure, that of the pulmonary capillary system is between 5-15 mmHg, which is well below the osmotic pressure of plasma proteins. Such conditions favor fluid absorption and ensure a minimum of interstitial fluid in alveolar walls [1].

2. The role of interstitial fluid pressure is less well understood, but from a variety of experiments it appears that it may be as low as 15 mmHg subatmospheric [38]. This negative pressure would tend to draw fluid from pulmonary capillaries and would favor the absorption of liquid from alveoli. Such interstitial fluid is subsequently drained away by pulmonary lymphatics.
3. As will be discussed below, the intrinsic permeability properties of the alveolar-capillary membrane are such that they serve to maintain a barrier at the air-blood interface.
4. Finally, the surfactant system, by reducing alveolar surface tension which would be transmitted through the alveolar wall, also counters the transudation of fluid into alveoli. The present discussion will be limited to the structural elements of the alveolar-capillary wall which subserve its barrier function.

Quantitative observations on the exchange of solutes across a generalized nonfenestrated capillary endothelium, are usually interpreted in terms of the pore theory of capillary permeability [1]. The latter states that the capillary endothelium behaves as though it were a semipermeable membrane which is penetrated by two sets of water-filled pores. The small pores, which have a radius of between 35 and 42 Å, allow the rapid exchange of small, water-soluble molecules across the capillary wall. As the molecular weight of the transported material increases, there is progressive restriction to passage through the small pores, so that substances with a molecular weight greater than 90,000 daltons cannot cross the endothelium by this route. Instead high molecular weight substances may pass through a sparser system of large pores having a radius of 250 Å. In nonfenestrated capillaries the "small pore" system has been postulated to be located in intercellular junctions between adjacent endothelial cells [18], while pinocytotic vesicles have been suggested as the morphological equivalent of the "large pore" system [39]. However, the anatomical site of these two pore systems remains a matter of controversy [69].

In the case of the alveolar-capillary wall, physiologic studies have suggested that it is the alveolar epithelium rather than the endothelium which determines the extent to which water-soluble solutes may enter the alveolus [40]. This was confirmed in studies employing cytochemical techniques for the demonstration of intravenously injected peroxidatic enzymes of varying molecular weight [17]. When mice were injected intravenously with horseradish peroxidase (HRP) (40,000 daltons), the enzyme rapidly leaked through endothelial junctions and permeated the surrounding basement membrane (Fig. 4). However, tight junctions between epithelial cells prevented the enzyme from entering the alveolar space. These morphological observations were supported by the physiological

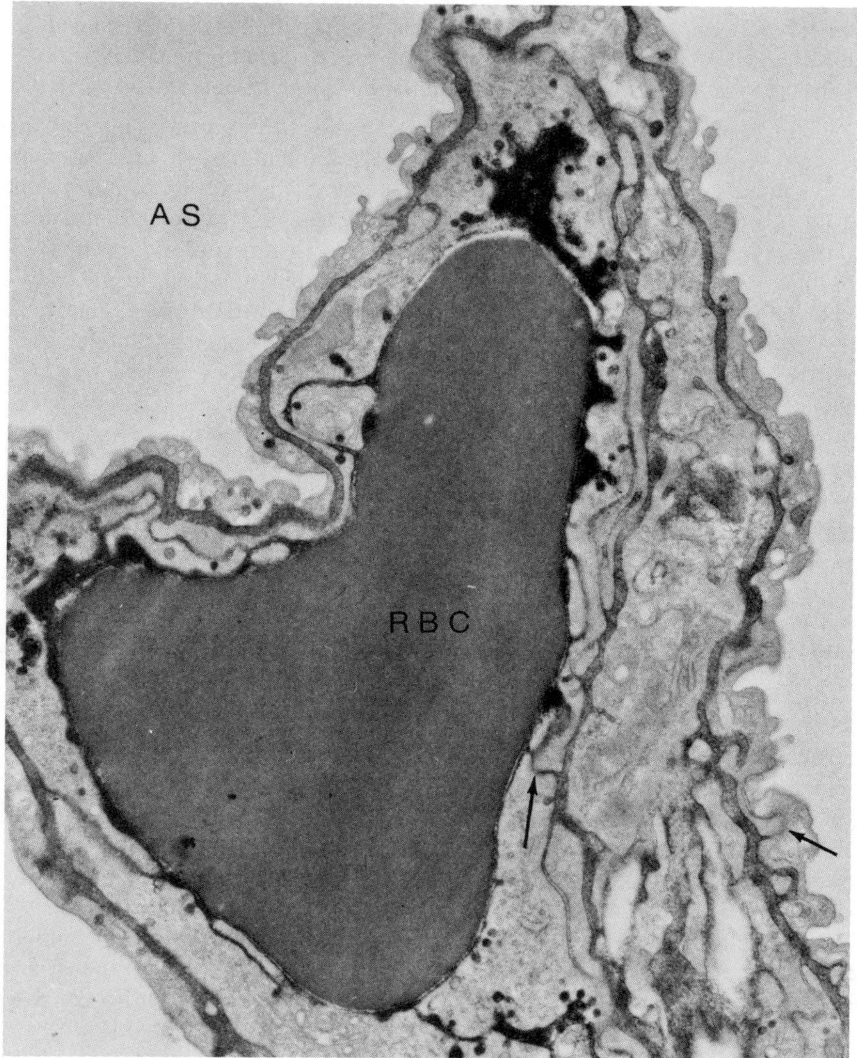

FIGURE 4 Newborn mouse lung 90 sec after the injection of horseradish peroxidase (HRP) in a volume representing 20% of the animal's blood volume. Reaction product fills the capillary lumen, and has permeated endothelial junctions (arrows) as well as the surrounding basement membrane. However, the enzyme is prevented from entering the alveolar space (AS) by tight epithelial junctions (arrow). Pinocytotic vesicles of both endothelial and epithelial cells contain reaction product. ×17,000.

studies of Taylor et al. [41] who, on the basis of experimentally determined reflection coefficients of a variety of substances, calculated a pulmonary endothelial pore radius of 40-58 Å, and a pulmonary epithelial pore radius of 6-10 Å.

In the above cytochemical tracer experiments the enzyme was injected in a relatively large volume (30% of the animal's blood volume) which may have temporarily but substantially increased the pressure in the pulmonary capillary lumen. Subsequent experiments using either HRP or hemoglobin (Hb) (64,500 daltons) in isolated perfused dog lungs, showed that with normal perfusion pressures (15-20 mmHg) both tracers remained confined to the capillary lumen. It was only when perfusion pressures were increased to 30 mmHg for HRP and 50 mmHg for Hb, that these two tracers leaked through endothelial junctions [42]. Further work with both adult and newborn mice confirmed the above observations [3]. HRP injected in a volume of saline representing about 3% of the animal's blood volume, remained confined to the capillary lumen, did not permeate endothelial junctions and gradually labeled endothelial pinocytotic vesicles (Fig. 5). These morphological observations lend support to the concept that endothelial pores may be labile and susceptible to stretching by increased intravascular pressure [43]. It also indicates that, while the endothelial junctions represent the site of diffusion of small water-soluble molecules, at normal capillary pressures, molecules the size of HRP and serum proteins are chiefly transported by pinocytotic vesicles.

Experiments with intravenously injected tracers have also shown that, whereas tight junctions between alveolar epithelial cells prevent the escape of protein tracers, even at elevated pressures, there is pinocytotic transport of protein onto the alveolar surface [2] (Fig. 6). Such pinocytotic transport appears to be of importance in delivering small quantities of serum albumin and immunoglobulins to the alveolar space. Indeed, the presence of IgG, IgA [44], and albumin [36,37], has recently been demonstrated in lower respiratory tract secretions. Pinocytotic transport may also explain the presence of α_1-antitrypsin (60,000 daltons) in human alveolar macrophages [45]. Admittedly, the inhibitor may have been taken up by macrophages before their migration into the alveolar space; however, its presence in normal alveolar secretions has recently been reported [46].

A number of studies have dealt with the effect of hypoxia, metabolic poisons [47], EDTA [48], or pharmacological agents [49] on the permeability of the alveolar-capillary membrane to albumin. From the results it was concluded that, while the permeability of the alveolar-capillary membrane is little affected by anoxia, its integrity does depend in part on metabolic processes [47]. No morphological changes were found to explain the increased capillary permeability to proteins during EDTA-induced pulmonary edema [48]. However, very few of these experimental models have been studied with the use of ultrastructural tracers. Such experiments would clearly be of interest in delineating not only

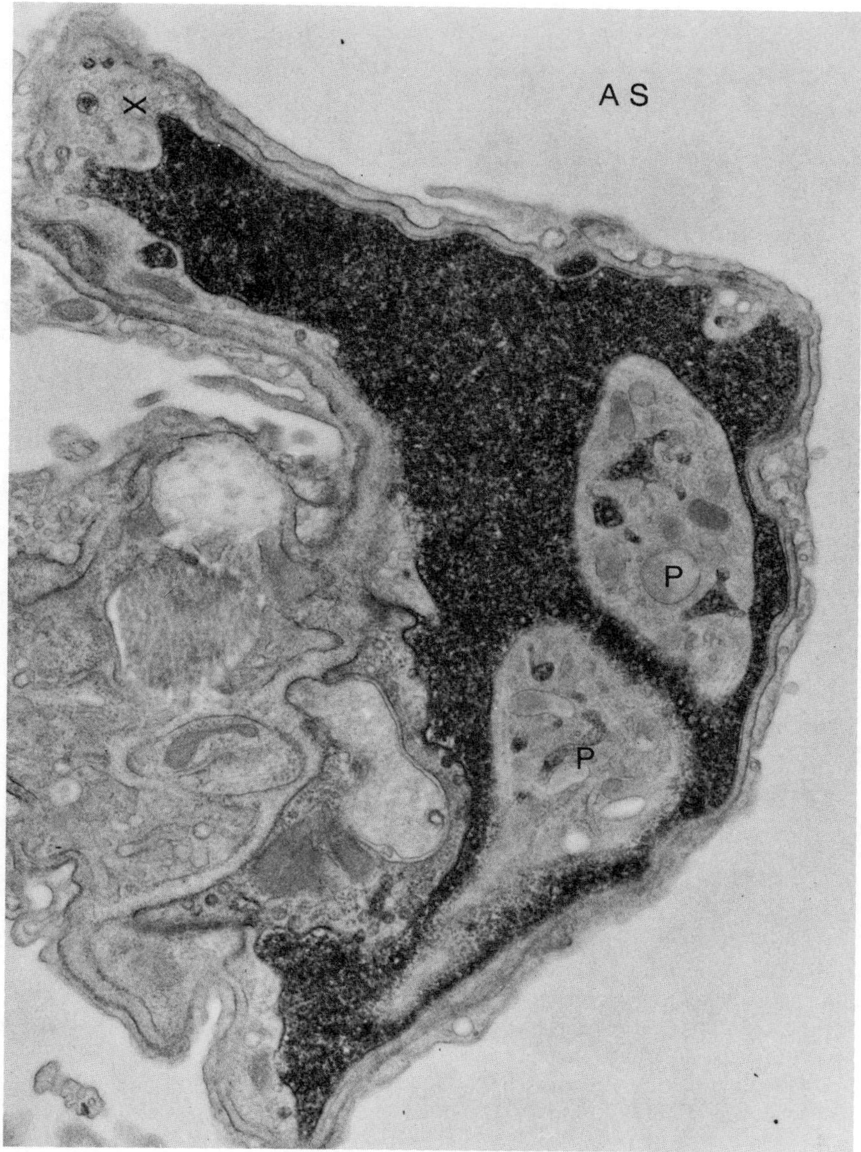

FIGURE 5 Adult mouse lung 6 min after injection of HRP in a volume representing 3% of the animal's blood volume. Reaction product remains confined to the capillary lumen and does not permeate endothelial junctions or the basement membrane. A few endothelial pinocytotic vesicles (X) contain reaction product. Two platelets (P) containing ingested enzyme are present in the capillary lumen. ×25,000.

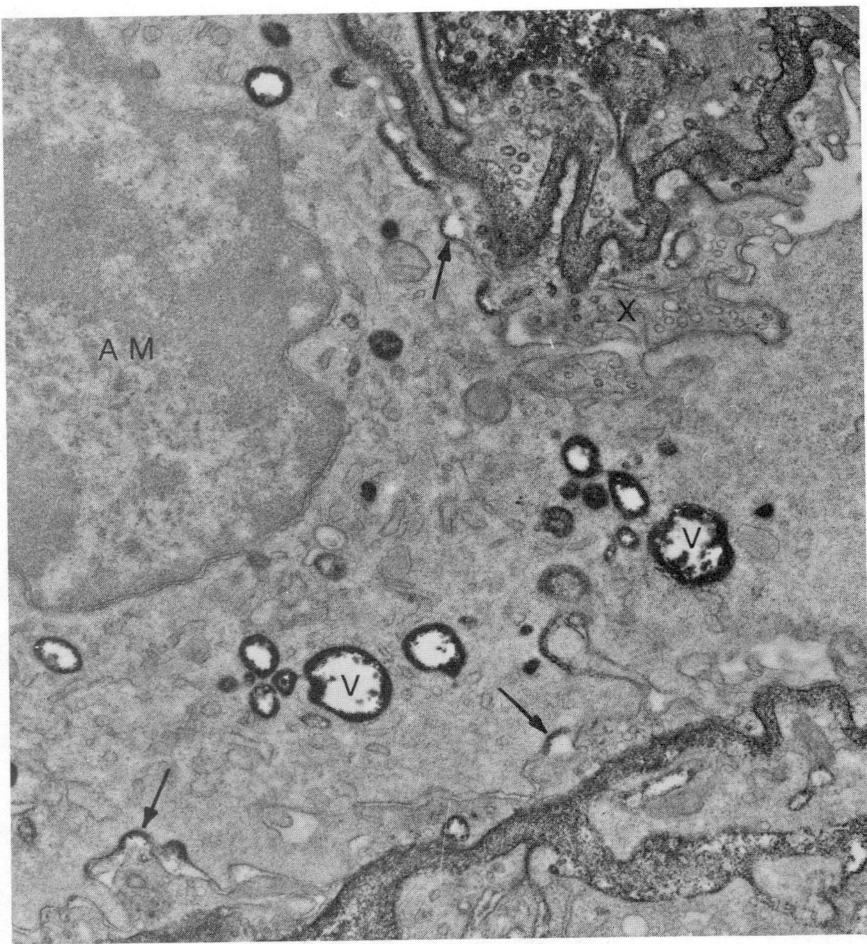

FIGURE 6 Mouse lung 2 min after the intravenous injection of HRP in 0.5 ml saline. An alveolar macrophage (AM) is closely apposed to two alveolar surfaces. Epithelial pinocytotic vesicles (X) contain reaction product. In the alveolar macrophage coated vesicles, at various stages of formation, are taking up the enzyme (arrows). Vacuoles (V) filled with reaction product are seen within the alveolar macrophage. ×21,000.

which layer of the alveolar-capillary membrane is chiefly affected by these various agents, but whether bronchial or pulmonary vessels are primarily involved. It has recently been shown, for instance, by Pietra et al. [20] and Gabbiani et al. [50], that it is the bronchial and not the pulmonary vessels which become leaky after exposure to histamine.

IV. Integrity and Absorptive Function of the Alveolar-Capillary Barrier to Intraalveolar Material

Inhaled, insoluble particles (up to 3 μm diam) reaching alveoli are phagocytized by alveolar macrophages which move along alveolar surfaces [51]. The uptake of particulate matter by alveolar epithelial cells, on the other hand, is less well understood. The early studies of Karrer [52], in which India ink was administered intratracheally to mice, showed that type I but not type II pneumocytes ingest a small amount of carbon. Corrin obtained similar results by giving thorium intratracheally to rats [5]. Interestingly, small amounts of thorium were released by type I pneumocytes into the underlying basement membrane, an observation which has recently been confirmed by Sorokin and Brain in mice after iron oxide inhalation [6]. Presumably particles released from epithelial vacuoles into the basement membrane are either taken up by interstitial macrophages or gradually swept toward pulmonary lymphatics by interstitial fluid. Pulmonary epithelial cells, therefore, are not an absolute barrier to inhaled particulate matter. However, the amount of material which is transported is probably small, due not only to the efficient phagocytic activity of alveolar macrophages, but also because, as mentioned above, alveolar epithelial cells do not readily take up particulate matter.

In contrast, the transport of protein (10,000-200,000 daltons) across alveolar epithelium is appreciable. It takes place not only during the resorption of intraalveolar edema fluid, but also during removal of lung liquid in the newborn period. The problem of protein absorption from alveolar spaces has been the subject of a number of studies [53-55]. Although it is generally thought to be a slow process with most of the absorbed protein returning to the lymphatic circulation [53,54], some experiments suggest that radioiodinated albumin leaves alveoli of dog lungs more rapidly than was previously appreciated [55]. After intranasal administration of small quantities of HRP in saline to adult mice, the epithelial intercellular junctions remain impermeable to the tracer [17]. Instead, small quantities of the enzyme are taken up by pinocytotic vesicles of type I pneumocytes. However, pinocytotic transport of this protein across the epithelium appears to be relatively slow: even 1 hr after administration of the enzyme, easily visualized quantities of the tracer remain in the alveolar space [17].

In the immediate newborn period, the absorption of lung liquid occurs during the first 5 hr after birth and is accompanied by a large increase in lymph flow from the lungs [56]. Although the protein concentration in lung liquid is low (0.3 mg/ml) [57], these macromolecules must traverse the alveolar epithelial layer during resorption. After the intranasal administration of HRP to newborn mice less than 1 hr old, the epithelial junctions, as in adult mice, are impermeable

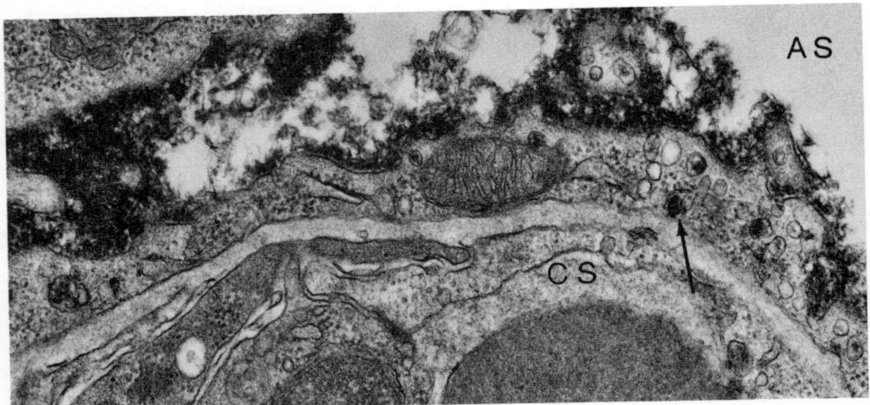

FIGURE 7 Lung from newborn mouse. A small amount of HRP was administered intranasally to the animal immediately after birth and the animal was sacrificed 1 hr later. In the air space (AS) a rim of reaction product coats the epithelial cell layer. Reaction product is present in epithelial pinocytotic vesicles one of which (arrow) appears to be releasing its contents on the basement membrane side. Although not shown, HRP does not permeate epithelial junctions. The capillary space (CS) is in the lower half of the electron micrograph. ×31,250.

to the tracer. Instead, uptake and release from pinocytotic vesicles appear to be the means of transport across type I pneumocytes, while type II pneumocytes do not participate in the uptake of HRP [3] (Fig. 7). These findings have recently been confirmed in newborn rabbits [4].

As compared to particulate matter and protein, the absorption from alveoli of small, lipid-insoluble and lipid-soluble molecules (60-250 daltons) is considerable. Indeed, it has been shown that the rate of absorption in the lung for such molecules is even greater than in the gastrointestinal tract [58,59]. Small lipid-insoluble molecules (e.g., p-aminohippuric acid, sulfanilic acid) appear to traverse the alveolar epithelial layer by a simple diffusional process, since the rate of disappearance is directly proportional to the concentration over a wide range. In addition, for molecules ranging in size from urea (60 daltons) to dextran (75,000 daltons), the rate of diffusion is directly proportional to the molecular weight [58]. The rate of absorption of lipid-soluble molecules, on the other hand, depends on their lipid/water partition coefficients. In general the greater the coefficient the more rapid the absorption rate [59]. The precise anatomical site in the lung where the transfer of both lipid-insoluble as well as lipid-soluble material takes place, remains to be established. However, the high absorptive capacity of the lung for certain solutes is of importance not only in environmental health and toxicology, but it may provide a means for the administration of therapeutic agents which are poorly absorbed from the gastrointestinal tract.

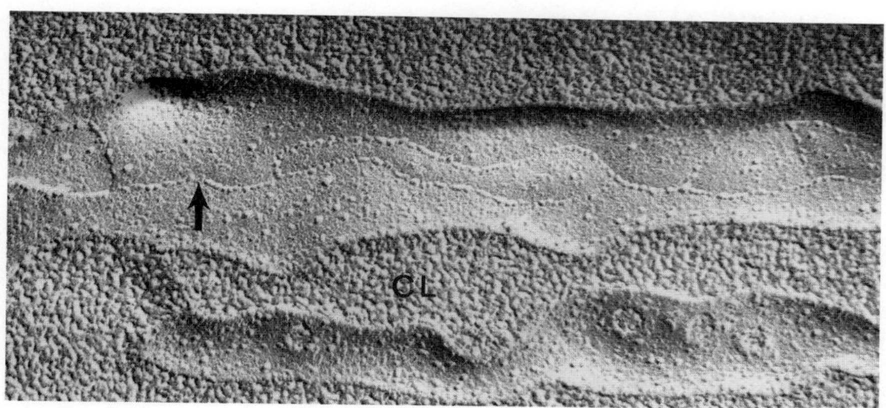

FIGURE 8 Freeze-fracture replica of a pulmonary capillary endothelial junction composed of 1 and 2 partially interconnected rows of particles showing a single discontinuity (arrow). The capillary lumen (CL) is at the bottom and the alveolar space at the top of the electron micrograph. ×82,500.

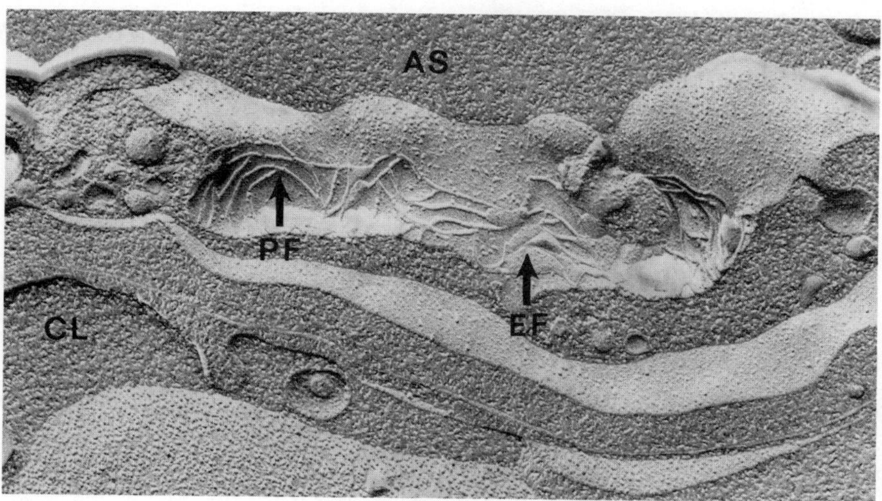

FIGURE 9 Freeze-fracture replica of an epithelial cell junction between type I pneumocytes. The junction consists of a continuous network of interconnected ridges on the protoplasmic face (PF) of the membrane and complimentary grooves on the half of the membrane facing the extracellular space (EF). The capillary lumen (CL) and alveolar space (AS) are indicated. ×50,000.

V. Filtering Properties of the Pulmonary Capillary Bed

As a consequence of both its location between the right and left sides of the heart, and its enormous capillary bed, the lung is uniquely suited to act as a trap for ridding the circulation of harmful emboli. Because of its dual blood supply (pulmonary and bronchial), the lung has the added advantage of being less susceptible than other organs to infarction. In addition, the sequestration of circulating granulocytes, lymphocytes, and megakaryocytes in the lung, suggests that it may play an additional role in regulating the number of circulating leukocytes and platelets [10-12]. It is these two filtering functions that will be dealt with in this section.

A. Trapping of Emboli

Depending on the size of the particle, there are a number of locations in the pulmonary vascular bed where trapping may occur. (a) Larger particles are apt to be caught in pulmonary arteries measuring 75-10 μm in diameter. At the level of the respiratory bronchioles, the pulmonary arteries taper down to 50 μm in diameter before breaking up into the capillary network [8]. These rapidly tapering arterioles have been designated "catch traps," as they are the sites where microemboli of glass beads are preferentially located after their injection into a number of different species [60]. (b) Pulmonary capillaries are also the site in which small emboli are trapped. In man, individual segments of the pulmonary capillaries measure between 6 and 13 μm in length and have an average diameter of 7-9 μm [15]. However, these dimensions are only an approximate guide as to what size particles will be trapped in the lung. This is due to a number of factors which include the rhythmic variation of capillary diameter during breathing, the interaction between surface charges on the particle and the endothelium, and the presence of arteriovenous communications which may allow the passage of larger particles through the lung [61].

In man, emboli from the systemic circulation, which may be trapped in the lung, are composed of a wide variety of substances. These include fragments of thrombi, fat, bone marrow, air, tumor cells, and, during pregnancy, placental tissue and amniotic fluid [62]. Depending on their size and number, these emboli may elicit few symptoms, or they may initiate a sequence of events beginning with bronchial constriction and pulmonary edema, and terminating in death.

Once trapped in pulmonary vessels, the lung must have effective mechanisms for ridding itself of emboli. That such mechanisms are operative has been shown by intravenously administering autologous thrombi to dogs in such amounts that a large part of the pulmonary vascular tree was involved. Within

2-6 weeks all evidence of these emboli had vanished from the lung, presumably as a consequence of fibrinolysis [9]. However, the proteolytic activity of the lung may not be limited to fibrinolysis: macroaggregates of serum albumin, for example, may disappear from the lung within hours after intravenous injection [63]. Pulmonary endothelial cells are capable of ingesting carbon after intravenous administration of low doses of this substance [50]. This suggests that, in addition to uptake by intravascular phagocytic cells, endothelial phagocytosis within the lung vasculature may also play a role in the removal of circulating particulate material.

B. Physiological Sequestration of Blood Cells in the Lung

On the basis of experiments which have shown that both lymphocytes and granulocytes are removed from the blood during its passage through the lung [10-12], it has been proposed that the lung may play a role in maintaining a stable level of circulating leukocytes. However, it is not clear at present whether this is simply effected by a temporary sequestration of these cells in pulmonary capillaries, or whether they return to the circulation by way of lymphatics. It is also possible that the trapped cells never return to the circulation, but rather enter into alveolar spaces, are transported to the bronchial system, and are eventually destroyed in the gastrointestinal tract [64]. Megakaryocytes, which are retained in the lung as physiological emboli from the bone marrow, appear to be an additional source of circulating platelets [11]. Indeed it has been estimated that from 7 to 17% of the body's platelets are released from pulmonary capillaries. However, the sequestration of leukocytes in pulmonary capillaries may not necessarily have a beneficial effect. It has recently been shown in monkeys that leukocyte trapping, induced by repeated endotoxin injections, results in widespread alveolar disruption [65]. This animal model may be of value in elucidating the mechanisms involved whereby emphysema develops in patients with α_1-antitrypsin deficiency.

The lodging of circulating macrophages within pulmonary capillaries has been observed in both normal [66] and experimentally manipulated lungs [67, 68]. The origin of these macrophages is not fully established since it is not known whether they represent monocytes from the bone marrow which are differentiating into alveolar macrophages, or whether under certain conditions they may represent migrating cells from the reticuloendothelial system [67]. Nevertheless, once they are trapped in pulmonary capillaries, these cells are capable of erythrophagocytosis and the uptake of circulating particulate matter [66]. As with leukocytes, the fate of these cells is uncertain, although there is evidence that some may gain access to the alveolar space and from there reach the gastrointestinal tract where they are eliminated [64].

VI. Summary

Though uniquely adapted to the rapid exchange of oxygen and carbon dioxide, the intrinsic properties of the alveolar-capillary membrane serve also to protect the organism from injurious, intra-alveolar agents and prevent the excessive leakage of liquid and protein into alveoli. Both physiological and ultrastructural studies indicate that it is the alveolar epithelium rather than the endothelium which acts as the chief barrier to diffusion of lipid-insoluble macromolecules. This is largely due to the fact that alveolar epithelial cells (type I and II pneumocytes) are held together by continuous, gasket-like tight junctions or zonulae occludentes, whereas endothelial cells are joined by discontinuous zonulae occludentes. While the epithelial tight junctions serve as barriers to the passage of lipid-insoluble macromolecules, the pinocytotic vesicles of type I pneumocytes transport material in a bidirectional fashion. These vesicles, therefore, afford a means of delivering salutary agents such as gamma globulins and α_1-antitrypsin into the alveolar space. Similarly, they play an active role in removing edema fluid proteins and, in the newborn period, lung liquid proteins from the alveolar space. Type II pneumocytes do not appear to participate in transporting material; rather, they are the site of surfactant synthesis and storage.

The combination of the low intravascular pressure prevailing in pulmonary capillaries and the colloid osmotic pressure of serum proteins, provides a large safety factor in keeping the lungs free of edema fluid. The areas between the discontinuous zonulae occludentes of pulmonary endothelial cells probably represent the small pore system of pulmonary capillaries. Under normal conditions, these are impermeable to most serum proteins and the endothelial pinocytotic vesicles provide the means of transporting serum proteins across the endothelium. However, endothelial junctions are susceptible to stretching when subjected to increased intravascular pressures, and under these conditions proteins the size of HRP have been shown to leak through endothelial junctions. This may be an important mechanism in the formation of interstitial edema.

The vast pulmonary capillary network also serves to trap emboli, thus protecting the systemic circulation from the injurious effects of embolism. Subsequently both phagocytic and proteolytic mechanisms aid in removing emboli from pulmonary vessels. Evidence also suggests that the pulmonary capillary bed may temporarily sequester leukocytes and megakaryocytes thus providing a means for regulating the level of circulating leukocytes and platelets.

References

1. E. M. Landis and J. R. Pappenheimer, Exchange of Substances through capillary walls. In *Handbook of Physiology*. Section II. Vol. 2. Edited

by W. F. Hamilton and P. Dow. Washington, D.C., American Physiological Society, 1963, pp. 961-1034.

2. E. E. Schneeberger, The permeability of the alveolar-capillary membrane to ultrastructural protein tracers, *Ann. NY Acad. Sci.*, **221**:238-243 (1974).
3. E. E. Schneeberger and M J. Karnovsky, The influence of intravascular fluid volume on the permeability of newborn and adult mouse lungs to ultrastructural protein tracers, *J. Cell Biol.*, **49**:319-334 (1971).
4. F. Gonzalez-Crussi and R. W. Boston, The absorptive function of the neonatal lung. Ultrastructural study of horseradish peroxidase uptake at the onset of ventilation, *Lab. Invest.*, **26**:114-121 (1972).
5. B. Corrin, Phagocytic potential of pulmonary alveolar epithelium with particular reference to surfactant metabolism, *Thorax,* **24**:110-115 (1969).
6. S. P. Sorokin and J. D. Brain, Pathways of clearance in mouse lungs exposed to iron oxide aerosols, *Anat. Rec.*, **181**:581-625 (1975).
7. Y. Susuki, J. Churg, and T. Ono, Phagocytic activity of the alveolar epithelial cells in pulmonary asbestosis, *Am. J. Pathol.*, **69**:373-388 (1972).
8. V. E. Krahl, The lung as a target organ in thromboembolism. In *Symposium on Pulmonary Embolic Disease.* Edited by A. A. Sasahara and M. Stein. New York, Grune and Stratton, 1964, pp. 13-22.
9. D. G. Freiman, Pathologic observations on experimental and human thrombo-embolism. In *Symposium on Pulmonary Embolic Disease.* Edited by A. A. Sasahara and M. Stein. New York, Grune and Stratton, 1964, pp. 81.
10. C. M. Ambrus and J. L. Ambrus, Regulation of the leukocyte level, *Ann. NY Acad. Sci.*, **77**:445-486 (1959).
11. R. M. Kaufman, R. Airo, S. Pollack, and W. H. Crosby, Circulating megakaryocytes and platelet release in the lung, *Blood,* **26**:720-731 (1965).
12. A. S. Weissberger, R. A. Guyton, R. W. Heinle, and J. P. Storaasli, The role of the lung in the removal of transfused lymphocytes, *Blood,* **6**:916-925 (1951).
13. B. Meyrick and L. Reid, The alveolar brush cell in rat lung–A third pneumocyte, *J. Ultrastruct. Res.*, **23**:71-80 (1968).
14. J. Gil, Ultrastructure of lung fixed under physiologically defined conditions, *Arch. Intern. Med.*, **127**:896-902 (1971).
15. E. R. Weibel, *Morphometry of the Human Lung.* New York, Academic Press, 1963, p. 101.
16. Y. Kapanci, A. Assimacopoulos, C. Irle, A. Zwahlen, and G. Gabbiani, "Contractile interstitial cells" in pulmonary alveolar septa: A possible regulator of ventilation/perfusion ratio? *J. Cell Biol.*, **60**:375-392 (1974).
17. E. E. Schneeberger and M. J. Karnovsky, The ultrastructural basis of alveolar-capillary membrane permeability to peroxidase used as a tracer, *J. Cell Biol.*, **37**:781-793 (1968).
18. M. J. Karnovsky, The ultrastructural basis of transcapillary exchanges, *J. Gen. Physiol.*, **52**:64S-95S (1968).
19. U. Smith and J. W. Ryan, Electron microscopy of endothelial and epithelial components of the lung: Correlations of structure and function, *Fed. Proc.*, **32**:1957-1966 (1973).

20. G. G. Pietra, J. P. Szidon, M. M. Leventhal, and A. P. Fishman, Histamine and interstitial pulmonary edema in the dog, *Circ. Res.*, **29**:323-337 (1971).
21. G. Majno, Ultrastructure of the vascular membrane. In *Handbook of Physiology*, Vol. III, Section 2. Edited by W. F. Hamilton and P. Dow. Washington, D.C., American Physiological Society, 1965, pp. 2293-2375.
22. D. Koffler, J. Sandson, R. Carr, and H. G. Kunkel, Immunologic studies concerning the pulmonary lesions in Goodpasture's syndrome, *Am. J. Pathol.*, **54**:293-300 (1969).
23. S. P. Sorokin, A morphological and cytochemical study on the great alveolar cell, *J. Histochem. Cytochem.*, **14**:884-897 (1966).
24. P. Petrik, Fine structural identification of peroxisomes in mouse and rat bronchiolar and alveolar epithelium, *J. Histochem. Cytochem.*, **19**:339-348 (1971).
25. E. E. Schneeberger, A comparative cytochemical study of microbodies (peroxisomes) in great alveolar cells of rodents, rabbit, and monkey, *J. Histochem. Cytochem.*, **20**:180-191 (1972).
26. E. E. Schneeberger, Development of peroxisomes in granular pneumocytes during pre- and post natal growth, *Lab. Invest.*, **27**:581-589 (1972).
27. F. B. Askin and C. Kuhn, The cellular origin of pulmonary surfactant, *Lab. Invest.*, **25**:260-268 (1971).
28. E. E. Schneeberger and M. J. Karnovsky, Substructure of intercellular junctions in freeze-fractured alveolar-capillary membranes of mouse lung, *Circ. Res.*, **38**:404-411 (1976).
29. J. B. Wade and M. J. Karnovsky, The structure of the zonula occludens. A single fibril model based on freeze fracture, *J. Cell Biol.*, **60**:168-180 (1974).
30. C. Kuhn, III, Cytochemistry of pulmonary alveolar epithelial cells, *Am. J. Pathol.*, **53**:809-833 (1968).
31. K. Hitchcock O'Hare, O. K. Reiss, and A. E. Vatter, Esterases in developing and adult rat lung. I. Biochemical and electron microscopic observations, *J. Histochem. Cytochem.*, **19**:97-115 (1971).
32. C. deDuve and P. Baudhuin, Peroxisomes (microbodies) and related particles, *Physiol. Rev.*, **46**:323-357 (1966).
33. C. deDuve, The peroxisome: A new cytoplasmic organelle, *Proc. R. Soc., Lond. [Biol.]*, **173**:71-83 (1969).
34. C. Kuhn, III, A comparison of freeze-substitution with other methods for preservation of the pulmonary alveolar lining layer, *Am. J. Anat.*, **133**:495-508 (1972).
35. T. E. Morgan, Pulmonary surfactant, *N. Engl. J. Med.*, **284**:1185-1193 (1971).
36. D. J. Klass, Immunochemical studies of the protein fraction of pulmonary surface active material, *Am. Rev. Respir. Dis.*, **107**:784-789 (1973).
37. E. M. Scarpelli, D. R. Wolfson, and G. Colacicco, Protein and lipid-protein fractions of lung washings: Immunological characterization, *J. Appl. Physiol.*, **34**:750-753 (1973).
38. A. C. Guyton, H. J. Granger, and A. E. Taylor, Interstitial fluid pressure, *Physiol. Rev.*, **51**:527-563 (1971).

39. R. R. Bruns and G. E. Palade, Studies on blood capillaries. II. Transport of ferritin molecules across the wall of muscle capillaries, *J. Cell Biol.*, **37**:277-299 (1968).
40. A. E. Taylor, A. C. Guyton, and V. S. Vishop, Permeability of the alveolar membrane to solutes, *Circ. Res.*, **16**:353-362 (1965).
41. A. E. Taylor and K. A. Gaar, Jr., Estimation of equivalent pore radii of pulmonary capillary and alveolar membranes, *Am. J. Physiol.*, **218**:1133-1140 (1970).
42. G. G. Pietra, J. P. Szidon, M. M. Leventhal, and A. P. Fishman, Hemoglobin as a tracer in hemodynamic pulmonary edema, *Science*, **166**:1643-1646 (1969).
43. H. H. Shirley, Jr., C. G. Wolfram, K. Wasserman, and H. S. Mayerson, Capillary permeability to macromolecules: Stretched pore phenomenon, *Am. J. Physiol.*, **190**:189-193 (1957).
44. W. L. Hand, J. R. Cantey, and C. G. Hughes, Antibacterial mechanisms of the lower respiratory tract, *J. Clin. Invest.*, **53**:354-362 (1974).
45. A. B. Cohen, Interrelationships between the human alveolar macrophages and alpha-1-antitrypsin, *J. Clin. Invest.*, **52**:2793-2799 (1973).
46. W. C. Tuttle and S. C. Westerberg, Alpha-1 globulin trypsin inhibitor in canine surfactant protein, *Proc. Soc. Exp. Biol. Med.*, **146**:232-235 (1974).
47. R. L. Goodale, B. Goetzman, and M. B. Visscher, Hypoxia and iodoacetic acid and alveolocapillary barrier permeability to albumin, *Am. J. Physiol.*, **219**:1226-1230 (1970).
48. T. Hovig, A. Nicolaysen, and G. Nicolaysen, Ultrastructural studies of the alveolar-capillary barrier in isolated plasma perfused rabbit lungs. Effects of EDTA and of increased capillary pressure, *Acta Physiol. Scand.*, **82**:417-432 (1971).
49. B. W. Goetzman and M. B. Visscher, The effects of alloxan and histamine on the permeability of the pulmonary alveolocapillary barrier to albumin, *J. Physiol.*, **204**:51-61 (1969).
50. G. Gabbiani, M. C. Badonnel, C. Gervasoni, B. Portmann, and G. Majno, Carbon deposition in bronchial and pulmonary vessels in response to vasoactive compounds, *Proc. Soc. Exp. Biol. Med.*, **140**:958-962 (1972).
51. J. D. Brain, Free cells in the lungs, *Arch. Intern. Med.*, **126**:477-487 (1970).
52. H. E. Karrer, Electronmicroscopic study of the phagocytosis process in lung, *J. Biophys. Biochem. Cytol.*, **7**:357-365 (1960).
53. C. K. Drinker and E. Hardenbergh, Absorption from the pulmonary alveoli, *J. Exp. Med.*, **86**:7-17 (1947).
54. A. L. Schultz, J. T. Grisner, S. Wada, and F. Grande, Absorption of albumin from alveoli of perfused dog lungs, *Am. J. Physiol.*, **207**:1300-1304 (1964).
55. E. C. Meyer, E. A. M. Dominquez, and K. G. Bensch, Pulmonary lymphatic and blood absorption of albumin from alveoli. A quantitative comparison, *Lab. Invest.*, **20**:1-8 (1969).
56. P. W. Humphreys, I. C. S. Normand, E. O. R. Reynolds, and L. B. Strang, Pulmonary lymph flow and the uptake of liquid from the lungs of the lamb at the start of breathing, *J. Physiol. (Lond.)*, **193**:1-29 (1967).

57. T. M. Adamson, R. D. H. Boyd, H. S. Platt, and L. B. Strang, Composition of alveolar liquid in the fetal lamb, *J. Physiol. (Lond.)*, **204**:159-168 (1969).
58. S. J. Enna and L. S. Schanker, Absorption of saccharides and urea from rat lung, *Am. J. Physiol.*, **222**:409-414 (1972).
59. S. J. Enna and L. S. Schanker, Absorption of drugs from the rat lung, *Am. J. Physiol.*, **223**:1227-1231 (1972).
60. G. C. Ring, A. S. Blum, T. Kurbatow, W. G. Moss, and W. Smith, Size of microspheres passing through pulmonary circuit in the dog, *Am. J. Physiol.*, **200**:1191-1196 (1961).
61. A. H. Niden and D. M. Aviado, Jr., Effect of pulmonary embolism on the pulmonary circulation with special reference to arteriovenous shunts in the lung, *Circ. Res.*, **4**:67-73 (1956).
62. T. M. Scotti, Disturbances of body water, electrolytes, and circulation of blood. In *Pathology*. Edited by W. A. D. Anderson. St. Louis, Mosby, 1966, p. 102.
63. G. V. Taplin, D. E. Johnson, E. K. Dore, and H. S. Kaplan, Lung photoscans with macroaggregates of human serum radioalbumin, *Health Phys.*, **10**:1219-1227 (1964).
64. T. Nichol and D. L. J. Bilbey, Elimination of macrophage cells of the reticuloendothelial system by way of the bronchial tree, *Nature*, **182**: 192-193 (1958).
65. E. H. Wittels, J. J. Coalson, M. H. Welch, and C. A. Guenter, Pulmonary intravascular leukocyte sequestration. A potential mechanism of lung injury, *Am. Rev. Respir. Dis.*, **109**:502-509 (1974).
66. K. Rybicka, B. D. T. Daly, J. J. Migliore, and J. C. Norman, Intravascular macrophages in normal calf lung. An electron microscopic study, *Am. J. Anat.*, **139**:353-368 (1974).
67. E. E. Schneeberger and E. J. Burger, Intravascular macrophages in cat lungs after open chest ventilation, *Lab. Invest.*, **22**:361-369 (1970).
68. S. W. Woo and J. Hedley-Whyte, Macrophage accumulation and pulmonary edema due to thoractomy and lung over inflation, *J. Appl. Physiol.*, **33**: 14-21 (1972).
69. N. Simionescu, M. Simionescu, and G. E. Palade, Permeability of muscle capillaries to small heme-peptides. Evidence for the existence of transendothelial channels, *J. Cell Biol.*, **64**:586-607 (1975).

Unit Five

THE ROLE OF PULMONARY MACROPHAGES

Nearly a century ago, the Russian zoologist Metchnikoff described large, phagocytic and ameboid cells (the macrophages) and demonstrated that they removed endogenous cell debris, "foreign bodies," and were involved in defending the organism against bacterial invasion. During the last two decades, there has been renewed interest in the structure, biochemistry, function, and origin of macrophages. The pulmonary macrophages defend humans against a wide variety of materials. No doubt their most serious challenge is a wide variety of pathogens, but they also prevent excessive antigenic stimulation. Their ability to identify and destroy neoplastic cells, thus preventing the development of cancer, has also been emphasized. In addition, inhaled particles, effete cells sloughed on to the respiratory surface, occasional red blood cells finding their way into the alveoli, and probably worn-out surfactant, are all ingested by the macrophage.

Unit Five deals comprehensively with the phagocytic functions within the lung. Chapter 19 discusses endocytosis, a primitive mechanism essential to single-celled organisms as they seek adequate nutrition. In addition to molecular transport mechanisms, endocytosis is another way of introducing essential materials into the cell. Even in humans, most cells exhibit some kind of endocytosis, whether it be phagocytosis, pinocytosis, or micropinocytosis. In the lung, alveolar epithelial cells and pulmonary capillary endothelial cells exhibit some endocytosis. Typically, however, we emphasize those cells specialized for phagocytosis. The granulocytic series, also known as the polymorphonuclear leukocytes or neutrophils, are indispensable in the response to infection. They are a mobile and easily recruitable force that deals aggressively with infection. Mononuclear phagocytes, on the other hand, are a resident population present even in the absence of infection or particulate challenge.

Pulmonary macrophages are adaptable both in terms of activity and number. Techniques for quantifying adaptive increases in number are discussed in Chapter 20. The origin and fate of pulmonary macrophages are also discussed. Then the general aspects of energy metabolism in these cells and the essential features of lipid, carbohydrate, and protein metabolism are presented. Next, the morphological, biophysical, and metabolic events which characterize endocytosis and ameboid movement in the macrophage are described. The migratory potential of macrophages and evidence relating to chemotaxis are discussed. The realization is growing that eating and crawling are variations on a single theme. Attention then turns to a variety of in vivo and in vitro models (with the limitations and virtues) for quantifying the lungs' ability to kill pathogens. A summary of environmental, physiologic, and clinical variables which alter this ability is followed by the essential details of the mechanisms of pulmonary microbicidal activity. Although emphasis is placed on intracellular killing mechanisms, external influences on macrophage function and possible extracellular killing mechanisms are also considered.

Chapter 21 discusses macrophage and pulmonary clearance as they defend the body against excessive antigenic stimulation. At other times clearance mechanisms may cooperate with the immune system. Thus, pulmonary macrophages may either suppress or enhance the immunogenicity of antigens. Chapter 26 discusses the pivotal role of macrophages in the pathogenesis of certain lung diseases.

Macrophages, emerging from their historically defined role as mere resident scavenger cells, are being recognized as mobile and versatile cells performing many functions essential to health. They are important to antimicrobial strategies, cell-mediated immunity, allograft rejection, delayed sensitivity reactions, and are involved in the pathogenesis of autoimmune diseases. They have extensive synthetic potential and may secrete such diverse substances as lysosomal enzymes, interferon, and certain components of complement. All these functions require full exploration.

The relationship between the alveolar lining fluid and macrophage function is little understood. The fluids contain not only surfactant but a variety of opsonins and other factors which may influence macrophage ingestion and killing. Is the fluid lining involved in adaptive changes? Mediators serving not only as chemotactic factors but as signals to stimulate increases in enzymatic content are likely present. Other agents may stimulate mitosis among macrophage precursors present in alveolar walls or more distant bone marrow.

Even basic quantitative questions about alveolar macrophage function remain unanswered. What is the average surface area monitored per alveolus and the average particle-to-macrophage distance? At what speeds do macrophages move in situ? Essential stages in the life history of macrophages remain undescribed. How and when do cells destined to become pulmonary macrophages move from the blood to the interstitium and then from the interstitium on to the alveolar surface? What is the role of the interstitial macrophage and how does it differ from the surface or alveolar macrophage? Along with awareness of these unanswered questions, there is the conviction that pulmonary macrophages have a central role in the maintenance of the lung as a clean and sterile surface suitable for gas exchange. Further research is needed since control of disease stems from the recognition of factors important to the defense of the organism.

Joseph D. Brain

19

Phagocytes in the Lungs
Incidence, General Behavior, and Phylogeny

SERGEI P. SOROKIN

Harvard University School of Public Health
Boston, Massachusetts

I. Enumeration of the Phagocytes

Having an extensive contact with the bloodstream and an intimate exposure to atmospheric gases, dusts, and airborne microbes, the lungs both require and obtain access to all the kinds of phagocytic cells that travel in the bloodstream, and all of them can be found in one pulmonary compartment or another at one time or another. Other cells more specific to the lungs variously contribute in great or small degree to the phagocytic capacity of the organ. Through ingestion and processing of undesirable foreign materials these phagocytic cells collectively contribute in a major way to the cellular defenses of the lungs, and only exceptionally do their actions make matters worse. All these phagocytic cells, their general properties and lineage, together with their interactions within compartments of the lungs, form the materials of this chapter. Further discussion of aspects of this broad topic will be found in other chapters of this monograph, whereas fuller consideration of the phagocytic leukocytes will naturally be found among extended writings on hematology [29,48].

Before the turn of the last century, Ilya Metchnikoff had recognized two principal phagocytes among the migratory cells of the blood: the microphages, or polymorphonuclear granulocytes (Figs. 1-4) and the macrophages, or phagocytic mononuclear cells; and the terms he used rank these cells in order of appetence. In mammals the former normally are the commonest leukocytes to be encountered in the bloodstream. The latter circulate in adults as monocytes, which are large rounded leukocytes with a reniform nucleus. Upon leaving the bloodstream they become transformed into macrophages. Since both types of cells are able to infiltrate pulmonary tissues, they serve as the chief phagocytes of extrinsic origin to be found in that organ.

Besides these two chief phagocytes, a second granulocyte, the eosinophil, engages in phagocytosis to a limited degree (Figs. 5,6). This was not appreciated by the great pioneer hematologists Paul Ehrlich and Metchnikoff, not because the cell was unknown [111], but, because when confronted with foreign particles or bacteria, these cells usually show little inclination to ingest either. Eosinophils are almost always present in the lungs even when they are absent from other organs of the body [9]; in the lungs they are usually confined to connective tissue surrounding the bronchial tree, which they share with mast cells and possibly basophils. The latter, respectively, connective tissue and circulating elements, are functionally related cells both capable of ameboid motion and phagocytosis but rarely observed to engage in them. Like the gamut of immunologically active leukocytes (large and small lymphocytes, plasma cells, etc.), the basophils (Fig. 9) and mast cells (Figs. 7,8) are more conspicuous for interacting with the principal phagocytes than for their own phagocytic actions. Their main preoccupations are with the synthesis and secretion of potent vasoactive agents.

Among phagocytic cells with a specifically pulmonary character, the alveolar macrophages occupy the first but not necessarily only place (Fig. 10). These cells display most of the traits typical of macrophages, but they also exhibit certain peculiarities that set them apart from other members of this class. Alveolar macrophages have an unusual propensity for functioning primarily on alveolar surfaces rather than within the tissues, and when studied biochemically are seen to require for phagocytosis a higher level of energy supplied through oxidative phosphorylation than is needed by comparable numbers of peritoneal macrophages [117,185]. Despite these and other distinguishing characteristics of alveolar macrophages, it is not certain whether they constitute a homogeneous population of similarly derived cells, or whether some originate, for example, from circulating monocytes and others from precursors within the lungs. Further discussion on this point is given in the succeeding chapter [36].

A second category of pulmonary macrophages inhabits the various connective tissue regions within the lungs. If these cells might share a common lineage with alveolar macrophages, they are to a degree distinguishable from them in a functional sense. Accordingly, the pulmonary connective tissue macrophages are here accorded an independent status, at least for purposes of discussion. It might be added that just as elsewhere in the body, fibrocytes in the lungs can be provoked to ingest small amounts of colloidal particles (trypan blue, india ink) if these are administered systemically long enough to exceed the collective storage capacity of resident macrophages and those widely scattered outside the lungs. Furthermore, they recently have been shown to ingest and digest collagen fibrils from their surroundings, thereby serving as a vector in the remodeling that accompanies normal growth [256].

As for the remaining cells of the lungs, modest endocytotic activity is attributable to some cells of the endodermal pulmonary epithelium, certainly to squamous alveolar epithelial cells and possibly to others in the bronchial and bronchiolar epithelium. Whether or not this activity strikes one as "phagocytosis" as originally understood (uptake and digestion of foreign materials by cells) may depend on one's understanding of the degree of digestion implied by the term. Among different cell types the ingestive, or endocytotic, phase of this process may be carried out at different scales; both liquids and solids may be taken up in relatively large or relatively small packets. Recognizing this, Komiyama and Spicer [127] propose using "macroendocytosis" to cover cellular ingestion whether of solids (phagocytosis) or liquids (pinocytosis) into cytoplasmic vacuoles having a diameter larger than 1000 Å and "microendocytosis" (microphagocytosis or rhopheocytosis and micropinocytosis) to cover incorporation into smaller vesicles. Apart from scale, there may be metabolic differences between these two processes (Ref. 205, p. 314), as well as between (macro)pinocytosis and phagocytosis, although these differences have been spelled out in only a few experimental cell systems and likely do not apply to all animal cells. Among the mammals, most cells seem to favor microendocytosis, but phagocytes favor macroendocytosis on the whole, even if macrophages engage in both. In the case of the bronchial epithelium, microendocytosis seems the appropriate term to use, whereas in squamous alveolar cells the truth might lie closer to the borderline between terms.

There are gaps in our knowledge of the phagocytic potential of endothelial cells that line the different divisions of pulmonary and bronchial blood vessels, for these are not all alike. Considerable experimental attention has been brought to the matter of transport across the pulmonary alveolar capillaries, which are lined by a nonfenestrated endothelium somewhat similar to the endothelium lining capillaries of muscle, and this is reviewed in detail by Schneeberger [218] elsewhere in this book. If some transcapillary transport of large molecules occurs through clefts between the cells, some involves the formation of microendocytotic vesicles and crossing of the endothelium, either within the vesicles or possibly through transitory pores formed by fusion of the vesicles into a continuous passageway across, as has been shown in capillaries of the diaphragm [226]. Within pulmonary lymphatics the clefts between endothelial cells are much larger than between alveolar capillaries, and so translymphatic exchange proceeds mainly by

FIGURE 1 Acid phosphatase in an unfixed smear of human blood (azo dye method, AS-TR phosphate). Both granular and diffuse reactions are present (black) and other cellular detail is somewhat suppressed. (A) Eosinophil with reactive lysosomes encircling the cell center, nucleus at upper right. (B) Basophil (?) with large reactive granules obscuring the nucleus. (C) Top: Neutrophil (microphage) with prominent nuclear lobes and inconspicuously reactive cytoplasmic granules; Below: Monocyte with strongly reactive cytoplasm both in granules and diffusely. (D) Top: Lymphocyte with diffuse and some granular reactivity (arrows), other lymphocytes may be unreactive; Below: A second monocyte, or possibly a large lymphocyte.

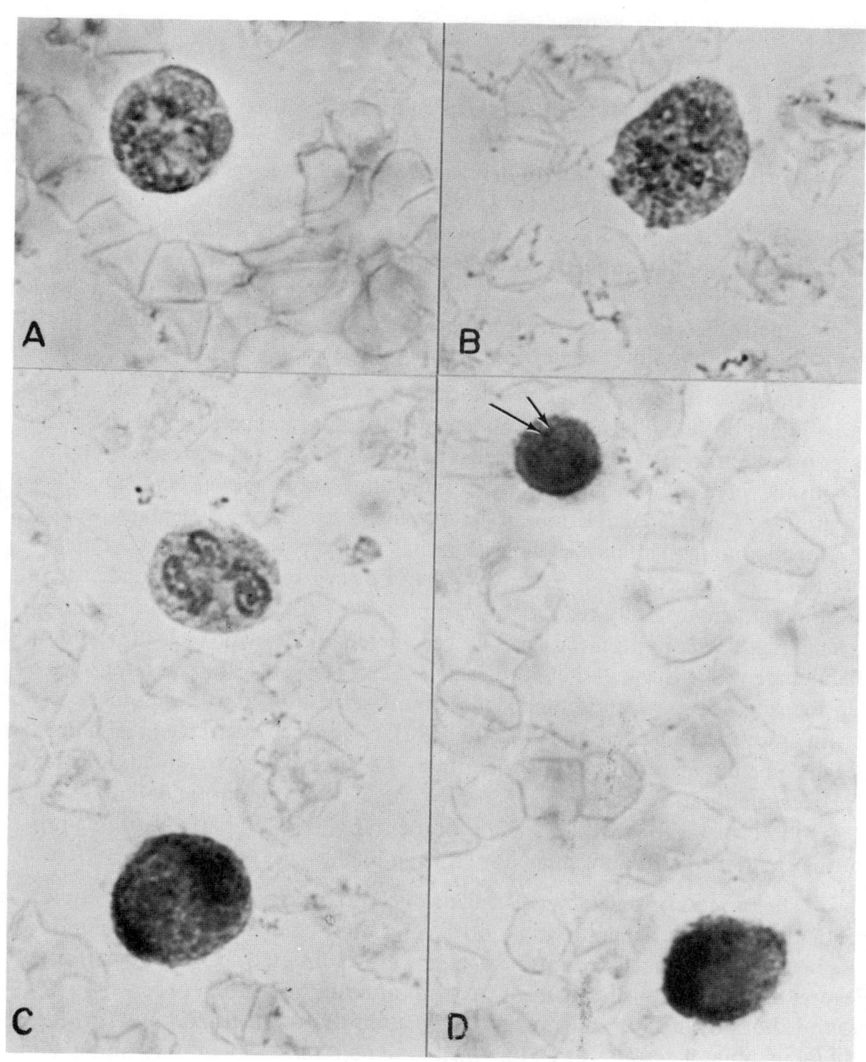
A
B
C
D

this route. Consequently, however tenuous the similarity might be between the processes of phagocytosis and transendothelial transport in the capillaries, it is still more remote in the lymphatics.

II. Functional Attributes of Phagocytic Cells

Metchnikoff observed that microphages and macrophages, the principal blood phagocytes, both struggle against a wide variety of foreign bodies and living organisms by attempting to ingest them and then to degrade them by intracellular digestion, and he understood these cellular actions to be the basis of an organisms's inflammatory response to wounding. This theory is brilliantly argued in Metchnikoff's *Lectures on the Comparative Pathology of Inflammation* [169], from which many points raised in succeeding pages are taken.

Among vertebrates, cellular defenses nonetheless are carried out in a milieu replete with both highly specific and less specific humoral agents, and the phagocytes use them to advantage. These agents act on noxious particles or infective organisms, serve to draw phagocytes to them, and assist these cells in subsequent reactions to the invaders. Humoral defense mechanisms are particularly well developed among mammals. The notion that they are important had arisen before the end of the eighteenth century when Edward Jenner [108] made use of a serum antigen-antibody reaction in demonstrating that acquisition of immunity to smallpox develops after patients are vaccinated with cowpox. By the end of the nineteenth century, earlier studies by Pasteur (1822-1895) and later ones by von Behring, Kitasato, and others had demonstrated the clinical usefulness of serum antibody reactions, and from the work of Ehrlich, their chemical nature began to be understood. At the same time, the discovery of serum complement [34] revealed that nonspecific agents also participate in humoral defenses. The interactions of these substances with phagocytes will only lightly be alluded to in this chapter, their importance notwithstanding.

The process of phagocytosis begins once the phagocytes reach the site of particulate or bacterial contamination as a result of chemotactic attraction or else because of chance encounters made during undirected scavenging patrols. Several distinct actions make up the entire process; these are in order, *recognition* of the foreign substance by the phagocyte followed by *attachment* to the cell membrane; *ingestion,* or endocytosis; and *digestion.* Sometimes undigested residues are excreted (exocytosis), but they often remain stored in the cytoplasm. Before phagocytosis begins, motile leukocytes may be drawn to the arena of struggle against invasive organisms by chemical attraction or chemotaxis, and a prerequisite to all the preceding is that phagocytes normally can invade body tissues because they do not possess the property of "contact inhibition" which brings about an arrest of motility after one cell with this property touches another. It is possessed by fibrocytes and other sessile cells of tissues but may be lost if the cells undergo malignant change into sarcomatous cells [11].

A. Aids to Phagocytosis: Chemotaxis

Many kinds of substances attract, or are positively chemotactic for phagocytes. As a result, cellular motion becomes polarized toward the attractant and increases in speed. As examples of agents exerting positive chemotaxis, Metchnikoff lists leucin, an oxidation product of albumin, solutions of gluten and casein, and various products of bacterial cells. Metchnikoff also recognized negative chemotaxis, or the repulsive action of agents on phagocytes, and among negatively chemotactic agents he includes virulent bacteria like those of chicken cholera, certain organic solvents, bile, and quinine. In our time we emphasize positive chemotaxis and prefer to explain away apparent cases of negative chemotaxis in other ways—for instance in terms of a bacterium's capacity to resist phagocytosis—or else to pay it little attention at all. Attractants evidently can have a variety of chemical configurations. Besides the above they include starch grains, paraffin oil, and many other carbohydrates, lipids, and proteins. Metchnikoff had seen that mammalian leukocytes in general are more sensitive to chemical excitation than are phagocytes of frogs, and we now realize that this reflects an amplification of chemical chemotactic effect by humoral mechanisms better developed in mammals than in amphibians. Furthermore, many substances are chemotactic only in the presence of plasma or serum. For years it was thought that the basic chemotactic response, either positive or negative, is the same in isolated microphages and macrophages; but at least after serum is added, differential phagocytic responses begin to be plain to see. Under these conditions *many substances either attract both of the major phagocytes or only the microphages* [229].

Substances have been tested for chemotaxis by placing them in a small chamber separated by a millipore filter from a suspension of the phagocytes being studied. Optimum pore sizes are 3 μm or more for microphages, 5 μm for eosinophils, and 8 μm for macrophages. After a time the number of cells to migrate through the filter can be counted on the filter surface facing the chemotactic agent, and this forms the basis for rough quantitation of the response [35]. In this way it has also been shown that microphages migrate and penetrate interstices most readily, peritoneal macrophages less readily, and alveolar macrophages scarcely at all [269]. At times, the alveolar macrophages seem more preoccupied with ingesting the filter than trying to migrate through it, and so data for migration rates might not fully reflect the cells' migratory capacity in vivo.

FIGURE 2 Microphage (polymorphonuclear granulocyte) in a pulmonary alveolar capillary. An intensely heterochromatic nucleus, a sparsity of granular endoplasmic reticulum together with a scattering of free ribosomes, a Golgi apparatus reduced to a small perinuclear remnant, and a heterogeny of smallish, ovoid, cytoplasmic granules characterize this postmitotic cell.

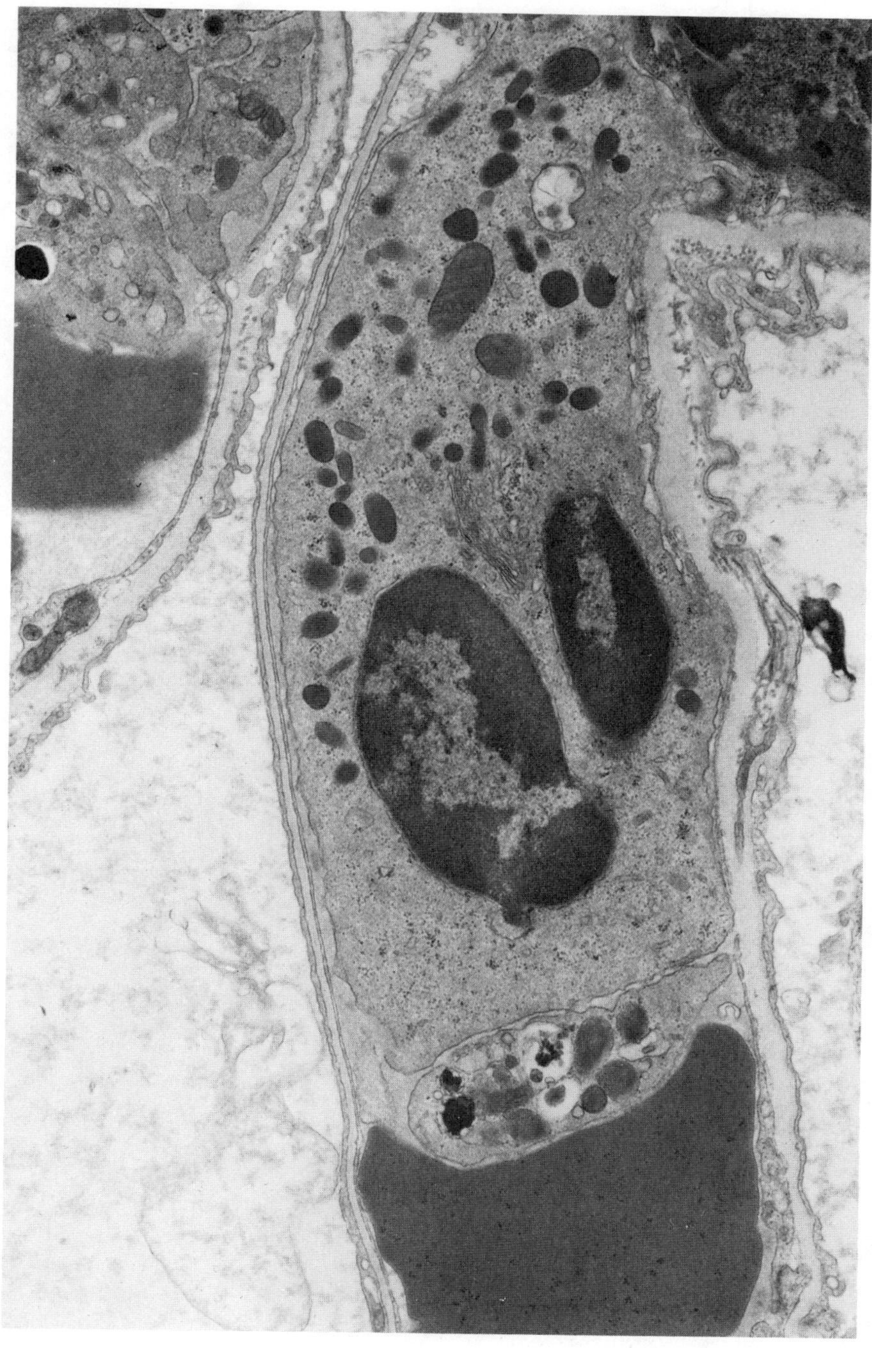

FIGURE 3 Microphage recovered from pulmonary lavage of a mouse some hours after exposure to an aerosol of iron oxide particles (black granules). The cell has taken up the iron but unlike alveolar macrophages does not convert any into ferritin, which otherwise would appear as a fine stippling in the cytoplasm. Compare with Figs. 12 and 18.

FIGURE 4 Detail of the perinuclear region in a microphage showing a centriole and other cytoplasmic detail. The outer membrane of the nuclear envelope has no ribosomes attached.

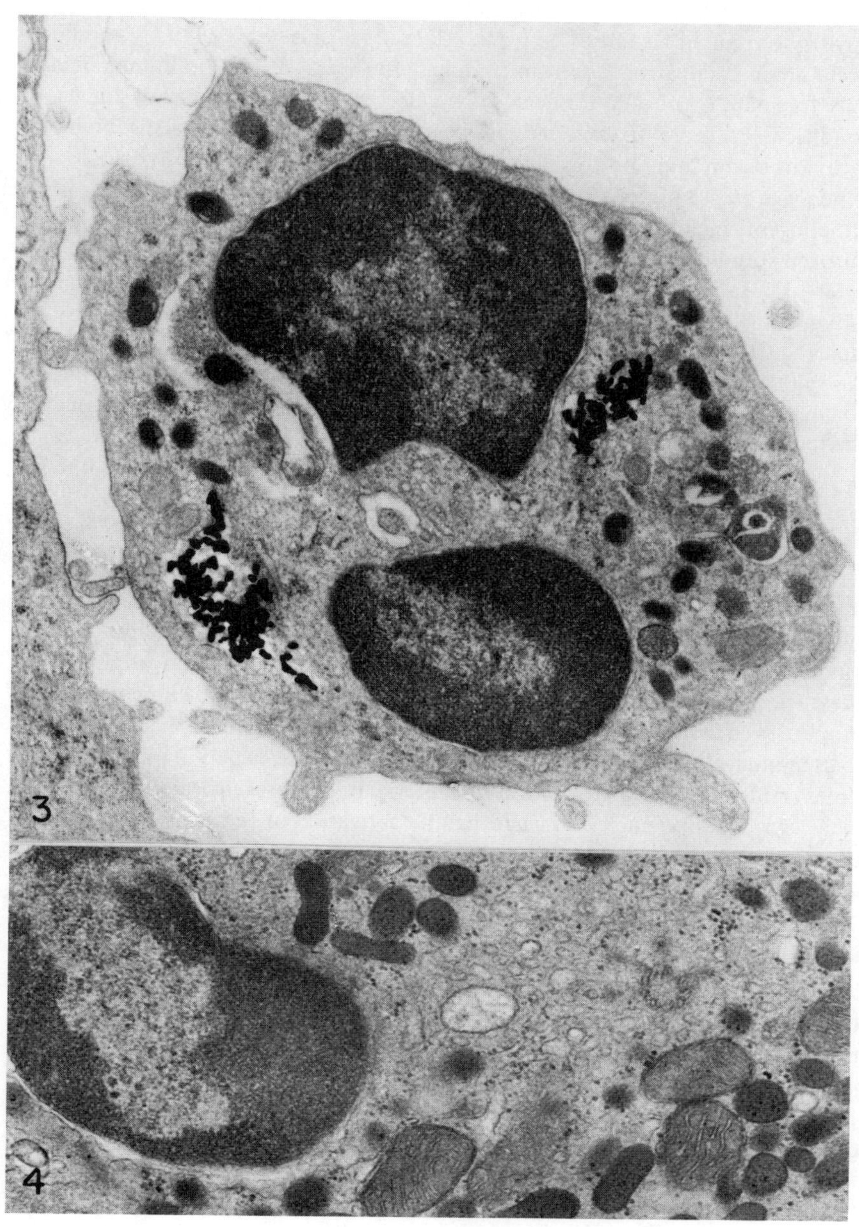

3
4

Recent studies on chemotaxis have focused on those agents chemotactic in vitro that might also be effective in intact organisms. Several likely candidates occur among derivatives of serum complement (Sec. II.B), but in human beings only fragment C3a has so far been shown effective under more-or-less clinical conditions. A more rigorous case has been made for agents formed by interaction of serum immunoglobulins IgG and IgM with a neutral sulfhydryl-dependent protease present in lysosome-like bodies (Sec. II.E) of leukocytes [94]. Other agents include a heat-stable (MW ~12,500) factor released by antigen- or mitogen-stimulated lymphocytes that is chemotactic only to homologous monocytes [3]. In vitro eosinophils respond to several factors, but in vivo they are drawn especially by antigen-antibody complexes in serum [215,237] and by a factor (ECF-A) apparently released by sensitized mast cells in the lungs [118]. Basophilic responses have not yet been adequately tested (Table 1). Among peculiarities of the in vivo response, once macrophages begin to arrive in quantity the microphages often stop coming.

B. Serum Complement: Promotion of Phagocytic Actions

Certain components of serum complement are among the most carefully scrutinized promoters of chemotaxis and phagocytosis. Operation of this humoral system unquestionably mediates much of the phagocytes' response to many kinds of antigen-antibody complexes, for the system becomes activated in the presence of these complexes, and some resulting products have chemotactic properties as indicated below. These generally produce a microphagic rather than monocytic response [229]. Chemotactic derivatives of complement sometimes result from the direct action of bacterial or cell proteinases on complement components (Table 2) rather than by activation of the entire system [271], but on the whole, complement-mediated reactions contribute a quantitatively uncertain proportion to the sum of chemotactic factors that act upon phagocytes in vivo.

Complement is a system of serum proteins whose concerted action serves in the capacity of a generalized humoral defense mechanism. It brings about the lysis of sensitized red blood cells or bacteria and participates in several of the humoral reactions that help to make up the inflammatory response to injury. In experiments using serum from goats immunized against cholera, Bordet [34] showed that if immune serum were heated to 58°C for 1 hr, it became incapable of preventing the growth of cholera subsequently seeded into it, but if the same serum were added to fresh, nonimmune guinea pig serum and the mixture were seeded, the bacteria rapidly became lysed. That is to say, a heat-labile but nonspecific serum factor (complement or "alexin") was necessary for the immune reaction to occur in lysis. More recent studies have used the lysis of

TABLE 1 Some Chemotactic Factors for Leukocytes[a]

1. Factors for microphages in vitro

   Complement derivatives C3a, C5a, $C\overline{567}$ (C3a also in vivo)
   Soluble products of bacterial metabolism
   Hydrolyzed fragments of collagen
   Factors released by antigen-stimulated lymphocytes
   Leucoegresin from action of leukocyte protease I and IgG (in vivo)

2. Factors for eosinophils in vitro

   Complement derivatives C3a, C5a, $C\overline{567}$ (C3a also in vivo)
   Soluble products of bacterial metabolism
   Product of antigen-stimulated lymphocytes made eosinophil-specific after interaction with relevant immune complexes
   Eosinophil chemotactic factor (ECF-A) released by lung tissue during anaphylaxis
   Specific factor produced through interaction of immune complexes and guinea pig serum (ECF-C)

3. Factors for monocytes in vitro[b]

   Complement derivatives C5a, C3a (C3a also in vivo)
   Serum factor (not $C\overline{567}$) produced by addition of immune complexes
   Soluble products of bacterial metabolism
   Monocyte-specific lymphokine from antigen- or mitogen-stimulated lymphocytes
   Cationic peptides (?) released by microphages
   Reaction product of microphage protease II and IgG (in vivo)

4. Factor for basophils in vivo (Sec. III.E)

   Basophil-specific lymphokine from antigen-stimulated lymphocytes

5. Factors for lymphocytes in vitro

   Lymphocyte-specific lymphokine from antigen-stimulated lymphocytes
   Reaction product of microphage protease II and IgM (in vivo)

[a]All examples, except no. 4 are based on data from Refs. 94 and 270 and others.
[b]Response varies depending on source of mononuclear cells and method of harvesting.

sensitized erythrocytes as an analytical model for the action of complement. In this, the "classic complement pathway," nine sequentially acting components have been identified. These consist of 11 proteins making up some 10% of the globulin fraction of normal serum. Most of them are β-globulins, although two

TABLE 2 Reactions of Complement

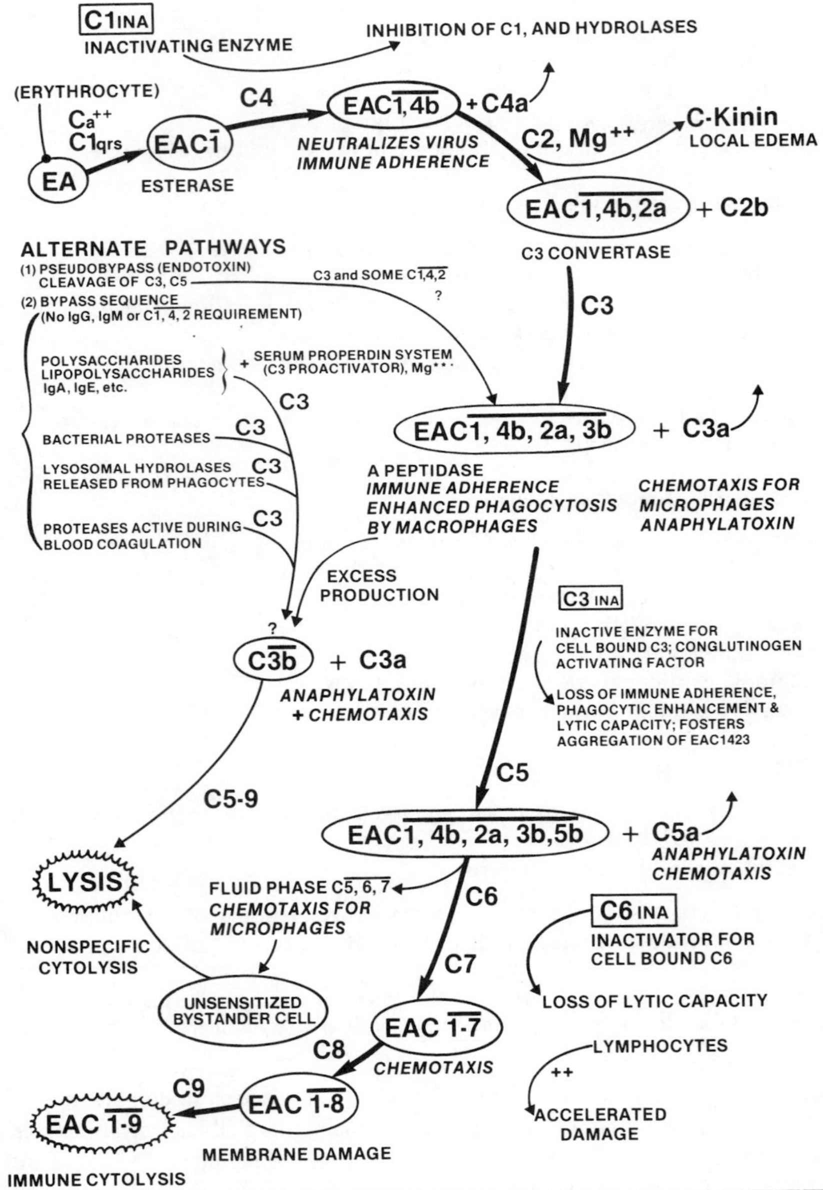

CLASSIC COMPLEMENT PATHWAY
Immune Complex via C1,4,2:
IgG or IgM ANTIBODY REQUIREMENT
C1INA
INACTIVATING ENZYME
INHIBITION OF C1, AND HYDROLASES
(ERYTHROCYTE)
Ca++
C1qrs
EA
EAC1
ESTERASE
C4
EAC1,4b
+C4a
NEUTRALIZES VIRUS
IMMUNE ADHERENCE
C2, Mg++
C-Kinin
LOCAL EDEMA
EAC1,4b,2a
+ C2b
C3 CONVERTASE
ALTERNATE PATHWAYS
(1) PSEUDOBYPASS (ENDOTOXIN) CLEAVAGE OF C3, C5
C3 and SOME C1,4,2
?
(2) BYPASS SEQUENCE
(No IgG, IgM or C1, 4, 2 REQUIREMENT)
POLYSACCHARIDES
LIPOPOLYSACCHARIDES
IgA, IgE, etc.
+ SERUM PROPERDIN SYSTEM (C3 PROACTIVATOR), Mg++
C3
BACTERIAL PROTEASES
LYSOSOMAL HYDROLASES RELEASED FROM PHAGOCYTES
PROTEASES ACTIVE DURING BLOOD COAGULATION
EAC1, 4b, 2a, 3b
+ C3a
A PEPTIDASE
IMMUNE ADHERENCE
ENHANCED PHAGOCYTOSIS
BY MACROPHAGES
CHEMOTAXIS FOR MICROPHAGES
ANAPHYLATOXIN
EXCESS PRODUCTION
C3 INA
INACTIVE ENZYME FOR CELL BOUND C3; CONGLUTINOGEN ACTIVATING FACTOR
LOSS OF IMMUNE ADHERENCE, PHAGOCYTIC ENHANCEMENT & LYTIC CAPACITY; FOSTERS AGGREGATION OF EAC1423
?
C3b
+ C3a
ANAPHYLATOXIN
+ CHEMOTAXIS
C5
C5-9
EAC1, 4b, 2a, 3b,5b
+ C5a
ANAPHYLATOXIN
CHEMOTAXIS
LYSIS
FLUID PHASE C5, 6, 7
CHEMOTAXIS FOR MICROPHAGES
C6
C6 INA
INACTIVATOR FOR CELL BOUND C6
NONSPECIFIC CYTOLYSIS
C7
LOSS OF LYTIC CAPACITY
UNSENSITIZED BYSTANDER CELL
EAC 1-7
C8
CHEMOTAXIS
LYMPHOCYTES
++
ACCELERATED DAMAGE
C9
EAC 1-8
EAC 1-9
MEMBRANE DAMAGE
IMMUNE CYTOLYSIS

are γ-globulins (C1q, one of 3 components of C1; and C8) and three are α-globulins (C1s, another component of C1; C1 inactivator, and C9). They range in molecular weight from 79,000 to 400,000. Some are enzymes, others are activators, and none have yet been fully characterized chemically. Their nomenclature is tentative and rather abstract, the numbering of the complement components being in order of discovery. As mentioned, activation usually is by soluble or cell-bound antigen-antibody complexes involving serum immunoglobulins of the IgG or IgM classes. In that case the reactions begin with the first component of complement, C1. Other normally occurring serum proteins like the β-globulin properdin [140], as well as certain proteolytic enzymes, sometimes activate other complement components, usually C3, thereby bypassing the initial reactions of the classical sequence; this entry into complement reactions is termed an alternate complement pathway. Once activated, whether through C1, C3, or possibly C5 [141], the reactions proceed from the point of activation to completion in the absence of cells or cell membranes. Several inactivating enzymes are normally present in the serum and interact with the system. The many steps in the sequence renders the system finely controllable through use of activators, inhibitors, and competitive reactions.

Classic and alternate complement pathways are schematized in Table 2; detailed discussion of the reactions can be found in thorough reviews written by "complementologists" [174,220]. The complete reaction sequence through C9 leads not only to lysis of sensitized eucaryotic cells but often to destruction of certain viruses as well. Terminal reactions lead to formation of ~80-100 Å holes in erythrocyte membranes. In the case of some bacteria this hole formation exposes the inner mucopeptide layer of the cell wall to the action of serum lysozyme, a hydrolytic enzyme produced by macrophages [241] and microphages as well, that splits the 1,4-glycoside bonds of the basic wall structure and converts the bacteria into spheroplasts. A process similar to lysis is used to destroy endotoxins [83], which are lipopolysaccharide complexes that make up part of the wall of gram-negative bacteria.

The importance of the complement system is not only for lysis but equally for the biological activities of cell-bound intermediates as well as of soluble derivatives that produce chemotaxis and promote the release of vasoactive agents (C-kinin, C3a, C5a). Fragments C3a and C5a sometimes are called anaphylatoxin, for they mediate the anaphylactic or toxic response to material against which the organism had previously become sensitized. They can be generated by both classic and alternate complement pathways [50,141]. Their appearance in the serum leads to degranulation and release of histamine and other vasoactive substances from mast cells and platelets, although the exact response varies considerably with the species [119]; in human beings, for example, both C3a and C5a are normally inactivated by a carboxypeptidase in the serum [33]. Histamine release in turn brings about an increase in vascular permeability in post-capillary venules and contraction of smooth muscle notably in the bronchi and alimentary canal. The contraction is blocked by the administration of antihistamines and characteristically diminishes after repeated exposures to the complement derivatives, eventually to reach a refractory state termed tachyphylaxis. Furthermore, through the binding of cell bound intermediates EAC $\overline{1,4b}$ and EAC $\overline{1,4b,2a,3b}$ to receptor sites on other nonsensitized cells, aggregation or *immune adherence* is produced. A similar reaction may result in the binding of particulate antigen-antibody complexes to nonsensitized erythrocytes, which is followed by phagocytosis and destruction of both cells and adherents by macrophages. Activation of C3 alone produces a fragment that also promotes immune adherence, although it is less effective than EAC $\overline{1\text{-}4}$. A derivative of activated C3 (C3b or C3o) in any case attaches itself to sensitized bacteria or cells and "opsonizes" them, coating them so as to enhance phagocytosis. Although other serum factors, notably IgG in high concentrations, opsonizes particles or cells, C3b is an important agent, because C3 is normally abundant in serum (900-1500 μg/ml), far ahead of all other complement factors in this respect [220].

If it is now clear that there are many ways to activate complement (Table 2), including activation of C3 by components of the blood coagulation mechanism, it also appears that complement sometimes initiates coagulation, and this complicates efforts to assess the magnitude of complement's role in defense. In the lungs all the preceding interactions naturally can occur in all vascularized compartments.

C. Phagocytosis: Recognition and Attachment

In order to be ingested by mammalian phagocytes, intrusive particles or cells frequently must first become coated, or opsonized, through interaction with serum. Both heat-stable (specific antibody) and heat-labile (complement) opsonins are recognized, and both make use of specific antigenic sites on the particles; the phagocytosis promoted has been termed immune phagocytosis. Such a thing as nonimmune phagocytosis also exists, and this is observable in many cells, notably protozoans, which lack any blood vascular system, let alone humoral factors. Chapman-Andresen [43] has described pinocytosis in detail in amebas, finding it similar in essentials to other ingestive processes, and this work is a cornerstone of modern studies on nonimmune endocytosis. Elements of the nonimmune mechanism as seen in amebas are retained in mammalian cells, as considerable experimental work attests. Finally, there is nonphagocytosis, which results from negative chemotactic factors released by certain infectious organisms, or else from chemical properties of their surface coats: The polysaccharide capsules of pneumococci, the superficial polypeptide coat-

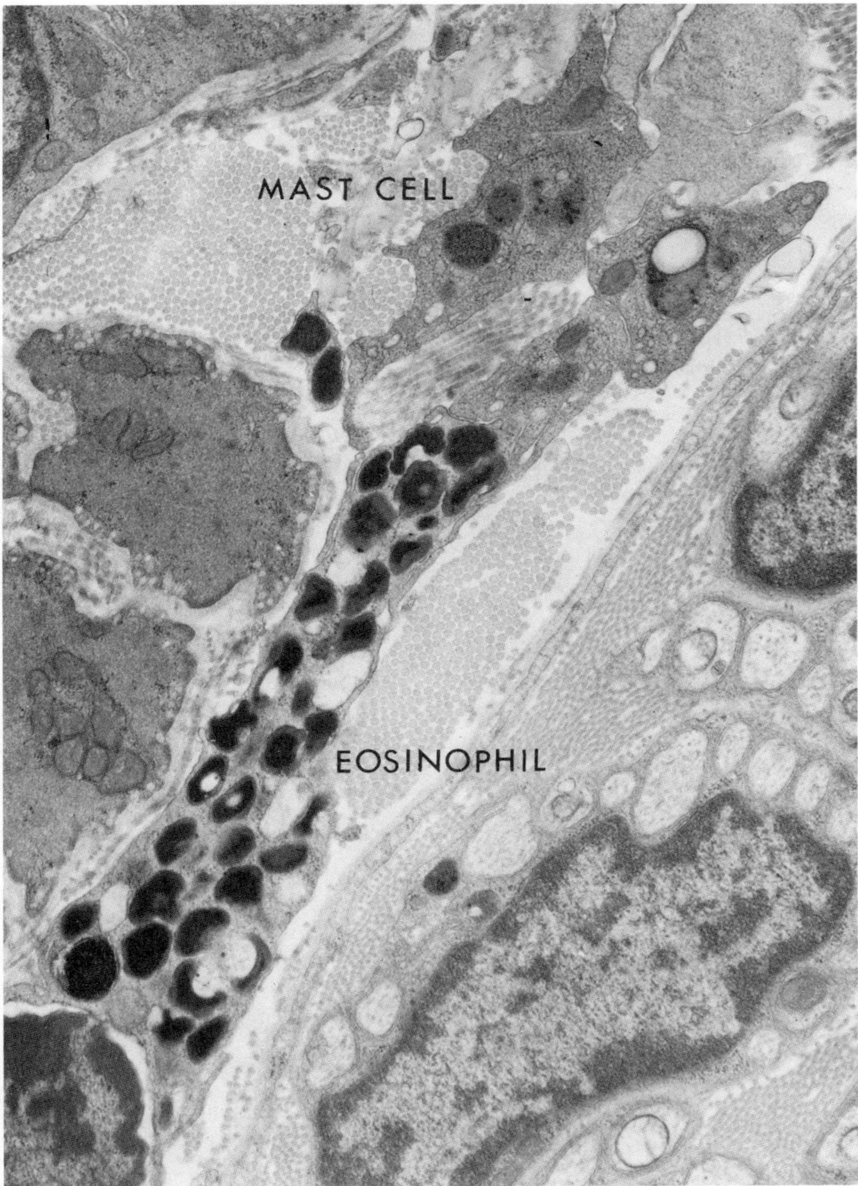

FIGURE 5 Eosinophil in bronchiolar connective tissue. In its characteristic intrapulmonary locus, the cell extends between smooth muscle (left) and an unmyelinated nerve (right) to contact processes from a mast cell. Specific granules of eosinophils are both larger and more uniform in size than those of microphages, and they have a dense core.

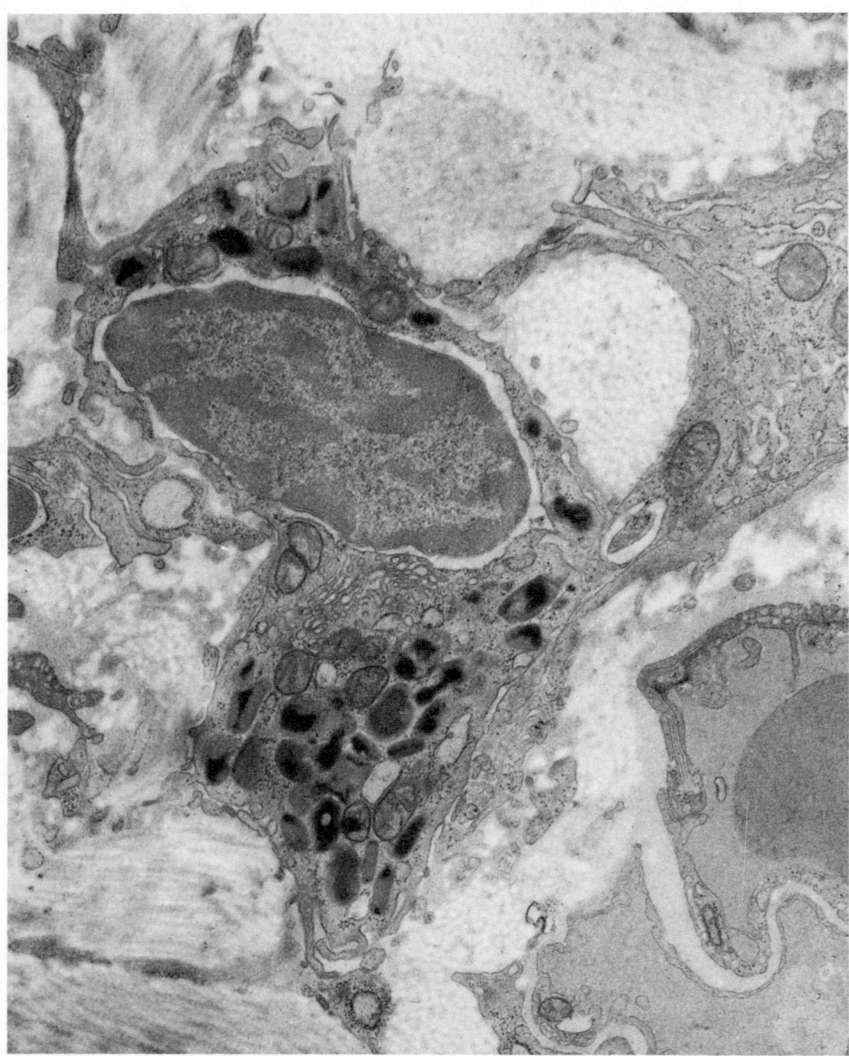

FIGURE 6 Eosinophils can penetrate even densely collagenous tissues and in passing frequently brush surfaces of the fixed cells they encounter, as shown here in the lungs.

ing of anthrax bacilli, and a variety of other substances in other organisms protect them from ingestion and place them in the class of extracellular pathogens.

Recognition of both solid particulates and dissolved matter is preceded by cell contact, and if endocytosis is to follow, the materials become attached to the cell surface, either directly onto the cell membrane or indirectly onto surface coatings. Functionally, "receptors" can be said to exist for materials taken in by both immune and nonimmune phagocytosis, and much effort has been directed toward determining the properties of these receptors. It is nonetheless difficult to integrate information on the receptors with other new-found knowledge about the structure and dynamics of the cell membrane (Sec. II.D). As our concepts about membrane organization—and even what is the "membrane" and what the "coating"—change almost daily, little written about them today will be credible tomorrow.

In immune or antibody-mediated phagocytosis, relatively few kinds of specific receptors serve to bind a wide variety of substances. A common coating by serum antibodies or complement proteins on dissimilar particles makes them all appear similar to the phagocytes, exciting them into a stereotyped response, which likely involves attachment of the particulate matter to the phagocytic surface at receptor sites specific for the antibody or complement moieties. That the cell membrane is involved in initial events of phagocytosis seems indicated by the finding that antimembrane antibodies to macrophages can bring about a decrease in the ingestion of IgG opsonized particles but not of yeast cell walls or polystyrene spheres which do not need to be opsonized by immunoglobulin to be taken up efficiently [101]. Another is that sensitized target cells either in the presence or absence of complement often surround a macrophage and closely contact its plasmalemma [42], providing an appearance suggestive of immunochemical binding. This type of rosette is less readily formed where microphages are substituted for macrophages.

Cytochemical techniques using antibodies labeled with fluorescein or peroxidase markers have begun to be used in research on the binding that precedes phagocytosis. For example, if IgG antibody-producing lymphocytes (B-lymphocytes) are incubated at 4°C with a marked antiimmunoglobulin IgG, the surfaces of the lymphocytes can be seen to become coated with the anti-IgG. If these cells are exposed to macrophages at 37°C, they are shortly ingested; but if they are first kept for a while at room temperature, the lymphocytes undergo "capping," when all sites binding the anti-IgG become concentrated at one pole (the uroid) due to translocation of peripheral portions of the plasma membrane. When these capped lymphocytes are given to the macrophages, the latter attach to the caps but do not ingest the lymphocytes [88]. Binding therefore can occur without subsequent phagocytosis. For this to occur, attachment must be made between many sites on the surface of the ingestible particles and on the macrophage.

As the preceding and earlier studies indicate, mammalian macrophages have immune receptors for the F_c segment of IgG (the carboxy terminal end of the molecule, opposed to the amino terminal ends that combine with antigen). They possess other receptors for complement factor C3b [95], and together these enable the cells to bind opsonized particles. Microphages apparently also have receptors for IgG, since they ingest erythrocytes opsonized with this antibody; however, macrophages require less IgG to do the same [135]. Macrophages also can bind free globulin when it is present in fairly high concentrations, but granulocytes cannot. Such bound antibodies are called cytophilic antibodies. They seem rather loosely attached to the cell surface, inasmuch as they readily exchange with antibodies of different specificity at 37°C [25], and they apparently have little to do with phagocytic activity. Indeed, membrane receptor sites for cytophilic and particle-associated (opsonizing) antibody may well be different, as Rabinovitch has suggested [204,205]. For all these and other reasons [243] it is prudent to make few generalizations about immune receptors until more comprehensive information is at hand.

Opsonization of nonsensitized materials can occur through immune adherence following activation of complement, and nonimmune animals sometimes opsonize materials if the alternate complement pathway becomes activated by bacterial polysaccharides or by immunoglobulins like IgA that do not activate the C142 pathway (Table 1). Being opsonized "by hook or by crook," such materials subsequently are bound to phagocytes and ingested using the mechanisms of immune phagocytosis. Mammalian phagocytes, particularly macrophages, also ingest materials in the absence of serum, when membrane receptors for IgG or complement are unlikely to be involved. In this case they take up much the same materials that fibrocytes do (a number of bacteria, polystyrene particles, metal oxides, silica, and cells "artificially opsonized" with tannic acid). Since the fibrocytes, unlike macrophages, respond to addition of antibody against particulate antigens by a decline in phagocytic activity, it seems that the basis for their recognition and binding of particles is other than through membrane receptors for immunoglobulin [204]. If mammalian phagocytes also possess a nonimmune mechanism for particle recognition like that of the fibrocytes, arguably they make little use of it while bathed in serum. It may be of some importance to macrophages out on alveolar surfaces and to phagocytes in complement- or immunoglobulin-deficient patients, when serum factors would be in short supply.

For many cells, phagocytes and nonphagocytes alike, the factors that promote nonimmune endocytosis are thought to be similar, although over the animal kingdom the various cells still exhibit different partialities as to material they will ingest, even where no immune mechanism can be suspected to participate in the process. In amebas as well as in mammalian cell cultures, macro-

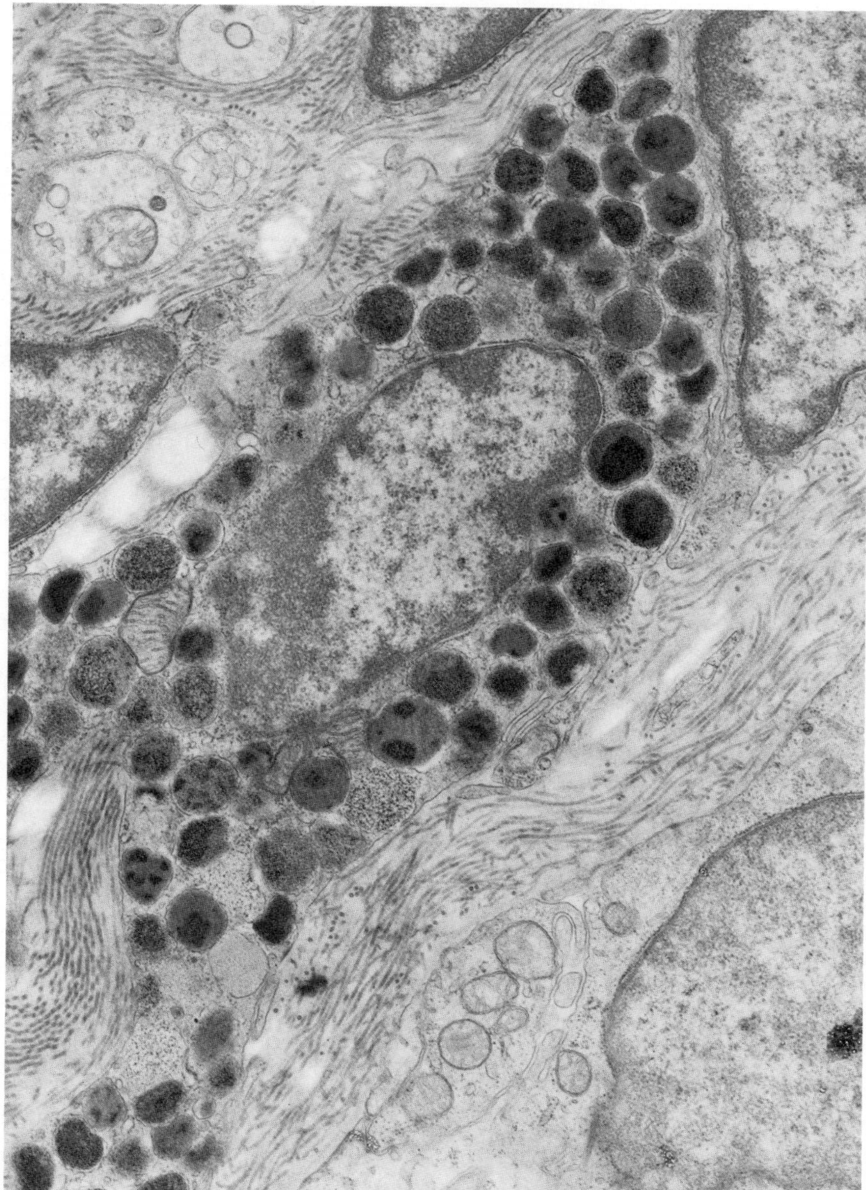

FIGURE 7 Mast cell in laryngeal connective tissue. In this cell the nucleus typically is ovoid and centrally located, while short processes extend from the cell margin. The specific granules are large and filled with material of varying density and often of a fibrillar texture.

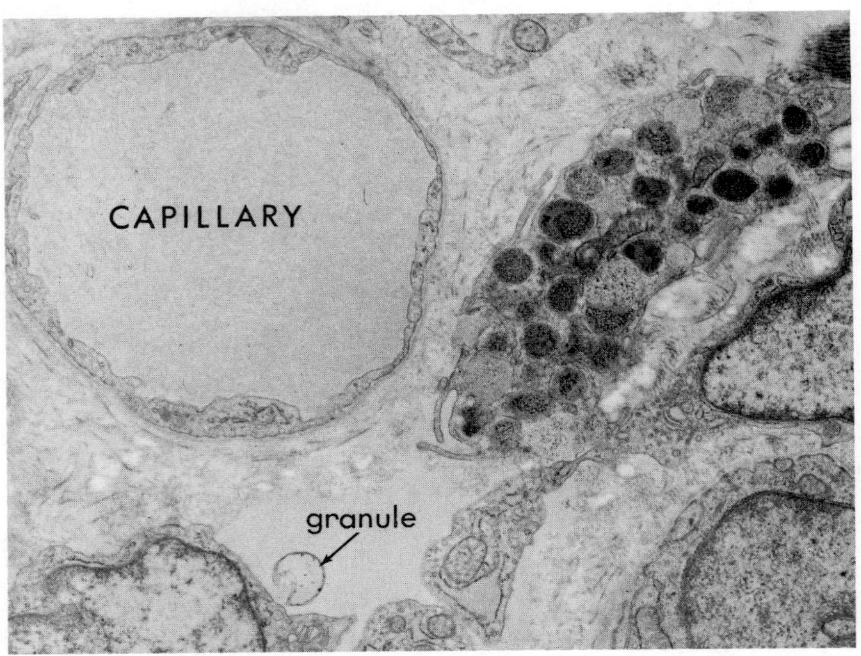

FIGURE 8 Mast cells slowly migrate through pulmonary connective tissues leaving behind a solvated passageway and sometimes a few granules as they move on.

pinocytosis or cell-drinking can be induced by adding suitable concentrations of inorganic ions or certain organic compounds to the medium; in macrophages this type of endocytosis is observable in the undulating processes located at the advancing end of the cell. Cohn and associates have listed a wide variety of organic molecules including proteins, nucleic acids, and polysaccharides that will stimulate endocytosis in mouse macrophages cultured in the absence of serum factors, finding the molecules to be negatively charged at physiological pH's and more effective if large and possessed of a high charge density [86]. The same generalizations hold if serum and presumably complement factors are present in the medium, only lower concentrations of the stimulating substances are necessary for uptake to occur. Other studies similarly suggest that the stimulating effect of various compounds is related to their surface charges, and the cellular response is also influenced by the pH and ionic composition of the medium in which the cells are bathed.

Whether macroendocytosis or microendocytosis is favored by a given cell, soluble materials including various macromolecules, are taken in, and if some of the material is identifiable by cytochemistry or by electron microscopy, further details of the endocytotic process can be visualized. For example, the water-soluble protein ferritin is identifiable under the electron beam because of its high content (~24%) of electron-dense iron in the form of micelles of ferric hydroxide-ferric phosphate. Prior to uptake it can be seen to become attached to a fuzzy coating (glycocalyx) comprised of glycosaminoglycans and glycoproteins and located on the outside surface of the plasmalemma. This material is stainable with alcian blue dyes 8GS/8GX [221,242], which are relatively specific for acid mucopolysaccharides; in the electron microscope the same coating is visualized using alcian blue complexed with lanthanum nitrate to achieve electron density [223], or using the hexavalent cation ruthenium red [151]. In amebas a surface coating is visible even without use of these special techniques but is enhanced by staining; in mammalian cells it is less conspicuous. Without special staining it can be seen in electron micrographs to cover the free surfaces of columnar absorptive cells in the intestines and to coat the plasmalemma delimiting the macroendocytotic and certain microendocytotic cavities of the phagocytes. Microendocytotic cavities or vesicles possessing the coat (coated vesicles or acanthosomes) are thought to be engaged in uptake of proteins or colloids. They are not uncommonly seen in phagocytes (Figs. 13 and 16) whereas in other cells they occur in far smaller numbers than uncoated vesicles, and they are rare indeed in endothelial cells like those of pulmonary capillaries, where the uncoated vesicles are associated with bulk fluid transport. In mammalian phagocytes stained for components of the glycocalyx, a fuzzy coating is perceptible covering the entire cell surface. It is thought that prior to internalization, many soluble as well as insoluble materials become bound to this coating rather than to the plasmalemma beneath, but it remains controversial as to precisely where on the cell surface each specific "receptor" is located (see further discussion in Sec. II.D).

The presence of divalent cations like calcium or magnesium often seems to foster attachment of particles to the glycocalyx, possibly through formation of bridges linking the negatively charged particles with the negatively charged surface. In their studies Cohn and associates found that addition of calcium or magnesium ions to the medium did not influence the macrophage response to anionic compounds [86], perhaps because these cations were already sufficiently abundant in the incubation media (TC-199 with 1% calf serum and balanced salt solution with 0.1 mg/ml bovine serum albumin). Other compounds like the congery of plant proteins called lectins apparently bind to saccharide groups present among components of this cell coating. After binding they frequently cause cells to agglutinate, and they can produce a reversible inhibition of phagocytosis [26]. Lectins have been widely used as a tool for investigating cell surface phenomena [179], but experimental results have not been easy to interpret. Two points nevertheless can safely be urged here: (a) *chemical interactions with cell surface coatings do occur,* and (b) *some can affect the cell's capacity for endocytosis.*

In the absence of serum factors, phagocytosis of objects is slow, but in the case of wandering phagocytes it is aided considerably if the cells work in a tissue environment where particles can be pushed up against fibers, a solid matrix, or sheets of cells, so that the phagocytes can flow around them and envelop them more readily. In this situation cell motility plays an important part in the preliminaries to phagocytosis; under laboratory conditions cell motions can be minimized, and the importance of attaching the ingestible materials to the phagocytes then becomes easy to see. When extensive enough, represented by a single particle about 0.03 μm in diameter or a number of smaller ones covering a certain minimum surface area, attachment triggers later phases of endocytosis and digestion [182].

D. Ingestion or Endocytosis

With endocytosis initiated in the phagocytes, their energy consumption rises. Whether derived from peritoneal lavage or from the circulation, microphages more than double their oxygen uptake and show a sixfold increase in oxidative activity for glucose. Resident peritoneal macrophages are less affected by phagocytosis, but macrophages freshly elicited from the bloodstream show over threefold increases in respiration and tenfold increases in oxidative activity toward glucose. Alveolar macrophages exhibit small increases during phagocytosis, but the resting respiratory rate of these cells is far ahead of the others, about three and nine times higher than elicited peritoneal macrophages and microphages,

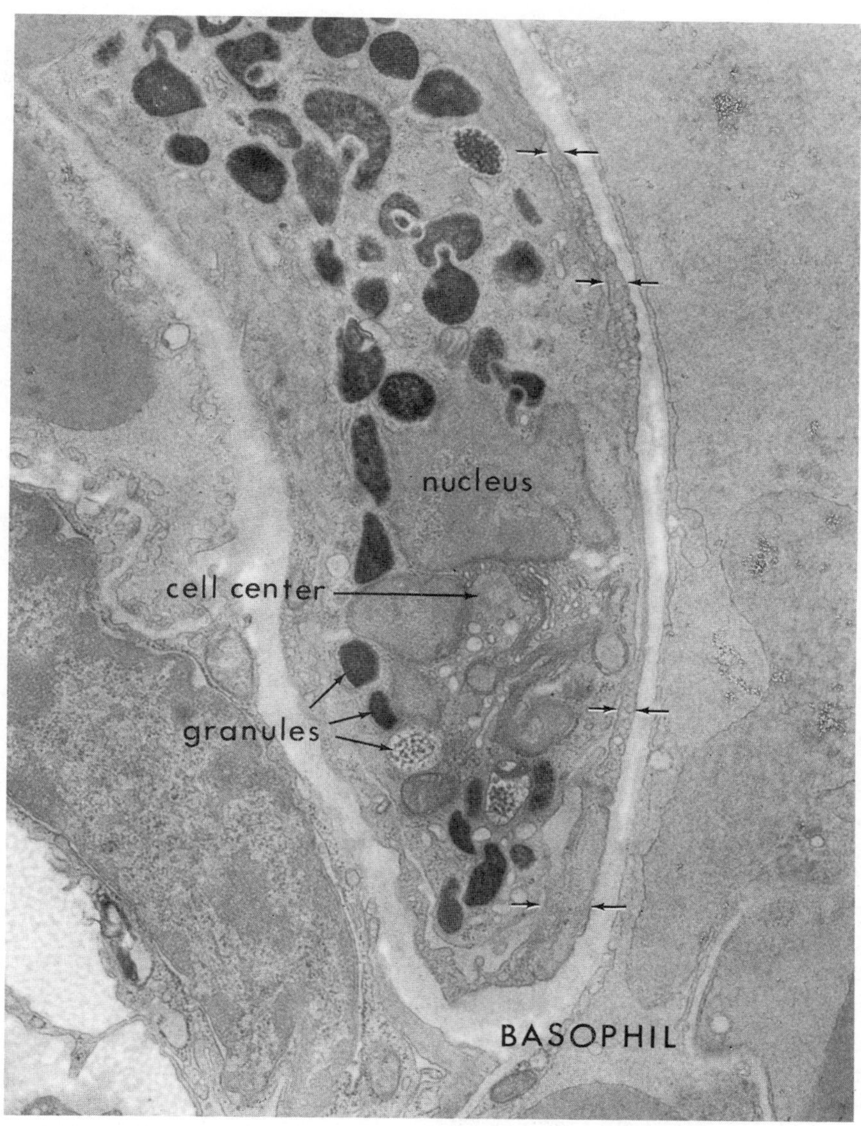

FIGURE 9 Basophil within the bronchial circulation near an alveolar duct. Basophils are rarely seen in the lungs owing to their scarcity in the circulation. This example is tightly fitted within a capillary whose endothelium can just be discerned (between paired arrows). The lobed nucleus descends to the left of the cell center with its centriole and Golgi membranes. Granular reticulum and free ribosome clusters are sparsely scattered throughout the cytoplasm dominated by markedly irregular but generally large and electron-dense specific granules. As a whole the cell is organized along granulocytic lines, although in many species granule contents resemble those of mast cells.

respectively [117,185]. Ribonucleic acid turnover and cholesterol and lecithin synthesis also rise during phagocytosis. Aside from the alveolar macrophage's obligate aerobism, another metabolic difference between phagocytes is the microphage's *myeloperoxidase-halide-peroxide system* [122], effective against many bacteria and fungi [46], and conspicuously absent from alveolar macrophages. Metabolic aspects of phagocytes are further discussed elsewhere in this monograph [81,159,176]. For the present it suffices to mention that during endocytosis, increases in cell motility, in the internalization of the surface membrane, and in its eventual replacement by newly synthesized membrane help to account for some energy spent. Other debits arise from the synthesis of new surface coatings, from the production of hydrogen peroxide, and possibly from the stimulus to certain active transport mechanisms involved in bactericidal causes.

Cellular movements related to endocytosis are not only those used to form and extend pseudopodia around ingestible particles, but also include movements that dimple the cell surface, draw the particles inside, seal them off in vesicles, and move these in and about the cytoplasm. All of these actions arise from changes in the disposition of the ectoplasm, which has a gelated consistency and appears replete with fine 50-60 Å microfilaments and devoid of most of the cytoplasmic organelles. These microfilaments are considered to be polymers of the contractile protein actin and have been proven so in a relatively few cases. While an alveolar macrophage goes about its scavenging activities its subplasmalemmal filaments undergo great upheavals in their concentration, orientation, and perhaps their state of polymerization as well (Figs. 12-16). Myosins and other components of an energy consuming contractile system similar to that of skeletal muscle have been sought and found in both microphages and macrophages. While it is a current pursuit to learn to what extent cell movement and the motions of endocytosis are comparable to contraction as it is understood in muscle [182,201,243], it is certain that a sliding-filament system identical to that of skeletal muscle does not occur in phagocytes.

The shifts in the surface contour and underlying ectoplasm of the phagocytes result in the formation and pinching-off of membrane-bounded cytoplasmic vesicles termed phagosomes [245] that contain the engulfed fluid medium and the particles, viruses, or bacteria. Endocytosis evidently occurs to some extent in all animal cells, but in phagocytes is a necessary prelude to enzymatic activity in the internal digestion of foreign matter. As described further along, the phagosome receives injections of digestive enzymes from the cell and subsequently serves as a digestive vessel within the cytoplasm, taking on a different appearance and new names as it does so. If the enclosed material is a pathogen like the tubercle bacillus or *Histoplasma capsulatum,* it may resist the destructive actions of the cell and multiply within the endocytotic vesicle eventually to burst out with destruction of its host. Other intracellular pathogens like viruses or

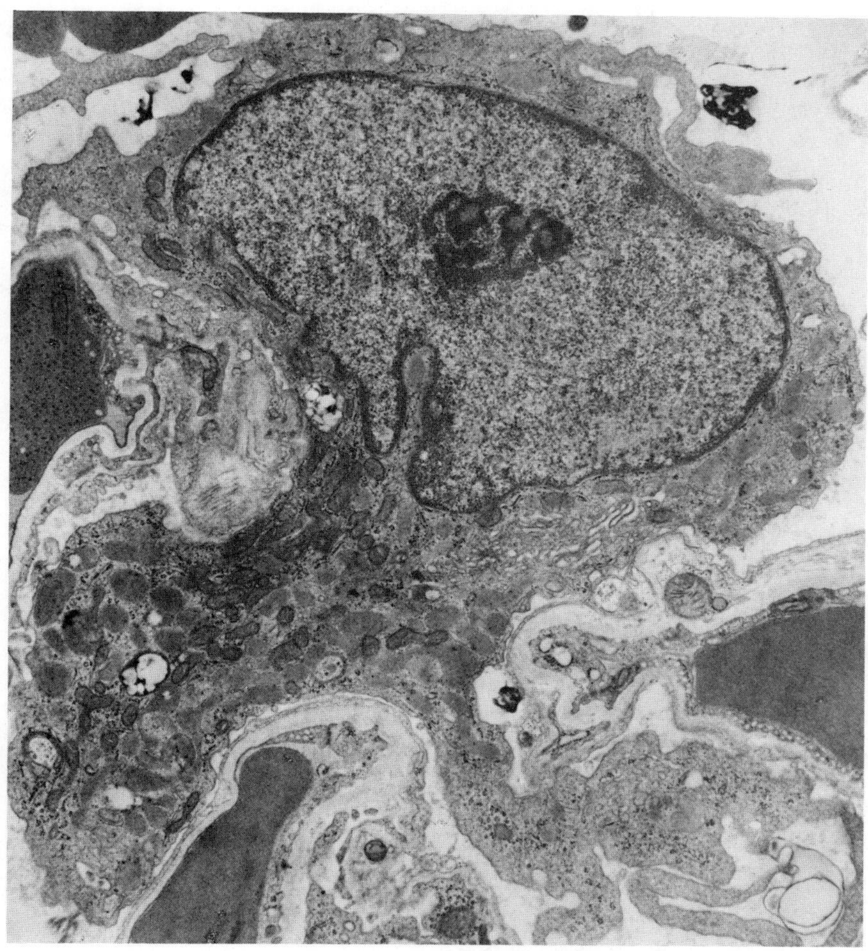

FIGURE 10 Alveolar macrophage in the alveolus of a vampire bat's lung. The cell extends between protruding capillaries, its advancing edge (ruffled membrane) at the lower right. A large nucleolus lies at the center of the nucleus; clustered mitochondria (left) and Golgi membranes (right) occupy the constricted region just beneath, while free and attached ribosomes (dark specks) and many indistinct heterolysosomes fill the remaining endoplasm.

FIGURE 11 Mouse lung previously exposed to an iron oxide aerosol. An alveolar macrophage (lower right) stores iron particles in heterolysosomes (dark granules) and after transformation into ferritin, in the cytoplasm. A Prussian blue reaction for iron gives the cell its grayish cast. A great alveolar epithelial cell (left adjacent) neither takes up nor breaks down the particles.

FIGURE 12 Electron micrograph of a region similar to that boxed in Fig. 11. The approximate boundary between the fibrillar ectoplasm and an organelle-rich endoplasm is indicated. Fine speckling (60 Å) is attributable to ferritin; fainter speckling (200 Å) to ribosomes, while the dense black particles are of iron oxide. The alveolar wall beneath does not contain ferritin.

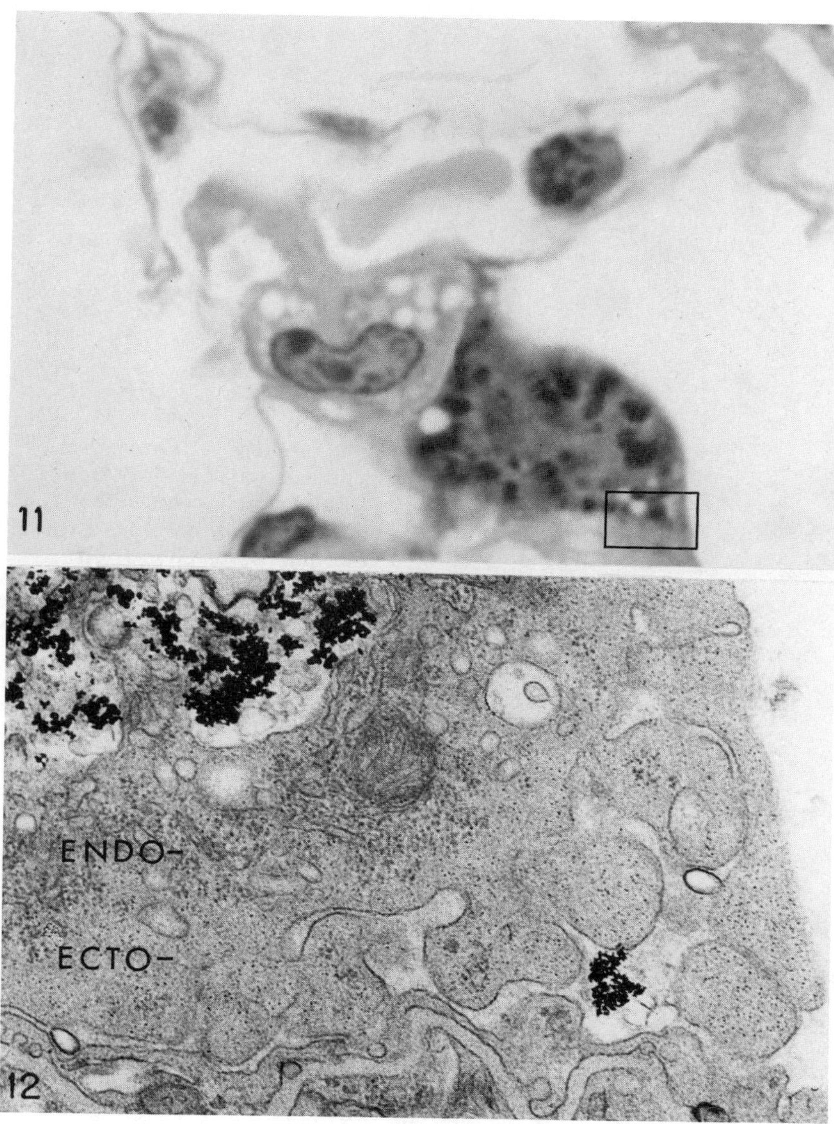
11
12
ENDO-
ECTO-

FIGURE 13 A macrophage in motion along the alveolar surface. The cell extends short pseudopods (large arrows) from the (myo)fibrillar ectoplasm, and these closely contact the epithelium subjacent. It is presumed that the ectoplasm then contracts, changing its configuration relative to these fixed points, which then break off to reform at new positions. The cell also exhibits formation of a microendocytotic vesicle (small arrows) and various organelles, the Golgi lamellae shown having little to do with formation of the many lysosomal structures present.

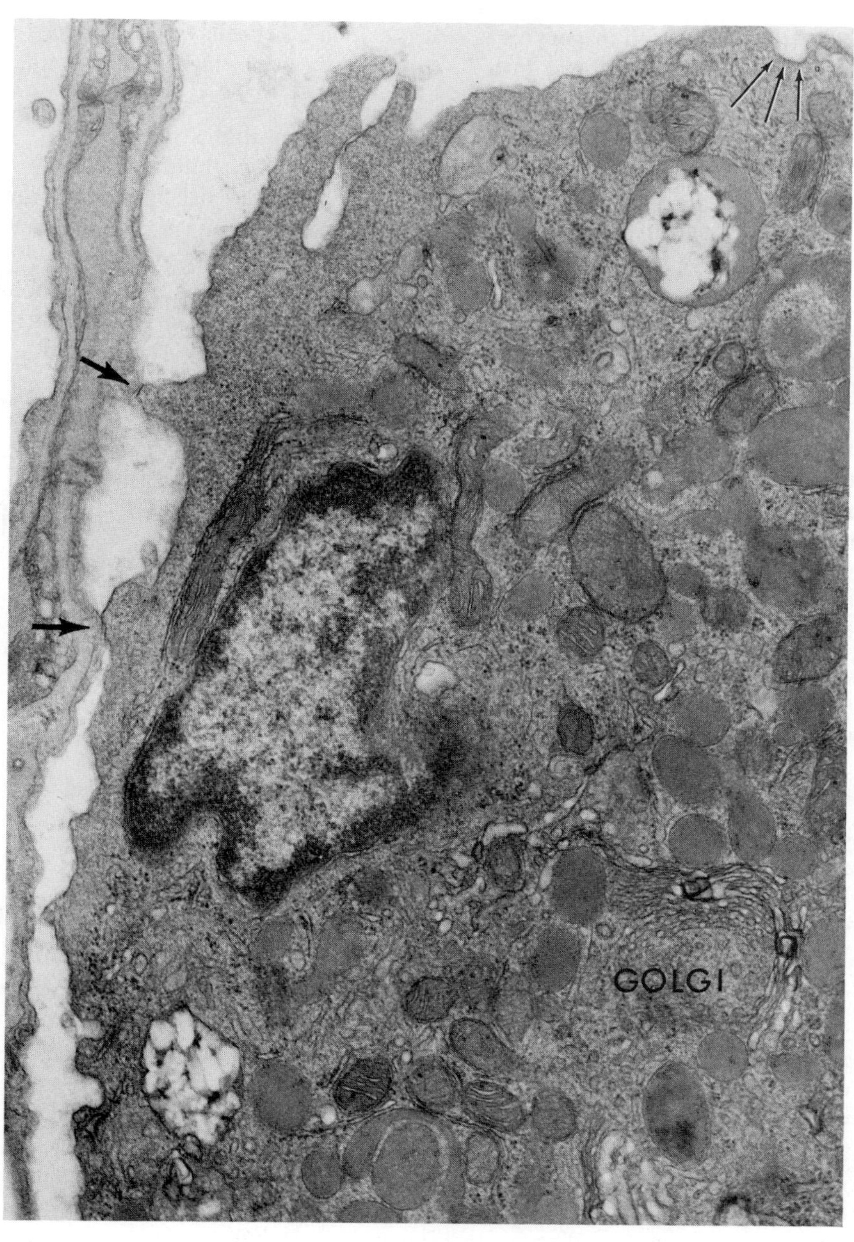
GOLGI

Rickettsiae may enter phagocytes as well as certain other cells through endocytosis, subsequently to break into the cytoplasm or nucleus where they normally multiply.

Phagosomes evidently can be formed at various positions along the surfaces of cells. They might appear at the tips of pseudopodia but more often form along relatively smooth contoured portions of the plasmalemma or between pseudopodia when large objects are being engulfed. They may be large (~1 μm) or small (600 Å), and several may combine into one large phagosome very shortly after they are formed (Fig. 24). By pulse-labeling the phosphatidylcholine of peritoneal macrophages with [^{3}H] choline, whence the label largely appeared over the cell periphery, and by following the cells subsequently, Gordon and Cohn [86] showed autoradiographically that in pinocytizing cells the interiorized membrane is actually derived (at least in part) from the surface membrane. By electron microscopy, the phagosomes of alveolar macrophages appear relatively clear (Fig. 19), but those that have been recently produced often have a fuzzy coating on their membrane similar to the coating present on the plasmalemma at the original site of vesicle formation (Fig. 13), and this gives one a little visual confirmation of the preceding. The coating is seen while large inorganic particles as well as colloids are being ingested, but it does not persist in interiorized phagosomes for long.

When cells imbibe fluid they form vesicles having one of roughly two sizes (600 Å, 1000 Å), whereas they may form these as well as much larger vesicles during attempts to phagocytose various particles or organisms. The shaping of these vesicles is influenced not only locally by changes in the cell membrane but also by changes in the conformation of the ectoplasmic gel which gives the cell its shape and typically differs in granulocytes and macrophages. The difference is particularly evident when these cells move, the granulocytes pouring themselves into a forward-directed pseudopod and the macrophages advancing as a triangle with sheets of hyaloplasm undulating near the peaks [28].

From the cell surface the new-forming phagosome is guided inward through the mediation of the cytoplasmic *centriolar-microtubular apparatus,* which serves as organizer for a variety of dynamic processes as well as for mitosis and is prominent in all phagocytic cells (Figs. 4, 9, 17, 18). The microtubules (~200 Å diam) radiate from the centrioles outward to the cell periphery, sometimes contact the phagosomes, and may form a scaffolding along whigh the phagosomes are drawn by contractile movements possibly originating from the microfilaments (~50-60 Å diam) (Fig. 24). Microtubules are said to be more prominent in phagocytizing as compared to resting human microphages, and when these are exposed to a variety of agents that disrupt microtubules, defects in the internal circulation of phagosomes and their sequelae soon appear [100]. In living granulocytes the complement of specific granules surround the centrosome with its centrioles and are drawn back and forth as the centrosome swings pendulum-fashion about the center of the cell [28]. Brusque displacements within the cell often affect a row of granules, as if all were being held in a channel encircled by microtubules.

As they are being drawn inward through the ectoplasm (Figs. 10 and 16), the phagosomes temporarily alter the arrangement of nearby ectoplasmic microfilaments, typically matted in parallel bundles, and in so doing bring about changes in the region somewhat reminiscent of changes seen during translational movements of the cell. As a macrophage moves or sends out a pseudopod, the adjacent ectoplasm seems transiently to be cleaved by planes temporarily lined by trilaminar plasma membranes (Fig. 15); and as the ectoplasm on one side slides past the ectoplasm on the other side, the membrane lining the cleavage plane between them is resorbed. Electron micrographs of active phagocytes leave the impression that ingestive as well as translational movements can be related to changes in the orientations and thickness of nearby microfilament bundles as well as to changes in the cell membrane, but this impression has yet to be analyzed systematically in any of the phagocytes.

There are suggestions if not proof that initial degradative steps are undertaken in phagosomes before digestive enzymes and other substances stored elsewhere are introduced. In many cells the earliest change thought to occur is a drop in pH. Metchnikoff [168,169] had observed that among a wide range of phagocytes some but by no means all could change the color of ingested litmus granules from blue to red; the point of color change in this indicator dye is rather imprecise (pH 6-4.5, depending on purity of preparation), but the dye is well tolerated by cells. Amebas and the plasmodium of myxomycetes exhibit such acid digestion, but the vacuoles found in macrophages of sponges do not, and in Metchnikoff's experience the leukocytes of vertebrates rarely did so. These studies and others on mammalian cells rarely have distinguished between the pH in the phagosome and that in the digestive vacuole (heterolysosome) the phagosome eventually becomes. Mandell [153] gives a range of pH 6.0-6.5 for the "intraphagosomal pH" of human microphages and attributes its acidity to the lactic acid production known to accompany phagocytosis. Use of various metabolic inhibitors as well as colchicine and hydrocortisone tend to support the supposition that intraphagosomal and not intraheterolysosomal pH was being measured, since in various ways these agents tend to prevent fusion of lysosomes with phagosomes and the attendant mixing of contents. Cline [47] attributed the early drop in pH to the action of carbonic anhydrase present on the surface membranes of leukocytes. A point to remember, however, is that in microphages intracellular digestion makes use of enzymes having both acid and alkaline pH optima.

FIGURE 14 A large macrophage sitting atop the alveolar epithelium in an opossum's lung. The nucleus is euchromatic and the cytoplasm replete with lysosomal bodies including large ones rich in triglycerides. The peripheral cytoplasm above and below is markedly homogeneous in comparison to that of the cell body.

FIGURE 15 Detail of a cell like that in Fig. 14. The peripheral cytoplasm is bisected by a row of vesicles partly fused into a pair of membranes that border a line or plane of cleavage. In forming or dissolving, these structures separate or bring together bundles of myofilaments in the ectoplasm and so affect movements of the cell.

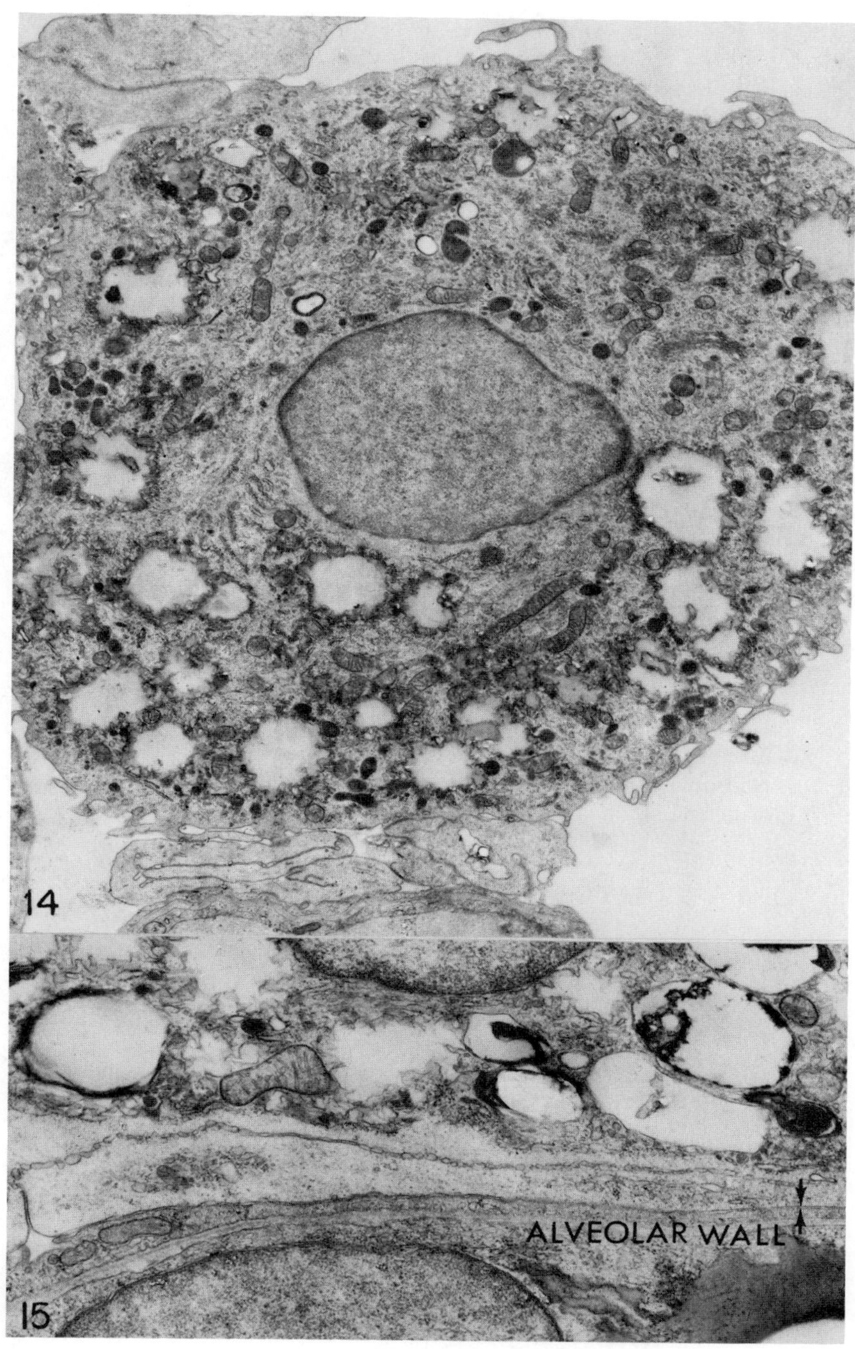
14
15
ALVEOLAR WALL

FIGURE 16 Peripheral hyaloplasm in a mouse alveolar macrophage. Pseudopods in this undulating margin advance and recede, exhibiting thickening of opposed plasmalemmas as adjacent cell processes are brought into fusion (arrows). Both microendocytotic and macroendocytotic vesicles seem to be forming, the former a "coated vesicle" (1) and the latter a pinosome (2). The endoplasm (lower left) contains both primary and secondary lysosomes.

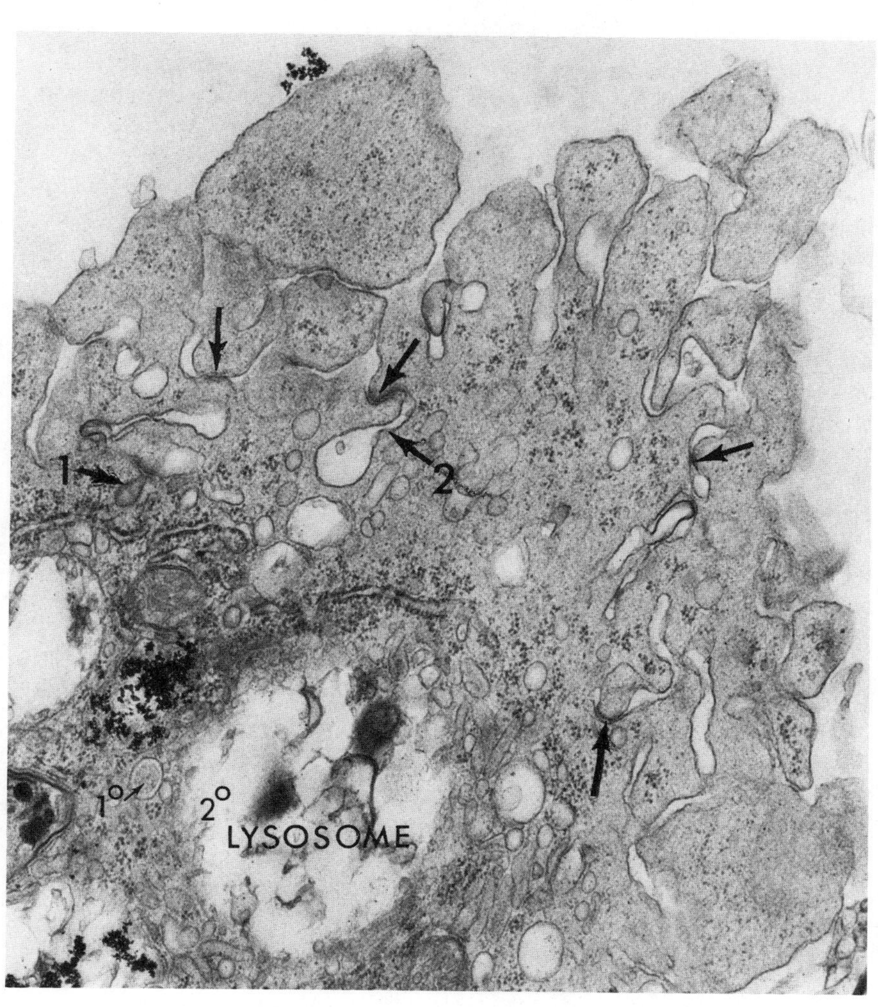
1
2
1°
2°
LYSOSOME

As seen in electron micrographs, ingested solids appear to become concentrated in phagosomes; hence, water and perhaps other substances pass from them into the cytoplasm as a consequence of cellular action.

Since cell membranes possess mechanisms for facilitated or active transport, they might retain these functions for some time after becoming internalized by endocytosis. Were such membrane-associated machinery present in phagosomes, it could well contribute toward pH and water regulation of the contents. As discussed immediately below and further on, this may be true for vesicles formed by *micro*endocytosis but may not be true long for phagosomes produced by *macro*endocytosis.

Electron-cytochemical studies indicate that in many endothelial cells employing microendocytotic vesicles in transport across cells, an "adenosine triphosphatase"—or more properly a nucleoside phosphatase [156,157]—is present on both surface and endocytotic membranes. This enzyme is able to hydrolyze ATP and certain other substrates, becomes activated by magnesium or calcium ions, is inhibited by adenosine diphosphate and sulfhydryl poisons, and is thought to play a role in active transmembrane transport of materials between the cytoplasm and either the cellular environment or the contents of the vesicles. In leukocytes of guinea pigs a similar enzyme is located on the cell surface and on the membrane of small, apparently new-formed cytoplasmic vesicles, but not in phagocytic vacuoles that have been separated for some time from the surface [181]. In these vacuoles, mediated transport sites with their enzyme carriers might not be taken in at all, or if taken in might be destroyed on contact with the lysosomal hydrolases. In endothelial cells the vesicles retain ATPase activity, perhaps because few lysosomal enzymes are made and hence could be on hand to destroy it.

Hydrogen peroxide has been localized in phagosomes of mammalian microphages using an elegant cytochemical technique that reveals peroxide in the presence of both the cell's myeloperoxidase and the reagent diaminobenzidine [39]. It is found both in fully formed and forming phagosomes that have not completely pinched off from the surface. Hydrogen peroxide is generated by a microphage mechanism that oxidizes reduced pyridine nucleotides NADH and/or NADPH; and, while NADPH oxidase activity has been found in the lysosomal granule fraction [192], an NADH oxidase has been localized cytochemically to the surface membrane. This enzyme is internalized during phagocytosis and remains able to function in the phagosome [38].

The preceding examples suggest ways in which phagosomes and their membranes may function prior to contact with lysosomes and their membranes. In seeking a better understanding of this and of other aspects of endocytosis, one must acquire a clearer picture of cell membrane structure and the localization of membrane-associated activities than is available to us from models currently proposed [27]. Concerning the early stages of recognition and attachment, for instance, it would be well to know more about phagocytic receptors and how they touch off endocytosis. Like the membrane-associated carriers of mediated transmembrane transport systems, both the specific and nonspecific receptors of phagocytosis are essentially "operational" conceptions, for their molecular configurations are largely unknown. It is therefore too early to fix them three-dimensionally in or upon the cell membrane with any certainty. Nevertheless, if surface membranes are examined after they have been prepared by freeze cleavage, certain irregularities are seen on the inner and outer leaflets of these trilaminar membranes, and they may represent sites of specialized function. In the somewhat atypical case of mammalian erythrocytes, cytochemical localizations for many cell surface components—antigen, anionic sites, binding sites for lectins (concanavalin A, phytohemagglutinin, etc.) and influenza virus—have all centered upon these intramembranous irregularities or "particles" [197,199, 200,260]. In other cells (see below) this may not be true.

From studies of Werb and Cohn [274], it seems that in cultured peritoneal macrophages a net increase in total cell cholesterol and phospholipid is measurable some 10-12 hr after the cells had been induced to begin phagocytosis, and the amount synthesized is directly related to the amount of membrane taken in. Prior to this little change is detectable in the amount of membrane-associated lipids. There is increased labeling of membrane-associated phosphoinositide and phosphatidylserine from inorganic [^{32}P] orthophosphate while microphages as well as stimulated peritoneal macrophages are phagocytizing, indicating an increased lipid synthesis or turnover in these cells; but the effect is not seen in alveolar macrophages [115,116]. As for enzymic sites on the surface membrane, the electron-cytochemical study of North [181] previously mentioned and the study by Werb and Cohn [274] indicate that certain plasma membrane "marker" enzymes, respectively, nucleoside phosphatase ("membrane ATPase") and 5′-nucleotidase, are absent or disappear from the internalized membranes; in the case of the biochemical study, the 5′-nucleotidase could be demonstrated in phagolysosomes shortly after phagocytosis began but declined thereafter according to a half-life of about 2 hr. Increases in the activity of this enzyme were detectable beginning some 6 hr after phagocytosis, were localizable entirely to the surface membrane, and attained prephagocytosis levels some 4 hr later. This study could be taken to indicate that during phagocytosis part of the surface membrane is simply rolled up inside the cell and that the loss of surface area resulting from the endocytic activity is made up by resynthesis later on. Nevertheless, in careful studies on phagocytosis of polystyrene beads by leukocytes and alveolar macrophages, Tsan and Berlin [261,262] obtained a somewhat different result: after the cells had taken up sufficient beads to result in 30-50% internalization of the cell surface, no change could be detected in the number of membrane carrier sites for transmembrane transport of lysine or adenine [93], sites normally associated with the surface membrane. On the other hand, when the experiment was repeated using cells exposed to colchicine or vinblastine prior to phagocytosis, the number of transport carriers for nucleosides and bases decreased in proportion to the extent of phagocytosis [263]. These studies have been taken to mean that the cell membrane is a mosaic whose transport sites are normally endowed with translational mobility. During phagocytosis these remain on the surface, while other components of the membrane, including phagocytic receptors, flow inward. Colchicine and vinblastine are known to disrupt microtubules, and Ukena and Berlin's [263] results were seen as indicating that mobility of transport carriers is determined in part by microtubular proteins [27], although no direct evidence for this was given. The findings of Werb and Cohn [274] and the associates of Berlin are not far apart if one concedes that after phagocytosis the internalized membrane need not consist of identical components laid out just as they are on the surface. Other possibilities remain to be explored; for example, that the internalized membrane in reality is newly assembled during phagocytosis from building blocks previously synthesized and stored, and that the increase in lipids seen 10-12 hr after phagocytosis merely reflects a replacement of this reserve. Clearly it is desirable to know more about the dynamics of membranes and how and where new membrane is added to old.

Other investigators have attempted to follow the flow of surface membranes during phagocytosis and other cellular activities by staining a component of the membrane or the glycocalyx and following subsequent changes using the stained component as a marker. The problem with this approach is not unlike the problem that arises in interpreting the previously cited work: no single marker necessarily tags "the cell membrane"; this has recently been very well demonstrated for the surface of *Entamoeba histolytica* [198]. In these Protozoa the freeze-etched intramembranous particles seem to correspond to acidic sites that are ionizable at pH 1.8 and bind colloidal iron; but they show no association with concanavalin A receptors, which normally bind to the peripheral membrane coating but in erythrocytes also bind to the particles. Furthermore, when living cells are exposed to low levels of concanavalin A-peroxidase, the concanavalin receptors are redistributed to a pole of the cell—the uroid. Other markers of the glycocalyx like ruthenium red do not follow this redistribution, while the intramembranous particles of these cells remain evenly distributed over the membrane surface except for the uroid, where they are absent. *The point is plainly that peripheral membrane components may move independently of the more central, integral membrane components, and that some of the peripheral markers may even move independently of each other.*

E. Intracellular Digestion: Lysosomes, Related Structures, and the Exoplasm Concept

The digestive actions so central to the operations of both microphages and macrophages and indeed all phagocytes are carried out by their intracellular digestive systems. In essence these consist of packets of hydrolytic enzymes functionally associated with a well-developed granular endoplasmic reticulum programmed in the phagocytes to synthesize these enzymes, as well as with the machinery of endocytosis, previously described. The Golgi apparatus in these cells serves as perhaps the first part of the digestive system, concentrating many of the newly formed enzymic products in vacuoles limited by essentially semipermeable membranes [66]. The term "lysosome" has often been applied to the packets of hydrolytic enzymes, and the term "lysosomal activity" to their activity. Biochemically or histochemically this is often estimated as the action of one constituent, acid phosphatase; but many varieties of hydrolytic enzymes having pH optima in the acid range are normally present in lysosomes, and the presence of any or all of them in these bodies implies previous and possibly continued action of the whole system in producing them. The most typical of these additional acid hydrolases are acid ribonuclease, acid deoxyribonuclease, β-glucuronidase, and cathepsin; certain other enzymes are found in association with these in some cells, and collectively they are able to degrade proteins, nucleic acids, polysaccharides, and lipids (Table 3). From the outset de Duve and his associates had considered the lysosomal enzymes to have essentially a degradative rather than a synthetic or transfer function and to be kept from destroying the cell by being held in a "latent" or inactive state, which was considered to result from their being sequestered within semipermeable lysosomal membranes.

A variety of enzyme-rich and membrane-bounded bodies have dimensions generally comparable with lysosomes (0.1-0.5 μm) and sediment with them in a cell fraction admixed with small mitochondria. The specific granules of granulocytes number among these and like them have a degradative function. Another class of granules, the microbodies or peroxisomes, may also be present; these are considered to be of nearly ubiquitous occurrence in eukaryotic cells and with some troubling exceptions [65] seem to contain catalase in association with D-amino acid oxidase, urate oxidase, or sometimes other flavin oxidases. Reducing equivalents are transferred to oxygen, producing hydrogen peroxide, which can be broken down in the presence of catalase. In leaves of plants these organelles are involved in complex photorespiratory reactions, and in germinating seedlings they help to convert fatty residues into sugars [165]. No such specific involvement of peroxisomes has been worked out in animals, but they are most

TABLE 3 Exoplasmic Activities of the Phagocytes Compared

	Macrophages	Alveolar macrophages	Microphages	Eosinophils	Basophils	Mast Cells
Phagocytosis	++++	+++++	+++	++	+	0
Microendocytosis	++++	++++	0	+	+	+
Content of lysosomal (azurophil) granules	*Preactivation (monocytic?) complement: minor* Acid hydrolases Acid phosphatase Aryl sulfatase Esterase, lipase 5-Nucleotidase RNAase, DNAase β-Galactosidase β-Glucuronidase Glucosaminidase Lysozyme Cathepsin Aminopeptidase Protease and proteinases Basic protein S-Mucopolysaccharide		*10-15% of granules* Acid hydrolases Acid phosphatase Aryl sulfatase Esterase 5-Nucleotidase RNAase, DNAase β-Galactosidase β-Glucuronidase Myeloperoxidase Lysozyme (1/3) Cathepsin Basic protein S-Mucopolysaccharide	*Minor component* Lysosomal enzymes (fate uncertain)	*Minor component* Lysosomal enzymes (see text)	*Minor component* Lysosomal enzymes (see text)
Content of specific granules	*Postactivation lysosomes: major store of digestive enzymes* (as above)		*85% of granules* Alkaline phosphatase Lysozyme (2/3) Phagocytin Lactoferrin Cationic proteins Acid mucosubstances	*Major component* Peroxidase (high) Acid phosphatase β-Glucuronidase ATPase Basic protein S-Mucopolysaccharide	*Major component* Acid phosphatase Heparin Histamine Other amines Basic protein	*Major component* Glucosaminidase Trypsin- and chymotrypsin-like alkaline proteases Heparin Histamine Other amines Basic protein

Tertiary granules	–	–	Acid phosphatase Acid mucosubstances	Acid phosphatase	–	–
Formation and disposition of granules	Single granules	Formed as reticulum of "wormy bodies" later becoming single	By fusion of small granules into larger single granule	By fusion into single granules	By fusion into single granules	By fusion into sets sharing a common membrane
Predominant site of digestion	Intracellular digestion		Intracellular	Intracellular	Intracellular	(Intracellular)
Retention of heterolysosomes	For extended periods (tattoos) throughout life and through cannibalism thereafter		Brief	Brief	Less than 24 hr	Granules retained over long period, although accessible from outside
Secretion of lysosomes or granules	Absent under optimal conditions		Agonal, or under special immunological conditions	Doubtful	Degranulation in anaphylaxis	Degranulation in anaphylaxis; physiological "exteriorization"
Clearance	By lysis and migration		By lysis	By lysis and migration	By lysis and migration	Slight; cells long-lived (see text)

abundant in metabolically active hepatocytes and kidney cells, and functional roles have been proposed [207]. On the whole these bodies do not seem to have a primarily "digestive" function, and where they may become confused with lysosome-like bodies is where the latter exhibit catalase or peroxidase activity, discussed further on.

Great variation is found among cells in the size of their digestive systems, the variety of hydrolases present, their pH optima, and their distribution within compartments of the system. In some cells it is notably dynamic, expanding or contracting to meet momentary functional needs, or in response to morbid outside stimulation [1]. The concept of an intracellular digestive system therefore embraces more than just the activities of the "classic" lysosomal hydrolases. Other enzymes stored within packets of their own may be handled similarly. Furthermore, mechanisms other than hydrolysis may be employed to serve the ends of the system. Strict usage of the terms, lysosome and lysosomal system, nevertheless applies only to the workings of the acid hydrolases. In reconciling earlier concepts of lysosomes with our gradually improving understanding of cell function, de Duve and other specialists on lysosomes have modified and broadened them, as the following paragraphs attempt to show. Some new terms have had to be added to accommodate the expanded viewpoint.

The phagocytes under survey all have extensively developed but not identical lysosomal and other degradative systems as befit cells with primary digestive roles. Cytoplasmic components of these systems in phagocytes do not greatly differ in functional organization from the organization found in exocrine cells like the pancreatic acinar cells which secrete digestive enzymes used in the duodenum. While both categories of cells are synthesizing these enzymes, they both exhibit an expansion of the granular endoplasmic reticulum within the *endoplasmic space,* which is the region of cytoplasm that surrounds the nucleus and serves as the place of origin for its anabolic reactions. The enzyme products are then transferred to an *exoplasmic space* through the Golgi apparatus, which acts as a point of demarcation between spaces. There the enzymes are packaged and concentrated within granules that are termed lysosomal or lysosome-like in the case of the phagocytes and zymogenic in the case of the pancreatic cells. The lysosomes or zymogen granules are stored until needed within the exoplasm, the enzymes remaining latent until called upon to act. One obvious difference between phagocytes and exocrine cells is that in phagocytes the enzymes digest their substrates inside the exoplasm, whereas in a pancreatic acinar cell the stored enzymes are released to the outside. Accordingly, in phagocytes the machinery for endocytosis is highly developed. In the pancreatic cell emphasis is placed on secretion rather than ingestion, and the mechanisms of surface transport are attuned toward exocytosis rather than endocytosis. In either case, exchanges with the outside are mediated in the exoplasm.

The exoplasm is conceived as the cytoplasmic space nearer the cell margin where catabolic reactions predominate. (In comparison, the older term *ectoplasm* refers simply to the peripheral cytoplasm, frequently gelled; it remains to see if usage will equate both words.) Various packaged cell products are stored in the exoplasm, and a great variety of interchanges are facilitated between or among lysosomes, endo- and exocytotic vesicles, secretory granules, and the plasma membrane [64]. Common to these exoplasmic entities is a membrane, conceived to be sufficiently similar to the plasma membrane as to permit fusion with it, while sufficiently dissimilar from endoplasmic membranes (nuclear envelope, smooth and granular reticulum, mitochondria, and part of the Golgi membranes) to prevent fusion with them. A changeover from the endoplasmic to the exoplasmic type of membrane is postulated to occur at the level of the Golgi apparatus, and this may be accompanied by a 25% increment in membrane thickness, attributable in part to the presence of a glycoprotein/lipid coating on the outer face of the exoplasmic but not endoplasmic membranes, as shown electron-cytochemically by lectin (ricin-ferritin) binding [77]. The effect of this change would be to permit products of anabolism to penetrate the catabolic (exoplasmic) compartment but to prevent a reverse penetration of the catabolic into the anabolic space. Within the exoplasm, however, fusion between any of its membrane-bounded bodies or between any of them and the plasma membrane would be feasible, subject to metabolic regulation and to control over encounters exerted by the centriolar apparatus.

In this interpretation of cytoplasmic organization, the "lysosomal system" represents that part of the functional exoplasm that has to do with degradative activities catalyzed by the lysosomal hydrolases. In phagocytes the predominant exoplasmic activities are those of endocytosis and digestion; other exoplasmic functions, such as secretion and cellular autophagy, may go on as well but are less prominently featured. Mammalian macrophages and granulocytes alike possess one or two contractile vacuoles per cell, and these exoplasmic structures have been observed to expel their fluid contents to the outside [28]; but if indigestible particles are taken up, they tend to remain inside these cells (Figs. 3, 11, 28). On the whole, compared to the phagocytes of many lower animals, mammalian phagocytes exhibit only a limited propensity for exocytosis. Among a wider range of cell types, whether emphasis is placed on endocytosis (phagocytes), exocytosis (pancreatic acinar cells), or else a neat balance in-between (thyroid follicular cells), the exoplasm consists of common elements, but among them the elements may be very differently emphasized, as if transformed in D'Arcy Thompson's [259] Cartesian nets.

F. Studying Lysosomes

Over the years since lysosomes first became subjects of intensive study [6,244], the heterogeneity of granule sizes and densities and the dynamic nature of lysosomal and related exoplasmic systems have given biochemists innumerable problems in interpreting experimental results obtained by cell fractionation and differential or density gradient centrifugation. It has been most helpful to have this work complemented by cytochemical and ultrastructural studies. To mention a few difficulties, lysosomal enzymes need not be localized exclusively to lysosomes, since like other proteins they are synthesized on ribosomes and hence are detectable at times in the microsome fraction of the cell. It is also possible that two or more enzymes, one lysosomal and the other(s) belonging to the supernatant, may react with the same substrate used in the analysis and so be taken for a single enzyme [177,178]. Activators and inhibitors, electrophoresis, or still other methods are then put to work to sort out the enzymes involved. Further discussion of these complexities and of lysosomal studies in general will be found in a number of excellent reviews [67,246].

G. Dynamics of Lysosomal Interactions

Because of their "latency" in lysosomes and lysosome-like granules, large stores of previously synthesized hydrolases or bactericidal agents can be maintained for days without damaging the cells that harbor them. For example, the classic lysosomes (azurophil granules) of microphages cease to be produced well before these cells are ready to be released from the bone marrow into the circulation, and they remain quiescent during this period (myelocyte-to-blood transit time), estimated to last for 10-12 days [41,62]. In other cells like macrophages, the lysosomal enzymes are largely synthesized after the phagocytes have resided for a time in the tissues and have become stimulated by exposure to casein, serum albumin, BCG (bacillus Calmette-Guérin), Freund's adjuvant (a mixture of paraffin oil, sorbitol laurate, and mycobacteria with bovine gamma globulin), triolein, or other substances. An added effect of such stimulation is that the newly or previously synthesized enzymes lose their latency and become available for interaction with their substrates. Some of the factors involved in the "activation" of latent lysosomes are known, but the process as a whole is imperfectly understood. The same can be said of a second aspect of activation, the stimulus to enzyme production. To what extent these two separate aspects of "activation" are related is scarcely known.

In his early work on lysosomes, de Duve considered that the basis for lysosomal enzyme latency lay in the separation of the enzymes from their substrates. Suspensions of purified lysosomal cell fractions show little enzymic activity until the lysosomal membranes are disrupted by freezing and thawing, sonication, exposure to surface-active agents, or other drastic treatment [66] whence the enzymes and substrates are brought into contact and interact at once. This loss of latency occurs nearly simultaneously for all the classic lysosomal hydrolases, which suggested to de Duve that all of them were packaged together. Under similar conditions in vitro, a different rate of "activation" observed for another latent enzyme might be explained by considering the enzyme to be housed in a separate granule. This is true for the alkaline phosphatase of microphages, as shown biochemically by means of zonal centrifugation and isopycnic equilibration [16], and cytochemically as well.

The membranes of lysosomes and similar granules are semipermeable, and within certain limits the bodies act as osmometers. On occasion living cells make use of lysosomes without first bringing them into apposition with other cellular bodies, as shown when they segregate vital dyes dissolved in the cell sap; but in accordance with more orthodox practice, the enzymes and substrates are brought together inside the phagosome by a fusion of lysosomal and phagosomal membranes to produce a new cytoplasmic entity, the heterolysosome (phagolysosome, secondary lysosome). This behavior makes it possible to add limited quantities of enzymes to the substrate while reserving the bulk for later needs. Previously synthesized lysosomal enzymes in any case undergo spontaneous degradation in time, and after activation further losses occur during catalysis, perhaps because some of the enzymes become inhibited allosterically by products of ingested microorganisms, or else because certain anionic molecules in the medium are taken up and become concentrated sufficiently in the phagosomes to inhibit enzyme action. This effect has been shown under laboratory conditions for substances like Suramin, dextran sulfate, and trypan blue [52].

Activation of latent lysosomes might not entirely be explained by the bringing together of enzymes and substrates. Even if it were, the fusion this necessitates between lysosomal and phagosomal membranes gives cytoplasmic mechanisms a chance to exert a regulatory influence on activation and intracellular digestion. For example, there is some basis for suggesting an involvement of the plasma membrane enzyme adenine cyclase and its product, cyclic adenosine 3′,5′-monophosphate (cyclic AMP), in the regulation of fusion between phagosomes and lysosomes of leukocytes, high intracellular levels of this substance tending to inhibit the discharge of lysosomal contents [100]. It also appears that the successful intracellular parasitism of *Mycobacterium tuberculosis* and *Mycobacterium microti* depend on their ability to produce sufficient quantities of cyclic AMP to prevent fusion of macrophage lysosomes with the phagosomes in which they reside [149]. Sufficiently stimulated, these bacteria apparently can produce enough cyclic AMP for this purpose, even though it is relatively poorly taken up from the medium (and phagosome?) by mammalian cells [252], and a concentration on the order of 10^{-4} M is necessary to show this effect. The effect of cyclic AMP on lysosome fusion has been considered to result from its influence on microtubule assembly

[280], presumably because assembled microtubules along with centrioles might be involved in guiding lysosomes to phagosomes (or vice versa); but cyclic AMP like cortisone is also one of a few agents known to stabilize lysosomal membranes in vitro, and so its effects may be several. This topic is further discussed by Gee and Khandwala [81]; they indicate it is too early yet to evaluate the role of cyclic nucleotides in the overall control of intracellular digestion.

Among other factors involved in the control of activation: *First,* there may be structural provisions for latency in lysosomes apart from that provided by their membranes. *Second,* certain intermediates may have to come from the phagosomal membrane in order to complete a complex reaction and so permit the action of the relevant lysosomal enzymes to be effective. The following gives some idea of what is known about these two possibilities.

1. Many believe that the lysosomal and related hydrolases as well as certain antibacterial basic proteins are contained within the matrix of lysosomes or lysosome-like granules and that the hydrolases take up only a small part of the space available. Much of it seems to be occupied by nonenzymic substances; and while some of them like the constituent phospholipids of the membrane may occur in all lysosomes, others are unique to lysosomes of certain cell types only. One has only to compare the cytochemical properties of the granules in the different blood leukocytes to see that this is so. These nonenzymic components include nucleotides, glycolipids, acidic mucopolysaccharides, and proteins [246]. Among these substances, an acidic glycoprotein may comprise about half of the total protein content. It has been postulated to function in binding the lysosomal enzymes ionically so as to bar access of substrates to catalytic sites on the enzymes and thereby assure latency until it is reversed by the action of cationic compounds [124], an elution effect similar to that used in column chromatography. To some extent, thiol groups on certain enzymes, by binding to matrix lipoproteins through links with the fatty acids or by disulfide bonds, may help to maintain latency; if cysteine speeds up proteolysis within heterolysosomes [167], it may act by cleaving the –S–S– links between enzymes and matrix. In this view the limiting membrane contributes to latency principally in restricting the diffusion of the polyanion matrix-enzyme complex. Others have considered that the enzymes are attached to the lysosomal membranes either as part of the envelope structure itself or else as a result of binding to membrane components after the manner proposed for binding to matrix elements. A criticism of the simple "osmotic bag" concept of lysosomes and a defense of the matrix-binding theory is given by Koenig [123], while arguments in favor of the membrane-binding concept are given by Lucy [150] in the symposium edited by Dingle and Fell. It can safely be concluded that the behavior of the lysosomal membrane differs from an ideal semipermeable membrane in some particulars and that the molecular architecture of the lysosomes has not yet been accurately mapped.

One of the most vexing problems with cytochemical determinations of lysosome or lysosome-related enzyme activities is that the level of reactivity may vary considerably following only minor variations in tissue handling or incubation technique, and it can vary perceptibly in day-to-day repetitions of palpably the same procedure using similar reagents and comparable biological material. In smeared cell preparations or in unfixed or possibly formalin-fixed frozen sections, the hazards to enzyme integrity brought about by preparative techniques would seem to lead the list of possible causes for inconstant readings of enzyme activity. Membrane rupture and enzyme loss may plague incubations of unfixed material, whereas use of formaldehyde, especially long-standing formalin solutions contaminated with formic acid, may inhibit enzyme activity variably from sample to sample. In electron-histochemical preparations, failures to demonstrate a known lysosomal constituent are often without cause attributed to denaturation of the enzyme by the preparative technique or else to failure of the reagents to penetrate the lysosome. Meanwhile, it could be that the enzyme had not been properly "activated" and hence could not react with the cytochemical substrate. Clearly, interpretive caution is called for.

Given the case where most of the acid phosphatase activity of eosinophils is localized within inconspicuous membrane-bounded bodies, while only a few of the conspicuous specific granules are reactive, it is difficult to decide what accounts for the unreactivity of the remainder. These might have failed to react because the reagents could not penetrate the limiting membranes, or equally because the few reactive granules had lost their latency, while the rest had retained theirs. Then too, the enzyme might normally occur in only a small part of the specific granule population, or else the reactive granules might have been exhibiting a false localization due to diffusion and adsorption of the cytochemical reaction product onto their surfaces, and so on. Choosing among these possibilities, Komiyama and Spicer [127] offer reason to believe that the reactive eosinophilic granules are activated and the remainder, while possessing the enzyme, are latent. While specific granules of microphages seem to become activated only after macroendocytosis and fusion with the phagosomes, a minority of the specific granules of eosinophils appear to become activated somewhat similarly, by fusion not with phagosomes but with microendocytotic vesicles. These specific granules strictly speaking then become heterolysosomes, although they continue to look essentially like their latent companions (primary lysosomes).

A way of further exploring this problem of latency is to use living preparations where cells can tolerate the cytochemical reagents awhile, and in a series of cautiously evaluated experiments to seek hints from lysosomal behavior under close to living conditions. A number of studies of this nature have been attempted with the aim to see if the latency of lysosomal granules is reversible or not in vivo and if it need always be associated with endocytosis. In cultures of mammalian cells, it seems that just prior to rupture of their membranes the lysosomes become reversibly permeable to substrates such as β-glycerophosphate [30] and the vital dyes euchrysine and neutral red [2]. In guard cells of angiosperm leaves *(Campanula persicifolia)*, a physiologically reversible activation and deactivation of acid phosphatase in lysosomes (spherosomes) is demonstrable and can be related to the normally large daily swings in the osmotic pressure of the cells (~5 atm). The lysosomes become active when the turgor drops and the cells enter a relatively catabolic phase of metabolism, and they become inactive when the turgor increases and the cells become more anabolic [230]. Such cells are confined by cellulose walls and are not phagocytic. Unlike animal cells, they contain few vesiculated structures describable as microendocytotic vesicles even though their vacuolar apparatus is highly developed; in any case, no such vesicles have been observed in the process of fusion with the spherosomes. Thus, as illustrated in plants, the processes of lysosome enzyme activation and inhibition at times are localizable to the lysosomes themselves and do not necessarily require prior stimulation by endocytosis or fusion between endocytotic and lysosomal vesicles. The enzymes themselves may play a broader role in cell metabolism than one exclusively tied to the breakdown of sequestered foreign or autophaged materials. To what extent metabolic shifts govern activation or inhibition of lysosomal enzyme activity in phagocytes is an interesting matter for speculation.

2. Certain digestive processes may require additional contributions to be made from phagosomal or other sources before otherwise activated lysosomal enzymes and substrates can interact optimally The myeloperoxidase antimicrobial system of microphages is a good example of this. In the presence of lysosomal myeloperoxidase, hydrogen peroxide and oxidizable cofactors such as halide ions, bactericidal action against *Escherichia coli* is much more pronounced than in the presence of only one or two of these components [122]. If hydrogen peroxide production in the microphage fails, some of its bactericidal capacity will be lessened except where it is brought to bear against peroxide-producing organisms or a mixed population of bacteria containing them. Normally hydrogen peroxide is generated by nonlysosomal components of microphages during a respiratory burst associated with phagocytosis. Other needed cofactors are obtained from the serum, the microphages in particular being able to concentrate iodide against an electrochemical gradient [224] and even to obtain it by deiodination of circulating thyroid hormones [130]. The feeding of these nonlysosomal contributions into phagosomes and heterolysosomes likely is regulated by mechanisms other than those used to remove latency from the lysosomes, but these mechanisms, broadly speaking, contribute to "activation" of the cell's digestive system. At times a single cause may underlie the activation of all these mechanisms: The generation of hydrogen peroxide proceeds

rapidly on stimulation of the plasma membrane by chemotactic or other factors that either irritate it or promote recognition [85,87] and is measurable before the lysosomes are stirred up. As seen above, however, activation of the lysosomes themselves need not be preceded by successful generation of peroxide.

The presence of heterolysosomes in the cytoplasm of phagocytes indicates that lysosomes in the cells had become activated; but after considering the findings on eosinophils just discussed [127], one would be careful not to say that all of the lysosomes necessarily had been. Furthermore, once the heterolysosomes have worked on their contents awhile, many become quiescent but remain charged with indigestible residues (Figs. 14, 16, 23, 25, 26) often whorls of lipid-rich matter and sometimes remnants of bacterial cell walls made indigestible by their coatings resistant to lysosomal hydrolysis. These heterolysosomes then become residual bodies, which may remain for a long time in the cytoplasm of macrophages. For example, tattoo inks are retained by them for the life of connective tissue macrophages, and the anchor or mermaid designs on the individual's skin change little in his lifetime even though the cells that originally ingested the inks eventually die and their contents are reingested by younger cells. The inert material in residual bodies evidently need not provide continuing provocation to the cell, and the lysosomal system of cells containing them may lapse into quiescence. In other macrophages nonmetabolizable but continually irritating materials like certain particulate carcinogens may provide a continued stimulus to the lysosomal system, perhaps through the agency of receptors on the heterolysosome membrane that resemble those on the cell surface concerned with mediating the recognition responses. It is not known whether or not these surface receptors survive the internalization of plasma membrane during endocytosis, nor is it known if similar but newly synthesized receptors replace them on heterolysosome membranes.

If cellular receptors are continuously being triggered by irritating materials in residual bodies, the effect would be to encourage continued synthesis of lysosomal enzymes and continued activation of other intracellular digestive functions. Among wandering phagocytes these events would normally be feasible in macrophages, for only they live to retain residual bodies for long and possess the reserve capacity to make new enzymes. Continued activation might also take place in some epithelial cells of the lungs. In bronchi or bronchioles this might result from microendocytosis of incompletely digestible irritants deposited and too slowly removed from the free surface of the epithelium [160], for apical vesicles, tubules, and the like are frequently seen in the ciliated cells (Fig. 35), and the cells have reasonably prominent digestive systems and contain numerous residual bodies in the cytoplasm (Fig. 34).

As indeed one might expect, the digestive systems of phagocytes are sufficiently versatile to be able to break down a wide variety of large molecules into compounds of smaller molecular weight, but differences in the capacities of these systems naturally occur among the various leukocytes and the alveolar macrophages (Table 3). Concerning digestion in macrophages, it has been interesting to learn whether these cells normally contribute to immunological defenses by ingesting and partially degrading bacterial and other cell products into still relatively large but manageable units that might be better antigens than the microorganism in its entirety. In addressing this question and more general ones about the digestive capacity of macrophages, Cohn and associates first determined that about 80-95% of iodinated albumin and a number of other proteins taken up by cultures of these cells were broken down into small molecules within about 20 hr after they were first administered; the reaction products were largely soluble in trichloroacetic acid, and monoiodotyrosine was recoverable from the incubation medium [70]. This suggests that the macrophages break down ingested proteins to amino acids and small peptides. To see if this occurs within heterolysosomes, Ehrenreich and Cohn [71] used these organelles as osmometers. They found that sucrose (MW 340) as well as certain tripeptides and large dipeptides of D-amino acids (MW >230) remained in the heterolysosomes once taken up by pinocytosis [53]. Since these compounds could not pass through the surrounding membrane, they drew in water, causing the organelles to swell. In the case of sucrose, administration of yeast invertase hydrolyzed the molecules into glucose and fructose (MW 180), which passed through and relieved the swelling. The same size limit applied to the peptides of the D-amino acids; the amino acids and many dipeptides got through but larger peptides did not. Use of D-amino acid isomers enabled these authors to determine the size limit for peptides; those of natural L-isomers of amino acids are broken down by lysosomal peptidases. *On the whole, these experiments indicate that hydrolysis of ingested protein can be carried to completion within heterolysosomes of macrophages.* It would seem doubtful that antigen-processing (see discussion in Ref. 195) is carried out in this manner.

Passage through the heterolysosomal membrane occurs either because it contains pores sufficiently large to admit molecules of the size of glucose, or else because the membrane contains "permeases" or mediated transport systems for these but not for sucrose or D-tripeptides. Tentative preference might be given the first explanation for reasons already discussed [262].

Inside the digestion vacuoles of mammalian phagocytes the pH has generally been found to be acid, although estimates vary. Rous [212] used litmus and some other substances as vital dyes by injecting them into the bloodstreams of mice and thereafter observed red litmus granules in the cytoplasm of abdominal macrophages. In dying cells these turned blue again. After administration of bromphenol blue (yellow at pH 3.0, blue at 4), he found that similar cytoplasmic granules became yellow, which indicated that the pH of their contents was somewhere near 3.0. Approaching this question in a different way, Mego [166] concluded the value for mouse liver heterolysosomes to be closer to pH 5. He measured the effects of various strengths of buffers at pH 4, 5, 7, and 8 on proteolytic activity and generally found inhibition increasing with buffer concentration at all values except pH 5. Preincubation in 0.2 M sodium bicarbonate inhibited hydrolysis, but the inhibition could be reversed by resuspending the particles in the pH 5 medium. The bicarbonate has no buffering capacity at a neutral pH but being a small molecule readily diffuses into the heterolysosomes and then acts to neutralize the pH inside until it is washed out once again by resuspending the particles. The presence of an internal buffering system rather than membrane impermeability to bases was therefore postulated to be the main provision for maintaining intravacuolar pH. Mego considered that this buffering system may consist of the same acidic lipoproteins that others have credited with keeping the enzymes latent inside lysosomes (p. 758). In heterolysosomes it would maintain optimum pH for enzymic activity and buffer the inhibiting effects of basic degradation products. He also mentioned that the acid pH optima of lysosomal hydrolases tend to minimize damage to the cell in the event the hydrolases escape into the cytoplasm. In the case of hydrolysis by nonlysosomal specific granules of microphages, however, more alkaline conditions and presumably different buffers might be necessary. It is not yet clear whether alkaline and acid hydrolysis in these cells takes place in the same or in separate digestion vacuoles, and if in the same, how the pH optimum for each type of hydrolysis might be maintained. Perhaps alkaline hydrolysis precedes the acid. In relation to acid hydrolysis, however, the repeated fusions that have been observed between lysosomal granules and the relatively long-lived heterolysosomes of macrophages might help to assure the continuing operation of these vacuoles as much by adding fresh buffer as by replenishing the enzymes.

Particulate materials are taken up and processed in a sequence of events that seem to differ little from that followed in processing invasive organisms. In the lungs, inhaled particles are taken up by microphages as well as alveolar macrophages whenever microphages are present on alveolar surfaces; normally few are. Some stages in the degradation of these particles can be seen in electron micrographs of these cells [235]. When alveolar macrophages ingest particulate iron oxide the particles remain recognizable for a time after segregation in lysosomal bodies (Fig. 28) but subsequently lose the shape they possessed while airborne and become progressively finer textured as they occupy progressively denser heterolysosomes. Some of the iron so sequestered is converted into ferritin, a natural storage form that accumulates in residual bodies as well as in the cytoplasm (Fig. 12). After microphages have taken up similar particles, the treatment accorded the particles is different, for ferritin does not accumulate in the cytoplasm, and many of the cell's cytoplasmic granules remain unfused with the iron containing vacuoles (Fig. 3). Although the specific granules of these cells possess lactoferrin, a protein that binds iron [15], that material is used as an antimicrobial agent, and the cells themselves do not seem comparably involved with iron conservation for the body as are most of the macrophages [79]. In certain cases therefore, it can even be seen in electron micrographs that microphages and macrophages have different capabilities for degradation.

In concluding this section on lysosomal interactions, it may be worth stressing that hydrolysis and peroxidation are only two of several defensive tacks that the digestive systems of phagocytes use against invasive organisms or ingested particles. Other substances effective against bacteria include the acid medium of the digestive vacuole; lysozyme, present in both micro- and macrophages as well as in the serum; lactoferrin and certain basic proteins present mainly in specific granules of microphages; and other materials produced by these and other cell types. Some lysosomal products of one or more of the phagocytes exert protective indirect actions in influencing vasoactivity or in contributing factors used in humoral defense mechanisms, and several of the leukocytes produce endogenous pyrogen which reacts centrally to produce a rise in body temperature.

H. Excretion

While many Protozoa have developed complex cellular mechanisms for excretion of undigested residues, few mammalian cells possess anything comparable; for if the unicellular organisms eject solids and make vigorous use of their contractile vacuole systems, mammalian cells go about these activities more timorously, and with passage of time a great many of them accumulate residual solids in the cytoplasm, variously called aging pigment, lipofuscin granules [183], or the debris of macrophages. Microphages are too short-lived to require a mechanism for release of these solids, and it is debatable whether the longer lived macrophages would benefit the organism by having one. This is because at a metazoan level of organization, the expulsion of residues from component cells merely passes the task of excretion on to other cells. As scavengers of these Metazoa, macrophages ingest dead and dying cells of all kinds and so ultimately receive almost all of their solid residues. To the organism these macrophages then become contaminants, and excretion is achieved by ejecting the cells, thereby purging the organism of undesirable matter. This metazoan excretory mechanism is known to exist in many phylogenetically unrelated animals including the ascidians [128] and the mollusks [240] as well as the mammals. In the last group the main route of egress is along the bronchial tree and out into the pharynx. It is used mostly by alveolar macrophages but is accessible to all of the leukocytes, and they most often leave the bloodstream to enter the pulmonary alveoli. The leukocytes also seem capable of leaving the body by crossing the bronchial, intestinal, or reproductive tract epithelia, but these routes are not taken by the majority of departing cells. Mammalian connective tissue macrophages, on the other hand, rarely migrate from their familiar haunts, but as they die their residues may be picked up by other cells, usually along the path of lymphatic drainage.

Where true exocytosis occurs, the process of expelling the residual bodies appears not to differ greatly from the process of merocrine secretion as seen in pancreatic zymogen cells. If this rarely occurs in macrophages, it does occur in great alveolar epithelial cells of the lungs, for to the lysosomist their surfactant-rich secretion granules (multilamellar bodies) easily qualify as residual bodies. In these cells the bodies pass toward the cell surface, and their membranes then fuse with the plasmalemma, to release their contents onto the alveolar surface. As it nears the cell periphery, and before fusing with the cell membrane, each residual body penetrates the region of (polyactin?) microfilaments and so becomes segregated from other cell organelles—possibly endocytosis in reverse. Centrioles frequently occur at the cell surface close by [232].

It is debatable to what extent excretion of lysosomes or phagolysosomes from leukocytes is a normal event [180], but it can be provoked experimentally by administration of cytochalasin B. This mold metabolite most often inhibits cell movements, supposedly by disrupting microfilaments and possibly by depolymerizing actin [201]. It has been reported to inhibit exocytosis in several endocrine cells but paradoxically seems to stimulate it in microphages [63,92]. Under more physiological conditions, rabbit microphages in vitro will release some of their granule contents upon reaction with immune complexes bound to a nonphagocytosable surface [96]; this insightful observation may explain why extracellular materials are sometimes digested in certain kinds of immunological disease (Sec. V.D).

III. Special Cytology of the Phagocytes

The purpose of this section is to describe functional characteristics of the separate mammalian phagocytes in more particular detail than has been presented in Sec. II. In that section, general points were most frequently documented from studies on microphages or macrophages, while other phagocytes were somewhat neglected. A correcting emphasis is given here, and comparisons and contrasts among all the phagocytes are drawn in closer relation to the cytology of these cells.

A. Microphages and Macrophages

In their common struggle against infection, the two principal classes of phagocytes show different responses to different bacteria. Metchnikoff observed in mammals that β-hemolytic streptococci and gonococci are taken up by microphages but not by macrophages, whereas the reverse is true concerning the mycobacterium of leprosy. Furthermore, the microphages, while present in the bloodstream, are not usually present in the tissues. They reach the tissues during an early or acute phase of an inflammation when large numbers migrate out of the bloodstream by active movement, or diapedesis, through vessel walls. In contrast to the microphages, small numbers of macrophages are normally demonstrable in the tissues before wounding occurs, but additional numbers arrive and cross over from the blood later on to initiate the chronic phase of inflammation. In the case of healthy lungs in normal but not germfree animals, alveolar macrophages are present on alveolar surfaces in some number, but the polymorphonuclear microphages arrive in quantity during acute pulmonary infections notwithstanding, and their appearance is followed in due course by the arrival of mononuclear cells from the bloodstream, just as normally occurs in many other tissues of the body. These mononuclear cells likely had been monocytes in the bloodstream, but it is conceivable that some of them had other previous histories. With evidence pro and con, there is still sufficient reason to believe that at times Kupffer's cells are released from the liver to circulate as macrophages of the blood and then to lodge in the pulmonary capillaries, ultimately to emerge on alveolar surfaces [219], but the numbers contributed to the alveolar macrophage pool in this manner are likely to be small. Mononuclear cells that arrive in the lungs become transformed into macrophages and usually blend imperceptibly into the wandering macrophage population there. The possibility that "alveolar macrophages" in reality consist of a mixed population of different types of macrophages will be discussed in Chap. 20.

The reasons for the normally early arrival of microphages and the later arrival of macrophages are not well understood but, as mentioned in Sec. II, could be related to the microphage's more rapid migration through vessel walls and the tissues as much as to differences in chemotactic responsiveness. Any macrophage presents a broader front than the microphage while it is migrating and this conceivably slows it down; Metchnikoff also believed that the multilobed microphage nucleus presents less of an impediment to passage between endothelial cells during diapedesis as compared to the single rounded macrophage nucleus, for so it appeared to him whenever he watched the migration of these cells under the microscope. Why macrophages predominate among very late arriving phagocytes is more readily explained by differential chemotaxis, particularly when sensitized T lymphocytes are on hand at the wounding site to release macrophage-attracting lymphokines (p. 795).

The metabolism of the microphage is suited to a cell that often serves as the first line of defense for the body, because the energy for phagocytosis is supplied by anaerobic glycolysis [185], and the cell enters the region of damaged tissue carrying its own store of glycogen. The mitochondria in these cells have been characterized as "really in terrible shape," whereas those of macrophages are "quite decent" [114]. Mitochondria of alveolar macrophages are still more impressive with a cytochrome system capable of sustaining the cells even where oxygen tensions are very low, and they normally make it possible for the cells to maintain Q_{O_2}'s of 22-25, oxidative activity levels comparable to neurons of the brain and other highly active cells. Other evidence indicates that when they enter the circulation, microphages are thoroughly ripened cells ready to expend their bactericidal armament and remaining energies and then expire; when released the cell is no longer capable of division, and the nucleus, besides being much lobated, shows considerable condensation of its chromatin—a shutdown of DNA transcription at gene loci. With further aging the nuclei become still more lobated. The presence of 5 or 6 lobes is the mark of a senile cell unless the occurrence is in large microphages, when it results from interference with nucleoprotein synthesis due to a deficiency of folic acid or vitamin B_{12}. Mature microphages have relatively large numbers of azurophil (lysosomal) and specific granules but little granular endoplasmic reticulum, evidence of a reduction in protein synthesis compared with what had passed while the cells were maturing in the bone marrow. The Golgi apparatus persists, while the centrosomes together with its centrioles and an aureole of microtubules show no evidence of degeneration (Figs. 1-4). Among different species the exact enzyme and matrix composition of the specific granules may differ as is evident from the varied coloration of these granules after staining with Romanovsky-type eosin-azure-methylene blue mixtures as well as from the cell's synonym of "heterophil."

In contrast, macrophages typically have a less condensed nucleus usually no more than simply lobated. Lysosomal granules of all kinds dominate a changeable cytoplasmic picture. The endoplasmic reticulum and Golgi apparatus are often prominent, although the granular reticulum never extends as much as it does in protein-secreting cells. The cell center, centrioles, and usually arrays of microfilaments are all conspicuous (Figs. 17 and 18). A peritoneal macrophage is often taken for a typical macrophage, since these cells are readily obtained by inducing a sterile inflammation in the peritoneum and lavaging its contents, and they are often studied. Alveolar macrophages are as easily recovered from lung washings and so their appearance is almost as well known. These and other regional macrophages share general features, although small differences in size, nuclear condensation, etc. sometimes help to distinguish one subtype from another. Greater differences are seen if macrophages are compared side by side with precursor forms, monocytes, and epithelioid and giant cell members of the macrophage family.

FIGURE 17 Centrioles encircled by Golgi lamellae in a mouse alveolar macrophage. Expansion of the Golgi compartment occurs in actively phagocytic cells, but the time of maximal expansion is better correlated with the time of peak phagosome rather than lysosome formation.

FIGURE 18 Centriole and radiating microtubules in a mouse alveolar macrophage that had ingested iron oxide dust. Ferritin (60 Å) particles are abundantly scattered in the cytoplasm.

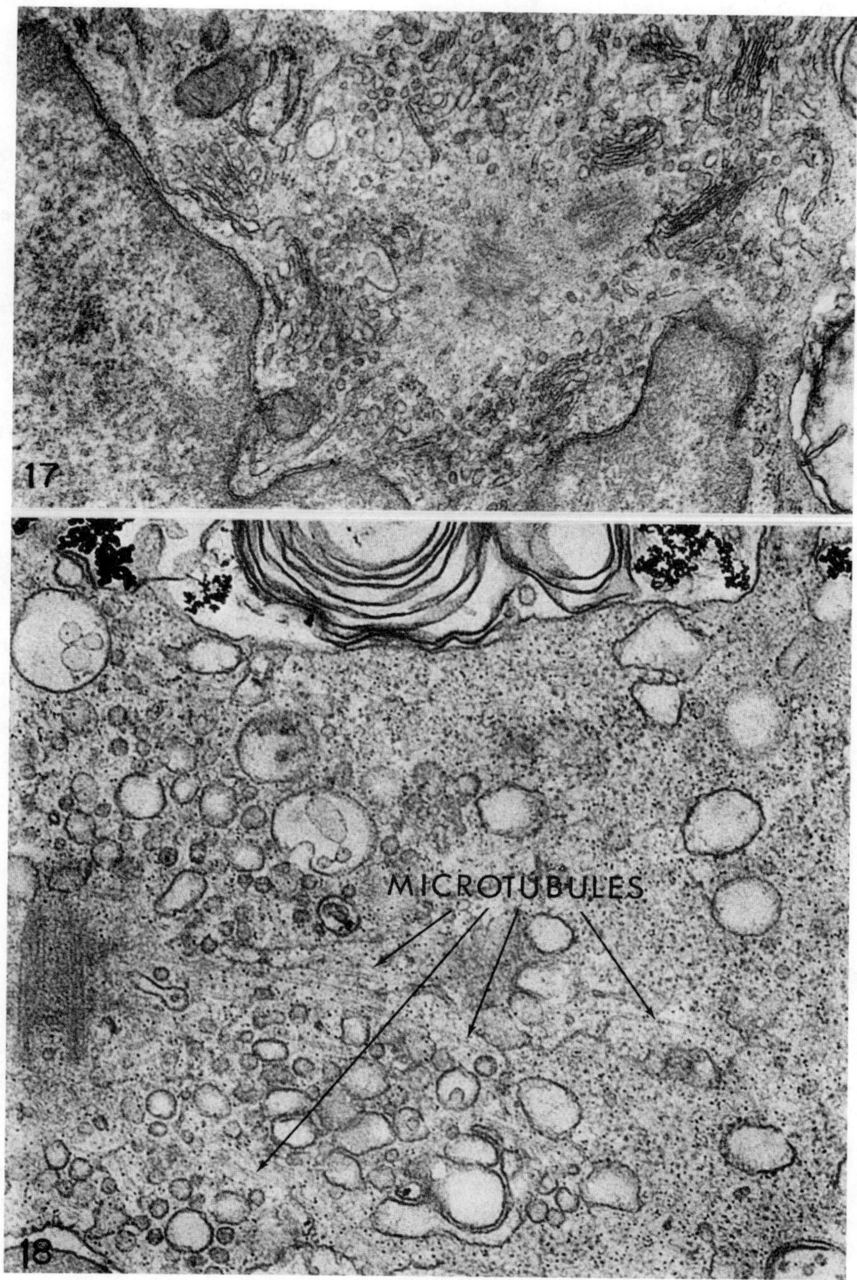
17
18
MICROTUBULES

Just what the precursor forms of macrophages are and where they are located remains controversial as further reading in this and the next chapter should indicate, but precursors of the circulating monocyte, the *monoblasts, promonocytes,* and *immature monocytes* have been described in the bone marrow of mice [76] and human beings [254], and it is possible to perceive them as forming a differentiating cell line, although it is far easier to perceive the stages in the differentiation of erythroid or granulocytic lines of vertebrate blood cells. All these monocytic cells share a certain undifferentiated appearance not unlike stem cells or "blast" forms of other blood lines: a fairly large nucleus with one or more nucleoli and a moderately basiphil cytoplasm containing mostly free polysome clusters together with scattered profiles of both granular and agranular reticulum, a compact Golgi apparatus, moderate numbers of short rodlike mitochondria, a few small vesicles both coated and uncoated, and a sparse assortment of 0.1-0.5 μm electron-dense and azurophil granules of a lysosomal character. The monoblast is considered to have the fewest granules and the most dispersed chromatin pattern of any of these cells, and as the path of differentiation is traced the chromatin becomes more clumped, granules and cytoplasmic membranes become more abundant, and the number of free polyribosomes declines. Centrioles are about equally prominent in these cells and the cytoplasm of all contains microfilaments. Immature human monocytes are considered by Tanaka and Goodman [254] to differ from myelo-(granulo-)blasts mainly in exhibiting nuclear indentation and more condensed chromatin, and from promyelocytes and myelocytes in producing fewer and less characteristic granules. All the cells of this series are phagocytic and have an irregular cell outline, whereas early granulocytes (promyelocytes) of mice are not phagocytic and have smooth outlines [76]. In this species both promonocytes and promyelocytes are reactive for peroxidase, although this enzyme is not active in macrophages; in guinea pigs, however, it is [217]. Circulating monocytes seem to vary in the number of lysosomal granules they carry, but in acid phosphatase preparations of peripheral blood, many of them are among the most reactive cells present (Fig. 1). The same is true of smears reacted for β-glucuronidase [147] and N-acetyl-β-glucosaminidase, the latter being only minimally reactive in human granulocytes [208]. The nucleus of a circulating monocyte is distinctly lobed or even horseshoe-shaped; it is heavily outlined by heterochromatin, and the nucleolus may be inconspicuous or absent. Upon reaching the tissues, monocytes undergo stimulation and become transformed into macrophages. Whatever lysosomal reserves the cell possessed as a monocyte are now supplemented by synthesis of new granules, and the cells become more aggressively phagocytic than monocytes could have been while suspended in the circulation, or than their relatives or precursors had been in the bone marrow. Many details in this process of transformation are well known, for it was carefully observed in many species long ago [142,162,163], although a purely monocytic and not a lymphocytic origin of transforming cells could not be established. In tissue cultures of chicken blood, transformation readily occurs, and it has been documented both cytochemically and morphologically at light and electron microscopic levels [251,273]: The cells become more mobile and increase in volume. The Golgi apparatus enlarges and lysosomal enzyme activity is enhanced. Later on the macrophages become more quiescent, and retaining many heterolysosomes but no longer engaging in phagocytosis, they become epithelioid cells. In still older cultures giant cells begin to appear, apparently more as a result of fusion of individual macrophages than as a consequence of repeated cell division (see Plate 2a). Two variant forms of macrophage-derived giant cells have long been recognized by pathologists, *the Langhans type* with multiple nuclei distributed peripherally or at the cytoplasmic poles and *the foreign body giant cell* with many, and sometimes hundreds of nuclei either scattered or centrally located. Both varieties are known to occur in the lungs under somewhat different circumstances (Sec. V).

In the tissues "activated" macrophages will give varying evidence of being engaged in new synthesis of lysosomal enzymes. Compared to monocytes there will be an expansion of the endoplasmic reticulum, an ultrastructurally visible enlargement of the Golgi apparatus, and increments in the cytoplasmic content of various membrane-bounded vesicles and vacuoles associated with endocytosis and internal digestion, notably phagosomes, heterolysosomes, some multivesicular bodies, and transitional lamellae (GERL) between the agranular reticulum and the Golgi apparatus. The nuclear chromatin pattern frequently seems more "open," that is, less condensed than in monocytes, and usually one nucleolus per cell is typical. Leake and Heise [137] have compared the cytology of alveolar and peritoneal macrophages in germfree rats, finding the former to be generally larger cells with rounder nuclei more frequently provided with a nucleolus; they found the peritoneal macrophages had more granular reticulum, a more extensive Golgi apparatus, and rather more elongated mitochondria than alveolar macrophages; but as noted, these cytoplasmic characteristics can differ from one cell to another and may vary in a given cell from time to time.

B. Alveolar Macrophages

Electron micrographs of alveolar macrophages show variable chromatin patterns in the nucleus depending on the cell's physiological state but also somewhat depending on the fixatives used to preserve them. The chromatin rarely exhibits marked condensation in keeping with the cells' undoubted capacity to divide, mitotic figures being relatively easy to find in lung washings or when one is scanning sections of lung (see Plate 1C). Cultures of peritoneal macrophages in contrast have been characterized as a nondividing population, remaining in the G_0 phase of the cell cycle until DNA synthesis is stimulated by exposing the

FIGURE 19 One of the smaller alveolar macrophages obtained by lavage of mouse lungs, this cell is considered to be recently "activated" into production of lysosomal enzymes but otherwise relatively immature. The outer nuclear membrane is studded with ribosomes (cf. Fig. 17) and at two places (arrows) is seen to continue into the granular endoplasmic reticulum, moderately expanded at this time.

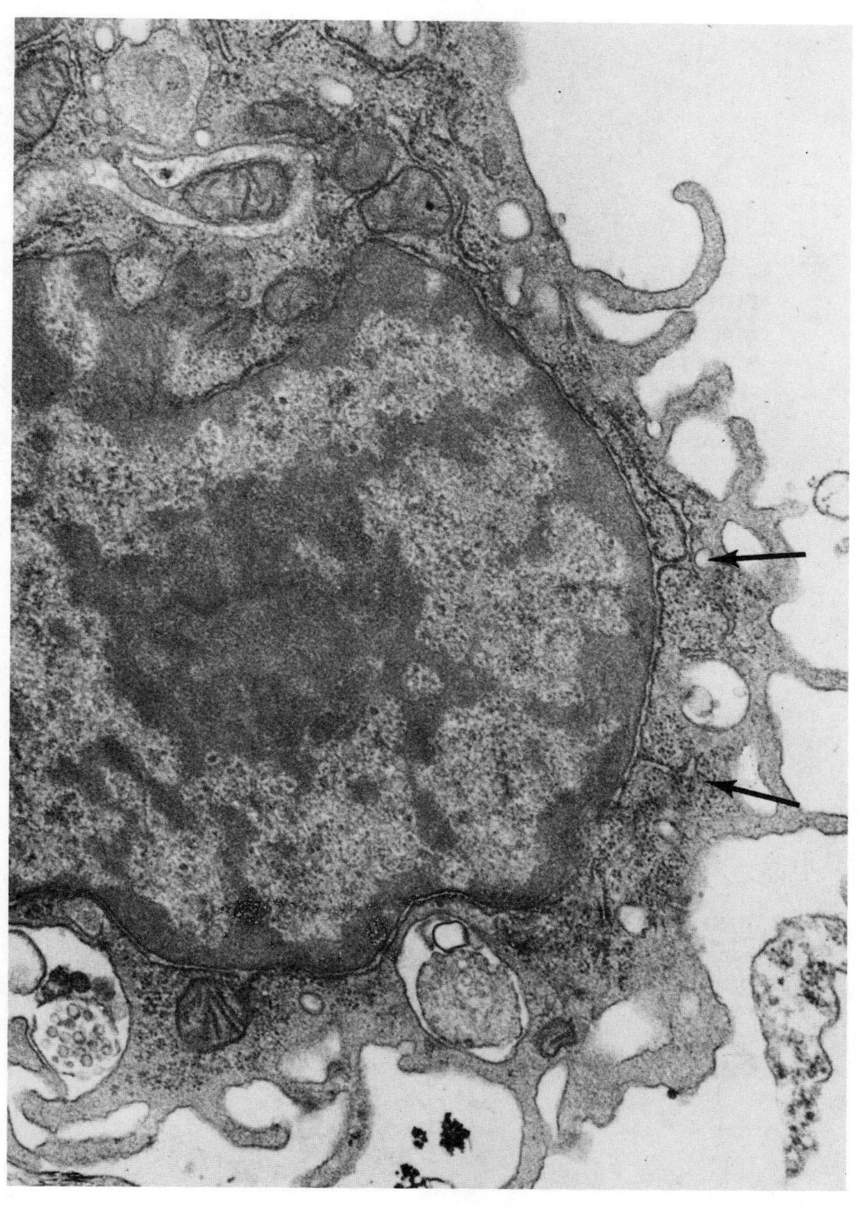

FIGURE 20 Mouse alveolar macrophage lavaged 3½ hr post-exposure to iron oxide dust. The perinuclear region is the site where primary lysosomes are formed. At first these structures appear rod- or wormlike in longitudinal section and rounded in cross section; in three dimensions they may exist awhile as a continuous network. (From Ref. 235.)

FIGURE 21 The "wormlike bodies" subsequently enlarge through accretion of electron-dense material within the core of the lysosome. Deposition is nodular rather than continuous, so that the lysosomes take on an irregularly rounded shape. (From Ref. 235.)

FIGURE 22 A more fully developed lysosome in an iron-exposed mouse macrophage. It opens out conidium-like at the end of a narrower channel (arrow); its contents are variably osmiophilic and, but for a trace of iron oxide present, might be taken for a mature primary lysosome.

FIGURE 23 One of the more unusual forms of heterolysosomes found in mouse macrophages. Iron oxide particles are present as well as tubules that encircle a densely osmiophilic region of the matrix.

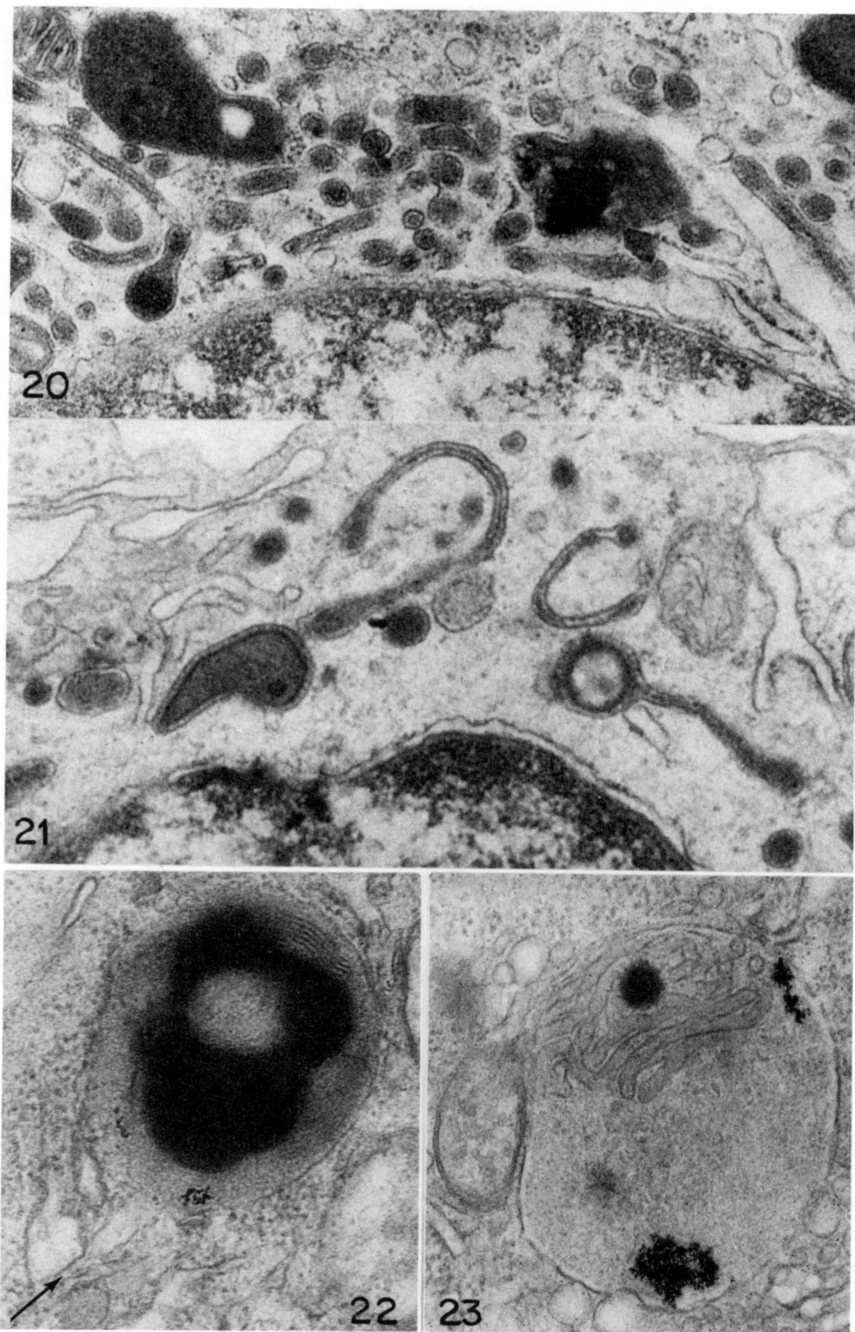
20
21
22
23

cells to a medium enriched with factors produced by other proliferating cells, for example, L-cell fibroblasts [86].

The cytoplasmic appearance of alveolar macrophages is as variable as it has been claimed for macrophages in general. Heterolysosomes and residual bodies become numerous after the cells are stimulated following introduction of inflammatory agents like BCG or inhalation of inorganic particles into the lungs; but even without this stimulation alveolar macrophages usually contain a number of them. Such bodies often give these cells a species-specific appearance: In rabbits the heterolysosomes typically contain dense, circular inclusions [55]; in cats they may have considerable lamellated material [54]; in opossums (Fig. 14) they may consist in large part of triglycerides [233], and so on. Often this reflects the usual pulmonary environment of these animals as much as it indicates differences in cellular contributions to the makeup of these bodies. For example, in man, typical heterolysosomes of alveolar macrophages are relatively electron-dense and uniform in appearance, but some are larger and contain ferritin or bacterial and alveolar cell debris, including lamellated materials presumably derived from secretions of the great alveolar cells; these contents are also seen in the alveolar macrophages of mice and rats, hamsters and bats (Fig. 25). In the lungs of smokers (Fig. 26) the macrophage heterolysosomes are larger, rather more elongated and denser than they normally are in nonsmokers [202].

Other cytoplasmic features of alveolar macrophages provide still clearer evidence that the cells undergo changes in activity. If the ribosomal arrays on the nuclear envelope are examined in a number of alveolar macrophages, they sometimes seem to provide a fairly uniform coating over the cytoplasmic surface, whereas at other times they are scarcely present at all. Most frequently they furnish a distinctly uneven or even a sparse covering (Figs. 17 and 28). In contrast, the outer nuclear membrane of microphages is usually without them, and this is nearly as true of eosinophils (Figs. 4 and 6). To some extent *these differences must reflect differences in the state of protein synthesis associated with the endoplasmic reticulum* (proteins destined for storage or secretion in an exoplasmic vesicle) in these cells, for as soon as a cell begins to synthesize an enzyme or other identifiable protein belonging to this class, that product first appears in the perinuclear cisterna (see Fig. 8 in Chap. 20). With expansion of synthesis, not only this portion but other parts of the endoplasmic reticulum become involved, and the product begins to accumulate extensively throughout the cisternae of the reticulum (see Fig. 9 in Chap. 20). Possibly the first association among the ribosomes that manufacture the protein, the ribonucleic acid messenger that contains its code, and the transfer RNAs takes place in the cytoplasm next to the nucleus (source of these RNAs); and as protein synthesis begins the elected ribosomes become ranged in polysomal clusters along the outer membrane of the nuclear envelope, which subsequently "unrolls" into the cytoplasm

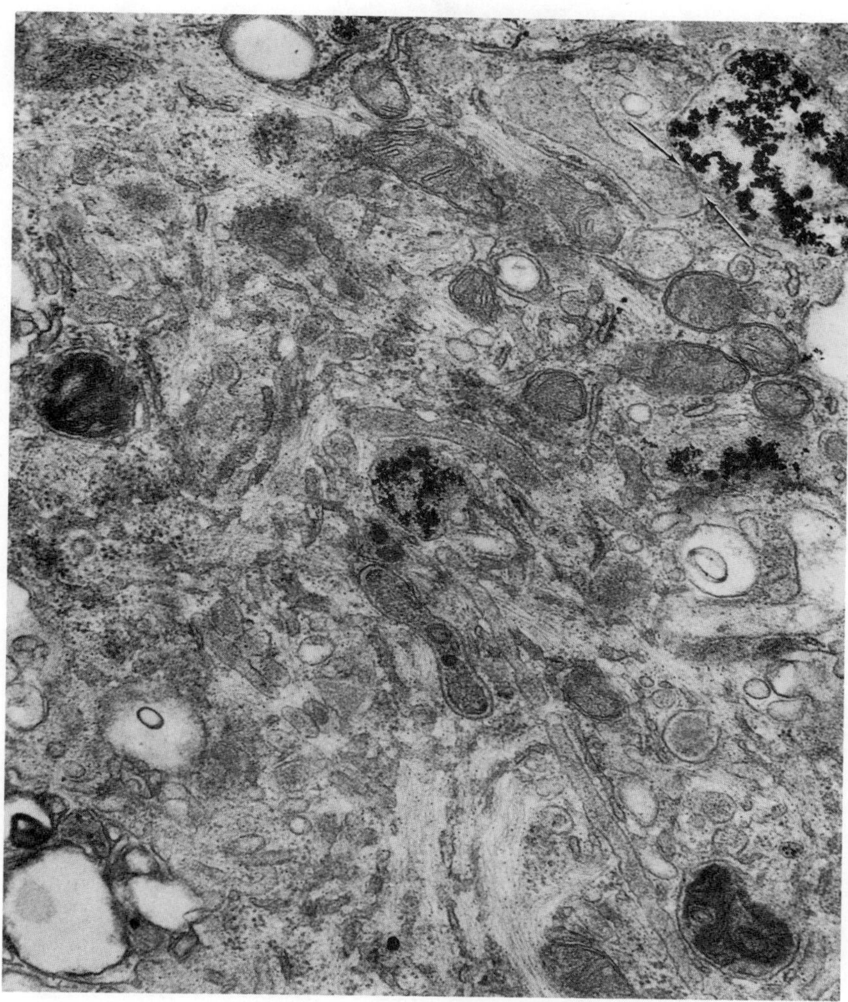

FIGURE 24 Cytoplasmic detail from a mouse alveolar macrophage exposed to iron oxide dust. Near the surface (upper right) a phagosome containing iron particles undergoes fusion with an enlarged primary lysosome (between arrows). Other more slender primary lysosomes (wormlike bodies) as well as heterolysosomes occur among mitochondria and profiles of endoplasmic reticulum, while the ground plasm is crisscrossed by many microfilaments and a few microtubules.

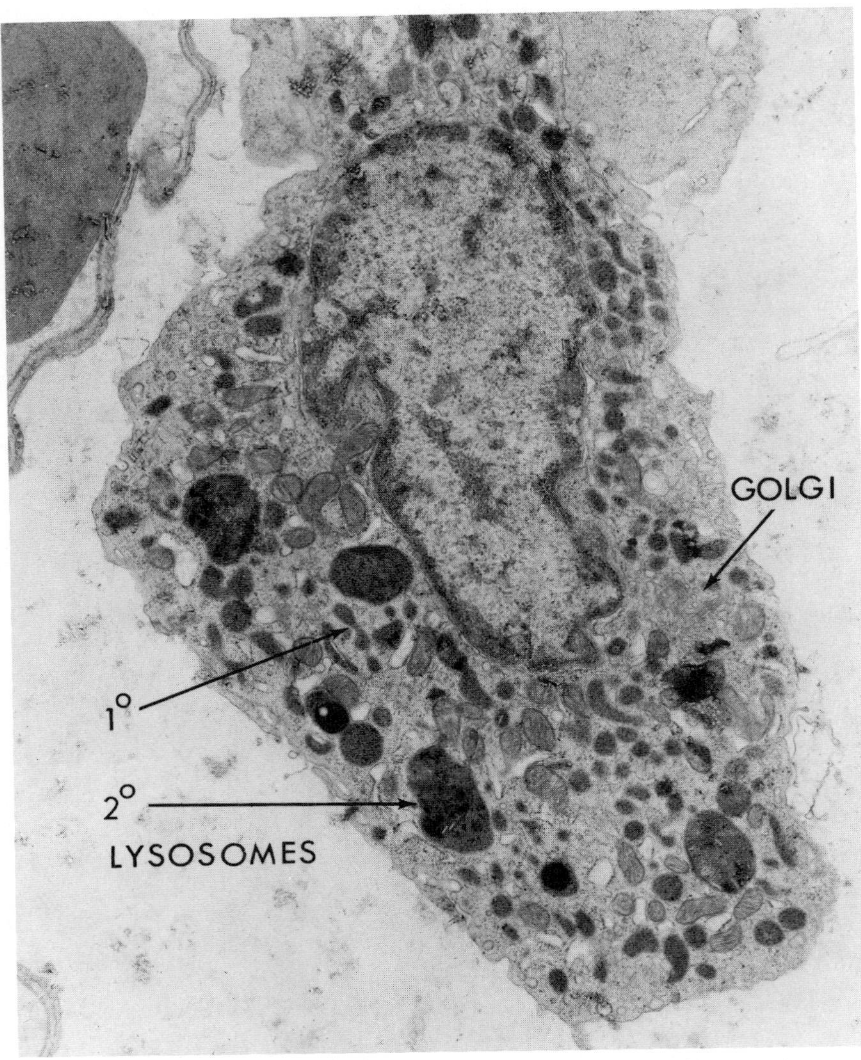

FIGURE 25 Alveolar macrophage in a bat's lung. The lysosomal system is interpreted as having been recently "activated." Nuclear envelope and cytoplasmic membranes retain moderate numbers of attached ribosomes. The wormlike primary lysosomes have expanded and spread throughout the cytoplasm. Most remain small, but some grade up to bodies with heterogeneous contents, the secondary or heterolysosomes. Few vesicles specifically identifiable as phagosomes are present, and the Golgi area is small.

and is replaced by newly assembled membrane to which new ribosomes adhere. The groupings of ribosomes visible on the outer nuclear membrane in electron micrographs represent the polysome clusters, and these are best seen in sections that graze the nuclear surface. From observing the clusters one may obtain further information on the protein synthesis under way. First, *the size of the clusters may reflect the molecular size of the protein,* since the strand of messenger RNA to which the ribosomes attach is longer the larger the number of amino acids in the protein; hence it can accommodate more ribosomes at one time, making a larger polysome cluster (assuming that free ribosomes are in excess and the rate of synthesis is to be maximized). Second, *from the density of polysomal studding on the nuclear membrane, one might obtain a crude indication of the level of synthesis recently initiated.* An alveolar macrophage with many polysomes adherent to the nuclear envelope but few attached to peripheral cytoplasmic membranes (Fig. 19) might be a cell in which synthesis of a certain protein had begun. Conversely, one with few polysomes on the nuclear membrane but some attached to peripheral cisternae might well be a cell in which the synthesis had peaked and is now waning (Fig. 28). The preceding would likely apply to the case of lysosomal enzymes as well as to secretory products, for these are synthesized by the granular endoplasmic reticulum; it would not apply to the case of proteins synthesized on polyribosomes unassociated with these membranes.

Often the alveolar macrophage with a heavy ribosomal coating on its nuclear envelope is a smallish cell with relatively little ingested material and few heterolysosomes—perhaps a recently "activated" cell. Those with a light ribosomal coating on this membrane are often more "experienced" cells whose cytoplasm contains a variety of phagosomes and primary and secondary lysosomes; collectively these details make up the image of a cell that has already responded to stimulation.

The Golgi apparatus of alveolar macrophages undergoes expansion and contraction during the life of these cells, but the meaning of these changes is scarcely understood. In mononuclear as well as granulocytic leukocytes, this organelle lies in the synthetic pathway leading to the azurophil lysosomes, but the nature of Golgi contribution(s) is only vaguely comprehended and is quantitatively if not qualitatively different in promonocytes from normal as compared to abnormal (Chédiak-Higashi syndrome) mice [184]. In the case of normal alveolar macrophages, this Golgi contribution may differ in lysosomes produced, respectively, before and after the cells became "activated" in the lungs:

If we grant that macrophages are derived from circulating monocytes or their precursors, we would expect that they reach the lungs already possessing azurophil lysosomes; these would constitute the first population of primary granules in these cells. They differ little from azurophil lysosomes synthesized by promyelocytes in the bone marrow [239], and apparently their manner of formation is similar. Both become electron-dense and peroxidase-positive. Using a marker for myeloperoxidase in the human neutrophilic line, Bainton et al. [19] implicated the perinuclear cisterna, the granular endoplasmic reticulum, and the Golgi apparatus in the synthetic pathway and characterized these three structures as the granule-producing apparatus. These lysosomal granules seem to be formed at the *inner face* of the Golgi apparatus [17]. During the myelocytic stage of development, specific granules begin to form and synthesis of the azurophil granules falls off; the new nonlysosomal granules contain alkaline phosphatase among other things [16] and first appear against the *outer convex surface* of the Golgi apparatus. Synthesis of these specific granules continues long after production of the lysosomes has ceased, and with continued cell division, the latter become reduced in number, while the former eventually amount to about 80% of the granules in the mature neutrophil. Whether or not a third type of granule, also lysosomal, exists in human neutrophils is controversial; such a granule appears in mature rabbit heterophils, is acid phosphatase-positive but peroxidase-negative, and is small but irregular in shape [16,275] (also see Ref. 254).

The main population of primary lysosomes arises in alveolar macrophages following stimulation in the lungs. If these macrophages are emigrants from the bloodstream, then the "intrapulmonary" lysosomes constitute a second lysosomal population in these cells; in any case they overshadow any earlier population present (see Plate 1b at end of chapter). The newly formed granules have lysosomal enzyme activity (Fig. 29) (see Plate 1d) but in rabbit macrophages tend to be less strongly azurophilic than typical lysosomes of bone marrow cells; and, while they arise in the perinuclear zone where the Golgi apparatus is generally located (Fig. 17), the evidence linking this organelle with their synthesis is tenuous. The first appearance of this new lysosomal population is striking: A single spot of acid phosphatase activity appears on one side of the nucleus (see Plate 1a). The enzymatic reactivity and the diameter of this spot increase from a region having a quarter of the diameter of the nucleus to one of half its diameter. Subsequently the enzymatic reactivity spreads round the nucleus and still later it extends to the periphery of the cell (see Plate 1d) when heterolysosomes have by then begun to form. As seen by electron microscopy, the structures that follow the changing localizations of acid phosphatase are certain rodlike, sometimes dumbbell-shaped and often wormlike bodies that are moderately but inhomogeneously electron-dense and are limited by membranes (Figs. 20 and 21). The smallest of these have dimensions similar to individual Golgi lamellae and are perhaps 700-800 Å thick, but at the least they differ in containing a dense central line that runs the length of the body. These rods frequently expand at their extremities when the dense line seems to split to enclose newly deposited material. When viewed in cross section, slightly expanded rods seem to have a

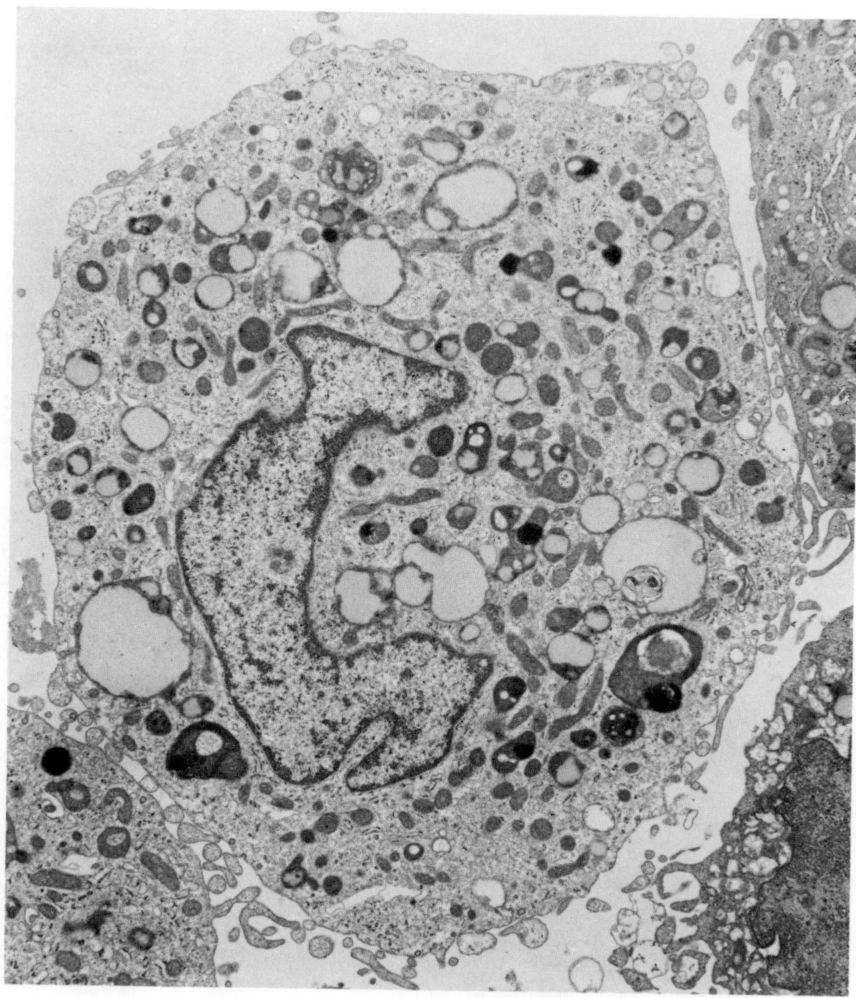

FIGURE 26 Human alveolar macrophage from a bronchial lavage of a smoker's lung. A later stage of the intracellular digestive process is pictured than is shown in Fig. 25. The expanded lysosomal compartment consists mainly of heterolysosomes, some possessing clear lipid rich centers. Most of the linear structures in the cytoplasm are mitochondria and not primary lysosomes. (Courtesy of A. J. Ladman, from work of Pratt, Smith, Ladman and Finley, Ref. 202.)

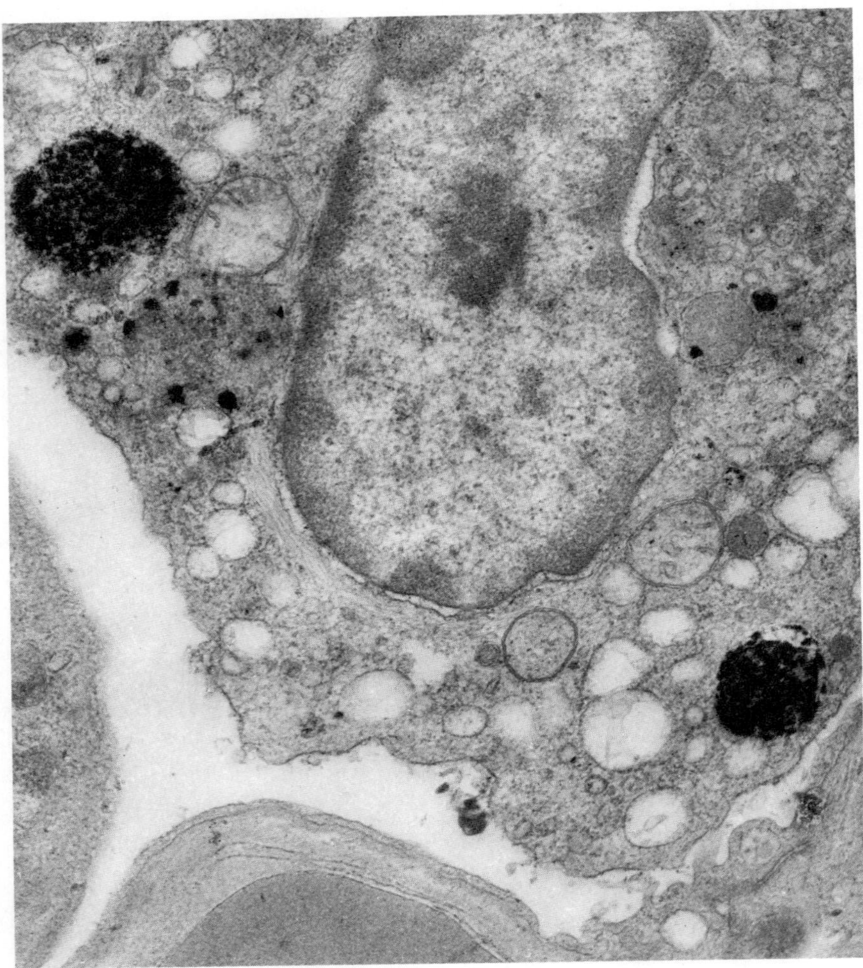

FIGURE 27 Electron-histochemical reaction for acid phosphatase in a bat's alveolar macrophage located in the lungs. Enzymatic activity (black deposit) is both in small circular profiles about the size of primary lysosomes viewed in cross section as well as in larger heterolysosomes. Gomori's method.

lighter "cortex" and a denser "medulla," which represents the thickened central line. These bodies eventually expand still further into rather ovoid to spherical lysosomes up to 0.5 μm or more in diameter, new material accumulating in the medulla. In these enlarged lysosomes a structure like the original central dense line often adheres to one side of the medullary region. Wormlike bodies like these have been observed to comprise the perinuclear "rosette" of lysosomes seen early in stimulated rabbit alveolar macrophages [138] as well as in mice [235]. Early in its existence the rosette may consist of a continuous tubular network which soon after becomes demarcated into segments and subsequently breaks up into individual wormlike lysosomes. Leake et al. [139] consider this tubular system to represent the Golgi apparatus as it appears in alveolar macrophages during the period of lysosomal synthesis, but it remains to show that it is not a specialized extension of the endoplasmic reticulum instead. Small bodies like these as well as larger heterolysosomes are reactive for acid phosphatase in electron-cytochemical preparations (Fig. 27). Continued growth of the primary lysosomes may result from fusions of several wormlike bodies, and until they fuse with phagosomes (Fig. 24) they interact relatively little with vesicular structures derived from the endoplasmic reticulum or Golgi apparatus. Well formed heterolysosomes sometimes have two or more of the primary lysosomes' dense lines incorporated into their structure, suggesting that several fusions may occur between the primary lysosomes and a phagosome or heterolysosome [235]; other heterolysosomes in the same cell may take on different aspects (Figs. 22-25).

Whatever the Golgi apparatus may have to do with the synthesis of this "second population" of lysosomes in alveolar macrophages, it seems to expand in relation to other cellular functions, since it is often enlarged when few wormlike bodies are in evidence (Fig. 17). In relation to its participation in lysosomal synthesis, the Golgi contribution might be more to matrix components and less to the enzymes. It is probable that the sulfated mucopolysaccharides and basic protein that account for the azurophilia of lysosomes in monocytes and granulocytes [102] are constituents requiring Golgi participation for their synthesis, since this organelle is known to play a role in the synthesis of mucopolysaccharides [196]. Furthermore, in having no azurophilia, the specific granules of microphages differ from the lysosomes in matrix as well as enzymatic constituents, and the manner of Golgi interaction differs during the genesis of each. Something similar might apply to the role of the Golgi apparatus in the synthesis of azurophil vs. later-formed lysosomes of alveolar macrophages—the Golgi apparatus being more deeply involved in production of the former as compared to the latter. Perhaps the azurophil materials confer on the lysosomes greater stability or "latency" than is possessed by the lysosomes formed by macrophages in direct response to stimulation and are only added at a late stage in the formation of these bodies.

C. The Essentially Different Life Patterns of Microphages and Macrophages

Although the macrophages and microphages carry out defensive actions that are more similar to each other than to actions of eosinophils or basophils, the latter cells are all granulocytes and share a life pattern that differs from that of the macrophages. An understanding of the dissimilarity between these will help to make clear why both microphages and macrophages are present in infected tissues. The life cycle of nearly all blood cells starts with a stimulus given to initiate division in a hematopoietic stem cell; and this beginning, the developmental potentiality of the cell at once becomes restricted to a greater or lesser degree, while "differentiated" characteristics gradually become manifest in successive generations of descendants. Looking back from a mature microphage, it is at first easy to trace the lineage of this cell through larger and less mature versions (metamyelocyte, myelocyte) with recognizably similar characteristics, but soon it is possible only to adjudge that the immature cell being examined is a precursor of some type of granulocyte (promyelocyte), and eventually only that it is some kind of primitive blood cell (blast). The lineage of eosinophils is also at first easy and then more difficult to trace back, while that of the basophils is at once difficult because relatively few of these cells are available for study and their specific or secondary granules are azurophilic like the primary granules of all the granulocytes. Among other blood cell lines in vertebrates, the erythrocytic and thrombocytic lines are as clearly traceable as the granulocytic lines, but the lymphocytic line is not, and the monocytic-macrophage line is only partly so. This is because there are *progressive changes* in the former lines: with maturation specific cell products appear (specific granules, hemoglobin, etc.), while basophilia, mitotic capacity, and cell size decline, and even enucleation occurs in the red cell line. The case of lymphocytes is confused by the possibility that a number of functionally different cells may share a similarly undifferentiated but repressed appearance (Fig. 32), while all the "stages" in the maturation sequence of monocytes and macrophages are not too far apart morphologically, representative cells being variable and unspecialized in appearance. One might say that a certain degree of cell multiplication but little differentiation of specific cytoplasmic structures or products occur while the cells reside in the hematopoietic tissues. A monocyte might be 3 to 4 generations away from a stem cell [276], whereas a microphage is an indeterminate number more. Development in the hematopoietic tissues is also accompanied by a degree of nuclear shutdown, so that monocytes enter the circulation in a somewhat repressed state that subsequently is reversed as the cells become transformed into macrophages, usually in the peripheral tissues and sometimes in the bloodstream. These differences between the developmental patterns of granulocytes and the monocyte-macrophage group argue toward understanding microphages as cells

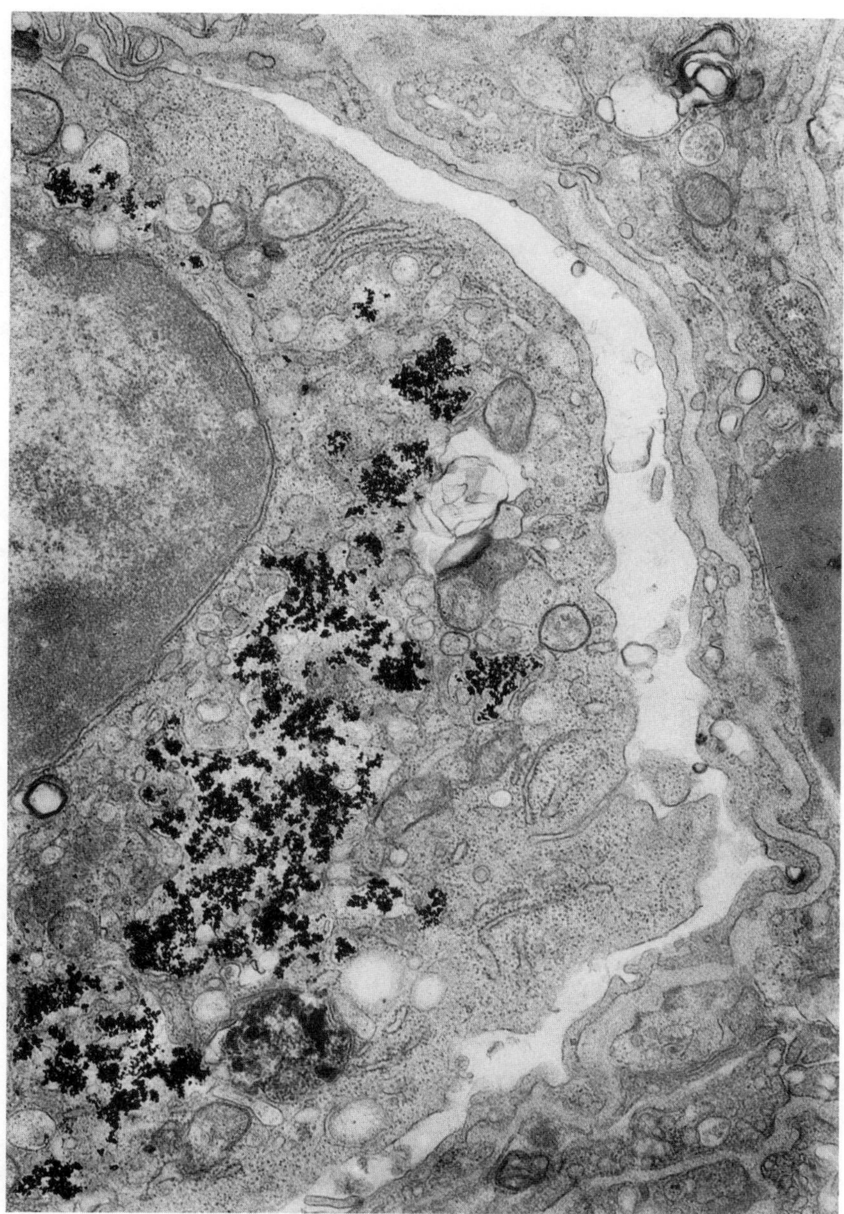

FIGURE 28 Mouse alveolar macrophage in situ 1 hr after a 3-hr exposure to an iron oxide aerosol. The particles, still recognizably in the form they had on emergence from the particle-generating furnace, are being concentrated in a large confluence of vesicles near the nucleus. Profiles of granular endoplasmic reticulum are seen in the periphery, but the outer nuclear membrane carries fewer ribosomes than it sometimes does. Compare with Fig. 19.

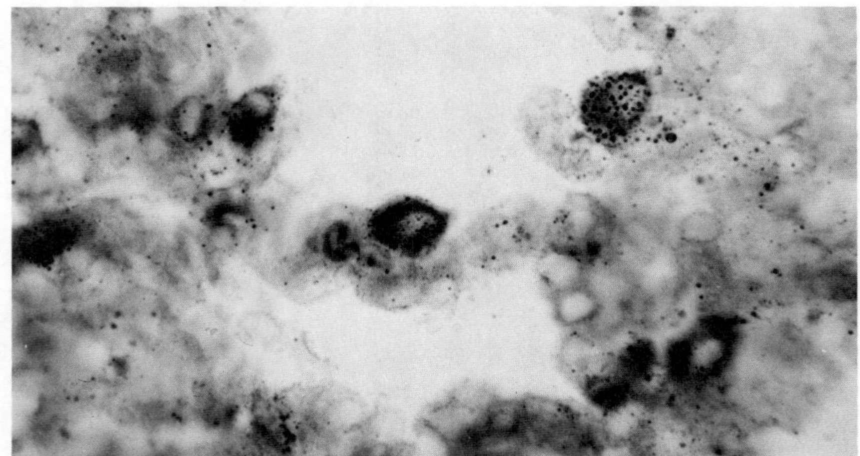

FIGURE 29 Nonspecific esterase in opossum lung. Alveolar macrophages are the most reactive cells shown in this frozen section. α-Naphthyl acetate method.

capable of immediate and powerful but rather stereotyped defensive responses and macrophages as equally potent in defense but more adaptable to changing circumstances. Once expended the microphages die and are replaced by new cells from a sizeable microphage pool [14,62], whereas macrophages do not accumulate in such maturation pools [265] but may continue for a long time in the tissues as more or less migratory cells, sometimes dividing, and sometimes, but not necessarily always, becoming epithelioid or giant cells, as they do in culture and often do in the lungs. Apart from their direct actions against ingested materials, these more flexible cells apparently contribute indirectly to defense in adding to circulating levels of interferon, pyrogen, and serum lysozyme [241].

D. Eosinophils

Eosinophils normally circulate in small numbers as they travel from the bone marrow to their accustomed habitat in the tissues. Some 200-300 are there for each cell in the circulation and they preferentially occupy loose connective tissue beneath an epithelium [214]. In the blood they number some 1-3% of the leukocytes, but in allergic states this may increase rapidly to 5-15%; consequently, it has long been suspected that eosinophils play a specific role in immunological reactions. Relatively recently these cells have been shown to respond chemotactically to antigen-antibody complexes, and in inflammatory exudates responding eosinophils exhibit striking attraction to certain of the mononuclear cells present [237], perhaps because of cytophilic antibody carried on their surface. By means of fluorescent and ferritin labeling techniques, eosinophils have been proven to take up complexes, or else antibody aggregates, formed with free (IgG, IgM) as opposed to cell-bound (IgE) immunoglobulins [148,215,279]. These are equally well taken up by microphages, but eosinophils have an advantage when it comes to soluble AgE-IgE complexes that have not become cell bound [103]. They are selective in their uptake of other substances, reportedly ingesting yeast cell walls (zymosan) and sensitized erythrocytes [7,8], but not commonly occurring microorganisms like *Escherischia coli, Micrococcus aureus* 502a, and *Candida albicans* [49]; notwithstanding, published illustrations show clearly that some bacteria are taken up by these cells [29].

In their appearance and general behavior, eosinophils are typical granulocytes; their cytological makeup is palpably similar to that of microphages (Figs. 5 and 6), and the movements and phagocytic actions of both are closely comparable [28]. The nucleus of circulating eosinophils is less segmented than that of microphages, being usually bilobed and rarely more than trilobed. The specific granules are eosinophilic in whatever species the cells occur, in contrast to the heterophilia of the microphages. In the bone marrow these cells first become distinguishable from other granulocytes during the myelocyte stage of development when azurophil granulogenesis declines and the specific granules begin to appear. As these mature they characteristically acquire electron-dense crystalloids within. Even though species variation occurs in the shape of these crystals, their presence is enough to identify the cells in electron micrographs. In man the crystals may take on any of several forms, but in cats they tend to be concentrically lamellated. By the time they circulate, eosinophils like microphages have passed their period of peak synthetic activity, but their mitochondria seem more robust and their nuclear chromatin is less condensed than those of microphages, perhaps because fewer generations separate mature eosinophils from their early ancestors. In any case the cells thereby seem less effete than microphages. Eosinophilic granules are both larger and more uniform than in microphages and characteristically are more regularly ordered in a radial fashion about the cell center.

Over the past two decades much effort has been made to identify the number and kinds of cytoplasmic granules in eosinophils and to localize specific cell products and enzymes in each. Both biochemically and cytochemically a range of "lysosomal" substances have been associated with the various granules present. They are rich in peroxidase and react cytochemically for mucopolysaccharides, but otherwise they contain most of the hydrolases present in granules of microphages (Table 3) excepting lysozyme and phagocytin [7,8]. In unfixed blood smears acid phosphatase is often demonstrable by azo-dye techniques in the large and presumably specific eosinophil granules (Fig. 1), although variability in staining is apparent [113]. In metal-salt (Gomori) localizations, only some of the large granules in rabbit eosinophils are reactive at their periphery, and most are unreactive, but additional activity is found in Golgi microvesicles. Exceptionally, all the specific granules in a given cell might be reactive [275]. Another lysosomal enzyme, β-glucuronidase, has also been localized to the specific eosinophil granules. The reaction is much enhanced if unfixed blood smears are pretreated with acetone, an effect particularly noticeable in eosinophils [147] and possibly consequent to damage of the granules' limiting membranes. On the basis of the preceding, the specific granules of eosinophils can be considered to be lysosomes. Since mature cells retain the azurophil lysosomes synthesized during premyelocytic stages of their development, at least two classes of primary lysosomes are present, the azurophil and the specific. Overall, the activity of lysosomal enzymes in mature eosinophils is close to the level seen in myelocytes and rather higher than that of mature microphages.

Recent work has demonstrated a third acid phosphatase-positive granule in human and rat eosinophils [127,191]. It is small, rarely over 0.5 μm in diameter, and contains no crystalloids. Enzyme activity is both uniform and strong in these granules as compared to specific granules. Nearby Golgi vesicles are reactive as well. After cells are exposed to colloidal gold, the marker becomes rather generally demonstrable in the small granules, whereas it only rarely penetrates the crystalloid-containing specific granules. The small ones consequently are heterolysosomes, apparently formed in response to microendocytosis (also see p. 759). They have their equivalents in macrophages and occasionally in lymphocytes as well, but they have not been noticed in microphages, which, as noted earlier, are thought not to engage in microendocytosis [182,186].

So far as this is known, phagocytosed materials are processed by eosinophils much as they are by microphages: specific granules empty their contents into phagosomes [61] even if their response to microendocytosis is problematical. In addition, the specific granules are sometimes released into the bloodstream, thereby adding to the pool of serum acid phosphatase otherwise derived largely from the platelets; Tanaka and Goodman provide an illustration of this in their atlas (Ref. 254, Fig. 3-37B). In allergic states, aggregation of eosinophils in the tissues may be followed by deposition of so-called Charcot-Leyden crystals at the site, the material being partly composed of the crystals present in the specific granules.

Whatever may be the significance of these actions, the overall effect of eosinophil action is antiinflammatory. Upon arriving at allergically reactive tissues, these cells remove antigen-antibody complexes that might otherwise bind to serum complement and so initiate inflammation [10]. Eosinophils are also drawn to sites occupied by basophils and mast cells (Sec. III.E) where they appear to counteract the inflammatory effect of secretions produced by these cells. It had been thought that the attraction resulted from the presence of histamine in these secretions [9], but when tested in Boyden chambers (Sec. II.A), histamine has no "eosinophilotactic" effect at all [228]; the attraction more likely results from release of an eosinophil chemotactic factor during anaphylaxis (ECF-A) and possibly from a complement-dependent factor (ECF-C) as well [118]. Just how eosinophils interact with basophils and mast cells is not certain, but some experimentation supports the idea that eosinophils release a soluble factor capable of inhibiting the release of histamine and other compounds stored in those cells [103].

One reason for uncertainty about some aspects of eosinophil behavior is that some tissue acidophils, similar to eosinophils by light microscopy, might really be distinct cells derived from mast cells or other basiphil precursors in the tissue and not from eosinophils of the blood. In rats two cellular species can be distinguished clearly because intravascular eosinophils have a ring-shaped nucleus, while tissue acidophils have a rounded one, but no such distinction exists in many other species. Whether of single or mixed origin, the tissue acidophils occur in the layer immediately beneath the epithelium in the alimentary, reproductive, and respiratory tracts, wherever penetration by foreign antigens is likely. In the lamina propria of the duodenum and presumably elsewhere, tissue acidophils increase while circulating levels of estrogen are elevated and decline when progesterone secretion becomes dominant [109,214], perhaps responding to changes in tissue susceptibility to infection during those states.

E. Basophils and Mast Cells

The basophil is the least well known of the granulocytes because it occurs in the smallest number, rarely exceeding 0.5% of the circulating leukocytes in normal human peripheral blood and scarcely appearing at all in the blood of mice. It had been characterized by Paul Ehrlich [72] as a blood mast cell because its cytoplasmic granules share staining properties with the better known mast cells of the tissues, but it nonetheless exhibits typical granulocytic cytology which tissue mast cells do not. Both basophils and mast cells store within somewhat variable-sized and irregular appearing azurophil and metachromatic granules (see Plate 2b) a wealth of acutely vasoactive agents like histamine, heparin, and (in rodents) serotonin, as well as other agents like SRS-A (slow-reacting substance), which exerts a vasodilatory action on blood vessels. In basophils these usually obscure the nucleus (Fig. 1) which is usually bilobed with its chromatin rather condensed in appearance; as in microphages the cytoplasm often stores glycogen particles. Though rare almost everywhere, through diligence basophils can be demonstrated in vessels of the lungs (Fig. 9), and they originate from precursors in the marrow.

Unlike basophils, mast cells [73,206] are not observable in the circulation even if they are found in extravascular spaces of the bone marrow [254], so that they are not considered blood leukocytes. They form a distinctive cell line of their own [222], possibly arising in situ from undifferentiated reticular cells or else from cells of the lymphocytic group that reach the extravascular tissue through blood or lymphatic channels and there undergo transformation into actively dividing blasts [171].

From this precursor stage onward, mast cells develop within connective tissue; in this sequence a mastoblast with a large nucleus, several nucleoli, and an abundant cytoplasm rich in polyribosomes gradually begins to accumulate granules that from the first are strongly basophilic and metachromatic. Granular endoplasmic reticulum and Golgi membranes then become more prominent, but with increasing granule content in maturing cells the membranes of granular reticulum and somewhat later of the Golgi apparatus are gradually withdrawn, and the mitotic rate falls off. The preceding is seen in rats subjected to infection by an intestinal nematode *(Nippostrongylus brasiliensis)* that stimulates mast cell development [172,173]; under other conditions mast cells of the same species may differ somewhat in details of granule formation [57]. Most significantly, the granule matrix remains unchanged during development of the helminth-stimulated mast cells but (if permitted further maturation?) changes its staining properties in mast cells located deeper in intestinal connective tissues [57], perhaps with full sulfation of the polysaccharide component, heparin, and addition of new matrix proteins to previously formed granules. In his preparations, Miller also found that the granules of developing mast cells stained more strongly with basic dyes than did granules from basophils also present in the tissue. This distinction aside, the general features of granulogenesis are fairly similar in mast cells and basophils [257,275].

Scattered in connective tissue but usually close to blood vessels, mature mast cells exhibit a rounded nucleus which retains a limited capacity for mitosis [31] and a cytoplasm containing an unremarkable development of organelles and some glycogen. They typically extend small projections from their margin (Fig. 7); microfilaments and microtubules are usually easy to find within the cytoplasm; and the cells are capable of ameboid motion (Fig. 8).

Despite differences in cell form, in place of origin, and even in the ultrastructure of their characteristic granules, basophils and mast cells nevertheless share a peculiar reciprocal relationship among several mammalian species so that where basophils are abundant in the bloodstream, the mastocytes are often scarce in the tissues and vice versa [209]. Most of the studies on the function of these cells have focused on the potent pharmaceuticals stored in the cytoplasm, but recent work has begun to explore how these materials are released and in what other ways these cells may interact with other tissue components.

Specific granules of basophils owe their periodic acid-Schiff reactivity and metachromasia to the polyanion heparin, but otherwise the cytoplasmic granules in these cells contains an acid phosphatase [126] and some of the other hydrolases present in granulocytes (Table 3). They appear to contain a perioxidase as well [247], and as a first approximation the granules might be regarded as lysosomal in character with some hydrolase capacity perhaps being masked by complex formation with heparin. The azurophilia of the specific granules hampers attempts to determine whether mature basophils contain one or more classes of granules; for though circulating cells are dominated by their specific granules, these stain similarly to the azurophil lysosomes present during myeloblastic and promyelocytic stages of basophil development, and the fate of these lysosomes is uncertain. Mast cell granules, like those of basophils, can be regarded with some ambivalence as partially lysosomal in character [152]. They consist of about a third heparin, a third basic protein, and the rest histamine, dopamine, proteolytic enzymes, and certain other ingredients [132]. While most of the "classic" lysosomal hydrolases are detectable in mast cells of rats, only N-acetyl-β-D-glucosaminidase and trypsin- and chymotrypsin-like enzymes with alkaline pH optima are localizable to the metachromatic mast cell granules;

and this supports belief that mast cells have two classes of granules, lysosomal and specific, much as microphages and eosinophils do. Granule contents and enzyme localizations differ considerably in nonmammalian vertebrates. For example, in frogs neither histamine, serotonin, catecholamines, nor the above alkaline proteolytic enzymes occur in mast cells; and if the metachromatic granules possess N-acetyl-β-D-glucosaminidase, other lysosomal enzymes are demonstrable elsewhere in the cytoplasm [45]. This would seem to argue no further for ascribing a lysosomal character to the mast cell granules. Nevertheless, the metabolic defect (Chédiak-Higashi syndrome) that leads to abnormal fusion of primary lysosomes in many other tissue and blood cells also affects mast cell granules [44] and quasi-lysosomal melanosomes of melanocytes, and as in basophils the heparin matrix conceivably might mask other enzymes present. It is perhaps fair to regard mast cell granules as exoplasmic structures under evolution away from a primitively lysosomal nature. In various species they sometimes differ in appearance as well as in water solubility [222]. Interspecies differences are also notable among granules of basophils and not surprisingly between granules of basophils and mast cells in the same species (Figs. 7 and 9). For example, in man the specific granules of basophils are finely granular by electron microscopy [254], whereas in mast cells they contain lamellae either laid out straight or rolled into scrolls and sometimes admixed with material in other configurations [272].

Heparin is produced in both basophils and mast cells by enzymes of the supernatant and then is stored in the granules. Mature mast cells exhibit only a slow turnover of $^{35}SO_2$ [112], indicating slow synthesis and sulfation of heparin; the same can be deduced by histochemical staining of the granules with a sequence of alcian blue and saffranin, for alcian blue (acid mucopolysaccharide) at first predominates and only gradually becomes masked by saffranin (sulfation) [58,170]. Histamine is produced in the supernatant by decarboxylation of L-histidine, and after production like serotonin becomes bound ionically to heparin, and so can be stored in the granules. These substances are more readily released than heparin because release is carried out through a cation exchange mechanism [119] and does not necessarily require degranulation or cell lysis which the release of heparin requires.

Whatever is known concerning the functions of basophils may well prove one-sided; because they are scarce and rarely increase in number except during myelogenous leukemia, many of their day-to-day activities may pass unnoticed. Like mast cells they are believed to discharge their function by releasing histamine or cytoplasmic granules into the extracellular space. As discussed below, both kinds of cells are excited into conspicuous activity during immunological reactions, when endocytosis as well as secretion may occur. Microendocytosis seems to be the scale usually favored [68,187], although basophils have been provoked into phagocytosis of sensitized red blood cells [216]. To judge from their granulocytic nature, basophils likely experience one peak of activity and then expire, whereas mast cells either give their all and die or else begrudge the ambient a few granules at a time and live on. Early work indicated that surviving mast cells are able to restock released histamine despite a cytological appearance that suggests little synthetic capacity, and indeed restitution of a degranulated population of mast cells may take several weeks [75]. Later work has provided confirmation that the turnover of histamine and 5-hydroxytryptamine [74] in rat mast cells is slow (half-life ~10 days) and that normal lifespan of the granules may be measured in terms of months rather than days [190]. All this points to the operation of an unusual secretory process as compared to those operating in many other cells.

Under carefully controlled conditions mast cell granules seem to be released individually and in their entirety [188,189], rather than all at once after damage to the cells. This view is all the more plausible because intact mast cell granules sometimes can be recognized within eosinophils or macrophages that had ingested them. At other times it seems that the granules are not fully released but instead are transferred to a membranous compartment confined to the cytoplasm but open to the outside; this can be demonstrated by vital staining of mast cells with ruthenium red, when granules released as well as exteriorized in the manner described will bind the dye, whereas intracytoplasmic granules will not [131]. Furthermore, some of the exteriorized granules appear to be taken up again, and this completes the provision of means for cyclical release and recharging of amines bound to the granular matrix (heparin and basic protein). Degranulation of the sort described can be provoked by administration of polymyxin B sulfate, and generalized degranulation may follow a variety of other stimuli such as the administration of ACTH or of certain snake venoms or after a drop in the pH of the environmental fluid; but it usually occurs in the course of a hypersensitivity reaction following the appearance of complement-derived anaphylatoxin (C3a, C5a) in the serum, or following the arrival of antigen against which a specific immunoglobulin (IgE), produced by plasma cells, previously had become bound to the basophils or mast cells.

Immediate or antibody-mediated hypersensitivity reactions (anaphylaxis) result from contact with an antigen to which the organism previously had been sensitized. Such reactions are often localized to sites where mast cells are abundant because the provoking antigen becomes bound to IgE antibody located on the surface of these cells, triggering release of vasoactive materials or degranulation, to produce a local response. It is also possible that the antigen may first bind to cytophilic antibody on macrophages or other cells in the tissue and subsequently become transferred to antibody on the mastocytes as they touch the other cells. If much vasoactive material is released and gains access to the circulation the reaction can become severe and general. Anaphylatoxin (C3a, C5a) derived from activated complement may help to secure large-scale degranulation. While basophils, platelets, and the gastric glands also produce histamine, the histamine and other agents derived from mast cells can be sufficient to sustain even generalized anaphylaxis. Among different species this reaction can vary in severity from organ to organ depending on both the local concentration of mast cells and their susceptibility to degranulating agents. In rats the "shock organ" is the gastrointestinal tract, in dogs it is the liver, in man it is the larynx and bronchi, and in guinea pigs it is the lung. Anaphylaxis has the following components [119]: dilatation and increased permeability of capillaries and especially of venules, contraction of smooth muscle, stimulation of gastric secretion, and inhibition of blood clotting. The last effect is attributed to the release of heparin, whereas the former effects can be simulated by administration of histamine. Slow reacting substance (SRS-A), an acidic lipid of low molecular weight, is released (by mast cells?) in the lungs during anaphylaxis. It produces a delayed and slow contraction of bronchial and visceral smooth muscle apparently of considerable importance in bronchial asthma [98], inasmuch as antihistamines are of little value in alleviating this condition. The action of SRS-A is opposed by the action of prostaglandins (see below) which is bronchodilatory, and in the lungs the two substances may even be competitively synthesized from the same precursors [268].

Systemic anaphylaxis is a complex reaction during which other compounds besides the above increase in the circulation and like them cause both vasodilatation and stimulation to smooth muscle. These include serotonin, present in rodent mast cells as mentioned but also found in platelets, the gut, and the brain (where it is used as a neurotransmitter); a number of vasoactive polypeptides related to bradykinin, a nonapeptide derived by hydrolysis from plasma proteins; and prostaglandins, phospholipids derived from the prostate gland, the lungs, and other organs. Consequently, the responsibility for anaphylaxis does not rest entirely with mast cells, and the extent to which it does clearly varies, being greater in guinea pigs and dogs and smaller in other species [119].

It has long been a question whether anaphylaxis confers any benefit on the organism forced to endure it. It may be of value in combatting intestinal infestation by certain nematodes. In this case a mast cell colony builds up and matures in the subepithelial tissue. Subsequent events coincide with the time when the worms are expulsed. Amine release, degranulation, and lysis occur, and surviving mast cells are said to transform into globule leukocytes, whose granules differ from those of mast cells in the texture of the matrix and in having little affinity for basic dyes [173]. A localized anaphylaxis results, the permeability of the epithelium increases, and antibodies produced by subepithelial plasma cells gain ready access to the worms in the intestinal lumen. Eosinophils are drawn into the field of conflict and may help to contain the reaction. Globule leukocytes characteristically occur in the epithelium of the intestine and sometimes in those of the reproductive tract [99] and the lungs [120], perhaps after anaphylaxis has occurred in the tissue beneath. Their relationship to mast cells is still a matter of conjecture; some consider them an independent cell line perhaps of a lymphoid kind [253]. Other possible mast cell functions have been discussed by Michels [171], and our certain knowledge of them has not greatly improved since then.

Basophils are known to behave somewhat similarly to mast cells in certain types of hypersensitivity reactions. To some extent they seem involved in reactions where antigens are carried in the serum [13], but their response is especially striking during cell-mediated hypersensitivity reactions [278], of which tuberculin sensitivity is the prototype. These are delayed in onset following exposure to antigen and are transferred not by serum but by immunologically competent T lymphocytes or by nonliving extracts of them that retain some antigenic specificity (transfer factor). The provoking antigen becomes bound to these lymphocytes and secures the release of a variety of mediators (lymphokines) that attract and perhaps "activate" macrophages, stimulate blastogenic transformation of B lymphocytes and themselves lyse cells (lymphotoxin) and prevent replication of viruses (interferon). The result is a mononuclear infiltrate at the reaction site [107].

Using single injections of a rat antihorseradish peroxidase gamma globulin as antigen, Strauss [247] obtained delayed-type skin reactions in the footpads of rabbits where the immunochemical events could be followed microscopically. Within 8-14 days following the sensitizing injection and 1-2 days after a second eliciting injection of antigen, specific antibody could be localized on the surfaces of lymphocytes and macrophages, in the cytoplasm of blastlike cells (immature plasma cells elicited from B lymphocytes), and in the perinuclear region of a few lymphocytes (T lymphocytes?); but antigen as well as antibody and antigen-antibody complexes could be identified in granules of basophils. This was seen in rabbits with a low titer of serum antibody, whereas in animals with a high titer, both antibody and antigen-antibody complexes occurred as well in heterolysosomal granules of macrophages and microphages. Where the serum antibody titer was low the reaction observed was of a fairly pure cell-mediated type, but where the serum titer was higher, the reactions seen were of a mixed type possessing characteristics of both cell-mediated hypersensitivity and cutaneous (Arthus) anaphylaxis. In Arthus-type lesions, serumborne antibodies (cytophilic antibodies), both those specific for the provoking antigen as well as others, coat the surfaces of lymphocytes, macrophages, all granulocytes, and fibrocytes. After some of these have combined with the antigen, the surface complexes might well be taken up and digested by the various phagocytes as the high-titer experiment suggested. On the other hand, ingestion of antigen-antibody complexes in cell-mediated immunity seemed to be the special province of the basophils. This might be explained by postulating: (a) on reexposure to antigen the sensitized cells (T lymphocytes) or possibly others release among other lymphokinins a mediator chemotactic to basophils; otherwise it would be difficult to understand how such rare cells could become congregated into the limited area of reaction. (b) Basophils and the plasma cells that produce the IgG or IgE antibodies used in this type of reaction [106] may interact more or less specifically so that the antigen-antibody complexes are taken up selectively by basophils, to be followed by release of histamine and other active agents in basophil granules; in any case, IgE has been localized to the surface membrane of basophils [250]. A special mechanism such as this might have evolved to obtain release of basophilic contents in situations typified by these cutaneous reactions where the main antibodies involved are not serumborne and hence might not be available to release histamine and other materials from mast cells, nor for that matter to activate complement into producing anaphylatoxin, or to obtain histamine from platelets or other similarly acting pharmacological agents through activation of Hageman factor, plasmin, and the bradykinin mediators. Whatever benefit the organism obtains from the release of such materials from mast cells would also be available from basophils, although elicited by a different mechanism.

From this viewpoint the basophil can be understood to function as a portable mast cell, transportable to far-flung reaches of the body that normally might have fewer resident mast cells than an emergency might require. If mast cells normally occur in the dermis near possible sites of cutaneous hypersensitivity reactions, their manner of increase is gradual, involving mitosis and cell differentiation, whereas the basophils cross over in number from the bloodstream and possess the granulocytic advantage that they are ready for action once they have arrived. As granulocytes, basophils may be subject to a different mode of regulation than is used to control mast cells, although it is apparent that basophils as well as mast cell precursors are attracted to regions of helminthic infection occurring in the intestine [172]. In any case, a gathering of basophils about cutaneous lesions has been noted before, and in guinea pigs a special "cutaneous basophil hypersensitivity" has been carefully described. As these cells congregate they take up antigen and perhaps antigen-antibody complexes [56,69]. Furthermore, the use of endocytosis in the course of obtaining histamine release has been better documented in these cells than it has yet been in mast cells.

IV. Phylogenetic Interrelationships

If our main interest in this section is to trace the lineage of the phagocytes that migrate through the lung, we cannot do this adequately without at least referring to the vascular systems of which they are part. Accordingly, both cells and systems are considered, even if this takes us away awhile from our main theme. The real point of introducing material on the vascular systems is to show that their phylogeny and that of the cells that circulate in the bloodstream have been distinct for long stretches of evolutionary history, although the two have come to be closely associated during the evolution of vertebrates. Just sufficient detail is given to make this clear.

A. The Blood Vascular Systems

It will be appreciated from study of the invertebrates that many diverging, some parallel, and a few converging pathways have been followed in developing the various blood vascular systems currently employed in the animal kingdom. No single evolutionary line leads to the blood vascular system of mammals. Many elements contribute to make up any such system, at the very least some blood cells, a fluid plasma, and the vessels through which the blood flows. To these some sort of heart and the means to regulate the circulation are added as the organism it serves becomes larger and more complex. Elaborate systems are correspondingly elaborate in these elements and present many new features besides, like separate blood and lymph channels and the means to filter them, as well as discrete tissues specialized in the production of only certain of an expanded range of blood cell types.

In any system made up of several components, evolutionary pressure may bear unevenly and with uneven effect on any single component or group of them; and in the blood vascular system few exhibit consistency of form or function throughout such a vast range of animal life as we survey here. For example, great variation is found in such things as the nature of the plasma; the presence or absence of respiratory pigments of different kinds, their occurrence in cells or in the plasma, and their representation among the various animal groups; the occurrence and characteristics of the various blood clotting mechanisms; the types of leukocytes formed in the organism; and the nature and locations of blood-forming tissues or organs.

To begin with the invertebrates, rudiments of a circulatory system are discernible in mesenchymal tissues of certain flukes (trematode platyhelminths), but the simplest closed circulatory systems occur among the rhynchocoels. In the basic plan, often elaborated in these animals, a pair of vessels runs longitudinally one on each side of the gut to join at the ends through mesenchymal lacunae lined by endothelium [22]. A variety of corpuscles are suspended in the blood which flows irregularly, aided by contractions of the larger vessels. The main similarities between this circulatory system and that of the trematodes are its bilateral symmetry and its orientation parallel to the midline digestive tube. Vascular systems of annelids are also closed off from the body cavity, but they are more highly developed than in the rhynchocoels and moreover are laid out according to a different plan whereby the dorsoventral axis is given emphasis and accommodation is made to the segmentation of the body. In mollusks the layout of the circuit again differs, and it is open to a greater or lesser degree, the blood being propulsed by a distinct heart into sinuses where cells of the body are bathed directly. Circulatory systems in arthropods are also open, although they are considered to have evolved away from a closed plan similar to that of the annelids. The dorsal vessel of these worms becomes a distinct heart in arthropods, consisting of one or more chambers arranged in linear order with lateral openings to receive blood from the surrounding sinus [264]. In Echinoderms the blood vascular (hemal) system is greatly reduced owing to the presence of a water vascular system and to extensive use of the body cavity for circulatory functions. Its form is adapted to the five-pointed symmetry of these organisms.

Among any of these invertebrate phyla the smaller animals may develop little in the way of any vascular system. At the other extreme the cephalopod mollusks, being large and having an elevated metabolism, not surprisingly possess the most highly developed of invertebrate systems complete with a closed circuit and an extensive capillary system. Blood pressure is maintained at elevated levels by contractions of a centrally located heart and an additional pair of branchial hearts placed just before the capillary beds of the gills. Some of the more complex invertebrates possess in addition to the basic elements a number of accessory structures associated with the circulatory system. Among these are spleen-like bodies that serve to filter the blood, such as the gills and the posterior salivary glands in the octopus, *Octopus* and *Elodone* [129,249], and the spleens of Kowalevsky present in a number of gastropod mollusks and arthropods [129]. The octopus also confines leukopoietic tissue within so-called "white bodies"; putting together these, the salivary glands, the blood phagocytes, and elements in the gills, Stuart [248] has argued that the assemblage constitutes a reticuloendothelial system for cephalopods palpably similar to the system of mammals [12].

Even the most superficial comparison of invertebrates will turn up examples that show the effects of selection pressure, the conservation of equally effective solutions, and parallel evolution during the development of the blood vascular system. All this makes it difficult to homologize many specifics of invertebrate blood systems with those of higher vertebrates, as the following may attest.

Among annelids, several glycerid and gephrean worms contain nucleated *(Glycera)* or, exceptionally, anucleate *(Thalassema* and *Magelona)* "erythrocytes" [125,211], even though the respiratory pigments (iron porphyrin proteins chlorocruorin, hemerythrin, and a variety of hemoglobins) when present are most frequently dissolved in the plasma. The erythrocytes may be discoid, when they possess a marginal band like mammalian erythrocytes; and except for *Magelona* they circulate in the coelomic fluid. Although the annelid circulation includes a well-developed system of vessels [91], the blood cells are produced by extra-vascular hemopoietic organs or peritoneal cells and after formation must migrate through the coelom and vessel walls in order to reach the bloodstream [5]. In *Glycera*, however, the vascular system is absent. In other forms, a cardiac body associated with the branchial heart seems to act as a spleen; it is composed of pigmented cells like those of chloragogen tissue from the peritoneum (the "liver") and may function as a center of intermediary metabolism. Furthermore, in most orders of leeches (Hirudinea) the ancestral annelid circulatory system is replaced by a new one formed from sinuses that come to occupy the coelomic cavity [154]. As a group the annelids seem to have explored nearly all workable ways of combining blood cells and vascular systems, as a detailed examination of only the polychaetes will show [211].

In mollusks as in arthropods the dominant respiratory pigment is hemocyanin, a copper containing, nonporphyrin protein. Hemoglobin nevertheless is found in a few representatives. Sometimes it is dissolved in the plasma (the gastropod *Planorbis*) and sometimes it is contained in corpuscles (the lamellibranchs *Arca* and *Lima*). Further complexities of relationship are found among the blood cells of these groups.

Basic features of vertebrate blood systems are scarcely discernible in urochordates, which have an extensively open circulation, but the general plan does become apparent in the cephalochordates despite the persistence of an open plan and hence an absence of capillaries. The plan is characterized by bilateral symmetry and a ventral heart and aorta connecting by aortic arches to a dorsal aorta that runs the length of the thorax and abdomen; this plan with various modifications serves all the vertebrates [210]. As in the case of the more complex of the blood vascular systems in invertebrates, those in vertebrates possess many special features like filters (spleen, liver), neurovascular bodies active in the regulation of blood pressure, and the like. Among the vertebrates, various evolutionary tendencies can be discerned among components of the vascular and hematopoietic systems; these can be seen as modifications of basic vertebrate structures, and so homologies are readily established among structures in various vertebrate species, whereas they are not easily made between one in a vertebrate and another in an invertebrate. Where they concern the defensive capacity of the vascular systems, these tendencies include: *(a) an internalization of elements of the tissue defense system within the vascular system; (b) the formation of specialized blood cell lines like the erythrocytes, the granulocytes, and the thrombocytes in addition to the undifferentiated leukocytes; and (c) the elaboration of complicated immunological defense mechanisms using protein and polypeptide components of the serum.* Among the latter, the antibody-complement system appears in one form or another in vertebrates more highly evolved than the cyclostomes [84] (Sec. IV.F). Furthermore, in teleosts and especially among land-based vertebrates, lymphatic systems become well developed. By "internalization" is meant the capture of blood-forming tissues and their confinement to compartments like the bone marrow and lymph nodes, so that the tissues become a contiguous part of the vascular system. Lymph nodes are almost uniquely mammalian features, and after they appear, the internalized hematopoietic tissue in mammals becomes more cleanly separable than in other vertebrates into *lymphoid tissue,* charged with the formation of thymocytes, lymphocytes, and plasma cells, and *myeloid tissue,* charged with the formation of erythrocytes, granulocytes, thrombocytes, and monocytes. Vertebrate blood is characterized first of all by an extensive development of erythrocytes which circulate in either nucleated or anucleate form, the most notorious exception being the teleost icefish *Chaenocephalus* [213] without any respiratory pigment whatever in its blood. In other vertebrates hemoglobin is used for this purpose almost without exception. Although hemoglobin and hemoglobin carrying blood cells occur among invertebrates, this probably cannot be taken to indicate any particularly close relationship between these animals and the vertebrates because heme molecules are ubiquitous in aerobic organisms and readily combine with globins to produce a great range of hemoglobins differing in amino acid sequence and molecular weight [37,105]. Those dissolved in the plasma are much larger than those confined within erythrocytes.

B. Phylogeny of Leukocytes

Many of the smaller invertebrate phyla can be said to possess little more than "hyaline" or nongranular leukocytes of one or more different sizes. These serve variously as stem cells or as macrophages and bear general resemblance to the "hemocytoblasts," the large lymphocytes, and the macrophages of vertebrates. In contrast, other phyla like the Arthropoda possess a cornucopia of additional blood cell types resplendent in variety and differing in assortment among arachnids, crustaceans, and insects [110]. Indeed, of the last group, it has been said that "each species appears to possess a unique set of blood cells" [60]. This wealth of material has as yet been insufficiently studied to enable hematologists to state their lineages with certainty, let alone to establish homologies among the greater part of them. Comparable difficulty exists with the blood cells of the lower chordates. Whereas cephalochordates have no blood-forming organs, and the blood cells present are of an undifferentiated, amoeboid type, the urochordates (tunicates) contain besides these colorless cells a variety of pigmented ones: a blue cell and an orange cell owing their colors to included particles, and a green cell owing its tint to a chromagen containing vanadium [97] which is kept in a reduced state by a high concentration of sulfuric acid in the cytoplasm.

Some of these unusual blood cells may resemble cells in the echinoderms, but they have no homologs in the chordates and few in any other group. This and some of the following material is discussed more fully in the monograph by Andrew [5].

Two evident points, however, are that *neither the development of large size nor complex organ systems need be accompanied by an elaborate blood picture:* Cephalopods are the largest and among the most highly organized invertebrates, yet undifferentiated amebocytes resembling monocytes are the only circulating cells in octopods [21,249].

C. Phylogeny of Granulocytes

Phylogenetically granulocytes are of more recent origin than macrophages, for at the most they occur among certain animals possessing a closed, or nearly closed, circulation, and they have no proven counterpart in the tissues of animals without one. Although cells with eosinophil, neutrophil, basiphil, or metachromatic granules have been described in representatives of many groups including the trematodes, rhynchocoels, mollusks, echinoderms, annelids, and arthropods, they are absent from the blood of many others in the same and in other groups. Consequently, it is not possible to envision a "line" of granulocytes extending from phylum to phylum across the animal kingdom, even if one accepted the basic homology of all these granular cells. Using additional criteria, one can doubt that cells strictly homologous with vertebrate granulocytes exist among the invertebrates. Among the granular cells in these spineless forms, few possess deeply lobed nuclei that no longer can divide, and few exhibit the behavioral patterns that characterize any of the three mammalian granulocytes (Sec. III). If it could be shown that the granules of invertebrate cells are stores of lysosomes or other enzyme-containing primary granules, and that they are housed within effete cells that appear as endpoints in the differentiation of certain blood cell lines, then some progress would have been made either toward establishing the relationship between the vertebrate and invertebrate cells, or toward proving a case of parallel evolution. Further resemblance between the granules in the two groups could be sought by comparing the specific forms and contents of the granules. The staining affinities mentioned give no hint as to enzymatic properties and little guidance as to other functional attributes of the granules; witness the variable affinity that vertebrate microphages have for eosin!

In some cases at least the granules in invertebrate leukocytes may represent ingested materials rather than primary cell products, and that seems to be true of the sometimes granulated phagocytes in Porifera; Metchnikoff mentions that paramylum grains and chloroplasts from ingested euglenae may remain in the phagocytes indefinitely (Ref. 169, p. 48). Persistent search sometimes turns

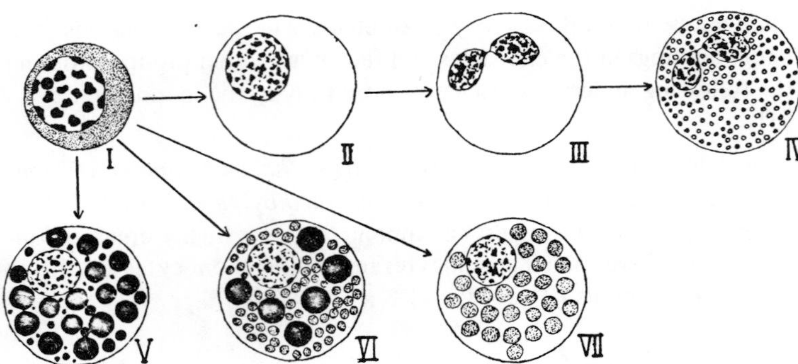

SCHEME 1 Evolution of invertebrate leukocytes. I. Hyaline leukocyte, stage I: Stem cell (hemoblast) with high nucleus/cytoplasm ratio, basophil cytoplasm, and frequent mitoses. II. Hyaline leukocyte, stage II: Spherical nucleus, pale or acidophil cytoplasm, and fewer mitoses. III. Hyaline leukocyte, stage III with polymorphous nucleus: Somewhat like a monocyte (end stage for gastropods, some insects, asteroids; in cephalopods preceding stages suppressed). IV. Granular leukocyte: Heterochromatic nucleus, granules usually acidophil or amphophil; retention of mitotic capacity (annelids). V. Adipohemocyte: Refractile granules (ascidians). VI. Adipospherule cell: Small nucleus, fat globules, and amphoacidophil granules (annelids and insects). VII. Spherule cell: Small nucleus and large albuminoid and amphobasophil granules; comparable to mast cell (many invertebrates). (From Ref. 125.)

up an invertebrate cell with more than one characteristic of vertebrate granulocytes—for example, an "eosinophil" in the gastropod *Busycon* shows little inclination for phagocytosis and may have a lobed nucleus [82]—yet many other granulated cells, especially the larger ones, behave more like macrophages. There is less argument about the origins of these granulated cells; like invertebrate "erythrocytes" they stem monophyletically from a lymphocyte-like hemocytoblast (Scheme 1) according to Kollmann [125], whose view finds modern champions [40].

From the preceding it seems that except for one or two varieties of nongranulated ameboid cells that provide a common denominator for many blood systems, few leukocytes of invertebrates or lower chordates are likely to bear close relation to the blood cells of vertebrates. As descendants of these undifferentiated cells, most blood cells become specialized along divergent lines and so are difficult to compare across phyla.

True microphages and eosinophils are first encountered with certainty in the blood of cyclostomes, and basophils first appear among the ganoids. Thrombocytes are also present, and in most respects the blood of these lowly fish exhibits typical vertebrate characteristics. Among these cells the microphages nearly always have the most highly segmented nucleus just as they do in mammals.

The overall blood picture is similar from one vertebrate group to another, and even where differences among the differentiated cells are present, they do not overstep the boundaries of the general class to which the cells belong. Among marsupials, however, a major shift occurs in the thrombocyte category, which moves away from a pattern of normal-sized, nucleated cells that circulate in the blood to one having megakaryocytes in the blood-forming tissues and platelets in the circulation. Differences that set apart the whole blood cell population of one group from another are rare. One of these is cell size: The blood cells of amphibians are larger than those in most of the other classes, but this reflects the number of generations circulating cells are removed from their progenitors as well as the general level of metabolism in these sluggish animals more than it does basic differences in phylogeny.

D. Phylogeny of Macrophages

Macrophages, unlike granulocytes, are identifiable in virtually all animals possessing a mesoderm with the notable exception of the nematodes; there phagocytosis is carried out by two pairs of enormous cells (3 × 5 × 0.3 mm) in the visceral cavity with a central nucleus, branching myofibrillar system, and peripheral phagocytic area [104]. In appearance and activity the more conventional macrophages can be compared with the more generalized types of ameboid protozoans, but in many respects of chemotaxis and phagocytic behavior they are also comparable to the plasmodium of *Myxomycetes,* when that organism's entire cell population has fused into one multinucleate mass and functions as an individual—a very large "giant cell." Among metazoans, living macrophages have been experimentally studied by Metchnikoff and many others in his time and since, sufficiently to justify belief that these cells are essentially similar whether present in simpler forms like the sponges and coelenterates or in more complex animals. This is not to say that these large mononuclear cells are everywhere identical in all respects; macrophages of invertebrates naturally lack receptors for mammalian immunoglobulin G or complement factors (Sec. II.C) and cytochemical behavior may differ among different macrophages, as it even does between human peritoneal and alveolar macrophages. The cell is not always clearly distinguishable from the hematopoietic stem cell (or cells) of many animals; for though the latter usually resembles the large lymphocyte of vertebrates [163], "hemoblasts" or "hemocytoblasts" of invertebrates are often more active phagocytes than they are among vertebrates, and so few reliable criteria remain to separate them from macrophages.

One concomitant of passing from a colony of similar cells through a two-layered body structure—present chiefly in embryos—and on to the three-layered organization (ectoderm, mesoderm, endoderm) present in even the simplest Metazoa is that the digestive and assimilative activity for the organism becomes the function of the endoderm (gastrodermis) that lines the gastrovascular cavity. This frees the macrophages, as the ameboid digestive cells of the mesoderm, to concentrate on defense against organisms that penetrate the outer or inner body walls. In echinoderms and urochordates some phagocytes apparently become specialized into "trephocytes" [144,145] or carriers of processed food to somatic or germ cells of the body, and so retain for blood cells (and the mesoderm) a nutritive role for the organism. There is little evidence that this tendency is carried over into vertebrate blood lines (mast cells?). Like the specialized trephocytes, however, the unspecialized macrophages possess great capacity for intracellular digestion wherever they are studied.

E. Evolution of Cellular Defense Mechanisms

Considered a while longer in terms of the well-known body layers, unusual phagocytic and digestive powers are often shared by many cells of the endoderm and mesoderm. In the mesoderm of simpler organisms this property and a responsibility for cellular defense are held almost exclusively by the macrophages, but in more complex organisms other cells in this compartment frequently become partners in these activities. In some cases, as in many mollusks, arthropods, and urochordates, more than one type of "macrophage"—one perhaps more differentiated than the other—may be present. In others distinct cells may share defensive functions with the macrophages, whether they be multinucleate cells in the pericardial tissue of certain insects [20], where the cells also serve as precursors to the blood cells, or true leukocytes and other elements of blood-vascular and lymphoid tissue. The latter mesodermal derivatives, which include both free cells and those fixed in the endothelium or extravascular tissues of blood-forming organs, gradually assume increasing importance in cellular defense as the "evolutionary ladder" is scaled.

Metchnikoff's own description [169] of the evolution of cellular defense systems remains the clearest yet written. Based on comparative studies on the reaction of cells to introduced pathogens and to tissue damage, it ascribed to macrophages the fundamental role in tissue defense and showed how with the development of blood, blood cells, and complete circulatory systems, new mechanisms came to be applied to the same end without preempting the macrophages from their ancient function. If macrophages are the only motile cells available for this purpose in the simplest Metazoa, they remain so in more advanced animals despite the emergence of a well-developed and closed circulatory system.

Indeed, in animals as well organized and "experimental" as the annelids, the only cells to respond to invasion by a parasite are the phagocytes arising from the peritoneal lining or suspended in the perivisceral fluid and not the cells in the blood (Ref. 169, pp. 67-72). Blood cells proper do participate in defensive reactions against bacteria and foreign bodies in many arthropods and mollusks as first shown by Haeckel [89] and later by Metchnikoff, Balbiani, Kowalevsky, Stuart [249] and others. Among the organized defenses of blood vascular systems requiring interaction to occur between the leukocytes and the vascular tissues, the reaction of diapedesis, or emigration of leukocytes from the bloodstream, is difficult to demonstrate in animals with open circulatory systems. The process can be inferred to take place in echinoderms because migratory cells are common to all three of these animals' fluid filled compartments while other equally free but nonmotile cells may not be [5]. The capacity to cross epithelial tissues is possessed by phagocytes in many organisms. For example, intracardiac injection of India ink in oysters (the lamellibranch *Ostrea virginica*) may result in partial occlusion of the circulation. In that case, amebocytes appear in the blood, ingest the ink particles, and emigrate through the vessel walls and the surface or intestinal epithelia, thereby eliminating themselves in the process of clearing the organism from the foreign particles [240]. Comparable results have been obtained in the snail *Bullia* after injection of thorotrast into the pedal sinus [40]. Self-sacrifice is a service rendered by many invertebrate hemocytes in the greater interest of the organism, and it is faintly echoed in mammals (Sec. II.H), where this biological mechanism seems to attract less attention than it deserves. The preceding indicates that more than one defensive attribute of vertebrate blood systems is present in lower forms.

F. Humoral Defenses

Vertebrate systems are far more advanced than invertebrate systems in areas of humoral and immunological defense. The process of blood coagulation has been less intensively investigated in invertebrates than in vertebrates, but indications are the mechanism involved is less complex when any exists at all. In several invertebrates it is calcium-dependent like the mammalian process, and in some echinoderms it operates by causing temporary agglutination of the blood cells [5]. Immunological reactivity is only modestly developed in invertebrates; lymphoid tissue is often poorly developed, and there is little evidence for the evolution of alternative sources of immunologically reactive materials. Some mollusks and arthropods possess bactericidins in blood fluids, but these do not resemble antibodies, and they are not important mediators of phagocytosis as antibodies are in mammals. Invertebrates also lack complement. Heat-labile agglutinins of high molecular weight are present in the serum of a number of crustaceans but are absent from the serum of the octopus [249]. At the least invertebrate cells are able to recognize foreignness, and annelids are said to exhibit graft rejection and to transfer transplantation immunity in lymphocyte-like "memory cells" [258].

Forerunners of truly mammalian kinds of humoral defenses are found in existing examples of primitive vertebrates. (a) Representatives of all classes of existing vertebrates produce high molecular weight circulating antibodies in response to foreign antigens, and these resemble the IgM antibodies of man. Antibodies of the IgG type are present in mammals and among certain therapsid reptiles, which resemble forms considered to be ancestral to mammals [155]. (b) A lytic and agglutinating system is present in the sea lamprey *Petromyzon marinus,* but it differs from the conventional antibody-complement system of mammals; this "first appears" in chondrosteans like the paddlefish *Polyodon.* Among sharks, whole complement activity occurs in some species, but only C1 or C3 activity can be demonstrated in others [84]. (c) Experimental studies on the development of various aspects of adaptive immunity, including the elaboration of humoral agents and the integration of their actions with those of leukocytes, once again brought honor to *Polyodon;* for this primitive fish exhibited "vigorous immunologic capacity and responded with production of circulating antibody to every antigen used," (*Brucella,* bovine serum albumin and γ-globulin in adjuvant, hemocyanin, and T_2 phage) as do most amphibians and reptiles [78]. In a series of vertebrates more primitive than this, the lamprey was found to have well-developed mechanisms for cellular immunity and a slight capacity for production of circulating antibody, whereas primitive sharks and rays, possessing both a thymus and spleen, were better able to produce antibody. More modern sharks were still keener producers of circulating antibody, and this seemed to be correlated with the presence of a distinct plasma cell system. In contrast, the lowly hagfish *Myxine* did not clear antigen from its circulation and showed no capacity for immune response in these experiments, although in earlier work by the same investigators it had been shown to respond to injection of complete Freund's adjuvant by a mild inflammation of mononuclear cells and "protogranulocytes." The hagfish has been defended on the grounds that by lacking alloantigenic diversity in its body it has had little stimulus to develop immunocompetence [258].

G. Continuing Evolution of Vertebrate Blood Vascular Systems

It has been mentioned that internalization of the tissue defense system within the vascular system is an important evolutionary feature of vertebrates; nevertheless, it appears that this continued tendency has not yet been brought to completion in even the highly developed systems of mammals. There are several reasons for thinking so: (a) The blood-forming tissues are superimposed onto existing organs such as the liver or kidney as frequently as they are segregated within special blood or lymph organs like the spleen or lymph nodes, and the exact choice of organs for this purpose varies considerably among different vertebrates and even so among different mammals. (b) In the ontogeny of an individual the sites of blood formation frequently shift, for example, from yolk sac to liver and thence to bone marrow. (c) Although lymphoid and myeloid tissues are better separated in mammals than in lower vertebrates, mammalian structures occasionally are found to possess characteristics of both tissues. For example, hemal (or hemolymph) nodes [32], best known in ruminants, are filters having an appearance intermediate between that of a lymph node and the spleen. Typically the sinuses within are supplied almost completely from the blood but in pigs are fed by both blood and lymph. Hemal nodes of deer seasonally may produce erythrocytes as well as lymphocytes. Furthermore, after substantial and chronic blood loss, even typical lymph nodes in man may exhibit hematopoiesis, although the change usually affects the spleen and liver first. Under those circumstances, mixed blood cell formation may occur as well at diverse sites in extravascular connective tissue normally active in this way only during embryonic life. This is to say that evolution in vertebrate vascular systems has reached the point in mammals where heredity provides specialized regions within the systems characterized by a reticular stroma and so favorable to hematopoiesis that stem cells of the blood tend to lodge and multiply there in preference to the extravascular connective tissue. These internalized regions become further specialized to favor the development of either lymphoid or myeloid elements. Nonetheless, because blood cell formation does occur outside of these tissues at various stages of life, and because the internalized sites set aside for lymphopoiesis can support myelopoiesis, a further development of existing evolutionary trends can easily be imagined.

If evolutionary pressure has tended to internalize hematopoiesis within the vascular system, its success in capturing the progenitors for all lines of differentiated and/or normally circulating blood cells appears to be unequal and incomplete. The blood-forming tissues of mature mammals may be regarded as having been seeded by hematopoietic stem cells (hemocytoblasts) whose ancestors originated from extraembryonic (yolk sac) or embryonic (body mesenchyme) mesoderm; these cells form a renewing population(s) of stem cells perhaps tending to become restricted into clones specialized for the production of erythrocytes, granulocytes, megakaryocytes, and so on. It is not controversial that some stem cells, defined as progenitors for certain differentiated cell lines, normally remain for example in the marrow and send out only *end products* of differentiation (granulocytes, platelets), while other stem cells now and then escape to carry out blood cell formation in extravascular connective tissues. To this category belong cells that in the guise of B lymphocytes travel to such sites and there undergo blastogenic transformation into progenitors for a line of plasmacytes. In a like manner, seeded stem cells possibly give rise to mast cells outside of the vascular system. What is more difficult to know is whether this extravascular tissue in mammals retains a renewing population of hemocytoblasts (or somewhat more committed precursors of macrophages) than it possessed early in embryonic life, or whether these reserves are lost with maturation, requiring the tissue to be reseeded repeatedly in order to maintain a functional population of macrophages. It is again not a question of whether formation of macrophages can occur in this connective tissue, for macrophages divide; but whether this dividing population can maintain itself there, and whether or not inactive reserves remain there besides.

Metchnikoff provided a partial answer to this question in amphibians by showing that a macrophage response to wounding could be elicited in the caudal fins of embryonic urodeles (axolotyl and *Triton*); it involved only connective tissue macrophages and did not involve the blood vessels, the nervous system, or the circulating leukocytes (Ref. 169, pp. 95-107). The reaction in these animals was found to be similar to the reaction Metchnikoff had observed in annelids. When similar experiments were performed on the tails of batrachian tadpoles *(Bombinator igneus),* the cellular reaction this time was attributable largely to the diapedesis of leukocytes which had access to the wounds owing partly to the greater vascularity of the tails and smaller sizes of the blood cells in the batrachian as compared to the urodele larvae. Locally produced connective tissue macrophages therefore still exist in these immature vertebrates just as they exist in simpler animals. As for mammals, the ontogenetic studies of Andersen and Matthiesen [4] in man somewhat favor the opposite view, arguing that macrophages do not appear in the tissues until they have become vascularized. Nevertheless, kinetic studies on peritoneal macrophages of mice prelabeled with [^{3}H] thymidine seem to rule out the possibility that all of these cells originate from blood monocytes [227]. Further discussion of experimental work on the questions of macrophage and alveolar macrophage origin will be found in the next chapter.

To the narrower question whether all macrophages are derived from monocytes, phylogeny teaches that the macrophages gave rise to the monocytes; and to the broader question whether all macrophages have a hematopoietic origin, it replies that the macrophages gave rise to the system.

H. Summary

The preceding sketch has tried to show that the evolution of vascular systems and blood cells have usually proceeded separately but that among vertebrates there has been a strong tendency to take in and compartmentalize blood cell-forming capacity, traditionally a property of generalized connective tissue, within the vascular system. It seems unlikely that this process has been completed; the blood vascular system after all is one of very few organ systems retaining considerable regenerative and transformative powers throughout life, and so by its nature may retain a certain ambiguity in the potentialities and distribution of its cell-forming tissues. This sketch has also contrasted the comparatively short phylogenetic history of the microphages and other granulocytes with the long history of macrophages. From this viewpoint the granulocytes can be understood to comprise a series of differentiated cells evolved in vertebrates for use in the more specialized of their defenses. These are immunological in nature, and granulocytic evolution has probably proceeded hand in hand with the development of immunological mechanisms. The macrophages, on the other hand, are basic ingredients of virtually all blood systems whatever their specific architecture and whatever other kinds of blood cells are present. They retain some capacity for further transformation but are far from being totipotent; only exceptionally do macrophages have unusual developmental potential, as in acoel, triclad, and polyclad flatworms (Turbellaria), where phagocytic "hémoblastes" appear to give rise to both germ and somatic cells [203]. As a stable line of *relatively undifferentiated* rather than primitive cells, macrophages number among the rare living things whose essential characteristics are preserved whatever else changes in the system to which they belong.

One might argue that a parallel situation to that between granulocytes and macrophages is to be found at a simpler level of organization among iron porphyrin proteins: in many animals using hemoglobin for oxygen transport, the globin molecules differ greatly from one to another, being selected to mediate optimally between the oxygen demands of the animal's tissues (first requirement) and the supply available from the ecological habitat occupied (second requirement). By way of contrast, in the enzyme cytochrome c, basic to the aerobic respiration of many organisms, the exact amino acid sequences are preserved along great lengths of the protein side chain wherever the enzyme occurs [158]. Among these proteins, as among the cells, the more basic entity is the one better protected from evolutionary pressure, whether this results from functional necessity or genetic conservatism.

V. Phagocytic Activity within Compartments of the Lungs

Like most other organs, the lungs can be divided into epithelial, connective tissue, lymphatic, and blood vascular compartments, and at various times wandering cells may be found in any of them as well as on the surfaces of alveoli and bronchial passages. The actual cell types present differ considerably under changing conditions of pulmonary health, and it is the purpose of this section to describe the changeable picture and to interpret it where possible in the light of what has been presented on the biology of these cells.

While normal tissue integrity is maintained, passage from one pulmonary compartment to another, easy for gases and small molecules but increasingly difficult for larger molecules [218], becomes impossible for all but wandering cells. Under conditions of mild acute inflammation, the integrity of vascular walls and pressure relationships in the vessels may change sufficiently to facilitate the passage of serum into the connective tissue, and under these circumstances the microphages find ready egress through clefts between endothelial cells and enter the connective tissue in significant numbers. They at once become the dominant cells of the immigrant population. Everyday conditions outside of a germfree environment can be considered equivalent to a state of mild chronic infection localized to tissues close to the bronchial passages, while alveolar surfaces remain sterile because of scavenging by alveolar macrophages. Connective tissues beneath pulmonary airways in this state always contain macrophages and a regular scattering of eosinophils as well, but microphages tend to remain confined to the blood vessels just as they do in other parts of the body constantly subjected to bacterial intrusion, at least until the invaders succeed in establishing a foothold. After considerable damage to the vessels, hemorrhage into the lung occurs, and then all compartments may become exposed to vascular contents.

In this section, most of the factual material on pulmonary disease has been obtained from standard works, primarily Spencer's *Pathology of the Lung* [238], to which acknowledgment is given.

A. Intravascular Phagocytes

At any moment most of the previously considered cells circulate in pulmonary vessels, but unless attached to a firm substrate they make inefficient phagocytes. Consequently, one might look to the endothelial cells bordering the bloodstream or to phagocytes deeper in the vessel walls in searching for possible scavengers of the intravascular compartment. If phagocytic pulmonary endothelial cells were present, they might resemble Kupffer cells of the liver and be as easily demonstrated by intravenous injections of suspended particles; but as yet no such proof has been offered. Certain venous endothelial cells and to a lesser extent those of small arteries may contain conspicuous membrane-bounded inclusions (Figs. 30 and 31), but by their homogeneous content these more likely are storage or secretory products rather than concentrations of microorganisms or particles filtered out from the blood stream. In mice at least, intravenously administered ferritin does not seem to accumulate in pulmonary endothelial cells of any sort, whereas it rapidly becomes trapped in the liver [235]. In other respects, the endothelium of large and small vessels in both the pulmonary and bronchial circuits is heterogeneous [234], but the meaning of this is unknown.

Pulmonary vessels possess deep-seated adventitial macrophages; they are drawn out between layers of extracellular fibers much like other pulmonary macrophages of connective tissue. Pericytes at times closely invest the capillary endothelium particularly in the bronchial circuit, but little is known about special functions they might carry on; some of them resemble smooth muscle.

Should stasis of blood flow follow embolization to the lungs, then bloodborne cells will attach to the vessel walls or to the embolus and set about ingesting materials in the vicinity of the lesion. The population of cells attracted will vary depending on whether the embolus is sterile, when it evokes a monocytic response, or infected, when the response may be predominantly granulocytic or mixed depending on the nature and severity of the infection. Septic emboli may originate from any vein, most frequently in cases of thrombophlebitis of the internal jugular veins or lateral sinus resulting from middle ear or peritonsillar infections. Infected emboli may also result from infected vegetations being released from the heart in cases of acute or subacute bacterial endocarditis. A marked granulocytic response follows embolization of amniotic fluid contents late in labor when lanugo hairs and meconium become lodged in the pulmonary vessels. A generalized granulocytosis is also apt to accompany the breakdown of any large single plug as well as multiple emboli. Rarely some saprophytic fungi occur among the obstructing materials, particularly after a primary infection had been treated by a long course of antibiotics; and these lesions may attract a variety of leukocytes. Marked eosinophilia of the blood accompanies the condition known as *tropical eosinophilic lung,* where circulating microfilarial parasites become trapped in small pulmonary vessels and give rise to a predominantly allergic reaction. Infections may also be transferred to thrombosed pulmonary vessels from the bronchi. Most of the many kinds of pulmonary thrombi or emboli are not infected, however. They are organized and resolved largely by the endothelium, which rapidly grows through fissures in the retracting clot to form many channels subsequently reorganized into one. The thrombus then becomes incorporated into one side of the vessel wall and usually leaves little more than a patch of intimal thickening to mark the spot. Less successful resolution of these emboli may contribute to the eventual development of serious obstruction in the pulmonary arteries and in turn to chronic pulmonary hypertension, particularly if the embolic showers continue over a long period.

One of the interesting responses occurring in the intravascular compartment follows embolization of non-infectious mineral or organic materials in the pulmonary vessels. This unusual disease entity has resulted from intravenous

FIGURE 30 Pulmonary arteriole in a bat's lung. Smallmembrane-bounded granules begin to appear in the endothelium of the smaller arterial vessels in this animal. Contrast with Fig. 31.

FIGURE 31 Small pulmonary vein in a bat's lung. The endothelial granules are larger and more numerous than in the arterial side of the circuit. As in other small mammals, cardiac muscle replaces the smooth muscle that invests the arteries.

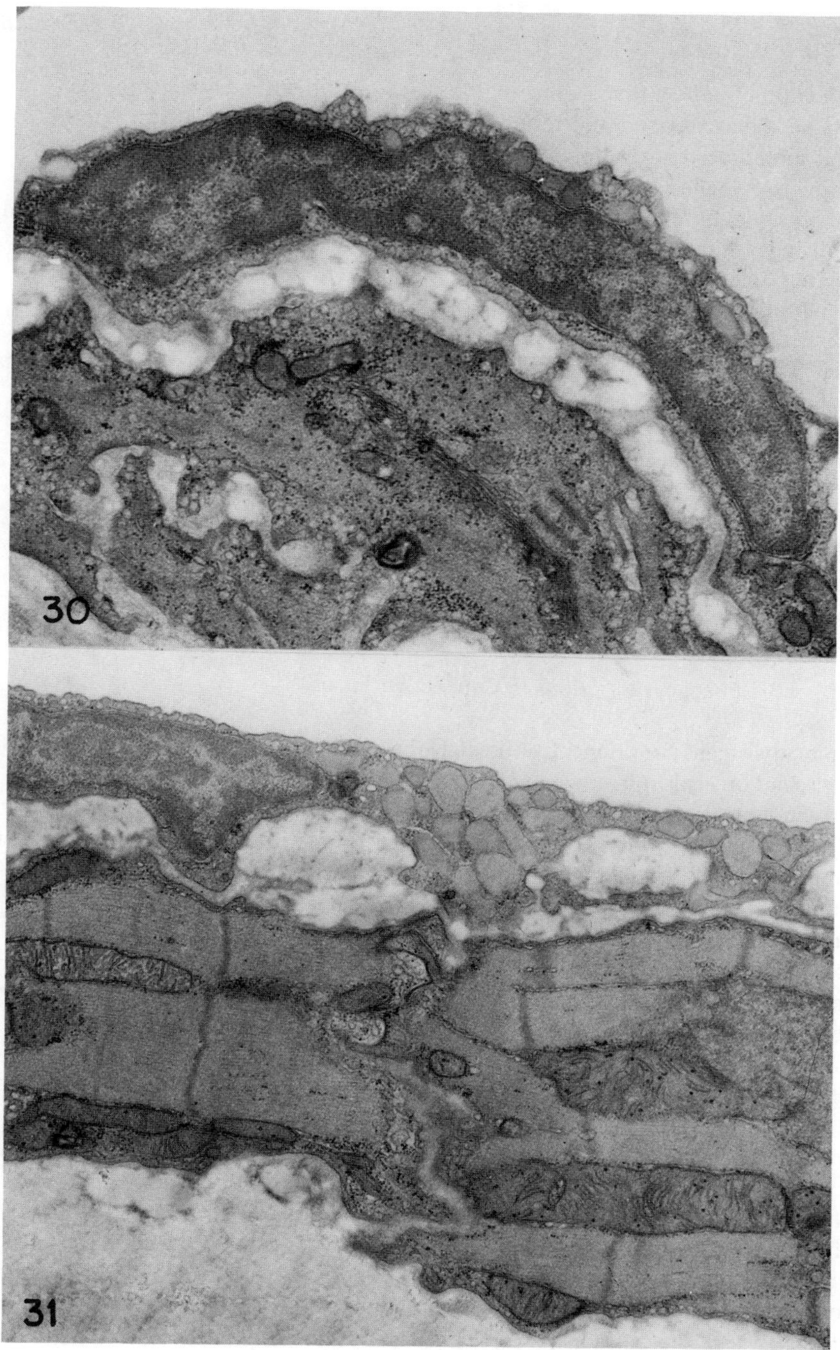
30
31

injection of cotton fibers along with medication when the cotton adhered to the needle used for administering the drug. This sometimes leads to arteritis and sometimes to granuloma formation [267]. A very similar condition has come to be called *blue velvet lung* because it commonly occurs among drug addicts who have injected a suspension of tripelennamine (blue velvet) absorbed onto talc, thinking to obtain the drug's central nervous system effects more acutely than could be achieved parenterally, the route of administration for which the pills were intended. The resulting sterile inflammation draws monocytes from the bloodstream; these become "activated" and infiltrate the embolus. The endothelium surrounding undergoes reactive hypertrophy, and the organizing lesion becomes incorporated into the intima. Gradually it works its way through the vessel to emerge in the lung [266], where it may provoke a new reaction among alveolar and perivascular macrophages, which migrate toward the lesion. The situation seemingly excites two separate macrophage responses: The first involves the transformation of blood monocytes and takes place in the intravascular compartment, while the second involves pulmonary macrophages and begins once the lesion reaches bona fide pulmonary tissues in the outer layers of the vessel.

B. Phagocytic Actions in Connective Tissue

In many organs the connective tissue is the main ground for collective phagocytic action against invasive organisms. It remains so in peribronchial regions of the lungs where connective tissue is abundant; and while phagocytes and other cellular responses to inflammation are not rare occurrences in perivascular and pleural tissues, they are not conspicuous features of these parts in normal lungs. In respiratory portions of the lungs, connective tissue is much reduced, and the scavenging action of macrophages on the alveolar surface does much to minimize the risk of airborne infections becoming established. In small mammals like mice or shrews or bats, the interposition of connective tissue between the alveolar epithelium and the pulmonary capillary endothelium is frequently so thin as to be incapable of holding a bacillus let alone serve as a field for macrophage maneuvers (Fig. 2); in larger mammals these walls and their connective tissue frameworks are thicker, but few walls are normally thick enough to contain or require lymphatic drainage. Even in these animals, *actively phagocytic* macrophages and other wandering cells are desultory inhabitants of this tissue at best. No animal in its accustomed haunts is ever completely free from exposure to antigenic stimulation and invasive organisms, and in alveolar connective tissue the main acknowledgment of this is in the isolated occurrence of a few lymphocytes and plasma cells. These may be found in niches where the pulmonary capillary loops and anastomoses leave a little connective tissue space between themselves and the overlying alveolar epithelium [233].

Connective tissue defenses are organized about several components. The wandering cells of the blood that enter this tissue as well as the tissue's own relatively fixed population of resident macrophages and mast cells share in coordinated protective efforts, notably during inflammation. The fibrocytes present serve as the main vehicle for repair and replacement of extracellular fibers and ground substance, and the ground substance itself in its firmer states of polymerization offers a component of resistance to bacterial extension. These defenses are closely adapted to existing patterns made by the networks of small blood vessels and lymphatics. This is most readily deduced from observing the purposeful distribution of mast cells ranged alongside vessels at the arteriolar end of small vascular circuits. This arrangement gives vessels excellent exposure to vasoactive agents released from mast cells and so facilitates their distribution throughout the region served by the local circulatory bed.

Mindful of this, one notes that the locations of mast cells in the lungs may differ considerably with the species. As a rule it seems there must be adequate connective tissue present before mast cells will appear in it. Certain regions in the lungs of larger animals may have them, whereas corresponding parts of smaller ones do not, and these differences in location of the cells must affect pulmonary defenses. Typically, as in man (and hamsters), mast cells are fairly extensively distributed in sublaryngeal and subbronchial connective tissues, but in mice scarcely extend beyond tissues surrounding the stem bronchi and major vessels near the hilum. In rats they extend alongside bronchi well inside the lungs and follow the branching of the vascular tree still further (see Plate 2b), but they sometimes occur as well at intervals in the pleura spaced a few alveoli apart. Degranulation of these pleural cells likely would produce its main effect elsewhere than on the smooth muscle of the airways; the local distribution of suspected cells and local circulatory patterns are best kept in mind while one goes about pinpointing pharmacological activity in the lungs.

The local circulation may also be affected by local release of additional pharmacological agents; for instance, from various components of the heterogeneous *small-granule cell complex* that occur in the laryngobronchial, bronchiolar, and even alveolar epithelium of man [90] and many other species [134]. By their content of characteristic cytoplasmic granules resembling variously the granules in catecholamine-secreting adrenal medullary cells and those in several distinct polypeptide hormone-secreting cells of the gut, by their innervation, and by apparent release of granules both intraepithelially and into the connective tissue beneath, these cells make likely candidates for effector roles in control of blood flow and/or secretion in parabronchial tissues. The defensive capability of the pulmonary connective tissue is influenced by regulation of the local circulation, for it affects the access circulating phagocytes and serumborne factors have to the region and is a factor in determining how much fluid becomes available from filtration of blood to drive secretion for mucociliary clearance mechanisms in the bronchi.

Connective tissue defenses are also organized with consideration being given the type and extent of lymphatic drainage in the region. In the lungs lymphatic drainage is both superficially across the visceral pleura to the hilar nodes, and deeply from just proximal to the alveoli along the bronchial tree, where bronchial lymphatic vessels are joined by others running in with the pulmonary veins and alongside pulmonary arteries. Apparently an undetermined but considerable proportion of the fluid produced by alveolar exudation drains into the parabronchial lymphatic network, where phagocytic and immunologically competent cells are positioned at intervals along the pathway to take up particulate material and to react to antigens received. Lymphoid tissue becomes established at many positions along the subbronchial drainage route and usually increases in extent during the lifetime of the individual, providing still finer monitoring of the lymph. At these positions the borderlands between the lymphoid cells and the regular connective tissue become rich in mast cells which loosely encircle the inner cords and sinuses just as they do in the larger and more formally organized lymph nodes located at the hilum and elsewhere in the body. Particle bearing macrophages that find their way into the general region are particularly conspicuous in these borderlands. There they often contact the mast cells, perhaps in order to transfer antigen carried on their surface (cytophilic) antibodies to cell-bound (IgE) antibodies on the mast cells. This type of activity is all the more apparent with the passage of time, after material cleared from the alveoli by this route (others being the bronchial airway and the bloodstream) gradually becomes concentrated in macrophages present in these areas, both in and around the lymphoid tissues [235].

The first immunological response to inhaled antigens may well take place in the upper respiratory tract and on the bronchial surface (Sec. V.F), yet most of the immunological reactions of the lungs occur in the connective tissues simply because the majority of cells capable of reaction reside there. Many of these cells are distributed alongside or else within the pulmonary lymphatic vessels; and since the lymphatic networks are best developed in the subbronchial tissue followed by the pleura and then by other locations, it is not surprising that the immunological activity of these different regions can be ranked in the same order. The important defensive roles of pulmonary lymphatics are further and more specifically discussed by Lauweryns and Baert [133] and by Leak [136] in this monograph.

C. The Connective Tissue in Diseased Lungs

Turning to more frankly pathological states, one observes that the normal infiltration of phagocytic cells seen in subbronchial and bronchiolar connective tissue is increased during localized infections of the bronchial tree (bronchitis and bronchiolitis). Microphages and edema fluid increase the size of this connective tissue compartment, and later on mononuclear infiltrates of chronic reaction rise. Damage to the epithelium may be severe, but unless it is frequently repeated, the regeneration that follows is usually complete. Meanwhile, in the underlying tissues lymphoid aggregations increase in volume. Laboratory animals like rats that are susceptible to chronic pulmonary infection usually have large quantities of subbronchial lymphatic tissue, while others less susceptible like hamsters have relatively less, and during chronic bronchitis in man the corresponding compartment enlarges partly for this reason and partly because the bronchial glands undergo hypertrophy.

More generalized pulmonary infection promotes infiltration of more phagocytes, and these enter additional connective tissue compartments of the lungs. Even the slender threads of connective tissue in interalveolar walls may become swollen by edema and emigration of cells from the blood. This stage is quickly passed during the development of pneumococcal pneumonia, when following leakage of serous fluid, microphages and erythrocytes pour into alveolar spaces and consolidation ensues; then the phagocytic populations both inside and outside of the connective tissue become similar. A later phase of resolution is marked by a large increase in the numbers of macrophages both inside and outside pulmonary walls. These must appear if resolution (fibrin absorption) and not fibrosis is to occur.

Although an early microphagic and later macrophagic response characterizes many acute bacterial pneumonias just as a predominantly mononuclear response typifies many viral infections, the picture in acute pneumonias is more variable than that, as a representative listing might show (Table 4). The various pneumonias often are marked by different clinical histories as well as by different phagocytic responses from those seen in the pneumococcal disease with which the word "pneumonia" is popularly linked. Among them, infections caused by many rickettsial and viral agents, as well as others resulting from chronic infective agents (syphilitic pneumonias), metabolic disease, or complex autoimmune reactions (rheumatic pneumonitis), bring on an *interstitial* type of pneumonia where the cellular response is generally tissue-bound and does not enter the alveoli. Interstitial pneumonias of viral, syphilitic, rheumatic, or some other type can usually be distinguished clearly from one another only on the basis of the total microscopic appearance; but, in the examples mentioned, differences in the connective tissue appearance alone would help to resolve a problem of

TABLE 4 Predominant Phagocytic Response in Selected Pneumonic Infections[a]

Bacterial Pneumonias	
Pneumococcal	Microphages, erythrocytes, and serous fluid in alveoli; macrophages in resolution phase
Micrococcal	Mild response by microphages and macrophages; venospasm and ischemia; focal abscesses with microphages
Streptococcal	Hemorrhagic edema with microphage and lymphocytic infiltrates; poorly localized infection with much epithelial damage and relatively few microphages in air passages
Friedländer's	Early mononuclear response with microphage reaction only after extensive alveolar necrosis
Aspiration	Little microphage response to ensuing putrefactive pneumonia unless hemorrhagic exudation is widespread
Pasteurella	Severe hemorrhagic pulmonary edema with fibrin; eventual appearance of micro- and macrophages with phagocytosis only by the latter
Anthrax	Macrophages ingest but do not destroy bacteria; little microphage response unless secondary infection
Tularemia	Predominantly mononuclear cell response surrounding focal lesions; absence of giant cells
Meningococcal	Bronchiolar and alveolar exudate containing actively phagocytic microphages
Coliform	Ingestion of bacteria by alveolar macrophages
Viral and Rickettsial Pneumonias	
Typical virus	Macrophage response; lymphoid cell infiltrates in connective tissue beneath infected epithelium
Q fever	Diffuse interstitial pneumonia with "chronic cell" infiltrates of lymphocytes, macrophages, plasma cells, and a few microphages
Influenza	Epithelial and interstitial mononuclear infiltrates with macrophages and lymphocytes in edematous alveoli

TABLE 4 (continued)

Viral and Rickettsial Pneumonias	
Psittacosis	Lymphocytic infiltrates and macrophage response in fibrin-rich, edematous alveoli
Measles	Lymphoid cell infiltrates with few microphages and giant cell transformation of epithelium
Pertussis	Heavy lymphoid infiltrates especially in airway connective tissues; mucopurulent exudate in lumen
Atypical virus	Pulmonary edema with erythrocytes and macrophages; focal lymphoid infiltrates in walls of alveolar ducts; transient areas of consolidation
Pulmonary Mycoses	
Mucormycosis	Little cellular response
Coccidiomycosis	Mixed and variable response may resemble that of lobar bacterial pneumonia except for increased mononuclear cell reaction surrounding lesions
Aspergillosis	Variable response depending on degree of hypersensitivity present; tuberculoid lesions have the organisms, mixed phagocytes, lymphocytes, and fibroblasts in the center and mononuclear and giant cells at the periphery, together with infiltrating and surface eosinophils
North American blastomycosis	Initial microphage response in alveoli and inter-followed by eosinophils, giant and mononuclear cells, and fibroblasts
South American blastomycosis	Initial macrophage response followed by microphages; small granulomas
Cryptococcosis	Local pneumonic lesions (torulomas) with mononuclear and giant cell reaction or acute bronchopneumonia with little phagocytic response
Histoplasmosis	Organism taken up by alveolar macrophages and other reticuloendothelial cells; these necrose and serve as foci of a chronic cell reaction

[a]Based on data from Ref. 238.

differential diagnosis: In viral pneumonias the connective tissue beneath an eroded bronchial epithelium is filled with lymphocytes which may extend into the interalveolar walls; in congenital syphilis the newborn lung exhibits diffuse interstitial thickening with fibrosis and a plasma cell and lymphocytic infiltrate; and in rheumatic pneumonia mononuclear cells infiltrate alveolar walls to the point of obscuring the capillaries, while the small vessels here and there undergo "fibrinoid necrosis," so called because of changes in the extracellular fibers and ground substance that give them staining properties similar to fibrin; and the alveoli and alveolar ducts become filled with a fibrinous edema fluid. Notwithstanding, a pathologist would scarcely ever rely on the changed appearance of only one pulmonary compartment in arriving at his diagnosis. Only rarely might a characteristic change be seen in the connective tissue; for example, the appearance of giant reticuloendothelial cells in pulmonary lymph nodules (Warthin-Finkeldey cells)—a cellular reaction to the intracellular virus—frequently completes the picture of mononuclear cell infiltration and giant cell formation at all levels of the epithelium that collectively characterize measles pneumonia. At other times a diagnosis can be suspected from the absence of phagocytic responses in the face of pulmonary damage. There could be many reasons for this; among them, some infectious agents might fail to elicit a chemotactic response, while others might resist phagocytosis and pass into the bloodstream to produce septicemia.

An illustration of the preceding was long ago provided by Tchistovich [255]. In studying cellular defensive actions in the lungs, he observed that after large doses of the bacteria were instilled into the bronchi of rabbits, vibrios of chicken cholera were not taken up even though they attracted a variety of phagocytic cells, and death came to the host a day later; but that anthrax bacilli were partially taken up and destroyed by alveolar macrophages forestalling death until 2½ days later; whereas the bacteria of swine fever were all taken up by macrophages and giant cells within 4 hr after introduction, leaving the host alive. That is, *different bacteria may elicit different phagocytic responses and successful resistance to the infection is partially correlated with successful phagocytosis.*

D. Immunological Reactivity in Pathological Pulmonary Connective Tissues

Cellular reactions to pulmonary disease are all carried out in conjunction with immunological mechanisms; nevertheless, hypersensitivity is of greater importance in some of these diseases than in others, and this frequently can be suspected from the presence of unusually large numbers of eosinophils and other features of the tissues [146]. In a few cases the diseases themselves result from defective or hyperactive immune mechanisms. McCombs [164] has discussed

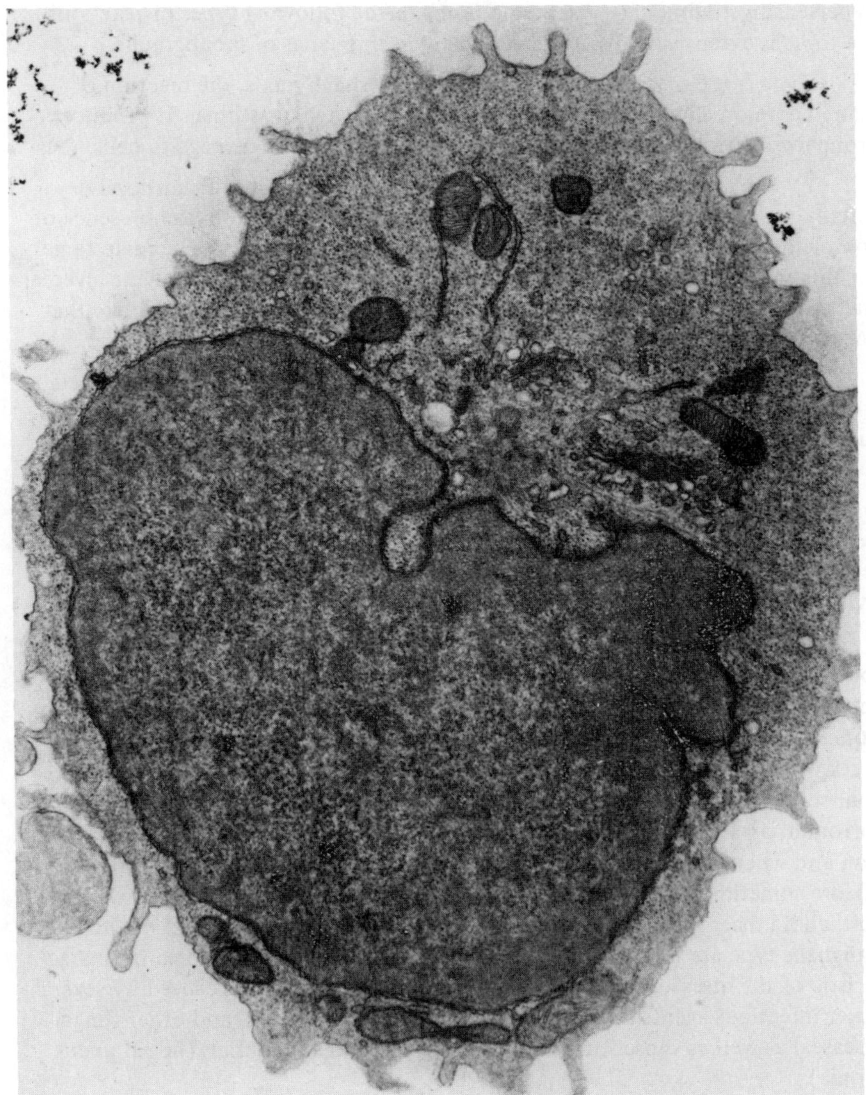

FIGURE 32 Lymphocyte recovered from pulmonary lavage of a mouse exposed to an iron oxide aerosol (dark specks in background). These cells do not take up the particles.

hypersensitive pulmonary diseases in terms of the following types of reactions; the topic is extensively discussed elsewhere in this series of monographs.

Type I, IgE-dependent hypersensitivity: Anaphylaxis, the reaction of many common allergies, is best represented by bronchial asthma. It produces bronchoconstriction and mucous hypersecretion but little damage to cells.

Type II, cytotoxic hypersensitivity involving tissue specific antibody: Circulating antibody reacts with cell- or tissue-bound antigen in the presence of complement to result in cell death or fragmentation of tissues. The main target for this autoimmune reaction in the lungs is extracellular material of the alveolar walls which undergoes degeneration (Goodpasture's syndrome) not unlike that occurring in the renal glomeruli during glomerulonephritis.

Type III, immune complex disease: Circulating antigens are complexed with IgG or IgM antibodies and sometimes become trapped in the tissues, activating complement, attracting microphages, and initiating hydrolytic reactions.

Type IV, delayed hypersensitivity reactions: These are mediated by T lymphocytes and do not involve circulating antibody unless a simultaneous type I or II reaction is present to similar antigens. These antigens are often the infectious organisms themselves–certain viruses, bacteria (tuberculin hypersensitivity), fungi, and eucaryotic parasites.

Granulomas frequently are seen in chronically infected lungs and are to some extent caused by type III reactions. They can occur intravascularly in reaction to a bloodborne agent as in tropical eosinophilic or blue velvet lung mentioned earlier, but more frequently they are formed in relation to airborne infection. In the course of their chronicity these become incorporated into the connective tissue. The predominantly mononuclear reaction in these lesions surrounds a variably necrotic center where giant cells frequently undergo formation and where causative agents, whether bacterial or viral [23,24] (histiocytosis X), are sometimes seen. The giant cells are surrounded by concentric layers of epithelioid macrophages in turn ringed by lymphocytes. Giant cells of the Langhans type are present in tuberculous granulomas and are said to be characteristic of the disease, but giant cells may occur in granulomas caused by several other infectious agents (the blastomycoses, coccidiomycosis, and other fungal diseases) as well as those formed in reaction to inhaled materials (lipoid pneumonia).

It is thought that the potential of immune complexes to cause disease is to some extent related to their "valence": a slight excess of antigen leaves the complex soluble so that it circulates and may reach even remote tissues. Combination with additional antibody makes the complex insoluble, an excess of antibody facilitating its ingestion by phagocytes but near-equivalence between antigen and antibody tending to promote granuloma and foreign body giant cell formation [164]. In this condition histamine is released, and with other factors released simultaneously (ECF-A?), eosinophils become attracted to the site of reaction.

Outside of granulomas, giant cells may form under conditions where the foreign objects are too large to be ingested by one macrophage; consequently they very frequently are seen in lungs affected by the pneumoconioses. As mentioned, certain viruses may bring about a giant cell response, but then additional cell types are often affected. Foreign body giant cells are to be distinguished as well from others originating from tumor cells (few nuclei markedly unequal in size) or those of reticuloses like Hodgkin's disease (small giant cells). Whether factors that promote giant cell formation in macrophages also help to promote it in other cell types is not known.

Some pulmonary mycoses bring about little cell reaction, whereas others like aspergillosis or North American blastomycosis often are accompanied by sizeable infiltrations of eosinophils. These cells characteristically are elevated in lungs infected by parasitic eucaryotes where they tend to concentrate in the connective tissue surrounding the organisms; in schistosomiasis they are especially numerous around dead flukes, the living ones exciting little reaction. These organisms usually occur as pulmonary emboli but may also be found in the lung tissue proper where they or else their ova incite granulomatous reactions. Another lesion tinged with eosinophils is the reticulosis, eosinophilic granuloma, which develops in the larger pulmonary connective tissue compartments beneath the bronchi, in the pleura, and about the blood vessels. Often it extends further with destruction of alveolar tissue. These granulomas are richly supplied with histiocytic and other cells of chronic reaction, but the eosinophilic infiltrate is usually so conspicuous as to make recognition easy; and like diseases with an allergic component in their etiology, this one is repressed by administration of cortisone.

Basophil reactions have not been clearly identified in the lungs owing to confusion between basophils and mast cells. A growing recognition that basophils may have special roles to play, particularly in cell-mediated hypersensitivity reactions, has tended to force reconsideration whether these cells undergo notable reactions in the lungs, and new information might be forthcoming.

E. The Epithelial Compartment

With tightly linked cells separated by little or no matrix, the pulmonary epithelium offers little accommodation for wandering phagocytes crossing over from the tissues to the epithelial surface. The alveolar epithelium is traversed fairly constantly as small numbers of cells leave the blood to enter the alveoli either directly [175] or after varying periods of residence in the connective tissue. This barrier is easily traversed, and cells may enter peripheral alveoli or else leave the bloodstream from vessels in the alveolar walls of respiratory bronchioles or alveolar ducts, and so come into the airway higher up. While phagocytes evidently can cross the bronchial and bronchiolar epithelium, more severe than normal conditions are required to demonstrate this. For example, Kilburn et al. [121] have published an electron micrograph showing microphages in the bronchial epithelium of a hamster as well as on the surface above and in the lamina propria beneath, but this documentation of migration was obtained from an animal exposed to an aerosol of cotton trash. On the other hand, where mice were exposed to a less stressful aerosol of iron oxide, no phagocytes were observed to enter the airway through the bronchial or bronchiolar epithelium, although a macrophage (but not a microphage) response evidently had occurred, causing emigration of cells into the alveoli [235]. Perhaps the demonstration of bronchial crossing is more easily made if an aerosol attractive to microphages is used, because of the facility these cells have for migration as compared to macrophages (Sec. II.A). Cells that do cross pass between the epithelial cells must unseal the tight junctions located near the apical surfaces. These maintain the integrity of the epithelial layer but readily reform once the phagocytes pass through. If phagocytes remained long in the epithelium they would undoubtedly have been observed there more frequently; nonetheless, a trained eye and thin microscopic sections both reduce the apparent rarity of such findings. One cell that has been seen in relatively unstressed lungs is the globule leukocyte (Sec. III.E), caught in the epithelium perhaps because it moves slowly, or perhaps because like lymphocytes it preferentially crosses the epithelium through the cytoplasm [94] rather than in-between the cells. Without being present in the epithelium, however, the phagocytes could still interact with it both immunologically and by transfer of ingested materials.

With an *endodermal* lineage, pulmonary epithelial cells inherit a phylogenetically proven capacity for endocytosis that persists to some degree in mammals; its vigorous expression nevertheless is to be found among the simpler invertebrates. In coelenterates, for example, digestion is a biphasic task involving different cells of the endoderm. In the extracellular phase, crustacean prey in the gastrovascular cavity are reduced to a soup by secretions of enzymatic cells; the bisque is then phagocytosed by nutritive-muscle cells, and digestion is completed intracellularly [22,80]. In newborn mammals intestinal absorptive cells engage in a more restrained kind of macroendocytosis, enabling infants to take up immunoglobulins in colostrum as well as milk proteins [59]. The yolk sac endoderm of many mammals possesses comparable ability and avidly absorbs large molecules as well as colloidal particles throughout most of its life [236, 277]. Ingestion by the mammalian cells does not involve formation of pseudopods as it does in *Hydra;* consequently, one might argue whether or not such mammalian activity should be called phagocytosis. In the pulmonary endoderm

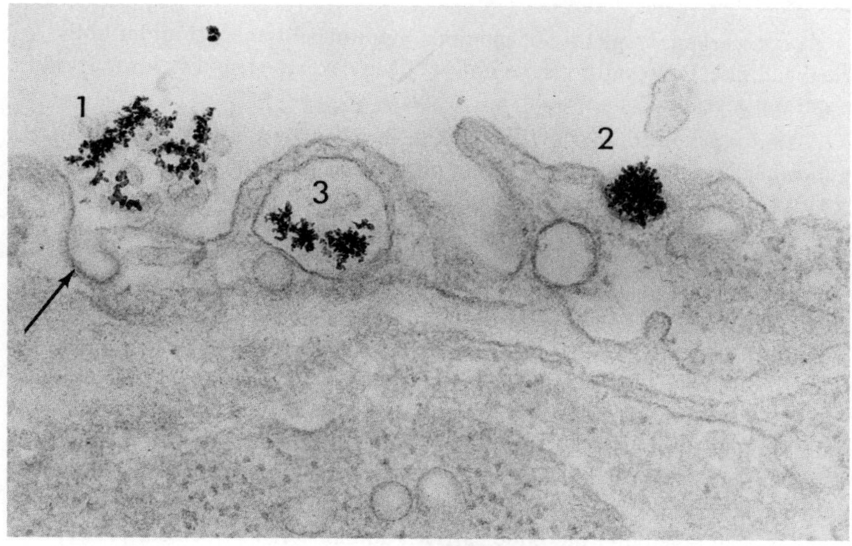

FIGURE 33 Attenuated portion of a squamous alveolar cell resting upon the epithelial basement membrane. Stages (1-3) in the uptake of iron oxide particles are shown. At the left a coated microendocytotic vesicle is visible (arrow).

the scale is further reduced (Secs. I, II,G; Figs. 33,34,35; also see Plates 3b and 4b), although epithelial cells possess undoubted ability to take up certain materials from the apical surface. Under none too drastic conditions it is easy to implicate a vesicle-transport mechanism in the uptake (Fig. 33) and transport of iron oxide particles across the alveolar epithelium, but this has not been proven as well for the airway epithelium. Where the cells are damaged, materials penetrate the epithelium more readily. Of course this is news only when the damage is not excessive, for dead cells do not exclude trypan blue (trypan blue viability test), and where the epithelium is denuded there can be no argument about its excluding anything!

A comprehensive picture of pulmonary epithelial transport under both normal and diseased conditions has not yet been developed, and so we must content ourselves with glimpses like the following:

After exposure to cigarette smoke, all levels of respiratory epithelium in guinea pigs could be seen to admit an intratracheally administered horseradish peroxidase tracer that had been excluded in nonsmoking controls [225]. The penetration first became evident in alveoli and bronchioles after 50 cigarettes and in the trachea after 270. As seen by electron microscopy, the tracer permeated the intercellular spaces, but the route of entry could not be determined with certainty, whether through an endocytotic mechanism or through rupture of epithelial tight junctions. After intratracheal administration, tantalum and hematite powder (smaller than 5 μm) are taken up in diminishing degree by the bronchial epithelium of monkeys, rats, and cats [160]. The uptake seems to occur only in regions where particles are retained for some time on the epithelial surface, and the ciliated cells appear to be the main ones affected. Much the same impression was gained in mice from study of regions where the bronchial epithelium had taken up iron oxide particles administered by aerosol [235].

F. Phagocytes on the Epithelial Surface

Among cells policing the interface between pulmonary tissues and the air, alveolar macrophages are awesomely preponderant. No credit is claimed for this "discovery" (see Ref. 231); something so long known benefits from repetition because many may have ceased to wonder at it or have simply forgotten the fact. *Alveolar macrophages greatly exceed the combined number of all other cells present, living or dead, and no one can seriously doubt but that most of these macrophages are "activated" and truculent while they remain on the surface* (see Plate 1). If they certainly form the first line of defense in the alveoli, they appear to continue in a defensive posture once they reach the surface of the bronchi and bronchioles [36], although other airway mechanisms then lessen the importance of the macrophages' contribution. The dimensions of macro-

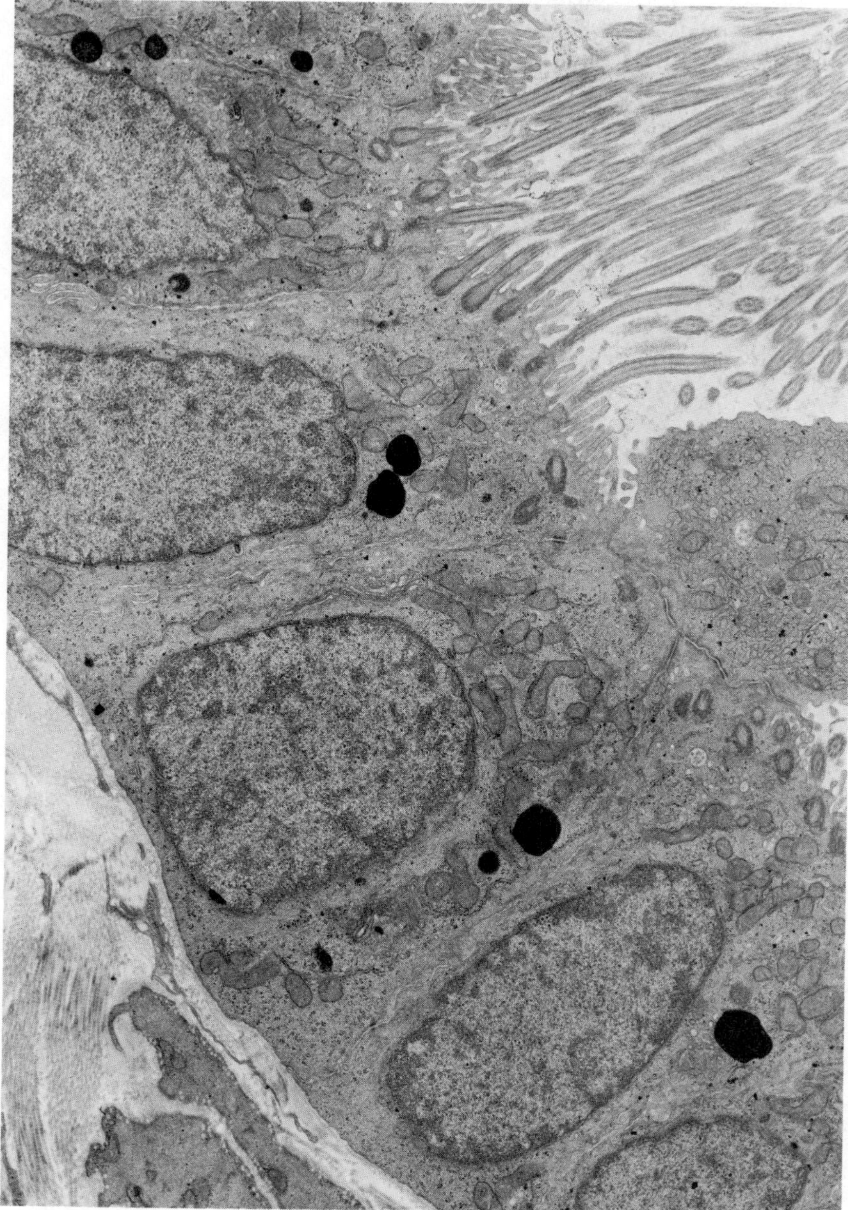

FIGURE 34 Bronchiolar epithelium of vampire bat lung showing large residual bodies (black) in the cytoplasm of the ciliated cells.

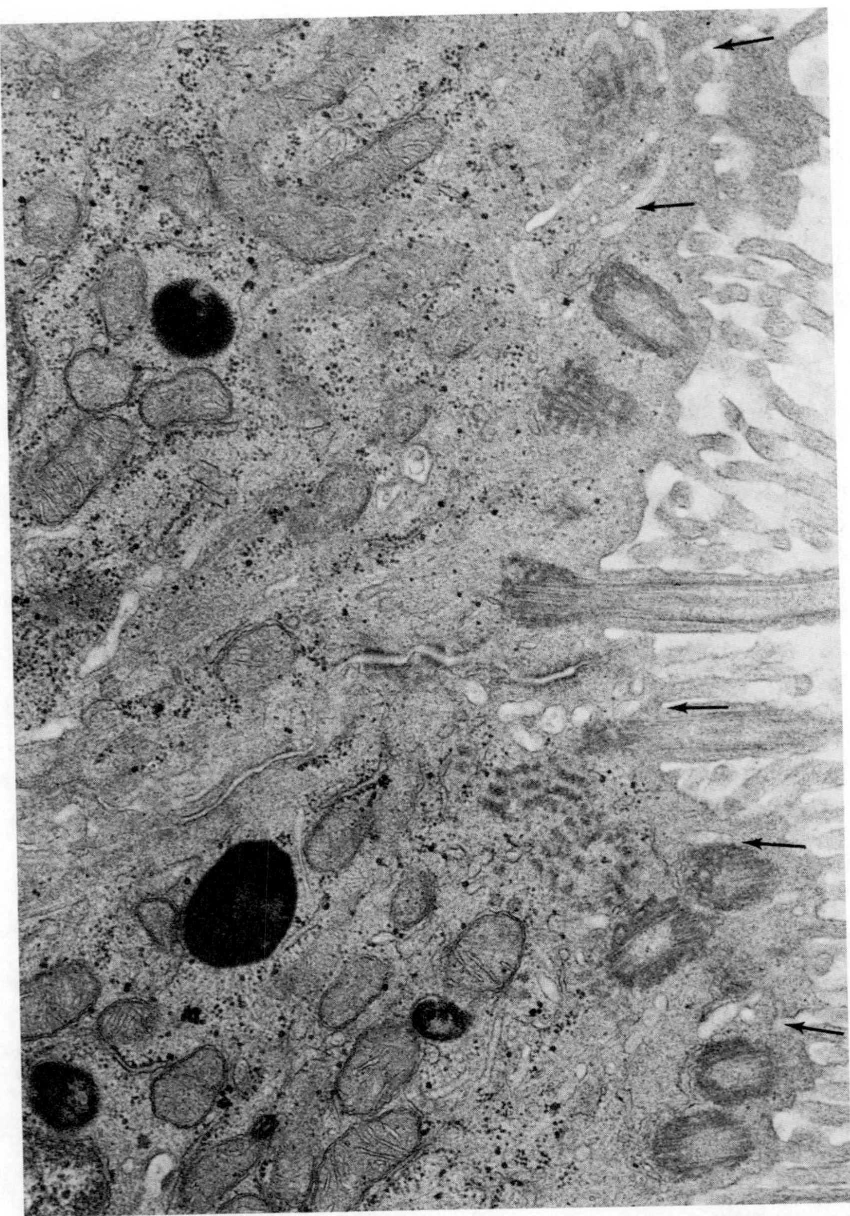

FIGURE 35 Apical cytoplasm of bronchiolar cells like those in Fig. 34. Tubular 600-1000 Å passageways (arrows) extend from the surface in-between the ciliary basal bodies; these indicate the scale of endocytosis normally associated with this epithelium. Being tortuous, the passages pass in and out of the plane of section.

phage action are less surely charted in the alveolar interstitium, although a case for activity can be made in diseased lungs where edema and cell infiltrates have swollen the alveolar walls and granulomas are under formation (Sec. V.C,D).

Besides alveolar macrophages, small numbers of microphages and eosinophils normally occur on pulmonary epithelial surfaces. The former increase in number when an acute infectious process is somewhere in the vicinity, and the latter increase when hypersensitivity is present. The absence of erythrocytes from this surface population is assurance that the granulocytes were responding to chemotactic attraction and were not simply being carried into the air space after damage to the epithelium and underlying blood vessels. Most frequently, lymphocytes (Fig. 32) rather than granulocytes are second to the macrophages in their contribution to the surface population. It is not yet possible to say whether these cells are B or T lymphocytes, nor whether they function normally at this location. Mast cells and/or basophils are such minor components of lung washings that they are often overlooked. Surface mast cells are likely to occur no farther down the bronchi than they extend in subepithelial connective tissue (Sec. V.B), and so their local concentration in the airway must be much higher than their insignificant percentage composition (well below 1%) in lung washings would indicate (Table 5). After harvesting by lavage in dogs and monkeys, these cells remain viable and release histamine as well as SRS-A when appropriately challenged [194]. Some of the IgE antibodies that mediate these reactions are produced in the lungs by plasmacytes and might well diffuse to the superficial histamine-releasing cells located in the trachea and bronchi, thereby turning them into early reactors for inhaled antigen [143,193]. Other materials in surface secretions include secretory IgA and the bacteriostatic protein lactoferrin, released by the bronchial glands [161].

In sum, many leukocytes that normally interact with macrophages occur as free cells on the epithelial surface, particularly in the conducting airways. Consequently, many of the interchanges needed for immunological reactions must take place there, even if serum factors are in shorter supply there than in the tissues, and even if the proportions of cells present are not as they tend to be in other pulmonary compartments.

VI. General Summary

This long chapter is only a short treatise on the basic cell biology of phagocytes occurring in mammalian lungs; that the cells discussed are those that hematologists write about should surprise no one, for the bloodstream is the source of most of the phagocytes in the lungs. As an introduction to a series of reviews on cellular defenses in this organ, the chapter offers a broad prospect of the func-

TABLE 5 Differential Counts of Cells Obtained from Canine and Rhesus Monkey Bronchi[a]

Animal no.	No. of cells/ml (millions)	Total number cells (millions)	Differential count (%)[b]							
			Mac	Epith	Lym	Eos	Neut	Unid	B	M
Rhesus monkey										
1	0.93	18.6	80.3	11.4	5.4	0.6	0	2.0	0	0.3
2	0.84	21.0	67.0	18.6	3.0	2.0	0	9.4	0.2	0
3	0.87	19.8	68.8	18.0	10.6	1.2	0.8	0.4	0.2	0
Ragweed-sensitive dogs										
1	0.48	13.4	37.7	18.1	6.0	44.2	0	2.7	0.5	0.8
	0.96	26.0	28.8	13.9	17.0	28.5	0.7	10.0	0.6	0.5
2	7.8	101.4	39.6	17.0	25.8	9.0	3.2	5.0	0.4	0
	2.6	46.8	40.4	28.5	26.0	0.6	0.7	3.5	0.2	0.1
3	2.4	48.0	27.3	50.3	15.0	3.4	0.9	2.9	0.1	0.1
	0.87	52.2	47.0	15.2	8.0	16.2	2.8	10.6	0	0.2
4	0.74	29.6	45.0	23.0	21.0	3.7	2.7	4.0	0.3	0.3
	0.52	28.08	41.0	24.0	20.7	2.1	1.5	10.0	0.5	0.2
Normal control dogs										
1	0.96	24.0	32.5	45.0	15.0	3.4	1.9	1.8	0.2	0.2
	0.64	19.2	40.9	38.5	7.8	7.1	1.2	4.2	0.2	0.1
2	0.43	15.02	30.0	34.2	22.1	7.6	0.7	4.5	0.4	0.5
	1.37	34.25	40.0	55.3	1.7	2.3	0	0	0.33	0.33
3	0.45	20.25	60.0	32.4	3.4	0.6	1.4	2.0	0.2	0
	0.86	21.50	32.2	57.2	1.8	1.2	4.4	3.0	0.2	0
4	0.92	30.80	48.0	6.0	21.0	18.0	2.0	5.0	0	0
	0.98	56.84	19.8	58.3	8.7	8.7	0.7	2.6	0.6	0.6

[a]From Ref. 194, with permission from *Clinical and Experimental Immunology*.
[b]Mac = macrophage; Epith = epithelial cell; Lym = lymphoid cell; Eos = eosinophil; Neut = neutrophil; Unid = unidentified cell; B = basophil-like cell; M = mast cell.

tional properties, the ontogenetic and phylogenetic histories, and the interactions of these cells; and it attempts to give phagocytes other than the alveolar macrophages their hour, for the accompanying chapters focus on the macrophages somewhat to the prejudice of these partners in defense.

At the least, all the intrapulmonary phagocytes are described and illustrated as they are found in the lungs. Among these, the alveolar macrophages stand out as particularly versatile cells, in character not far removed from primitive leukocytes and possessed of an appearance to match. The illustrating photo- and electron micrographs bear strongly on this theme. In later pages, all these cells are reconsidered in terms of their occurrence and characteristic associations in the vascular, connective tissue, and epithelial compartments of the lungs, as well as on the epithelial surface. The populations change considerably in the presence of disease.

Having assimilated the materials presented here, a nonspecialist can then turn to the other chapters in this book and read them with comprehension and profit. This chapter will have served its educational purpose even if the reader turns to the more specialized chapters with only the aim to discover how erroneous some of my assertions might be; for these I can offer ignorance tempered with assurance that much of what we "know" about the phagocytes today will be disproven before long.

Recent Developments

Three references touching aspects of the maturation of alveolar macrophages have been selected from a larger number on pulmonary phagocytes that have appeared since this chapter was completed in 1975 [281-283]. Fortunately for the author who strives to keep his work current while it is in press, truly new concepts emerge more slowly than new papers.

References

1. A. C. Allison, Mechanisms of macrophage damage, death, and of some pulmonary diseases. In *Respiratory Defense Mechanisms.* Edited by J. D. Brain, D. F. Proctor, and L. Reid. New York, Marcel Dekker, 1977, Chap. 26.
2. A. C. Allison, and L. Mallucci, Hisotchemical studies of lysosomes and lysosomal enzymes in virus-infected cell cultures, *J. Exp. Med.*, **121**:463-476 (1965).
3. L. C. Altman, R. Snyderman, J. Oppenheim, and S. E. Mergenhagen, A human mononuclear leukocyte chemotactic factor: characterization, specificity and kinetics of production by homologous leukocytes, *J. Immunol.*, **110**:801-810 (1973).
4. H. Andersen and M. E. Matthiessen, The histiocyte in human foetal tissues. Its morphology, cytochemistry, origin, function and fate, *Z. Zellforsch.*, **72**:193-211 (1966).
5. W. Andrew, *Comparative Hematology.* New York, Grune and Stratton, 1965.
6. F. Applemans, R. Wattiaux, and C. de Duve, Tissue fractionation studies. 5. The association of acid phosphatase with a special class of cytoplasmic granules in rat liver, *Biochem. J.*, **59**:438-445 (1955).
7. G. T. Archer and J. G. Hirsch, Isolation of granules from eosinophil leucocytes and study of their enzyme content, *J. Exp. Med.*, **118**:277-286 (1963).
8. G. T. Archer and J. G. Hirsch, Motion picture studies on degranulation of horse eosinophils during phagocytosis, *J. Exp. Med.*, **118**:287-294 (1963).
9. R. K. Archer, *The Eosinophil Leucocytes.* Oxford, Blackwell, 1963.
10. R. K. Archer, The eosinophil leucocytes, *Ser. Haematol.*, **I**(No. 4):3-32 (1968).
11. P. B. Armstrong and J. M. Lackie, Studies on intercellular invation in vitro using rabbit peritoneal neutrophil granulocytes (PMNs). I. Role of contact inhibition of locomotion, *J. Cell Biol.*, **65**:439-462 (1975).
12. L. Aschoff, Das reticulo-endotheliale System. *Ergeb. Inn. Med. Kinderheilkd.*, **26**:1-118 (1924).
13. P. W. Askenase, J. D. Haynes, D. Tauben, and R. De Bernardo; Specific basophil hypersensitivity induced by skin testing and transferred using immune serum, *Nature,* **256**:52-54 (1975).
14. J. W. Athens, Granulocyte kinetics in health and disease, *Natl. Cancer Inst. Monogr.*, **30**:135-156 (1969).
15. M. Baggiolini, C. de Duve, P. L. Masson, and J. F. Heremans, Association of lactoferrin with specific granules in rabbit heterophil leukocytes, *J. Exp. Med.*, **131**:559-570 (1970).
16. M. Baggiolini, J. G. Hirsch, and C. de Duve, Resolution of subcellular components of rabbit heterophil leukocytes into distinct populations by zonal sedimentation and density equilibration. In *Biochemistry of the Phagocytic Process.* Edited by J. Schultz. Amsterdam, North-Holland Publ., 1970, pp. 131-142.

17. D. F. Bainton and M. G. Farquhar, Origin of granules in polymorphonuclear leukocytes. Two types derived from opposite faces of the Golgi complex in developing granulocytes, *J. Cell Biol.*, **28**:277-301 (1966).
18. D. F. Bainton and M. G. Farquhar, Segregation and packaging of granule enzymes in eosinophilic leukocytes, *J. Cell Biol.*, **45**:54-73 (1970).
19. D. F. Bainton, J. L. Ullyot, and M. G. Farquhar, The development of neutrophilic polymorphonuclear leukocytes in human bone marrow. Origin and content of azurophil and specific granules, *J. Exp. Med.*, **134**: 907-934 (1971).
20. M. Balbiani, Etudes bactériologiques sur les Arthropodes, *C. R. Acad. Sci. (Paris)*, **103**:952-954 (1886).
21. V. C. Barber and P. Graziadei, The fine structure of cephalopod blood vessels, *Z. Zellforsch.*, **66**:765-781 (1965).
22. R. D. Barnes, *Invertebrate Zoology, 2nd ed.* Philadelphia, Pa., Saunders, 1968.
23. F. Basset and C. Nezelof, L'histiocytose X. Microscopie électronique. Culture in vitro et histo-enzymologie. Discussion à propos de 21 cas, *Rev. fr. Et. Clin. Biol.*, **14**:31-45 (1965).
24. F. Basset and J. Turiaf, Identification par la microscopie électronique de particules de nature probablement virale dans les lésions granulomateuses d'une histiocytose X pulmonaire, *C. R. Acad. Sci. (Paris)*, **261**:3701-3703 (1965).
25. A. Berken and B. Benacerraf, Properties of antibodies cytophilic for macrophages, *J. Exp. Med.*, **123**:119-144 (1966).
26. R. D. Berlin, Effect of concanavalin A on phagocytosis, *Nature [New Biol.]*, **235**:44-45 (1972).
27. R. D. Berlin and J. M. Oliver, Membrane transport of purine and pyrimidine bases and nucleosides in animal cells, *Int. Rev. Cytol.*, **42**:287-336 (1975).
28. M. Bessis, Microscopie de phase et microscopie électronique des cellules du sang, *Biol. Med. (Paris)*, **46**:239-288 (1957).
29. M. Bessis, *Cellules du Sang, Normal et Pathologique.* Paris, Masson, (1972).
30. L. Bitensky, The reversible activation of lysosomes in normal cells and the effect of pathological conditions, *Ciba Found. Symp.*, pp. 362-375 (1963).
31. W. K. Blenkinsopp, Mast cell proliferation in adult rats, *J. Cell Sci.*, **2**: 33-37 (1967).
32. W. Bloom and D. W. Fawcett, *A Textbook of Histology*, 9th ed. Philadelphia, Pa., Saunders, 1968, Chap. 8.
33. V. A. Bokisch and H. J. Müller-Eberhard, Anaphylatoxin inactivator of human plasma: its isolation and characterization as a carboxypeptidase, *J. Clin. Invest.*, **49**:2427-2436 (1970).
34. J. Bordet, Les leucocytes et les propriétés actives du sérum chez les vacinés, *Ann. Inst. Pasteur,* **9**:462-506 (1895).
35. S. Boyden, The chemotactic effect of mixtures of antibody and antigen on polymorphonuclear leukocytes, *J. Exp. Med.*, **115**:453-466 (1962).

36. J. D. Brain, J. J. Godleski, and S. P. Sorokin, Quantitation, origin, and fate of the pulmonary macrophage. In *Respiratory Defense Mechanisms*. Edited by J. D. Brain, D. F. Proctor, and L. Reid. New York, Marcel Dekker, 1977, Chap. 20.
37. G. Braunitzer, Structure and evolution of hemoglobin. In *Conference on Hemoglobin, Arden House, Harriman, New York*. New York, Columbia University Department of Medicine, 1962, pp. 267-273.
38. R. T. Briggs, D. B. Drath, M. L. Karnovsky, and M. J. Karnovsky, Localization of NADH oxidase on the surface of human polymorphonuclear leukocytes by a new cytochemical method, *J. Cell Biol.*, **67**:566-586 (1975).
39. R. T. Briggs, M. L. Karnovsky, and M. J. Karnovsky, Cytochemical demonstration of hydrogen peroxide in polymorphonuclear leukocyte phagosomes, *J. Cell Biol.*, **64**:254-260 (1975).
40. A. C. Brown and R. J. Brown, The fate of thorium dioxide injected into the pedal sinus of *Bullia* (Gastropoda: Prosobranchiata), *J. Exp. Biol.*, **42**:509-519 (1965).
41. G. E. Cartwright, J. W. Athens, and M. M. Wintrobe, The kinetics of granulopoiesis in normal man, *Blood*, **24**:780-803 (1964).
42. V. C. Chambers and R. S. Weiser, The ultrastructure of target cells and immune macrophages during their interaction in vitro, *Cancer Res.*, **29**: 301-317 (1969).
43. C. Chapman-Andresen, Studies on pinocytosis in amoebae, *C. R. Trav. Lab. Carlsberg*, **33**:73-264 (1962).
44. E. Y. Chi and D. Lagunoff, Abnormal mast cell granules in the beige (Chédiak-Higashi Syndrome) mouse, *J. Histochem. Cytochem.*, **23**:117-122 (1975).
45. H. Chiu and D. Lagunoff, Histochemical comparison of frog and rat mast cells, *J. Histochem. Cytochem.*, **19**:369-375 (1971).
46. M. Cline, Myeloperoxidase deficiency: A genetic defect associated with diminished leukocyte bactericidal and fungicidal activity. In *Biochemistry of the Phagocytic Process*. Edited by J. Schultz. Amsterdam, North-Holland Publ., 1970, pp. 111-114.
47. M. Cline, Mechanism of acidification of the human leukocyte phagocytic vacuole, *Clin. Res.*, **21**:595 (1973) (abstract).
48. M. Cline, *The White Cell*. Cambridge, Mass., Harvard University Press, 1975.
49. M. Cline, J. Hanifin, and R. I. Lehrer, Phagocytosis by human eosinophils, *Blood*, **32**:922-934 (1968).
50. C. G. Cochrane and H. J. Müller-Eberhard, The derivation of two distinct anaphylatoxin activities from the third and fifth components of human complement, *J. Exp. Med.*, **127**:371-386 (1968).
51. Z. A. Cohn, Lysosomes in mononuclear phagocytes. In *Mononuclear Phagocytes*. Edited by R. van Furth. Philadelphia, Pa., F. A. Davis, 1970, pp. 50-58.

52. Z. A. Cohn, Comment. In *Mononuclear Phagocytes.* Edited by R. van Furth. Philadelphia, Pa., F. A. Davis, 1970, p. 132.
53. Z. A. Cohn and B. A. Ehrenreich, The uptake, storage, and intracellular hydrolysis of carbohydrate by macrophages, *J. Exp. Med.,* **129**:201-226 (1969).
54. A. J. Collet, Fine structure of the alveolar macrophage of the cat and modifications of its cytoplasmic components during phagocytosis, *Anat. Rec.,* **167**:277-290 (1970).
55. A. J. Collet, J. C. Martin, C. Normand-Reuet, and A. Policard, Recherches infrastructurales sur l'evolution des macrophages alvéolaires et leurs reactions aux poussières minérales. In *Inhaled Particles and Vapours II.* Edited by C. N. Davies. Oxford, Pergamon, 1967, pp. 155-163.
56. R. B. Colvin, V. W. Pinn, B. A. Simpson, and H. F. Dvorak, Cutaneous basophil hypersensitivity. IV. The "late reaction," *J. Immunol.,* **110**: 1279-1289 (1973).
57. J. W. Combs, Maturation of rat mast cells. An electron microscope study, *J. Cell Biol.,* **31**:563-575 (1966).
58. J. W. Combs, D. Lagunoff, and E. P. Benditt, Differentiation and proliferation of embryonic mast cells of the rat, *J. Cell Biol.,* **25**:577-592 (1965).
59. R. Cornell and H. A. Padykula, A cytological study of intestinal absorption in the suckling rat, *Am. J. Anat.,* **125**:291-316 (1969).
60. M. M. Costin, Histochemical observations of the haemocytes of *Locusta migratoria, Histochem. J.,* **7**:21-43 (1975).
61. R. S. Cotran and M. Litt, The entry of granule-associated peroxidase into the phagocytic vacuoles of eosinophils, *J. Exp. Med.,* **129**:1291-1306 (1969).
62. E. P. Cronkite and P. C. Vincent, Granulocytopoiesis, *Ser. Haematol.,* **II**(No. 4):3-43 (1969).
63. P. Davies, A. C. Allison, R. I. Fox, M. Polyzonis, and A. D. Haswell, The exocytosis of polymorphonuclear leukocyte lysosomal enzymes induced by cytochalasin B, *Biochem. J.,* **128**:78P-79P (1972).
64. C. de Duve, The lysosome in retrospect. In *Lysosomes in Biology and Pathology 1.* Edited by J. T. Dingle and H. B. Fell. Amsterdam, North-Holland Publ., 1969, pp. 3-40.
65. C. de Duve, Biochemical studies on the occurrence, biogenesis and life history of mammalian peroxisomes, *J. Histochem. Cytochem.,* **21**:941-948 (1973).
66. C. de Duve and R. Wattiaux, Functions of lysosomes, *Annu. Rev. Physiol.,* **28**:435-492 (1966).
67. J. T. Dingle and H. B. Fell, *Lysosomes in Biology and Pathology,* Vol. 1, 1969; Vol. 2, 1969; Vol. 3, 1973. Amsterdam, North-Holland Publ.
68. A. M. Dvorak, H. F. Dvorak, and M. J. Karnovsky, Uptake of horseradish peroxidase by guinea pig basophilic leukocytes, *Lab. Invest.,* **26**:27-39 (1972).
69. H. F. Dvorak, A. M. Dvorak, B. A. Simpson, H. B. Richerson, S. Lesko-

witz, and M. J. Karnovsky, Cutaneous basophil hypersensitivity. II. A light and electron microscopic description, *J. Exp. Med.,* **132**:558-582 (1970).

70. B. A. Ehrenreich and Z. A. Cohn, The uptake and digestion of iodinated human serum albumin by macrophages in vitro, *J. Exp. Med.,* **126**:941-958 (1967).
71. B. A. Ehrenreich and Z. A. Cohn, The fate of peptides pinocytosed by macrophages in vitro, *J. Exp. Med.,* **129**:227-243 (1969).
72. P. Ehrlich, Über die specifischen Granulationen des Blutes, *Arch. Anat. Physiol. (Physiol. Abtl.),* **3**:571-579 (1879).
73. P. Ehrlich, Beitrag zur Kenntnis der granulirten Bindegewebszellen und der eosinophilen Leukocythen, *Arch. Anat. Physiol. (Physiol. Abtl.),* **3**:166-169 (1879).
74. L. Enerbäck and J. Jarlstedt, A cytofluorometric and radiochemical analysis of the uptake and turnover of 5-hydroxytryptamine in mast cells, *J. Histochem. Cytochem.,* **23**:128-135 (1975).
75. D. W. Fawcett, An experimental study of mast-cell degranulation and regeneration, *Anat. Rec.,* **121**:29-52 (1955).
76. M. E. Fedorko and J. G. Hirsch, Structure of monocytes and macrophages, *Semin. Haematol.,* **7**:109-124 (1970).
77. M. E. Feigenson, H. P. Schnebli, and M. Baggiolini, Demonstration of ricin-binding sites on the outer face of azurophil and specific granules of rabbit polymorphonuclear leukocytes, *J. Cell Biol.,* **66**:183-187 (1975).
78. J. Finstad and R. A. Good, Phylogenetic studies of adaptive immune responses in the lower vertebrates. In *Phylogeny of Immunity.* Edited by R. T. Smith, P. A. Miescher, and R. A. Good. Gainesville, Fla., University of Florida Press, 1966, pp. 173-188.
79. H. W. Florey and M. A. Jennings, Chemotaxis, phagocytosis, and the formation of abscesses. The reticulo-endothelial system. In *General Pathology.* Edited by H. W. Florey. Philadelphia, Pa., Saunders, 1970, pp. 124-174.
80. G. F. Gauthier, Cytological studies on the gastroderm of *Hydra, J. Exp. Zool.,* **152**:13-40 (1963).
81. J. B. L. Gee and A. S. Khandwala, Motility, phagocytosis and pinocytosis in lung defense cells. In *Respiratory Defense Mechanisms.* Edited by J. D. Brain, D. F. Proctor, and L. Reid. New York, Marcel Dekker, 1977, Chap. 22.
82. W. C. George and J. H. Ferguson, The blood of gastropod molluscs, *J. Morphol.,* **86**:315-327 (1950).
83. H. Gewurz, The immunologic role of complement, *Hosp. Pract.,* **2**(No. 9): 45-56 (1967).
84. H. Gewurz, J. Finstad, L. H. Muschel, and R. A. Good, Phylogenetic inquiry into the origins of the complement system. In *Phylogeny of Immunity.* Edited by R. T. Smith, P. A. Miescher, and R. A. Good. Gainesville, Fla., University of Florida Press, 1966, pp. 105-116.

85. E. J. Goetzl and K. F. Austen, Stimulation of the human neutrophil hexose monophosphate shunt (HMPS) by purified chemotactic factors, *Fed. Proc.*, **32**:973 (1973).
86. S. Gordon and Z. A. Cohn, The macrophage, *Int. Rev. Cytol.*, **36**:171-214 (1973).
87. R. C. Graham, Jr., M. J. Karnovsky, A. W. Shafer, E. A. Glass, and M. L. Karnovsky, Metabolic and morphological observations on the effect of surface-active agents on leukocytes, *J. Cell Biol.*, **32**:629-647 (1967).
88. F. M. Griffin, Jr., J. A. Griffin, and S. C. Silverstein, Distribution of anti-immunoglobulin IgG determines whether or not B lymphocytes are ingested by macrophages, *J. Cell Biol.*, **67**:145a (1975).
89. E. Haeckel, *Die Radiolarien (Rhizopoda radiaria). Eine Monographie*, Vol. 1. Berlin, Georg Reimer, 1862, pp. 104-105.
90. E. Hage, Electron microscopic identification of several types of endocrine cells in the bronchial epithelium of human foetuses, *Z. Zellforsch.*, **141**:401-412 (1973).
91. J. Hanson, The histology of the blood system in Oligochaeta and Polychaeta, *Biol. Rev.*, **24**:127-173 (1949).
92. D. Hawkins, Neutrophilic leukocytes in immunologic reactions in vitro. Effect of cytochalasin B, *J. Immunol.*, **110**:294-296 (1973).
93. R. A. Hawkins and R. D. Berlin, Purine transport in polymorphonuclear leukocytes, *Biochim, Biophys. Acta*, **173**:324-337 (1969).
94. H. Hayashi, The intracellular neutral SH dependent protease associated with inflammatory reactions, *Int. Rev. Cytol.*, **40**:101-151 (1975).
95. P. M. Henson, The adherence of leucocytes and platelets induced by fixed IgG antibody or complement, *Immunology*, **16**:107-121 (1969).
96. P. M. Henson, Interaction of cells with immune complexes: adherence, release of constituents, and tissue injury, *J. Exp. Med.*, **134**:114S-135S (1971).
97. M. Henze, Untersuchungen über das Blut der Ascidien. Die Vanadiumverbindung der Blutkörperchen, *Hoppe-Seylers Z. Physiol. Chem.*, **72**:494-501 (1911).
98. H. Herxheimer and E. Stresemann, The effect of slow-reacting substance (SRS-A) in guinea-pigs and in asthmatic patients, *J. Physiol. (Lond.)*, **165**:78P-79P (1963).
99. A. P. Hoffer, D. W. Hamilton, and D. W. Fawcett, The ultrastructure of the principal cells and intraepithelial leucocytes in the initial segment of the rat epididymis, *Anat. Rec.*, **175**:169-202 (1973).
100. S. Hoffstein, R. B. Zurier, and G. Weissmann, Mechanisms of lysosomal enzyme release from human leucocytes. III. Quantitative morphologic evidence for an effect of cyclic neucleotides and colchicine on degranulation, *Clin. Immunol. Immunopathol.*, **3**:201-217 (1974).
101. P. Holland, N. H. Holland, and Z. A. Cohn, The selective inhibition of macrophage phagocytic receptors by antimembrane antibodies, *J. Exp. Med.*, **135**:458-475 (1972).
102. R. G. Horn and S. S. Spicer, Sulfated mucopolysaccharide and basic protein in certain granules of rabbit leukocytes, *Lab. Invest.*, **13**:1-15 (1964).

103. T. Hubscher and A. H. Eisen, A possible immuno-pharmacological role of human eosinophils in allergic reactions. In *Mechanisms in Allergy.* Edited by L. Goodfriend, A. H Sehon, and R. P. Orange. New York, Marcel Dekker, 1973, pp. 413-437.

104. R. Hurlaux, La cytologie des cellules "phagocytaires" de l'Ascaris, *Bull. Soc. Zool. France,* **67**:188-193 (1942).

105. V. M. Ingram, *The Hemoglobins in Genetics and Evolution.* New York, Columbia University Press, 1963.

106. K. Ishizaka, H. Tomioka, and T. Ishizaka, Mechanism of passive sensitization. I. Presence of IgE and IgG molecules on human leukocytes, *J. Immunol.,* **105**:1459-1467 (1970).

107. E. Jawetz, J. L. Melnick, and E. A. Adelberg, *Review of Medical Microbiology,* 11th ed. Los Altos, Calif., Lange Medical Publ., 1974.

108. E. Jenner, *An Inquiry into the Causes and Effects of the Variolae Vaccinae.* Soho, London, Sampson, Low, 1798.

109. S. M. Johnson and J. E. Nellor, Changes in numbers of acidophilic and basophilic connective tissue granulated cells in the intestine of the rat during the estrous cycle, *Anat. Rec.,* **183**:449-457 (1975).

110. J. C. Jones, Current concepts concerning insect hemocytes, *Am. Zool.,* **2**:209-246 (1962).

111. T. W. Jones, The blood corpuscle considered in its different phases of development in the animal series. Memoir I, Vertebrata, *Phil. Trans. Soc. Lond.,* **1**:63-87 (1846).

112. J. E. Jorpes, E. Odeblad, and H. Boström, An autoradiographic study on the uptake of S^{35} labelled sodium sulphate in the mast cells, *Acta Haematol. (Basel),* **9**:273-276 (1953).

113. L. S. Kaplow and M. S. Burstone, Cytochemical demonatration of acid phosphatase in hematopoietic cells in health and in various hematological disorders using azo dye techniques, *J. Histochem. Cytochem.,* **12**: 805-811 (1964).

114. M. L. Karnovsky, Discussion. In *Mononuclear Phagocytes.* Edited by R. van Furth. Philadelphia, Pa., F. A. Davis, 1970, pp. 118-119.

115. M. L. Karnovsky and D. F. H. Wallach, The metabolic basis of phagocytosis. III. Incorporation of inorganic phosphate into various classes of phosphatides during phagocytosis, *J. Biol. Chem.,* **236**:1895-1901 (1961).

116. M. L. Karnovsky, A. W. Shafer, R. H. Cagan, R. C. Graham, M. J. Karnovsky, E. A. Glass, and K. Saito, Membrane function and metabolism in phagocytic cells, *Trans. NY Acad. Sci., [Ser. II],* **28**:778-787 (1966).

117. M. L. Karnovsky, S. R. Simmons, E. A. Glass, A. W. Shafer, and P. D'Arcy Hart, Metabolism of macrophages. In *Mononuclear Phagocytes.* Edited by R. van Furth. Philadelphia, Pa., F. A. Davis, 1970, pp. 103-117.

118. A. B. Kay, D. J. Stechschulte, and K. F. Austen, An eosinophil leukocyte chemotactic factor of anaphylaxis, *J. Exp. Med.,* **133**:602-619 (1971).

119. R. Keller, *Tissue Mast Cells in Immune Reactions.* Basel, Karger, 1966.

120. J. F. Kent, Distribution and fine structure of globule leucocytes in respiratory and digestive tracts of the laboratory rat, *Anat. Rec.,* **156**: 439-454 (1966).

121. K. H. Kilburn, W. S. Lynn, L. L. Tres, and W. N. McKenzie, Leukocyte recruitment through airway walls by condensed vegetable tannins and quercetin, *Lab. Invest.,* **28**:55-59 (1973).

122. S. J. Klebanoff, Myeloperoxidase-mediated antimicrobial systems and their role in leukocyte function. In *Biochemistry of the Phagocytic Process.* Edited by J. Schultz. Amsterdam, North-Holland Publ., 1970, pp. 89-110.

123. H. Koenig, Lysosomes in the nervous system. In *Lysosomes in Biology and Pathology 2.* Edited by J. T. Dingle and H. B. Fell. Amsterdam, North-Holland Publ., 1969, pp. 111-162.

124. H. Koenig and A. Jibril, Acidic glycolipids and the role of ionic bonds in the structure-linked latency of lysosomal hydrolases, *Biochim. Biophys. Acta,* **65**:543-545 (1962).

125. M. Kollmann, Recherches sur les leucocytes et les tissus lymphoides des invertebrés, *Ann. Sci. Nat. Zool. [Ser. 9],* **8**:1-240 (1908).

126. A. Komiyama and S. S. Spicer, Ultrastructural localization of a characteristic acid phosphatase in granules of rabbit basophils, *J. Histochem. Cytochem.,* **22**:1092-1104 (1974).

127. A. Komiyama and S. S. Spicer, Microendocytosis in eosinophilic leukocytes, *J. Cell Biol.,* **64**:622-635 (1975).

128. A. O. Kowalevsky, Einige Beiträge zur Bildung des Mantels der Ascidien, *Mem. Acad. Imp. Sci. (St. Petersbourg),* **38**(10):7 (1892).

129. A. O. Kowalevsky, Etudes expérimentales sur les glandes lymphatiques des Invertebrés. Communication préliminaire, *Mélanges Biol. Bull. Acad. Imp. Sci. (St. Petersbourg),* **13**:437-459 (1894).

130. G. S. Kurland, M. V. Krotkov, and A. S. Freedberg, Oxygen consumption and thyroxine deiodination by human leukocytes, *J. Clin. Endocrinol. Metab.,* **20**:35-46 (1960).

131. D. Lagunoff, Vital staining of mast cells with ruthenium red, *J. Histochem. Cytochem.,* **20**:938-944 (1972).

132. D. Lagunoff and E. P. Benditt, Proteolytic enzymes of mast cells, *Ann. NY Acad. Sci.,* **103**:185-197 (1963).

133. J. M. Lauweryns and J. H. Baert, The role of the pulmonary lymphatics in the defenses of the distal lung: Morphological and experimental studies of the transport mechanisms of intratracheally instillated particles, *Ann. NY Acad. Sci.,* **221**:244-275 (1974).

134. J. M. Lauweryns, M. Cokelaere, P. Theunynck, and M. Deleersnyder, Neuroepithelial bodies in mammalian respiratory mucosa: Light optical, histochemical and ultrastructural studies, *Chest,* **65**:22S-29S (1974).

135. W. H. Lay and V. Nussenzweig, Receptors for complement on leukocytes, *J. Exp. Med.,* **128**:991-1007 (1968).

136. L. V. Leak, Pulmonary lymphatics and interstitial fluid. In *Respiratory Defense Mechanisms.* Edited by J. D. Brain, D. F. Proctor, and L. Reid. New York, Marcel Dekker, 1977, Chap. 17.
137. E. S. Leake and E. R. Heise, Comparative cytology of alveolar and peritoneal macrophages from germfree rats. In *The Reticuloendothelial System and Atherosclerosis.* Edited by N. R. Diluzio and R. Paoletti. New York, Plenum, 1967, pp. 133-142.
138. E. S. Leake and Q. N. Myrvik, Rosette arrangement of electron-dense structures in granulomatous alveolar macrophages, *J. Reticuloendothel. Soc.,* **12**:305-313 (1972).
139. E. S. Leake, W. A. Sorber, and Q. N. Myrvik, Conglomerates of tubular structures in BCG-induced alveolar macrophages by negative staining, *J. Reticuloendothel. Soc.,* **15**:371-386 (1974).
140. I. H. Lepow, The properdin system: a review of current concepts. In *Immunochemical Approaches to Problems in Microbiology.* Edited by M. Heidelberger and O. J. Plescia. New Brunswick, N.J., Rutgers University Press, 1961, Chap. 19, pp. 280-294.
141. I. H. Lepow, W. Dias da Silva, and J. W. Eisele, Nature and biological properties of human anaphylatoxin, In *Biochemistry of the Acute Allergic Reactions.* Edited by K. F. Austen and E. L. Becker. Oxford, Blackwell, 1968, pp. 265-280.
142. M. R. Lewis, The formation of macrophages, epithelioid cells and giant cells from leucocytes in incubated blood, *Am. J. Pathol.,* **1**:91-100 (1925).
143. P. Lieberman, J. Ricks, L. W. Chakrin, J. R. Wardell, and R. Patterson, Immunoglobulins in respiratory secretions obtained from the canine tracheal pouch, *Proc. Soc. Exp. Biol. Med.,* **135**:713-716 (1970).
144. E. Liebman, On trephocytes and trephocytosis; a study on the role of leucocytes in nutrition and growth, *Growth,* **10**:291-330 (1946).
145. E. Liebman, The leucocytes of *Arbacia punctulata, Biol. Bull.,* **98**: 46-59 (1950).
146. A. A. Liebow and C. B. Carrington, Hypersensitivity reactions involving the lung, *Trans. Stud. Coll. Physicians Phila.,* **34**:47-70 (1966).
147. P. Lorbacher, L. T. Yam, and W. J. Mitus, Cytochemical demonstration of β-glucuronidase activity in blood and bone marrow cells, *J. Histochem. Cytochem.,* **15**:680-687 (1967).
148. M. Litt, Studies in experimental eosinophilia. VI. Uptake of immune complexes by eosinophils, *J. Cell Biol.,* **23**:355-361 (1964).
149. D. B. Lowrie, P. S. Jackett, and N. A. Ratcliffe, *Mycobacterium microti* may protect itself from intracellular destruction by releasing cyclic AMP into phagosomes, *Nature,* **254**:600-602 (1975).
150. J. A. Lucy, Lysosomal membranes. In *Lysosomes in Biology and Pathology 2.* Edited by J. T. Dingle and H. B. Fell. Amsterdam, North-Holland Publ., 1969, pp. 313-341.
151. J. H. Luft, Ruthenium red and violet. I. Chemistry, purification,

methods of use for electron microscopy and mechanism of action, *Anat. Rec.,* **171**:347-368 (1971).

152. M. A. Lutzner, Enzymatic specialization of organelles of blood cells, mast cells and platelets, *Fed. Proc.,* **23**:441 (1964).
153. G. L. Mandell, Intraphagosomal pH of human polymorphonuclear neutrophils, *Proc. Soc. Exp. Biol. Med.,* **134**:447-449 (1970).
154. K. H. Mann, *Leeches (Hirudinea), Their Structure, Physiology, Ecology, and Embryology.* New York, Pergamon, 1962.
155. J. J. Marchalonis and J. L. Atwell, Phylogenetic emergence of distinct immunoglobulin classes. In *Colloque. L'Etude Phylogénique et Ontogénique de la Réponse Immunitaire et Son Apport à la Theorie Immunologique.* Soc. Franc. Immunol., Paris, Ed. Inserm, 1973, pp. 153-162.
156. V. T. Marchesi and R. J. Barrnett, The demonstration of enzymatic activity in pinocytotic vesicles of blood capillaries with the electron microscope, *J. Cell Biol.,* **17**:547-556 (1963).
157. V. T. Marchesi and R. J. Barrnett, The localization of nucleosidephosphatase activity in different types of small blood vessels, *J. Ultrastruct. Res.,* **10**:103-115 (1964).
158. E. Margoliash, Discussion. In *Oxygen in the Animal Organism.* Edited by F. Dickens and E. Neil. Oxford, Pergamon, 1964, pp. 137-140.
159. R. J. Mason, Macrophage metabolism. In *Respiratory Defense Mechanisms.* Edited by J. D. Brain, D. F. Proctor, and L. Reid. New York, Marcel Dekker, 1977, Chap. 21.
160. R. Masse, P. Fritsch, R. Ducousso, J. Lafuma, and J. Chrétien, Retention de particules dans les cellules bronchiques, relations possibles avec les carcinogènes inhalés, *C. R. Acad. Sci. [D] (Paris),* **276**:2923-2925 (1973).
161. P. L. Masson, J. F. Heremans, J. J. Prignot, and G. Wauters, Immunohistochemical localization and bacteriostatic properties of an iron binding protein from bronchial mucus, *Thorax,* **21**:538-544 (1966).
162. A. A. Maximow, Cultures of blood leucocytes. From lymphocyte and monocyte to connective tissue, *Arch. Exp. Zellforsch.,* **5**:169-268 (1928).
163. A. A. Maximow, The lymphocytes and plasma cells. The macrophages or histiocytes. In *Special Cytology,* Vol. 2, 2nd ed. Edited by E. V. Cowdry. New York, Hoeber, 1932, pp. 601-650; 709-770.
164. R. P. McCombs, Diseases due to immunologic reactions in the lungs, *N. Engl. J. Med.,* **286**:1186-1194; 1245-1252 (1972).
165. E. McGroarty and N. E. Tolbert, Enzymes in peroxisomes, *J. Histochem. Cytochem.,* **21**:949-954 (1973).
166. J. L. Mego, The effect of pH on cathepsin activities in mouse liver heterolysosomes, *Biochem. J.,* **122**:445-452 (1971).
167. J. L. Mego and J. D. McQueen, The uptake and degradation of injected labeled proteins by mouse liver particles, *Biochim. Biophys. Acta,* **100**: 136-143 (1965).
168. I. Metchnikoff, Recherches sur la digestion intracellulaire, *Ann. Inst. Pasteur,* **3**:25-29 (1889).

169. I. Metchnikoff, *Lectures on the Comparative Pathology of Inflammation.* London, Kegan Paul, Trench, Trübner, reprinted by Dover, New York, 1968.

170. S. L. Meyer and A. M. Saunders, Cytofluorometric study of mast cell polyanions. II. Adult rat peritoneal mast cells regenerating after polymyxin treatment, *J. Histochem. Cytochem.,* **17**:56-61 (1969).

171. N. A. Michels, The mast cells. In *Handbook of Hematology,* Vol. I. Edited by H. Downey. New York, Hoeber, 1938, pp. 232-372.

172. H. R. P. Miller, Immune reactions in mucous membranes. II. The differentiation of intestinal mast cells during helminth expulsion in the rat, *Lab. Invest.,* **24**:339-347 (1971).

173. H. R. P. Miller, Immune reactions in mucous membranes. III. The discharge of intestinal mast cells during helminth expulsion in the rat, *Lab. Invest.,* **24**:348-354 (1971).

174. H. J. Müller-Eberhard, Chemistry and reaction mechanisms of complement, *Adv. Immunol.,* **8**:1-80 (1968).

175. G. F. Murphy, A. R. Brody, and J. E. Craighead, Monocyte migration across pulmonary membranes in mice infected with cytomegalovirus, *Exp. Mol. Pathol.,* **22**:35-44 (1975).

176. Q. N. Myrvik and J. D. Acton, Antimicrobial activities: extracellular influences and intracellular mechanisms. In *Respiratory Defense Mechanisms.* Edited by J. D. Brain, D. F. Proctor, and L. Reid. New York, Marcel Dekker, 1977, Chap. 24.

177. M. W. Neil and M. W. Horner, Studies on acid hydrolases in adult and foetal tissues. Acid p-nitrophenyl phosphate phosphohydrolases of adult guinea-pig liver, *Biochem. J.,* **92**:217-224 (1964).

178. M. W. Neil and M. W. Horner, Studies on acid hydrolases in adult and foetal tissues. 2. Acid phenyl phosphomonoesterases of adult mouse liver, *Biochem. J.,* **93**:220-224 (1964).

179. G. L. Nicolson, The interactions of lectins with animal cell surfaces, *Int. Rev. Cytol.,* **39**:89-190 (1974).

180. R. J. North, The localization by electron microscopy of acid phosphatase activity in guinea pig macrophages, *J. Ultrastruct. Res.,* **16**:96-108 (1966).

181. R. J. North, The localization by electron microscopy of nucleoside phosphatase activity in guinea pig phagocytic cells, *J. Ultrastruct. Res.,* **16**: 83-96 (1966).

182. R. J. North, Endocytosis, *Semin. Hematol.,* **7**:161-171 (1970).

183. A. B. Novikoff, P. M. Novikoff, N. Quintana, and C. Davis, Studies on microperoxisomes. IV. Interrelations of microperoxisomes, endoplasmic reticulum and lipofuscin granules, *J. Histochem. Cytochem.,* **21**:1010-1020 (1973).

184. C. Oliver and E. Essner, Formation of anamalous lysosomes in monocytes, neutrophils, and eosinophils from bone marrow of mice with Chédiak-Higashi syndrome, *Lab. Invest.,* **32**:17-27 (1975).

185. R. A. Oren, E. Farnham, K. Saito, E. Milofsky, and M. L. Karnovsky, Metabolic patterns in three types of phagocytizing cells, *J. Cell Biol.,* **17**:487-501 (1963).

186. J. Padawer, Ingestion of colloidal gold by mast cells, *Proc. Soc. Exp. Biol. Med.,* **129**:905-907 (1968).
187. J. Padawer, Uptake of colloidal thorium dioxide by mast cells, *J. Cell Biol.,* **40**:747-760 (1969).
188. J. Padawer, Cytological studies on normal and surviving mast cells in vitro, *Am. J. Anat.,* **127**:159-179 (1970).
189. J. Padawer, The reaction of mast cells to polylysine, *J. Cell Biol.,* **47**: 352-372 (1970).
190. J. Padawer, Mast cells: extended lifespan and lack of granule turnover under normal in vivo conditions, *Exp. Mol. Pathol.,* **20**:269-280 (1974).
191. R. T. Parmley and S. S. Spicer, Cytochemical and ultrastructural identification of a small type granule in human late eosinophils, *Lab. Invest.,* **30**:557-567 (1974).
192. P. Patriarca, R. Cramer, P. Dri, L. Fant, R. E. Basford, and F. Rossi, NADPH oxidizing activity in rabbit polymorphonuclear leukocytes: Localization in azurophilic granules, *Biochem. Biophys. Res. Commun.,* **53**:830-837 (1973).
193. R. Patterson and J. F. Kelly, Animal models of the asthmatic state, *Annu. Rev. Med.,* **25**:53-68 (1974).
194. R. Patterson, Y. Tomita, S. H. Oh, I. M. Suszko, and J. J. Pruzansky, Respiratory mast cells and basophiloid cells. I. Evidence that they are secreted into the bronchial lumen, morphology, degranulation and histamine release, *Clin. Exp. Immunol.,* **16**:223-234 (1974).
195. N. N. Pearsall and R. S. Weiser, *The Macrophage.* Philadelphia, Pa., Lea and Febiger, 1970.
196. M. Peterson and C. P. Lebond, Synthesis of complex carbohydrates in the Golgi region as shown by autoradiography after injection of labeled glucose, *J. Cell Biol.,* **21**:143-148 (1964).
197. P. Pinto da Silva, S. D. Douglas, and D. Branton, Localization of $A_{(1)}$ antigen sites on human erythrocyte ghosts, *Nature,* **232**:194-196 (1971).
198. P. Pinto da Silva, A. Martínez-Palomo, and A. Gonzalez-Robles, Membrane structure and surface coat of *Entamoeba histolytica, J. Cell Biol.,* **64**:538-550 (1975).
199. P. Pinto da Silva, P. S. Moss, and H. H. Fudenberg, Anionic sites on the membrane intercalated particles of human erythrocyte ghost membranes. Freeze-etch localization, *Exp. Cell Res.,* **81**:127-138 (1973).
200. P. Pinto da Silva and G. L. Nicolson, Freeze-etch localization of concanavalin A receptors to the membrane intercalated particles of human erythrocyte ghost membranes, *Biochem. Biophys. Acta,* **363**:311-319 (1974).
201. T. D. Pollard and R. R. Weihing, Actin and myosin and cell movement, *CRC Crit. Rev. Biochem.,* **2**:1-65 (1974).
202. S. A. Pratt, M. H. Smith, A. J. Ladman, and T. N. Finley, The ultrastructure of alveolar macrophages from human cigarette smokers and nonsmokers, *Lab. Invest.,* **24**:331-338 (1971).
203. M. Prenant, Recherches sur le parenchyme de Platyhelminthes. Essai d'histologie comparée, *Arch. Morphol. Exp. Gen.,* **5**:1-175 (1922).

204. M. Rabinovitch, Phagocytic recognition. In *Mononuclear Phagocytes.* Edited by R. van Furth. Philadelphia, Pa., F. A. Davis, 1970, pp. 299-313.
205. M. Rabinovitch, Comment. In *Mononuclear Phagocytes.* Edited by R. van Furth. Philadelphia, Pa., F. A. Davis, 1970, p. 314.
206. F. von Recklinghausen, Ueber Eiter- und Bindegewebskörperchen, *Virchows Arch. [Pathol. Anat.]*, **28**:157-197 (1863).
207. J. K. Reddy, Possible properties of microbodies (peroxisomes): Microbody proliferation and hypolipidemic drugs, *J. Histochem. Cytochem.*, **21**:967-971 (1973).
208. C. E. Reed and J. M. Bennett, N-acetyl-β-glucosaminidase activity in normal and malignant leukocytes, *J. Histochem. Cytochem.*, **23**:752-757 (1975).
209. J. F. Riley, *The Mast Cells.* Edinburgh, Livingstone, 1959.
210. A. N. Romer, *The Vertebrate Body.* Philadelphia, Pa., Saunders, 1962.
211. M. Romieu, *Recherches histiophysiologiques sur le sang et sur le corps cardiaque des Annélides polychètes.* Paris, Librarie Octave Douin, 1923, pp. 1-339.
212. P. Rous, The relative reaction within living mammalian tissues. II. On the mobilization of acid material within cells, and the reaction as influenced by the cell state, *J. Exp. Med.*, **41**:399-411 (1925).
213. J. T. Ruud, Vertebrates without erythrocytes and blood pigment, *Nature*, **173**:848-853 (1954).
214. T. Rytömaa, Organ distribution and histochemical properties of eosinophil granulocytes in the rat, *Acta Pathol. Microbiol. Scand.*, **50** (Suppl. 140):1-118 (1960).
215. S. S. Sabesin A function of the eosinophil: Phagocytosis of antigen-antibody complexes, *Proc. Soc. Exp. Biol. Med.*, **112**:667-670 (1963).
216. D. Sampson and G. J. Archer, Release of histamine from human basophils, *Blood*, **29**:722-736 (1967).
217. E. E. Schneeberger, Unpublished work, 1973.
218. E. E. Schneeberger, The integrity of the air-blood barrier. In *Respiratory Defense Mechanisms.* Edited by J. D. Brain, D. F. Proctor, and L. Reid. New York, Marcel Dekker, 1977, Chap. 18.
219. E. E. Schneeberger and E. J. Burger, Intravascular macrophages in cat lungs following open chest ventilation: An electron microscopic study, *Lab. Invest.*, **22**:361-369 (1970).
220. D. R. Schultz, *The Complement System.* Basel, Karger, 1971.
221. J. E. Scott and H. Guilford, Alcian blue 8GX: investigation of structural details using nuclear magnetic resonance and mass spectrometry, *J. Histochem. Cytochem.*, **20**:387-390 (1972).
222. H. Selye, *The Mast Cells.* Washington, D.C., Butterworths, 1965.
223. S. M. Shea, Lanthanum staining of the surface coat of cells. Its enhancement by the use of fixatives containing alcian blue or cetylpyridinium chloride, *J. Cell Biol.*, **51**:611-620 (1971).
224. E. Siegel and B. A. Sachs, In vitro leukocyte uptake of ^{131}I-labeled

iodide, thyroxine, and triiodothyronine, and its relation to thyroid function, *J. Clin. Endocrinol. Metab.*, **24**:313-318 (1964).

225. A. S. Simani, S. Inoue, and J. C. Hogg, Penetration of the respiratory epithelium of guinea pigs following exposure to cigarette smoke, *Lab. Invest.*, **31**:75-81 (1974).

226. N. Simionescu, M. Simionescu, and G. E. Palade, Permeability of muscle capillaries to small heme-peptides. Evidence for the existence of patent transendothelial channels, *J. Cell Biol.*, **64**:586-607 (1975).

227. C. E. Slonecker, B. Roos, B. Sordat, M. W. Hess, and H. Cottier, Kinetic studies on peritoneal macrophages and lymphoid cells in mice prelabelled with ^{3}H-thymidine. In *Mononuclear Phagocytes.* Edited by R. van Furth. Philadelphia, Pa., F. A. Davis, 1970, pp. 233-239.

228. E. Sorkin, Discussion. In *Mononuclear Phagocytes.* Edited by R. van Furth. Philadelphia, Pa., F. A. Davis, 1970, p. 421.

229. E. Sorkin, J. F. Borel, and V. J. Stecher, Chemotaxis of mononuclear and polymorphonuclear phagocytes. In *Mononuclear Phagocytes.* Edited by R. van Furth. Philadelphia, Pa., F. A. Davis, 1970, pp. 397-418.

230. H. P. Sorokin and S. P. Sorokin, Fluctuations in the acid phosphatase activity of spherosomes in guard cells of *Campanula persicifolia, J. Histochem. Cytochem.*, **16**:791-802 (1968).

231. P. A. Sorokin, *Fads and Foibles in Modern Sociology and Related Sciences.* Chicago, Ill., Regnery, 1956, Chap. 1, Amnesia and New Columbuses.

232. S. P. Sorokin, A morphologic and cytochemical study on the great alveolar cell, *J. Histochem. Cytochem.*, **14**:884-897 (1966).

233. S. P. Sorokin, Properties of alveolar cells and tissues that strengthen alveolar defenses, *Arch. Intern. Med.*, **126**:450-463 (1970).

234. S. P. Sorokin, The cells of the lungs. In *Morphology of Experimental Respiratory Carcinogenesis.* AEC Symposium Series 21. Edited by P. Nettesheim, M. G. Hanna, Jr., and J. W. Deatherage, Jr. CONF-700501, U. S. Atomic Energy Commission Division of Technical Information. Springfield, Va., National Technical Information Service, 1970, pp. 3-41.

235. S. P. Sorokin and J. D. Brain, Pathways of clearance in mouse lungs exposed to iron oxide aerosols, *Anat. Rec.*, **181**:581-626 (1975).

236. S. P. Sorokin and H. A. Padykula, Differentiation of the rat's yolk sac in organ culture, *Am. J. Anat.*, **114**:457-478 (1964).

237. R. S. Speirs and Y. Osada, Chemotactic activity and phagocytosis of eosinophils, *Proc. Soc. Exp. Biol. Med.*, **109**:929-932 (1962).

238. H. Spencer, *Pathology of the Lung (Excluding Pulmonary Tuberculosis).* Oxford, Pergamon, 1962.

239. S. S. Spicer and J. H. Hardin, Ultrastructure, cytochemistry, and function of neutrophil leukocyte granules, *Lab. Invest.*, **20**:488-497 (1969).

240. L. A. Stauber, The fate of India ink injected intracardially into the oyster, *Ostrea virginica* Gmelin, *Biol. Bull.*, **98**:227-241 (1950).

241. V. J. Stecher, Synthesis of proteins by mononuclear phagocytes. In *Mononuclear Phagocytes.* Edited by R. van Furth. Philadelphia, Pa., F. A. Davis, 1970, pp. 133-147.

242. H. F. Steedman, Alcian blue 8GS: A new stain for mucin, *Q. J. Microsc. Sci.*, **91**:447-479 (1950).

243. T. P. Stossel, Phagocytosis, *N. Engl. J. Med.*, **290**:717-723; 774-780; 833-839 (1974).

244. W. Strauss, Isolation and biochemical properties of droplets from the cells of rat kidney, *J. Biol. Chem.*, **207**:745-755 (1954).

245. W. Strauss, Colorimetric analysis with N,N-Dimethyl p-phenylenediamine of the uptake of intravenously injected horseradish peroxidase by various tissues of the rat, *J. Biophys. Biochem. Cytol.*, **4**:541-550 (1958).

246. W. Strauss, Lysosomes, phagosomes and related particles. In *Enzyme Cytology*. Edited by D. B. Roodyn. New York, Academic Press, 1967, pp. 239-319.

247. W. Strauss, Immunocytochemical observations on hypersensitivity skin reactions to horseradish peroxidase and to antihorseradish peroxidase-γ-globulin, *J. Histochem. Cytochem.*, **22**:303-319 (1974).

248. A. E. Stuart, The reticulo-endothelial system of the Lesser Octopus, *Elodone cirrosa*, *J. Pathol. Bact.*, **96**:401-412 (1968).

249. A. E. Stuart, Phylogeny of mononuclear phagocytes. In *Mononuclear Phagocytes*. Edited by R. van Furth. Philadelphia, Pa., F. A. Davis, 1970, pp. 316-334.

250. A. L. Sullivan, P. M. Grimley, and H. Metzger, Electron microscopic localization of immunoglobulin E on the surface membrane of human basophils, *J. Exp. Med.*, **134**:1403-1414 (1971).

251. J. S. Sutton and L. Weiss, Transformation of monocytes in tissue culture into macrophages, epithelioid cells and multinucleated giant cells, *J. Cell Biol.*, **28**:303-332 (1966).

252. M. Szabo and G. Burke, Uptake and metabolism of 3′,5′-cyclic adenosine monophosphate and N^6,$O^{2\prime}$-dibutyryl 3′,5′-cyclic adenosine monophosphate in isolated bovine thyroid cells, *Biochim. Biophys. Acta*, **264**:289-299 (1972).

253. A. Takeuchi, H. R. Jervis, and H. Sprinz, The globule leucocyte in the intestinal mucosa of the cat: A histochemical, light, and electron microscopic study, *Anat. Rec.*, **164**:79-100 (1969).

254. Y. Tanaka and J. R. Goodman, *Electron Microscopy of Human Blood Cells*. New York, Harper and Row, 1972.

255. N. Tchistovich, Des phénomènes de phagocytose dans les poumons, *Ann. Inst. Pasteur*, **3**:337-361 (1889).

256. A. R. Ten Cate and D. A. Deporter, The degradative role of the fibroblast in the remodelling and turnover of collagen in soft connective tissue, *Anat. Rec.*, **182**:1-14 (1975).

257. R. W. Terry, D. F. Bainton, and M. G. Farquhar, Formation and structure of specific granules in basophilic leukocytes of the guinea pig, *Lab. Invest.*, **21**:65-76 (1969).

258. G. H. Thoenes, The hagfish at the phylogenetical juncture towards immunological response. In *Colloque. L'Etude Phylogénique et Ontogenique de la Réponse Immunitaire et Son Apport à la Théorie Immunologique.* Soc. Franc. Immunol., Paris, Ed. Inserm, 1973, pp. 69-74.

259. D'Arcy W. Thompson, *On Growth and Form.* Abridged edition edited by J. T. Bonner. London, Cambridge University Press, 1961.
260. T. W. Tillack, R. E. Scott, and V. T. Marchesi, The structure of erythrocyte membranes studied by freeze-etching. II. Localization of receptors for phytohemagglutinin and influenza virus to the intramembranous particles, *J. Exp. Med.,* **135**:1209-1227 (1972).
261. M.-F. Tsan and R. D. Berlin, Membrane transport in the rabbit alveolar macrophage. The specificity and characteristics of amino acid transport systems, *Biochem. Biophys. Acta,* **241**:155-169 (1971).
262. M.-F. Tsan and R. D. Berlin, Effect of phagocytosis on membrane transport of nonelectrolytes, *J. Exp. Med.,* **134**:1016-1035 (1971).
263. T. E. Ukena and R. D. Berlin, Effect of colchicine and vinblastine on the topographical separation of membrane functions, *J. Exp. Med.,* **136**: 1-7 (1972).
264. A. Vandel, Généralitiés sur les Arthropodes. In *Traité de Zoologie.* Edited by P. Grassé. Paris, Masson, 1949, pp. 79-158.
265. R. van Furth, The origin and turnover of promonocytes, monocytes, and macrophages in normal mice. In *Mononuclear Phagocytes.* Edited by R. van Furth. Philadelphia, Pa., F. A. Davis, 1970, pp. 151-165.
266. W. C. Von Glahn and J. W. Hall, The reaction produced in the pulmonary arteries by emboli of cotton fibers, *Am. J. Pathol.,* **25**:575-595 (1949).
267. W. C. Von Glahn, J. W. Hall, and S.-C. Sun, Arteritis in guinea pigs, produced by emboli of cotton, resembling the arteritis of hypersensitivity, *Am. J. Pathol.,* **30**:1129-1139 (1954).
268. J. L. Walker, The regulatory function of prostaglandins in the release of histamine and SRS-A from passively sensitized lung tissue. Symposium on Prostaglandins, *Adv. Biosci.,* **9**:235-240 (1973).
269. P. A. Ward, Chemotaxis of mononuclear cells, *J. Exp. Med.,* **128**:1201-1221 (1968).
270. P. A. Ward, Chemotactic factors for neutrophils, eosinophils, mononuclear cells and lymphocytes. In *Biochemistry of the Acute Allergic Reactions.* Edited by K. F. Austen and E. L. Becker. Oxford, Blackwell, 1971, pp. 229-237.
271. P. A. Ward, J. Chapitis, M. C. Conroy, and I. H. Lepow, Generation by bacterial proteinases of leukotactic factors from human serum, and human C3 and C5, *J. Immunol.,* **110**:1003-1009 (1973).
272. A. Weinstock and J. T. Albright, The fine structure of mast cells in normal human gingiva, *J. Ultrastruct. Res.,* **17**:245-256 (1965).
273. L. Weiss and D. W. Fawcett, Cytochemical observations on chicken monocytes, macrophages, and giant cells in tissue culture, *J. Histochem. Cytochem.,* **1**:47-65 (1953).
274. Z. Werb and Z. A. Cohn, Plasma membrane synthesis in the macrophage following phagocytosis of polystyrene latex particles, *J. Biol. Chem.,* **247**:2439-2446 (1972).
275. B. K. Wetzel, S. S. Spicer, and R. G. Horn, Fine structural localization of acid and alkaline phosphatases in cells of rabbit blood and bone marrow, *J. Histochem. Cytochem.,* **15**:311-334 (1967).

276. D. W. Whitelaw, The intravascular lifespan of monocytes, *Blood,* **28**:455-464 (1966).

277. K. E. Williams, E. M. Kidston, F. Beck, and J. B. Lloyd, Quantitative studies of pinocytosis. II. Kinetics of protein uptake and digestion by rat yolk sac cultured in vitro, *J. Cell Biol.,* **64**:123-134 (1975).

278. P. Wolf-Jürgensen, The basophilic leukocyte, *Ser. Haematol.,* **I** (No. 4): 45-65 (1968).

279. D. Zucker-Franklin, The phagosomes in rheumatoid sinovial fluid leukocytes: A light, fluorescence, and electron microscope study, *Arthritis Rheum.,* **9**:24-36 (1966).

280. R. B. Zurier, G. Weissmann, S. Hoffstein, S. Kammerman, and H.-H. Tai, Mechanisms of lysosomal enzyme release from human leukocytes. II. Effects of cAMP and cGMP, autonomic agonists, and agents which affect microtubule function, *J. Clin. Invest.,* **53**:297-309 (1974).

281. B. A. Nichols, Normal rabbit alveolar macrophages. II. Their primary and secondary lysosomes as revealed by electron microscopy and cytochemistry, *J. Exp. Med.,* **144**:920-931 (1976).

282. S. P. Sorokin, A labyrinthian precursor of primary lysosomes in alveolar macrophages, *J. Cell Biol.,* **70**:381a (1976).

283. B. J. Zeligs, L. S. Nerurkar, J. A. Bellanti, and J. D. Zeligs, Maturation of the rabbit alveolar macrophage during animal development. I. Perinatal influx into alveoli and ultrastructural differentiation, *Pediat. Res.,* **11**:197-208 (1977).

PLATE 4

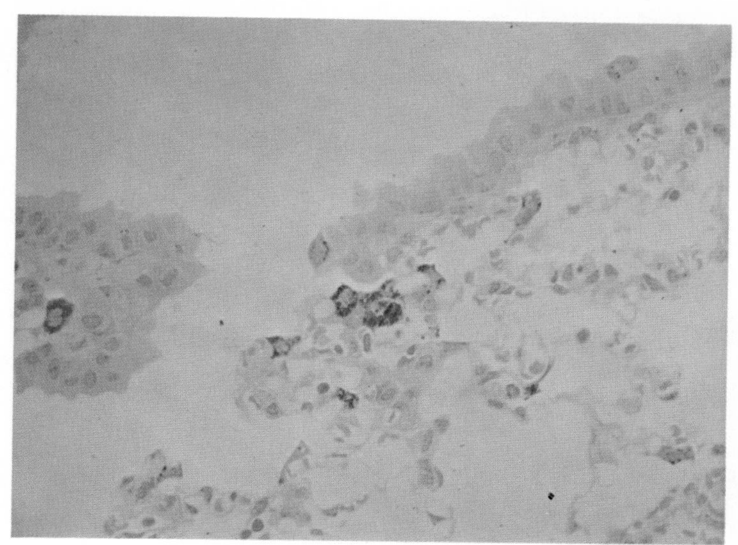

(a)

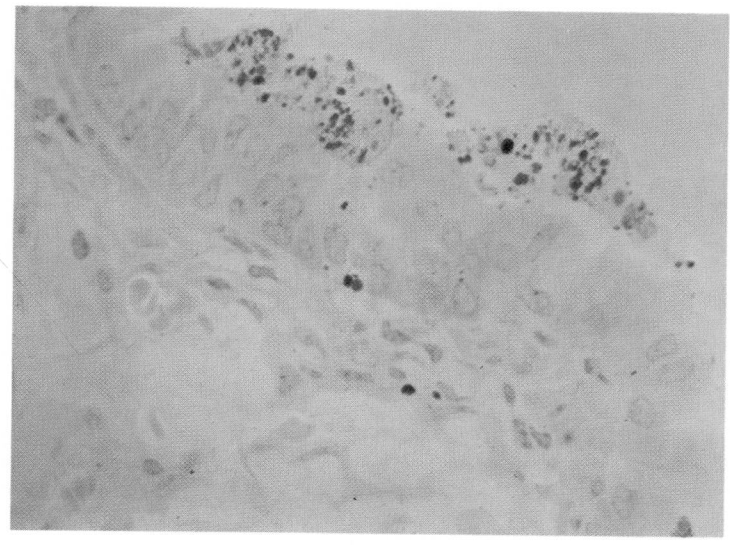

(b)

PLATE 4 (continued)

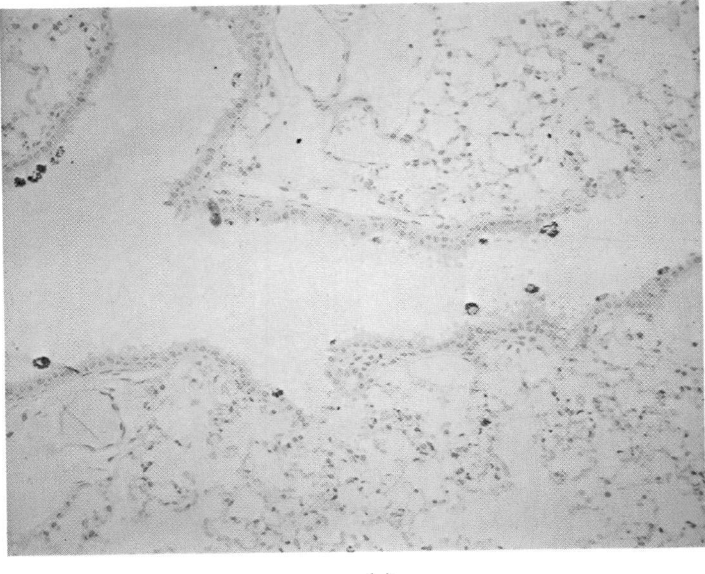

(c)

PLATE 4

(a) Particle-containing macrophages at the alveolar-bronchiolar junction. Such cells appear to congregate near the beginning of the bronchiole and appear to be migrating toward the bronchiolar surface. Two have ascended onto the bronchial epithelium. Glycol methacrylate sections of mouse lungs 21 days after a 3 hr exposure to ferric oxide. Prussian blue counterstained with basic fuchsin. ×250.

(b) Adherent airway macrophages on the bronchial epithelium. Diffuse and granular Prussian blue staining is present in the macrophages, in the bronchial epithelium, and in the connective tissue beneath suggesting transepithelial transport. Glycol methacrylate sections. Prussian blue stain and basic fuchsin. ×450.

(c) Numerous iron-filled macrophages are present on the bronchial epithelium 30 hr after a 1 hr exposure to iron oxide. Thus particles are concentrated above selected areas of the epithelium leading to "hot spots." Glycol methacrylate sections. Prussian blue stain and basic fuchsin. ×150.

20

Quantification, Origin, and Fate of Pulmonary Macrophages

JOSEPH D. BRAIN

Harvard University School of Public Health
Boston, Massachusetts

SERGEI P. SOROKIN

Harvard University School of Public Health
Boston, Massachusetts

JOHN J. GODLESKI

Medical College of Pennsylvania
Philadelphia, Pennsylvania

I. Introduction

A. Definition of Pulmonary Macrophages

Chapter 19 considered the wide range of phagocytic cells in the lung and presented both similarities and differences among them. In this chapter, we will focus on pulmonary macrophages, and examine certain aspects of their quantification, origin, and fate. It is important, however, to realize that even here we are dealing with a diverse group of cells. Pulmonary macrophages differ with respect to their anatomical location and perhaps in their basic cell biology as well. Pulmonary macrophages consist of at least three distinct types: the most prominent member of the pulmonary macrophage family is the *alveolar macrophage* and, at times, the terms are used interchangeably. Alveolar macrophages are large, mononuclear, phagocytic cells found on the alveolar surface (see Plate 3a). They do not form part of the continuous epithelial layer, which is made up of pulmonary surface epithelial cells (type I pneumonocytes) and great alveolar cells (type II pneumonocytes); rather, the alveolar macrophages rest on this lining.

Another important subdivision of pulmonary macrophages is the *airway macrophage* (see Plate 3b). These mononuclear cells are present in the conducting airways, both of large and small caliber. They may be present as passengers on the mucus escalator, or they may be found beneath the mucus lining, apparently adhering to the bronchial epithelium [87]. These airway macrophages most likely represent the result of alveolar-bronchiolar transport of alveolar macrophages, although it has been suggested that they are the product of direct migration of cells through the bronchial epithelium [21,53].

The third subdivision of pulmonary macrophages is *interstitial macrophages* (see Plate 3c) found in the various connective tissue compartments of the lung. These include alveolar walls, sinuses of the lymph nodes and nodules, and peribronchial and perivascular spaces. Connective tissue macrophages have been considered in some detail by Sorokin and Brain [87]. Nai-sun Wang [99] also observed numerous macrophages subjacent to the mesothelial cell layer of the visceral pleura, particularly in the Kampmeier foci (small white patches found in the pleural folds of the lower mediastinum). These interstitial macrophages vary in appearance and, no doubt, in function as well; their relationship to other cells and tissues also exhibits considerable variety. In addition to these primary compartments, other minor macrophage compartments exist. For example, macrophages are found in the pleural space where they not only serve a defensive role, but also act as miniature "roller bearings" facilitating movements between the parietal and visceral pleura [2].

All pulmonary macrophages are usually considered to be relatives of macrophages throughout the body [59] (see Sec. IV). This extended family includes the Kupffer cells of the liver, the free and fixed macrophages in the spleen, lymph nodes, bone marrow, the peritoneal macrophage of the serous cavity, and the osteoclasts of bone. They share certain common morphological characteristics, such as the ruffling of the plasma membrane which reflects their active participation in endocytosis. Other criteria, such as their capability for avid phagocytosis and pinocytosis, as well as their firm attachment to glass surfaces, are also useful hallmarks.

B. Role of Pulmonary Macrophages

The physiological role and significance of pulmonary macrophages are detailed in the following chapters and have been reviewed elsewhere [8,13]. Therefore, they will be mentioned only briefly here.

Although large numbers of infectious particles are continuously deposited in the lungs, the alveolar surface is usually sterile [60]. It is the phagocytic and lytic potential of the alveolar macrophages that provides most of the known bactericidal properties of the lungs. Like other phagocytes, alveolar macrophages are rich in lysosomes. The lysosomes attach themselves to the phagosomal membrane surrounding the ingested pathogen. Then the lysosomal membranes become continuous with the phagosomal membrane and the lytic enzymes kill and digest the bacteria. Specific bactericidal mechanisms are discussed in some detail in Chap. 24. Among the hydrolases they are known to contain are proteases, deoxyribonuclease, ribonuclease, β-glucuronidase, and acid phosphatase [73].

Pulmonary macrophages also ingest nonliving, insoluble dust and debris. Particles which remain on the surface of the alveoli, either within free alveolar macrophages or on the fluid surface, may be removed to the ciliated part of the lung. The speed of clearance is determined by the rate of macrophage migration and by the mouthward flow of alveolar capillary transudate mixed with alveolar cell secretions.

However, not all deposited particles remain on the internal surfaces of the lungs. Some cross the alveolar or bronchial lining, become sequestered in interstitial tissues, or enter the lymphatic tissue. Once particles leave the alveolar surface and penetrate the fixed tissues subjacent to the air-liquid interface, their removal from that compartment is less predictable.

Macrophages ingest almost any foreign material reaching the alveoli, such as aspirated cod liver or mineral oil. They may also engulf endogenous materials such as red cells which may be present following pulmonary hemorrhage caused by increased pulmonary capillary pressure subsequent to left heart failure. In fact, an early synonym for alveolar macrophages was "heart failure cells." Finally, macrophages may ingest endogenous cells and materials even without pathological provocation. Effete epithelial cells and excess or inactive pulmonary surfactant are also probably ingested and degraded by macrophages. It is likely that alveolar macrophages even ingest other dead or damaged macrophages.

II. Harvesting Techniques

Research on pulmonary macrophages often depends on our ability to isolate pure populations of macrophages from the lungs of animals and man. But, success in isolating pulmonary macrophages depends on the particular subclasses involved. Alveolar macrophages, for example, represent a relatively accessible and homogeneous cell population. Unfortunately, not all categories of pulmonary macrophages can be recovered with the same ease and purity. To our knowledge, no investigator has been able to prepare a pure suspension of interstitial pulmonary macrophages. Techniques for dissolving the lung and liberating individual cells are being developed and intensive efforts are underway with regard to separation of isolated lung cells [49]. However, interstitial macrophages are less numerous and little is known about the existence of unique physical or chemical properties which could be exploited in separating these cells. Conceivably, their proclivity for attachment to glass or the identification of a specific surface receptor could be exploited. If a lung, well washed to eliminate airway and alveolar macrophages, was dispersed, presumably those cells attaching to glass would be a relatively enriched population of interstitial macrophages. Airway macrophages may be procured with somewhat greater ease. Isolated lengths of airways can be gently rinsed to recover the free cells present on airway surfaces. This technique is adequate for recovering cells for counting or for morphological or histochemical analyses, but insufficient quantities are recovered for most biochemical or physiological studies. One can also attempt to lavage the airways and not the parenchyma. If the lungs are gas-freed and then carefully rinsed with small volumes of saline (1 to 3 times the volume of the dead space), then it is mainly the airways that are rinsed. Appreciable interfacial tension between the injected saline and the airway surface, and the very modest inflating pressures associated with the small volumes injected, make it unlikely that little saline will reach the parenchyma.

Airway macrophages can also be recovered by collecting the free cells leaving the lungs via the trachea. Spritzer et al. [88] cannulated the esophagus and collected all swallowed material in a polyethylene bottle attached to a rat's flank. They recovered between 1.24 and 2.47×10^6 macrophages per hour. Brain [13] developed a technique which permits the collection of diluted respiratory tract fluid from cats. Between 1.87 and 5.07×10^6 macrophages per hour were recovered from the lungs.

Finally, as will be pointed out in the next section, the first few washes of pulmonary lavage samples, using a balanced salt solution including divalent cations, are more heavily weighted with airway macrophages than are the later washes. Regardless of the technique, however, it is essential to recognize that the initial product is never pure. Desquamated epithelial cells, both ciliated and nonciliated, erythrocytes, neutrophils, and lymphocytes may be present in varying numbers. Thus, differential counts should always be performed and for some applications, macrophages should be purified by adhesion to glass or by isopycnic density gradient centrifugation.

Alveolar macrophages are traditionally recovered by lung lavage procedures. But not all free cells recovered by lung lavage meet the theoretical definition of alveolar macrophages discussed in the Introduction. Some type I and type II pneumonocytes, airway epithelial cells, and contaminating blood cells may also be harvested. Airway macrophages are always present, being more prevalent in the initial washes, less so in the later washes. Lung lavage or washing to recover macrophages was first used by Gersing and Schumacher [36], and has been used extensively since [57,58,72]. Brain and Frank [15,17] attempted to make the technique more sensitive and reproducible by utilizing multiple lung washings and by controlling the factors influencing the washing procedure. Their technique is as follows.

Anesthetized animals are exsanguinated by excising both kidneys or by cutting the aorta. A pneumothorax is produced by cutting the diagram, the chest cavity is opened, and the trachea is ligated to prevent blood from entering the lungs. The lungs are dissected free of other tissues and examined for evidence of disease. Following gas-freeing, the trachea is cannulated with polyethylene tubing. The tubing is filled with saline to prevent injection of air into the lungs. Physiological saline (0.85% sodium chloride) flushes are begun to collect the free cells from the lungs. In each washing 5 ml saline/g lung are used. Each wash takes approximately 1 min. The procedure is repeated six or more times. During the washing procedure, the excised lungs are suspended in physiological saline to eliminate hydrostatic gradients which might lead to uneven filling. When the washings are completed, the lungs are fixed, sectioned, and stained for histological examination.

In eight mammalian species studied, they generally obtained yields of between 3 and 15 million cells/g lung when the lungs were washed 12 times. As shown in Fig. 1, the cumulative yield continued to increase, demonstrating that macrophages are harvested even in the later washes. If lung washes are being used to assay the pool size of macrophages where it is necessary to obtain quantitatively consistent cell recoveries, it is essential to standardize all aspects of the

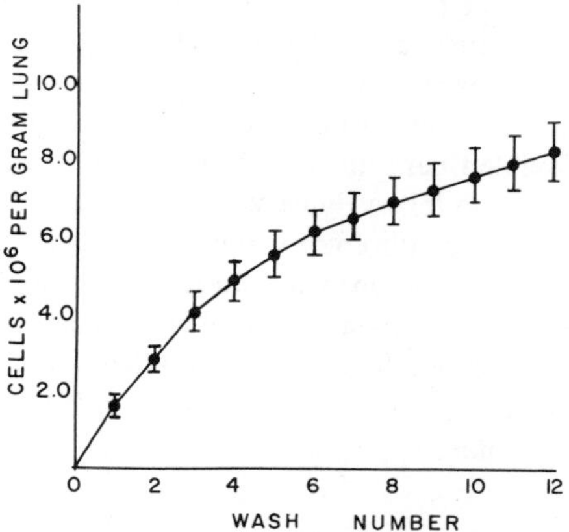

FIGURE 1 Cumulative yield of cells recovered from cat lungs by repeated washings, showing arithmetic means and standard errors from 13 lungs. 0.85% NaCl used as the lavage fluid.

washing procedure. Some procedural variables and their effects on macrophage recovery will be discussed later in this chapter.

Macrophages may also be harvested from lungs in situ by the same wash technique. In such experiments, it is impossible to express cell yields in numbers per gram lung (thus reducing variability), but the time saved is considerable. If washed in situ, the possibility of causing leaks in the lungs is also reduced. Following exsanguination, the neck is opened and the trachea cannulated. The chest wall can be opened to allow the lungs to empty themselves of as much air as possible. Washes are then carried out as described above.

Lungs of living animals may also be lavaged. Following induction of anesthesia, a cuffed endotracheal tube is introduced through the larynx and placed in the left or right bronchus. The cuff is then inflated to create a tight seal. The lung is gas-freed, if desired, by ventilating the lung with pure oxygen for 15-20 min, producing a low lung volume by making the airway pressure negative (~ -5 cmH_2O) and then occluding the airway. After a few minutes the remaining oxygen will be absorbed. The intubated lung may then be lavaged while the remaining lung meets the ventilatory demands of the animal. Animals will tolerate the procedure better if the left lung is lavaged, since the right lung comprises about 60% of the total lung tissue. Smaller subdivisions of the lung may be lavaged by using smaller caliber endotracheal tubes; tubes without inflatable cuffs may be simply wedged in an appropriately sized airway. Recoveries of injected saline may be low in animals possessing considerable collateral ventilation (i.e., dog). Instilled saline not recovered will be absorbed into the capillaries.

A number of investigators have used similar procedures to recover macrophages from human subjects [79]. For more than a decade, bronchopulmonary lavage has been used to remove unwanted cells and secretions from small airways and parenchyma. Studies have shown that the clinical status of patients with alveolar proteinosis and possibly cystic fibrosis is often improved by lavage. With the advent of flexible fiberoptic bronchoscopy [82], access to the lower respiratory tract has become relatively easy and nontraumatic. Segmental lobes can be lavaged to obtain cytopathologic material and bacteriologic specimens. Typically, a fiberoptic bronchoscope is introduced following premedication with atropine, meperidine, or diazepam, and topical anesthesia of the respiratory tract with a 2% lidocaine spray. Sterile saline can then be instilled and recovered through the bronchoscope placed in a pulmonary segment. The lavage procedure may be repeated several times.

III. Quantitation

Quantitative assessment of macrophage pool size can provide important information regarding the state of the pulmonary parenchyma. Changes in the numbers of free cells can be used as an indicator of adaptation in response to inhaled particles, gases, or pathogens [14] or can be used to chronicle the sequence of events in lung injury [20].

A. Morphometric Techniques

Before discussing lung lavage as a technique for estimating macrophage pool size, we will mention another approach, that of morphometric analysis of histological sections. Weibel [102] pioneered rational, quantitative approaches for measuring pulmonary dimensions and the frequency of various cell types. Others, although with less rigor, attempted to count macrophages in histological sections. For example, LaBelle and Brieger [56] counted the numbers of phagocytic cells in lung sections using the light microscope to estimate changes in the macrophage population. Pinkett et al. [77] used a similar technique to estimate the numbers of macrophages removed by their washing procedure.

Yet, at the light microscope level, it is often difficult to identify many of the free cells in the lungs. If the cells have ingested visible amounts of particles or if the histological procedures have caused them to detach and "round up," they are easily recognized. But, if unexposed animals are used and if the alveolar macrophage is still applied to the alveolar wall, it is difficult to eliminate error in distinguishing alveolar macrophages from great alveolar cells. If the electron microscope is used, it is certainly possible to identify free cells correctly. Unfortunately, the procedures are tedious and the problems of adequate sampling are troublesome. These techniques, however, do have the advantage of making regional measurements of macrophage numbers and correlating those numbers with other variables, e.g., airways vs. parenchyma, patterns of particle deposition, or disease status.

B. Lavage Techniques

Unlike morphometric techniques, bronchopulmonary lavage samples relatively large volumes of lung, and recovers cells not easily related to specific lung regions. Unless special care is taken, airway macrophages cannot easily be distinguished from alveolar macrophages. It is unknown to what extent macrophages are recruited by changes in lung volume and other consequences of the washing procedure. The efficiency of the harvesting procedure is also difficult to assess.

In spite of these reservations, lavage remains a useful way to follow changes in lung free cells. The composition (or contents) of lavage fluid can yield other valuable information regarding the state of the pulmonary parenchyma. It can be analyzed physically and biochemically for pulmonary surfactant, for the presence of serum proteins (indicating pulmonary edema), for airway mucus, or for secretory immunoglobulins.

C. Importance of Procedural Variables

To obtain quantitatively consistent recoveries of free cells it is necessary to control all aspects of the harvesting procedures. Brain and Frank [15] examined the effects of gas-freeing the lungs, of the length of the postmortem delay time, wash volume, leakage, pathological changes, and of the number of washes. Another paper reported the effects of age, sex, lung weight, and body weight on the numbers of free cells recovered [16]. Additional observations [17] dealt with the effects of wash osmolarity and temperature, and duration of the washing cycle. Mechanical factors are also involved in the recovery of free cells from the alveolar surface and airways. When excised rat lungs are washed with 0.85% NaCl, the yield of cells is more than doubled by gently massaging the lungs with the fingertips for a 30-sec period between instillation and withdrawal of the saline. Increases due to massage also occur when the washing fluid is a complete balanced salt solution (BSS) and in a variety of other species [14].

Many of the variables affecting harvest efficiency are simply procedural and should be controlled if consistent results are desired. Some investigations, however, have provided clues to more fundamental physiological questions. For example, experiments with varied washing fluid compositions have given insight into the surface forces existing between the alveolar macrophage and the alveolar wall [17]. Those experiments show that Ca^{2+} and Mg^{2+} ions are responsible for the differences in cell yields between BSS and physiological saline. Apparently Ca^{2+} and Mg^{2+} critically influence the adhesive forces which exist between alveolar macrophages and the alveolar wall. This effect of divalent cations is particularly prominent in small rodents such as rats, hamsters, and mice but is also seen in cats and rabbits. Figure 2 shows the shape of the washout curve for hamsters washed with either 0.85% NaCl or BSS. Unlike Fig. 1, which plots the cumulative yields, Fig. 2 shows the numbers of macrophages recovered per wash. The shapes of the washout curves are clearly influenced by the composition of the wash solution used.

Lung lavage is often used to quantify changes in macrophage pool size following aerosol challenge, lung infection, or lung injury. The lung lavage technique cited above is more reliable and sensitive with repeated washings. In most experiments, the mean cumulative yield increases at a faster rate than does the standard error. Even though individual washes vary, differences tend to cancel each other so that the cumulative total yield becomes less variable. Therefore, the coefficient of variation, 100 × standard deviation/mean, generally decreases with increasing numbers of washes. When the pool sizes of two different treat-

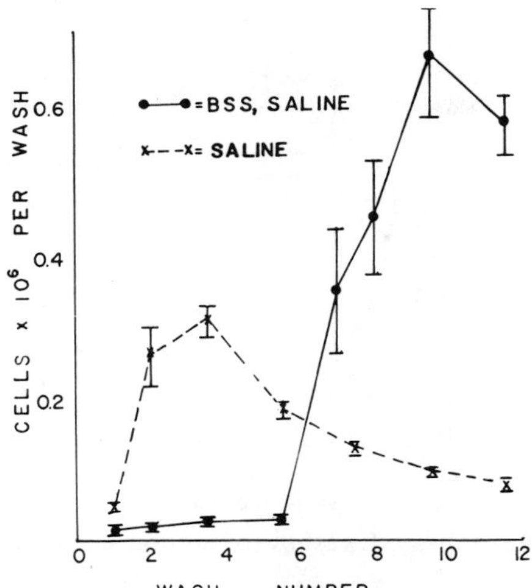

FIGURE 2 Yield of cells per wash recovered from hamster lungs washed with either saline (0.85% NaCl) or BSS (balanced salt solution containing Ca^{2+} and Mg^{2+}). The means are shown with their standard error.

ment groups are compared, there is an increasing t value (Student's t-test) and, hence, an increasingly significant difference as the number of washes increases. For example, in 14 different experiments, the value of t was calculated for the difference in cumulative pool size between the control and experimental groups at each wash number [14]. The average t values (±SE) for all 14groups are shown in Fig. 3. Also shown is the corresponding value of P, the probability of the observed difference occurring by chance. It is apparent that as the lung is repeatedly washed, the differences between groups become increasingly significant and hence the technique becomes more sensitive. The data suggest that lungs should be washed at least six times to achieve maximum sensitivity.

A final point regarding procedure is that for each exposure situation, it is essential to examine control animals simultaneously. We find that free cell recovery from groups of control animals of the same species vary by as much as 60%. This may be due to genetic differences, seasonal rhythms, changes in humidity or temperature, or perhaps undetected disease. Controls sacrificed at other times should not be used for comparison.

D. Adaptive Changes in Pool Size

It is not surprising that a cell system so intimately involved with the disposal of inhaled materials responds to the quantity of particles presented to it. Nearly

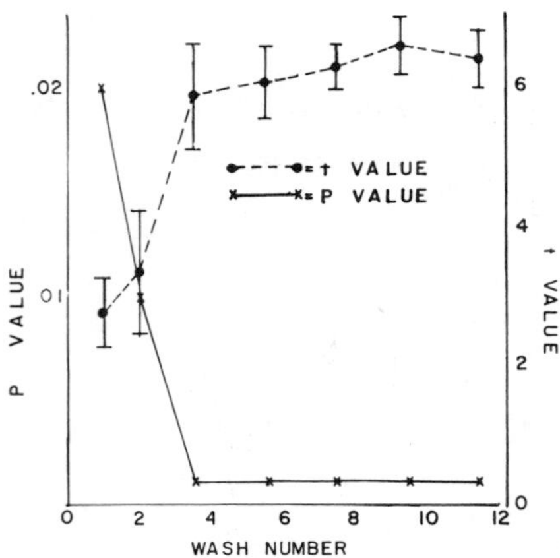

FIGURE 3 Relation of repeated washes to method sensitivity.

60 years ago, Permar [76] stated that foreign particulate material introduced into the lungs increased the rate of production of phagocytes. "The rate of the proliferative reaction depends entirely on the need for phagocytes as determined by the quantity of foreign particulate material to be removed from the air spaces. The contrast between the number of these cells appearing in the normal lung and that found after the introduction of foreign particulate matter is marked."

Carleton [23] gave intratracheal instillations of olive oil to dogs and rabbits and noted a swelling and release of alveolar cells. Drinker and Hatch [28] stated that, "Within the alveoli are phagocytes, which are brought out in vast hordes by the stimulus of foreign bodies, such as dust particles, which they engulf." More recently, LaBelle and Brieger [57,58] showed that inhalation of dust can increase the number of free cells. Yevich [104] reported an increase in the number of rat alveolar spaces which contained macrophages after exposure to aerosols of oil or diatomaceous earth. Ferin and coworkers [30-32] presented indirect evidence that trypan blue and titanium dioxide can influence the numbers of macrophages in the lungs. Bingham et al. [7] reported that exposure to lead sesquioxide resulted in decreased numbers of alveolar macrophages. Gross et al. [43] reported significant increases in pulmonary macrophages following massive intratracheal instillations of silicon dioxide and antimony trioxide.

Brain exposed hamsters and rats [13,14] and cats [12] to a wide variety of particulates, including carbon, coal dust, barium sulfate, triphenyl phosphate, chrysotile, iron oxide, and cigarette smoke. Particles were administered by inhalation or by intratracheal instillation. For each particle type, at least two parameters can be varied independently and thus the following questions can be answered: first, how does the response vary as a function of the magnitude

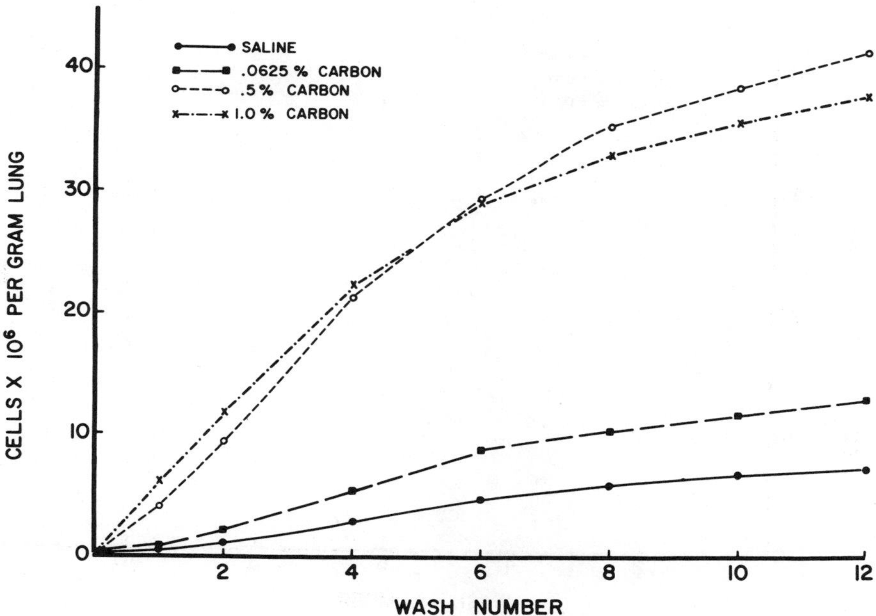

FIGURE 4 Number of free cells harvested from hamster lungs by repeated lung washings. All animals received intratracheally 0.15 cm^3 of a suspension of carbon particles per 100 g body weight. The concentration of carbon was 0.0%, 0.0625%, 0.5%, and 1.0%. All animals were sacrificed 1 day after the injection. All points are based on six or more animals.

of the exposure; second, how does the response vary as a function of the time elapsed since the exposure? To explore these dose-response and time-response relationships, Brain [14] instilled suspensions of carbon particles in saline intratracheally in over 70 hamsters. Figure 4 shows the results obtained from hamsters instilled intratracheally with a suspension of carbon particles 1-3 μm in size ultrasonically dispersed in physiological saline. All animals were killed 1 day following the intratracheal instillation. The total cell yields from the animals injected with carbon (0.0625%) are significantly greater ($P < 0.05$) than those from the controls injected with saline. All points on the curves for the 0.5% and 1.0% suspensions are significantly greater than the control points ($P < 0.005$).

The time-response relationships for carbon are displayed in Fig. 5 for hamsters receiving the 0.5% carbon suspensions. Animals were sacrificed at 4 hr, 1 day, and 3 days following intratracheal instillation. Control hamsters (not shown in Fig. 5) were injected with 0.15 ml saline/100 g body weight and were sacrificed at the same three times. The total cumulative yield at the end of the 12 washes was 10.54 ± 1.51 (SE) $\times 10^6$ cells/g lung for the 4-hr controls; 9.35 ±

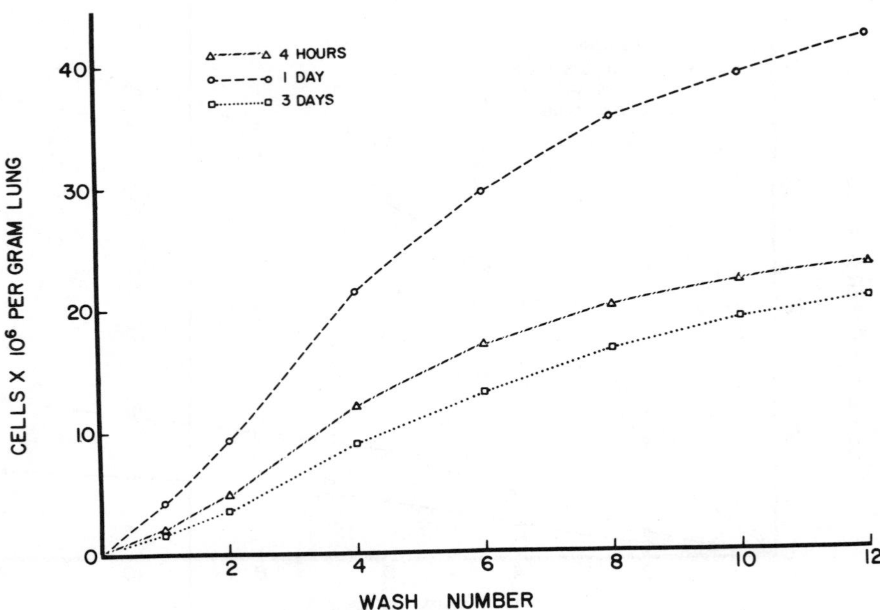

FIGURE 5 Number of free cells harvested from hamster lungs by repeated lung washings. All animals received intratracheally 0.15 cm^3 af an 0.5% suspension of carbon particles per 100 g body weight. The times shown represent the interval between the injection and the time of sacrifice. Control hamsters were injected with 0.15 cm^3 saline/100 g body weight. All of the saline control groups (not shown) for the three times had total yields of less than 10.6 $\times 10^6$ cells/g lung. All points are based on six or more animals.

0.84 (SE) $\times 10^6$ cells/g lung for the 1-day controls; and 8.54 ± 131 (SE) $\times 10^6$ cells/g lung for 3-day controls. Figure 5 shows how the yield of macrophages changes as a function of time after injection. The response is maximal 1 day after the injection, but it is also elevated above control levels at 4 hr and at 3 days.

Although considerable variation in both the dose-response and time-response relations for various particles exists, generalizations regarding the role of particles in recruiting macrophages can be made. In the absence of an acute inflammatory response (characterized by large numbers of red and white blood cells in the lavage fluid), a maximal response is usually seen at four to seven times the resting levels of alveolar macrophages. As shown in Fig. 4, further increases in dose yield no increases in response (compare 0.5 with 1.0% carbon). Typically, the greatest yield is obtained approximately 1 day following an acute exposure to particles. We have also observed that smaller particles tend to be more effective stimuli than larger particles. Thus the numbers of macrophages released may be related more to particle numbers or to particle surface area than to particle mass. In experiments with coal dust suspensions instilled into hamsters, identical masses of particles smaller than 0.053 mm produced twice the response of particles larger than 0.25 mm [14].

E. Problems in Interpretation of Pool Size

When attempting to interpret these changes in the numbers of free cells present in the lungs, one must be aware of the assumptions implicit in the lung washing technique and hence realize the limitations of the method. The efficiency of the harvesting technique is assumed to be constant. The fraction of all free cells present that are recovered is usually assumed to be the same in controls and in experimental exposure groups, but the possibility always exists that the experimental treatment has influenced the efficiency of recovery. If the experimental procedure provokes an inflammatory response or atelectasis, altered cell harvest efficiency may occur. Gross et al. [43] point out that severe pneumoconstriction, atelectasis, or fibrosis induced by large doses of particles are likely to affect the efficiency of the washing procedure.

One should also remember that the pool size of free cells, like any other biological pool, is dynamically determined. The equilibrium number of cells present at a point in time is a function of the input and output history of the pool. For example, if the pool size decreases, it may be due to decreased production, or recruitment of free cells, or accelerated clearance of free cells from the lungs. If input and output of free cells both increase, the pool size will remain constant in spite of increased release of alveolar macrophages onto the lung surface. Accelerated or depressed lysis of macrophages also influences the equilibrium number of free cells.

It is necessary to characterize the morphological, functional, and histochemical properties of the population of free cells recovered from control and exposure groups. The composition of the altered pool depends on the stimulus used. Although lung washings from animals exposed to some particulates (ferric oxide and carbon) contain mostly mononuclear alveolar phagocytes, highly irritating or infectious particles provoke an inflammatory reaction. This is usually characterized by a local exudation of blood cells, mostly polymorphonuclear leukocytes, as well as considerable numbers of red blood cells and plasma or edema fluid.

Long ago Lemon [61] pointed out that the lungs respond to different types of foreign particles in different ways. When he injected tubercle bacilli into the lungs, he found that the alveoli rapidly filled with polymorphonuclear leukocytes. When silica was injected there were essentially no polymorphonuclear leukocytes; the silica was ingested almost entirely by the mononuclear alveolar phagocytes. Using lung lavage in humans, Pratt et al. [79] demonstrated that free cells recovered from smokers had a higher percentage of macrophages than free cells recovered from nonsmokers. Thus, each experimental exposure produces its own profile of cell types in the lung washing.

What is the functional significance of increased numbers of free cells? Greater numbers of macrophages increase the probability that particles will be phagocytized and thus removed from direct contact with the alveolar surface. Schiller [83] maintained that only free particles penetrate the walls of the alveoli. Schiller, and later Sorokin and Brain [87], found little evidence that phagocytes laden with dust can reenter the alveolar wall. Thus, phagocytosis plays an important role in preventing the entry of particles into the fixed tissue of the lung. Once particles leave the alveolar surface and penetrate the fixed tissues subjacent to the air-liquid interface, their removal is slowed. Pathological processes, such as fibrosis, may further slow the clearance of particles from this compartment. Morrow et al. [70] emphasized the importance of the in vivo solubility of particles. In any case, the probability of a particle entering a fixed tissue where it would have a long biological half-life is reduced if the particle is phagocytized by a free cell.

Some experiments support these ideas. LaBelle and Brieger [56,57] demonstrated a high positive correlation between the amount of dust cleared from the lungs and the number of phagocytic cells counted. The fraction of the original lung burden excreted during the first day was related to the number of alveolar macrophages available to act as carriers. Ferin [31] reported that increased numbers of macrophages correlate with an increased fraction cleared rapidly via the airways. Since increased numbers of macrophages lead to increased particle removal, these experiments suggest that macrophages prevent the penetration of particles into lymph nodes and interstitial spaces.

IV. Origin and Maturation

Determining the origin of pulmonary macrophages is complex and consequently cannot be resolved in any simplistic way; it has withstood experimental probing over many years. It is not simply a question of whether macrophages originate from cells in the circulating blood or from cells living in the lungs, for even this formulation at once becomes more complex: one immediately asks, which cells in the bloodstream and which in the lungs? Is there any connection between these cells? It remains uncertain whether all macrophages in the lungs belong to the same cellular pool, or whether some have independent origins and means of maintaining their populations. Although the studies to be summarized here emphasize macrophages lavageable from the lungs, remember that macrophages not only reside on alveolar and airway surfaces, but are also found in connective tissue throughout the lung. It is reasonable to wonder if these diverse macrophage populations differ in their reproductive patterns and preferred locations for cell turnover. Possibly one type is more restricted to the lungs than is another. The question of macrophage "origin" then becomes a matter of determining how much of the functional phagocyte pool in each compartment originates from immediate precursors in the lung and how much from elsewhere, such as from monocytes in the blood.

A. History

In 1927, Foot [33] reviewed the origin of the pulmonary macrophages. He cited more than 30 papers specifically dealing with this subject and reviewed evidence which supported the capillary endothelium, the alveolar lining, the blood monocytes, and histiocytes from the alveolar wall as possible sources. He naturally concluded that the subject was unsettled and proceeded to report his own experimental work. Based on light-microscopic observations, he postulated the origin to be circulating monocytes, "with tissue histiocytes playing some part in their production." Interestingly, the next paper in the same journal was also a report on the origin of pulmonary macrophages. In this study, Gardner and Smith [35], using supravital staining and light microscopy, concluded that extravascular monocytes give rise to "septal cells" (histiocytes), which in turn migrate to the alveoli. If these studies are subjected to current interpretation, Foot suggested a dual origin of pulmonary macrophages: blood monocytes and an independent, self-replicating population of cells in the lung. Gardner and Smith suggested a single origin, the blood monocyte, which migrates through the lung interstitium to the alveolar surface and gains characteristics specific for alveolar macrophages during this passage. The difference between these possibilities continues to be a source of controversy.

There is a long history of claims and counterclaims concerning intrapulmonary sources of macrophages in the lungs. In the first place, there is the pulmonary epithelium, particularly the alveolar epithelium to consider, for the most persistent epithelial pretender has been the great alveolar cell (granular pneumonocyte, type II cell). It is fair to state, as will be seen below, that recent evidence does not support the notion that these cells transform into phagocytes; moreover, as mentioned in the previous chapter, these cells engage in no phagocytosis and precious little microendocytosis while they are attached to the epithelium. Nevertheless, this idea has had strong support by microscopists and tissue culturists of past generations, as a review of this literature shows [6]. Much of this literature is nearly impossible to evaluate today, due to uncertainty about which cells in the pulmonary alveoli were studied. A clean-cut identification of all the cells present in alveoli is rarely possible when using live or conventionally fixed paraffin sections as materials for study. The continuity or discontinuity and the embryological origin of the alveolar epithelium were also issues of concern in the older literature; opinions on these matters colored the interpretation of some observations. It is now accepted that this epithelium is continuous and of endodermal origin; this was shown by early electron microscopists [46,64] and other observers who reinvestigated its development during pulmonary organogenesis [85]. Until the advent of electron microscopy in the early 1950s, however, many supported the idea that the alveolar epithelium was of mesodermal origin. To some this gave the epithelium a better likelihood of harboring potential macrophages among its constituents, because macrophages generally have a mesodermal affiliation. Assignment of this epithelium to the endoderm does not rule out the possibility that macrophages could arise from it, for, as mentioned in the previous chapter, macrophages sometimes have an endodermal origin as well. Nevertheless, if the possibility that great alveolar cells or other epithelial cells can become macrophages has not been conclusively refuted, little in the recent literature supports it.

The experimental design used in studying pulmonary macrophage origin has been critically important. Gardner and Smith [35] began their paper with the statement, "So much has been written on the origin of the alveolar phagocyte that it would be useless to offer further discussion of the problem, unless approached from an entirely new angle." The work of Ungar and Wilson [91] is of historical interest since they pointed out that for one to confirm the presence of an extrapulmonary source of macrophages, these cells would have to be marked so that their progress from the source of supply to the pulmonary surface could be followed. To do this, they labeled exudative peritoneal macrophages of the guinea pig with carbon, harvested these cells, eliminated unphagocytized particulates, and then injected the cells intravascularly into other guinea pigs. By histologic observation, these cells were found in capillaries, in the pulmonary interstitium, and on the alveolar surface. They concluded that pulmonary macrophages are derived largely from monocytes of the circulating blood. Although their work emphasized the need for specifically marked, identifiable cells, their model was not entirely adequate. Peritoneal macrophages may die, disintegrate, and release their particles to be ingested by other cells. The ideal marker should be an integral constituent of progenitor cells which is easily identified, and not even theoretically transferrable to other cells.

B. Current Evidence: Chromosomal and Antigenic Markers

Pinkett et al. [77] made a notable advance by using a marker chromosome to specifically identify cells. CBA mice were irradiated (900 R) and given injections of bone marrow cells from histocompatible homozygous T_6 strain mice. These cells are easily differentiated from those of the host by chromosome analysis of cells in metaphase, since T_6 cells carry a recognizable chromosome marker. Six hours before sacrifice, the mice were injected with colchicine to produce metaphase arrest. In 15 of 19 chimeras, the T_6 markers were present in all of the observed spleen and bone marrow mitoses. Of cells lavaged from the lung, only 152 were found to be undergoing cell division in 19 animals. The percentage of those dividing cells with T_6 marker mitoses ranged from 64 to 78%. The authors concluded that two-thirds of alveolar macrophages are of hematopoietic origin and one-third of pulmonary origin, "derived presumably from the alveolar epithelial lining or from mesenchymal wall cells." But their conclusion must be accepted with some reservations. It should be noted that this technique assigns an origin only to lavageable cells which have entered metaphase during the last 6 hours of the procedure, not to all free cells present in the lung washing. Only a very small, highly selected population was examined (a mean of eight cells per mouse); it is also difficult to identify the cells selected as macrophages since they were examined in a metaphase spread. Furthermore, since only 6 hours elapsed between the colchicine injections and the lung washings, it is possible that other precursors of macrophages within the interstitium of pulmonary tissue were arrested in metaphase but were never released onto the alveolar surface during this period.

Another complication is introduced by the use of radiation. It is likely that whole-body exposure of this magnitude (900 R) would eliminate bone marrow cells, circulating monocytes and pulmonary interstitial cells capable of division. Thus, the ability of pulmonary tissues to serve as a source of alveolar macrophages may become compromised. Furthermore, the injection of replacement bone marrow introduces plenipotentiary cells which may not only "home" to the bone marrow but may also enter other tissues to replace lethally irradiated macrophage populations that normally reside and reproduce there. Thus, one still does not learn from studies of this kind whether the recovered tagged cells had originated directly from injected bone marrow cells or from monocytes that arose from them, or even from cells that had gone through an intermediary residence period in some pulmonary tissue compartment. Furthermore, pulmonary epithelial cells also appear to be more radioresistant than mesodermal derivatives of embryonic mouse lungs [1]. A dose of 1100 rads to cultures of fetal rat lungs does not affect the ability of its epithelium to form centrioles or undergo ciliogenesis, even though it completely depresses mitotic activity in all pulmonary cells for several days postirradiation [86]. If alveolar macrophage precursors existed in such lungs, they probably would not divide after exposure to 1100 rads.

Virolainen [97] also used the T_6 chromosome system in radiation chimeras to study the origin of macrophages. However, to assure that all cells studied were macrophages, he cultured cells in vitro (with macrophage growth factor) and then determined the presence of T_6 marker. In lethally irradiated animals, all explanted dividing macrophages from the peritoneum, lung, spleen, bone marrow, and thymus contained the T_6 chromosomes. In sublethally irradiated animals, a portion of the cells contained the marker; this proportion was the same in the lung as in other tissues. On the basis of these results, he concluded that all macrophages are ultimately of hematopoietic origin. This study used the selective pressures of growth in culture to eliminate extraneous cells, but in so doing produced a highly selected population of cells. The use of both lethal and sublethal irradiation in these experiments lessens to some extent the previous objections to studies using lethal irradiation.

Two major objections to the T_6 chimera model are that cell populations are selected by the need for cell division and that there are no morphological means to evaluate the cells studied. These objections were overcome by Godleski and Brain [38] who used a naturally occurring immunologic marker. This same approach was used earlier by Balner [3] and Goodman [41] to determine the origin of peritoneal macrophages. Mouse radiation chimeras were prepared in which the marker to identify the cellular origin of individual cells was a single known antigenic difference between donor bone marrow cells and recipient somatic cells. By using cytotoxic monospecific antibody to identify donor cells, it was possible to study large numbers of free cells obtained by lung washing and at the same time observe the cellular morphology to be certain that only mononuclear macrophages were studied. In addition, white blood cell count, pulmonary macrophage number, macrophage morphology, and lung morphology were monitored in the animals studied.

Mouse irradiation chimeras were sacrificed for analysis at 7, 14, 21, 28, and 35 to 50 days after lethal irradiation and bone marrow replacement. The relationships between time and percent of lung cells and percent of bone marrow cells of donor origin are shown in Fig. 6. The average kill by the cytotoxic test of marrow cells from donor control animals was 86% and of lung macrophages, 84%. The mean kill of marrow cells from recipient controls was 10% and of lung macrophages, 14%. At 7 days after irradiation, 60% of the marrow was replaced by donor cells, while 36% of the lung macrophages were of donor origin. At 14 days, marrow replacement had increased to 72% and lung macrophages of donor origin had increased to 57%. At 21, 28, and 35 to 50 days, the percent kill of marrow cells and of lung macrophages did not differ significantly. Also, percent kill at these periods was not significantly different from the percent kill in the donor control animals, indicating essentially complete replacement of recipient hematopoietic tissue by donor bone marrow. Chimeras were studied up to 10 months after irradiation and bone marrow injection; in all cases the difference between the percent kill of lung cells and marrow cells was not

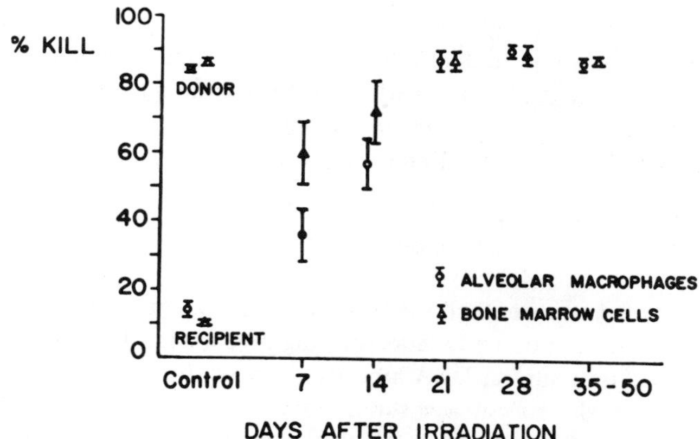

FIGURE 6 Percent kill in alveolar macrophages and bone marrow cells, as a function of time after irradiation and transplantation. The mean of eight animals studied ± SE are displayed. In each animal a minimum of 200 cells were counted at several antibody dilutions. (Reprinted from Godleski and Brain [Ref. 38; p. 633] by courtesy of the publisher *Journal of Experimental Medicine.*)

significant. In all animals studied, it was found that by 28 days after irradiation and injection of bone marrow, white blood cell count, pulmonary macrophage number and morphology, and lung morphology examined by light microscopy in all animals studied were the same as that of the nonirradiated control animals. It was therefore concluded that the ultimate origin of pulmonary macrophages in radiation chimeras is the hematopoietic system.

Although the studies of Godleski and Brain [38] circumvented some of the difficulties associated with previous chimeric studies, the progressive steps from bone marrow to alveolar surface were not delineated. Also, a study of the lungs of chimeras by electron microscopy would have helped to determine the extent of damage to pulmonary cells caused by the irradiation.

Brunstetter et al. [22] used another variation of the radiation chimera approach, an esterase marker. Their studies also support a primary ultimate hematopoietic origin. But, the problems associated with radiation were also present in their studies and qualitative electrophoretic analysis of esterase required pooling of cells recovered by lavage. The esterase content and hence the origin of individual cells was not determined.

The chimera studies reviewed here present strong evidence for the ultimate hematopoietic nature of lavageable macrophages. The strategy of these studies has been to show that injection of bone marrow cells with an identifiable marker gives rise to macrophages with that same marker. These studies have not yet been extended to show the progressive steps from bone marrow to alveolar surface. Nor were they designed to determine whether the lung is seeded continuously by bone marrow-derived cells, or whether it is seeded once after irradiation by the injected bone marrow cells with subsequent division of that local population. Labeling with nuclear material may answer some of these kinetic questions.

C. Current Evidence: DNA Labeling Techniques

Many investigators have approached the study of macrophage origin and turnover by using tritiated thymidine to label dividing precursors. Tritiated thymidine is incorporated into nuclear DNA by cells preparing for division and remains in these cells and in their progeny as a stable label. Labeled cells can be identified using autoradiographic techniques which also permit morphologic evaluation to be carried out on the same material. Volkman and Gowans [98] used this technique to show that monocytic precursors in bone marrow of rats give rise to monocytes which accumulate and form macrophages in the skin. Van Furth and Cohn [93] employed similar methods to identify promonocytes in the bone marrow of mice and to follow these cells as peripheral blood monocytes. It was found that a sterile inflammation in the peritoneal cavity results in rapid entry of labeled monocytes from the blood to this area. van Furth [92] found that 6% of the pulmonary macrophages were labeled at a time when 85% of the circulating monocytes were labeled. Both of these percentages then decreased with time. These data do not verify that monocytes go directly from the bloodstream to the alveolar surface. If that were the case, then the number of labeled alveolar macrophages should increase as the labeled monocyte population decreased; this was not seen.

Van Furth [92] also labeled mononuclear phagocytes in vitro (Table 1) by incubating them with tritiated thymidine for 24 hr; 50% of the promonocytes synthesized DNA but, in this study, no monocytes had this capability. Of the alveolar macrophages obtained by lavage, only 2.3% synthesized DNA in vitro. He concluded that pulmonary macrophages are usually nonproliferating cells under normal conditions, and probably are derived from peripheral blood monocytes. Although his data are consistent with this hypothesis, proof is lacking. Alternatively, it may simply indicate the promonocytes divide more rapidly than alveolar macrophages. The experimental design also fails to measure the possible incorporation of thymidine in local pulmonary self-replicating cell populations. Although Van Furth's in vitro studies showed 2.3% tritiated thymidine incorporation by lavageable macrophages, macrophages unobtainable by lavage (in the interstitium or alveolar wall) were not studied. In addition, studies [26] showing biochemical differences between blood monocytes and alveolar macrophages do not support rapid, direct emigration of monocytes to the alveolar surface under normal circumstances.

TABLE 1 In Vitro Labeling of Mononuclear Phagocytes[a]

Origin	Labeled cells (%)
Promonocytes	50.3
Peripheral blood monocytes	0
Peritoneal macrophages	2.2
Alveolar macrophages	2.3

[a]In medium with 0.1 μCi/ml [^{3}H] thymidine for 24 hr.
(Adapted from van Furth [92], by courtesy of the author and publisher.)

Bowden et al. [10] focused on the immediate precursors of pulmonary macrophages in the lung interstitium rather than on their ultimate origin. They administered 650 rads of whole-body radiation to mice. Chlortetracycline was given to inhibit infection. Over a 28 day postirradiation period, the DNA concentration in the lung and liver did not change. In the bone marrow, DNA content dropped precipitously by the second day, and returned to control levels by the fifth day. Lymphocytes, polymorphonuclear leukocytes, and monocytes fell to their lowest numbers in the peripheral blood on the second and third day, and then slowly returned to normal levels. The pool size of alveolar macrophages estimated by lavage did not decrease at any time, but on the twenty-first day showed a threefold increase. To determine the source of this increase, tritiated thymidine was injected 2 hr before sacrifice. Sections of lung were studied with light microscopy and results confirmed by electron microscopy. Figure 7 shows the radiographic index, a measure of cell proliferation within the lungs, and macrophage counts plotted on the same time scale. Following irradiation, DNA synthesis remained low for a few days and then rose to its highest point at 10 days. This peak immediately preceded the rise in the number of free macrophages recovered from the lungs. The following hypothesis was proposed: Pulmonary macrophages have their ultimate origin in bone marrow stem cells. Precursors are transported in the blood as monocytes which enter the lung interstitium where they are capable of division and also undergo maturation involving the development of enzymatic and other biochemical features peculiar to the pulmonary macrophage. Following this period, the mature cells then migrate to the alveolar surface.

The studies of Bowden and Adamson [9] further supported this hypothesis. Mouse lungs were excised and then perfused with medium to remove circulating blood cells. Finally, pieces of lung were cultured in vitro with tritiated thymidine. Their results are outlined in Table 2. It can be seen that there is initial interstitial cell DNA synthesis followed by labeling of free macrophages. Identification of cell types was made using both light and electron microscopy. Another recently published study of cultured explants of murine lungs also lends support to these hypotheses [9a]. Consistent with Bowden's proposed scheme is the

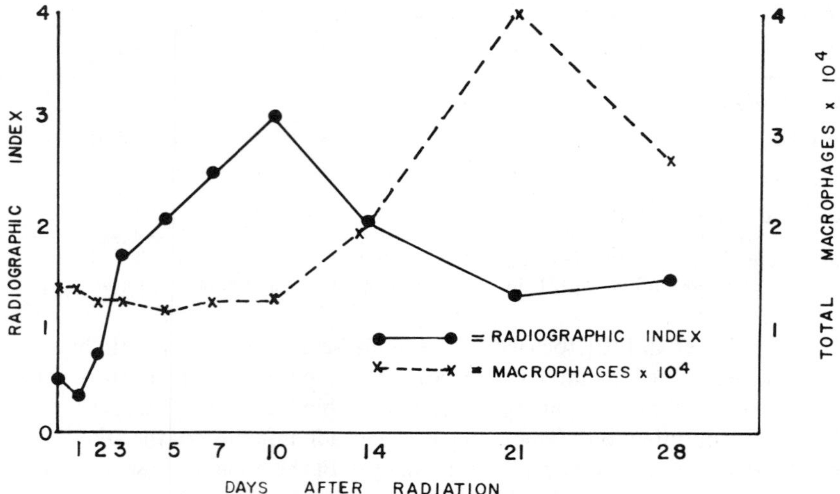

FIGURE 7 Radiographic indices of alveolar cells in lung sections (circles) and output of lung macrophages following 650 rad whole body radiation. Macrophages in washings $\times 10^4$ are indicated by X's. (Reprinted from Bowden et al. [Ref. 10, p. 543], by courtesy of the author and publisher.)

TABLE 2 Differential Counts of Labeled Cells in the Interval Label Study[a]

Time after 2 days of thymidine labeling (Days)	Labeled cells (%)			
	Interstitial	Free macrophages	Epithelial	Not identified
0	73	2	16	9
1	11	70	11	8
2	12	63	12	13

[a]Explants cultured for 2 days in media containing [^{3}H] thymidine, then transferred to unlabeled media.

(Adapted from Bowden and Adamson [9], by courtesy of the authors and publisher.)

work of Vijeyaratnam and Corrin [95] who treated rats with iprindole, an antidepressant drug which causes increased numbers of alveolar macrophages. Using light and electron microscopy, they found that interstitial cells increased and that they divided more rapidly. The pulmonary macrophages resulting from the iprindole stimulus possessed the usual enzymatic, ultrastructural, and phagocytic characteristics [96]. The maturation process of macrophages in the interstitium appears to involve increased protein synthesis and a gradual movement of the manufactured enzymes throughout the cell. Schneeberger (personal communication), for example, studied the distribution of peroxidase activity in guinea pig lung, focusing on its localization within alveolar wall cells that appear to be alveolar macrophage precursors and on the free alveolar macrophages themselves. As shown in Fig. 8, the interstitial macrophage is apparently immature with peroxidase activity limited to the perinuclear cisterna. A more mature macrophage (Fig. 9) found on the alveolar epithelium exhibits more widespread peroxide activity. The reaction product can now be seen in the endoplasmic reticulum extending throughout the cytoplasm.

Relevant to Bowden's concepts is the study by Golde et al. [40]. It is significant on two points: first, it approaches the study of pulmonary macrophage origin in man, and second, it further supports the concept of a replicating local pulmonary population of macrophages. Three patients with acute leukemia were studied. Although no monocytes were detectable in the peripheral blood of two of these patients, the number of pulmonary macrophages in all were similar to control subjects. Furthermore, these cells exhibited normal morphologic and functional characteristics. This work supports the concept of a pulmonary secondary cell renewal system, perhaps ultimately derived from bone marrow and monocytes, but potentially independent of it. Also of interest is a recent study by Volkman [97a]. He used parabiotic pairs of rats and concluded that resident macrophage populations in the unstimulated peritoneum and liver appear to be self-sustaining and do not necessarily have blood monocytes as their immediate precursors.

D. Origin During Stress

The studies reviewed up to this point dealt with the origin of pulmonary macrophages when the distal lung was not challenged by pulmonary infection or inhaled aerosols. As detailed earlier in this chapter, inhalation of some particulates brings about an increase in the number of macrophages on the alveolar surface. Pulmonary infection or inflammation also may be accompanied by increased surface and interstitial macrophages. The macrophage population may be composed of cells from different origins under various clinical circumstances.

Godleski and Brain [38] exposed mouse irradiation chimeras to an iron oxide aerosol and used immunologic techniques to study macrophage origins following the resulting increase in cell numbers. These animals demonstrated almost a twofold increase in macrophage numbers, yet the percent of cells containing the hematopoietic marker continued to be the same in both lung and bone marrow. This suggests that the increased cells ultimately derive from the hematopoietic system.

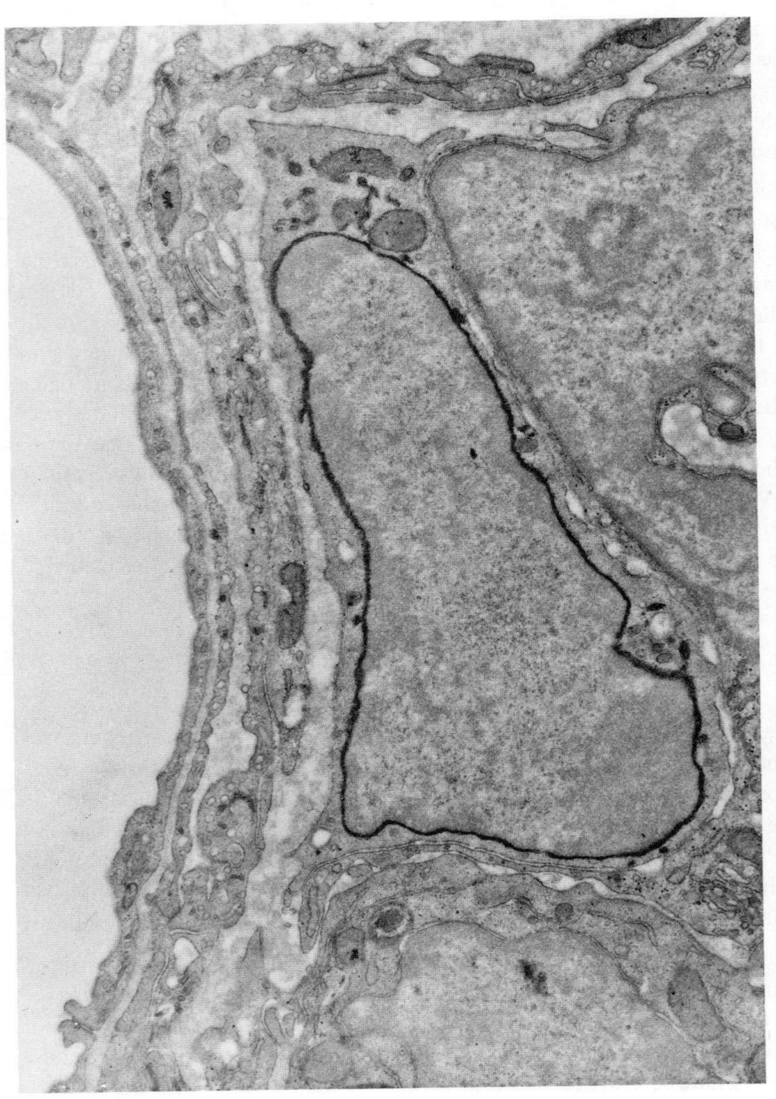

FIGURE 8 An interstitial cell in the guinea pig alveolar wall. The diaminobenzidine reaction has been used to reveal the distribution of peroxidase activity. This cell, with sparse cytoplasm and thought to be a precursor of the alveolar macrophages, exhibits peroxidase activity confined to the perinuclear cisterna. X12,000. (Courtesy of Dr. Eveline Schneeberger.)

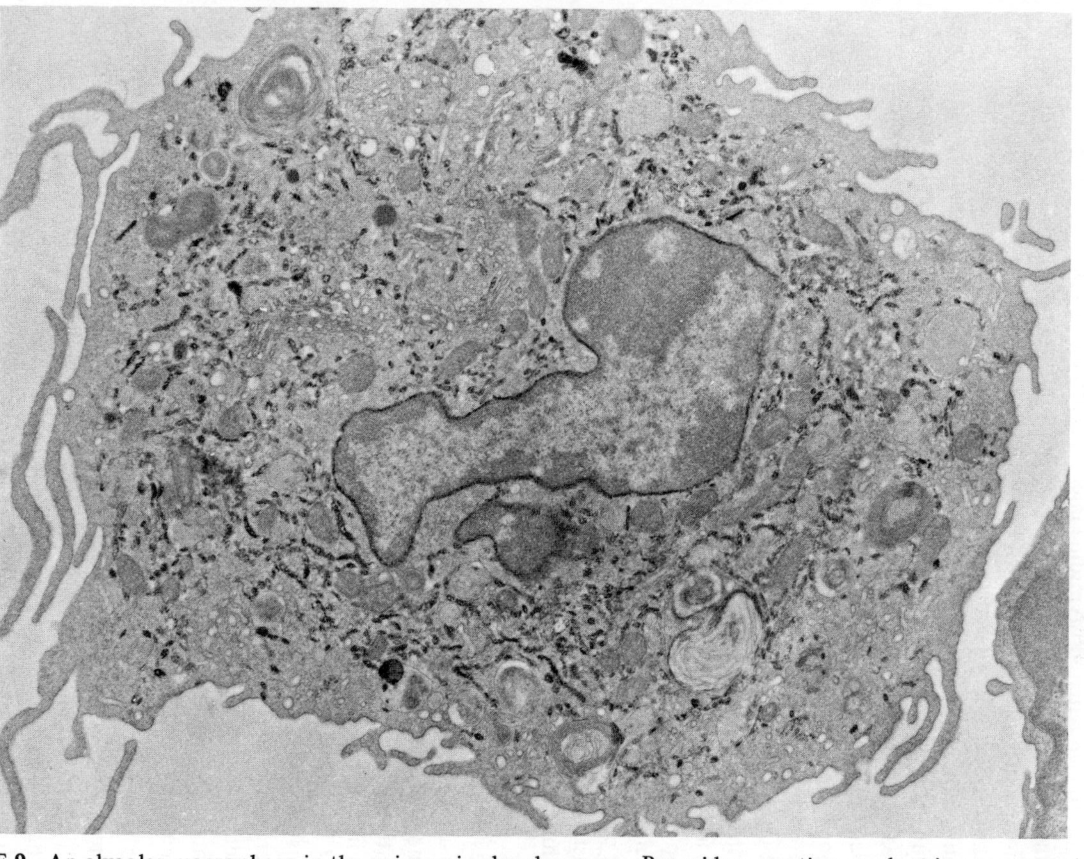

FIGURE 9 An alveolar macrophage in the guinea pig alveolar space. Peroxidase reaction product is now extensively distributed throughout the cisternae of the rough endoplasmic reticulum in a more abundant cytoplasm. The peroxidase reaches the periphery of the Golgi apparatus (center, above nucleus), but lysosomal bodies are unreactive. X12,000. (Courtesy of Dr. Eveline Schneeberger.)

Velo and Spector [94] studied the origin of pulmonary macrophages in mice and rats with experimental pneumonia produced by intratracheal instillation of bacillus Calmette-Guérin vaccine (BCG), Freund's adjuvant, or carrageenan. In vivo tritiated thymidine injections produced a parallel increase in labeling of blood monocytes, pulmonary macrophages in lung sections, and pulmonary macrophages obtained by lavage. Interestingly, only with carrageenan did the number of labeled macrophages in lung sections increase as the number of labeled monocytes decreased. This suggests that monocytes immigrating into the lung may account for the increase. Another explanation is that carrageenan decreases the emigration rate of labeled macrophages from the lung. However, labeled pulmonary macrophages obtained by lavage paralleled the labeled blood monocytes in all studies. By using thoracic irradiation and shielding of the bone marrow of the lower extremities, a delayed but normal response to the irritants used was seen in the lung. However, in these animals blood monocytes were not studied. In studies of pulmonary macrophages labeled with tritiated thymidine as well as carrageenan, the generation time for mature macrophages to develop from precursors was 2-3 days. A direct monocyte to alveolar surface route was not demonstrated. Velo and Spector [94] suggested that these data show that precursors of pulmonary macrophages originate in the bone marrow, are transferred to the lung via the blood, and undergo mitosis and maturation within the lung before entering the lavageable macrophage pool.

Using electron microscopy, Moore and Schoenberg [69] observed monocytes emigrating through capillary walls into the lung interstitium as early as 15 min after the intravenous injection of complete Freund's adjuvant in the rabbit. Mononuclear cell migration between alveolar epithelial cells was also noted. In addition, mitotic figures were seen in mononuclear cells in the interstitium. It was impossible to determine whether these mitoses were in monocytes or resident interstitial cells present before the injection. Kilburn [52,53] exposed hamsters and guinea pigs to cotton trash; these animals showed an increase in macrophages and other free cells in alveoli and distal airways. Neutrophils were observed sieving through the epithelium of the distal bronchioles in exposed animals. No evidence was presented showing that macrophages may have a similar entrance pathway.

Monocyte migration from capillaries to the alveolar surface has been reported in recent studies in a mouse model system [18,71], and in human lungs with interstitial pneumonitis [19]. This mouse model was devised to study the pathogenesis of pulmonary cytomegalovirus infections. During innoculation with antilymphocyte serum, the mice were injected subcutaneously with cytomegalovirus. In this immunosuppressed state, viral particles were found in monocytes from the 12th through the 37th day postinnoculation. An increase in both infected and uninfected monocytes was seen in the pulmonary vasculature, with infected cells visible in the lung interstitium and on the alveolar surface. The authors state, however, that although it is assumed that these monocytes migrated from the vessels to the alveoli, transitional stages indicative of cells crossing anatomic barriers were rarely observed. Further studies of this material [71] revealed passage of infected monocytes from the interstitium through the basement membranes of the bronchioles and alveoli. The development of zonulae adhaerentes was noted between monocytes and epithelial cells followed by separation of epithelial cells and emigration of the monocyte into the air spaces. A similar pattern of migration of mononuclear cells was observed in biopsy material of diseased human interstitial lung tissue. These studies would present strong evidence that macrophage precursors are dependent on monocytes if one could be certain that viral particles were only transferred from the subcutaneous infection site to the lung intracellularly and that the viral particles were integral, nontransferable markers.

Cell division of pulmonary macrophages has also been studied in the rat after exposure to 15-17 ppm NO_2 for 48 hr [29]. Dividing pulmonary macrophages were localized in alveoli near the openings of terminal bronchioles. The percent of labeled macrophages 1 hr after tritiated thymidine injection was 0.23% in controls and 10.3% in exposed animals. Duration of the cell cycle was calculated to be 9.2 hr in exposed animals. A study of dust-exposed rats by Casarett and Milley [25] showed a doubling of mitotic figures in the alveolar walls as compared to that of control animals. The relative contribution of increased cell division to pulmonary macrophage pool size has not been determined. However, the macrophage pool size can double in 4 hr in a stimulated animal. It is unlikely that this increase results solely from cell division if the time for completion of a cell cycle is 9.2 hr. It may also reflect release of cells from a preexisting reservoir.

E. Macrophage Transformation

The progression of pulmonary macrophages to other distinctive morphologic forms has been the subject of much speculation. In certain pathologic and experimental situations these cells have been reported to transform into epithelioid cells, multinuclear giant cells and fibroblasts [8]. Shima et al. [84] studied granulomatous lesions produced in rabbits with BCG. Macrophages developing into epithelioid cells were capable of division, but mature epithelioid cells were not. Also, macrophages incorporating bacilli did not divide within the lesion. The epithelioid cell has been studied in detail by Papidimitriou and Spector [75], but these studies utilized subcutaneous sites and peritoneal macrophages rather than pulmonary cells. Studies showing transformation of macrophages into giant cells [24,80] also employed peritoneal cells or subcutaneous sites. It is likely that pulmonary macrophages are also capable of this transformation. The development of fibroblasts from macrophages has been reported in the peritoneal cavity [55]. These transformations remain controversial at this time.

F. Origin and Maturation: Conclusions and Caveats

Few of the studies reviewed deal with normal animals or man. Models using irradiation, drugs, or patients with leukemia all lead to admittedly tentative conclusions. However, in toto the accumulated evidence in these model systems leads one to the following tentative conclusions:

1. In higher mammals, most macrophages are ultimately hematopoietically derived cells. Current evidence lends little support for epithelial, endothelial, or lymphatic origins.
2. The promonocyte of the bone marrow is a dividing cell which gives rise to circulating monocytes.
3. Monocytes leave the bloodstream at a rapid exponential rate. Half-time has been shown to be 3 days in the rat [104], 22 hr in the mouse [94], and 8.4 hr in man [67].
4. The monocyte can enter the pulmonary interstitium.
5. A population of mononuclear cells in the pulmonary interstitium is capable of mitosis, and these cells have been traced onto the alveolar surface. These interstitial cells are likely derived from monocytes but intrapulmonary origins cannot be completely excluded.
6. Some alveolar macrophages are capable of cell division.

These conclusions are not dogma and several qualifying statements should be added. For example, the discussion of the phylogeny of macrophages presented in the preceding chapter offers few reasons to believe that precursors of pulmonary macrophages must necessarily have a single locus. Rather, phylogeny reveals that the macrophage developed before the hematopoietic system. Furthermore, macrophages traditionally are associated with mesodermal tissues of which the vascular system is only a part. Finally, although there has been a tendency to "internalize" the blood cell-forming tissues within the vascular system, this tendency is expressed to different degrees in different vertebrate and even mammalian groups. What is proven true for one species does not necessarily apply to another.

In mammalian lungs, there can be no argument that monocytes leave the blood and enter the lungs. They can transform into macrophages and thus contribute to the pool of macrophages that police the alveoli. Yet it is not certain that monocytes are the only cells that contribute to the alveolar macrophage pool; there may be other contributors as well in the blood or in the lungs. Also uncertain is whether the relative contribution to the macrophage pool by the various precursors is always the same. Perhaps the monocytic contributions increase during emergencies such as lung infection just as the intrapulmonary populations of macrophages or eosinophils fluctuate with demand. As mentioned earlier, in some stimulated animals, specific locations where macrophages enter the alveoli or airways have been observed. Thus, during stimulation macrophage populations may be more dependent on an influx of circulating monocytes and less dependent on local intrapulmonary cell renewal systems.

We also need to determine if the monocytic contribution to pulmonary connective tissue macrophages is meted out according to the same rules that govern its donation to the alveolar. Current experimental work on the origins of pulmonary macrophages has sometimes stressed the importance of extrapulmonary hematopoietic origins of the lavageable macrophage populations. But, there remain questions regarding intrapulmonary residence requirements; presumably cells must first reside in mesodermally derived compartments of the lung, before the cells can emerge onto the alveolar surface as full-fledged alveolar macrophages. These compartments include the alveolar interstitium as well as other pulmonary connective tissues, the muscles, and the vessels. If the extravascular spaces are seeded early in development by bloodborne cells which then undergo repeated divisions, these cells would not be very different from the macrophage population derived from mesodermal cells which differentiated in the extravascular spaces in the first place. Therefore, the importance of the distinction between extrapulmonary and intrapulmonary "connective tissue" origin of the alveolar macrophages diminishes. If to these early pulmonary residents, new seedings from the bloodstream were added from time to time as needed, then there may be multiple origins of alveolar macrophages—some from intrapulmonary and some from extrapulmonary sources. Given our present understanding this is likely the situation.

It should also be noted that alveolar macrophages encompass cells of varying morphology and activity. We have little insight as to what subpopulations make up the range of cells functioning as alveolar macrophages. In appearance lavaged alveolar macrophages are strikingly less uniform than cells obtained by peritoneal lavage. This suggests greater variability in the functional readiness and metabolic activity of pulmonary macrophages, as compared with the peritoneal macrophage population. Presently unknown is whether the variability of alveolar macrophages may be correlated with different origins or perhaps different residence times in maturation compartments.

In 1969 a conference on mononuclear phagocytes was held in Leiden [59] and some of the conferees concluded that current knowledge of morphology,

TABLE 3 Mononuclear Phagocyte System[a]

Promonocyte (bone marrow)
↓
Monocyte (blood)
↓
Macrophage (tissues)
highly phagocytic

Connective tissue (histocyte)
Liver (Kupffer cell)
Lung (alveolar macrophage)
Spleen (free and fixed macrophage, sinusoidal lining cell)
Lymph node (free and fixed macrophage)
Bone marrow (macrophages, sinusoidal lining cell)
Serous cavity (peritoneal macrophage)
Bone tissue (osteoclast)
Nervous system (microglia?)

[a](Adapted from Langevoort et al. [59], by courtesy of the authors and publisher.)

function, and kinetics made it possible to place all highly phagocytic mononuclear cells and their precursors in one system called the mononuclear phagocyte system (Table 3). The most specific morphologic characteristic of these cells by this system is a ruffling of the plasma membrane. Functionally, all these cells avidly phagocytose material and firmly attach to a glass surface. The generalizations implicit in this table are useful and have been widely embraced. They emphasize the essential unity of mononuclear cells widely scattered throughout the body. At the same time they are an oversimplification, ignoring some of the possibilities and subtleties discussed here. To that extent, some of the generalizations may be premature and should not become dogma supressing research in an important area.

Placing all macrophages in a single system also tends to encourage extrapolation of data from one macrophage cell to others. This is often useful, but sometimes inaccurate. Despite obvious similarities between macrophages, there are notable differences. Oren et al. [74] showed that pulmonary macrophages depend primarily upon oxidative phosphorylation to provide energy for phagocytosis, while stimulated peritoneal macrophages depend only on glycolysis. Dannenberg et al. [26] showed higher levels of cytochrome oxidase, aminopeptidase, acid phosphatase, esterase, and succinic dehydrogenase in pulmonary macrophages than in peritoneal macrophages. Different responses to migration inhibitory factor (MIF) are seen in guinea pig peritoneal and alveolar macrophages

[63]. Alveolar macrophages from this species lack the surface receptors which enable peritoneal macrophages to bind MIF. However, two studies [4,101] have shown that human pulmonary macrophages respond to MIF, but the response varies. Pollock et al. [78] and Leu et al. [62] have also contrasted the in vitro migration of alveolar and peritoneal macrophages in response to chemotactic factors.

Perhaps the most perplexing differences among alveolar and peritoneal macrophages and blood monocytes are the demonstrated antigenic differences. Montfort and Perez-Tamayo [68] prepared antibody to rat peritoneal macrophages. This cross-reacted with peritoneal macrophages, bone marrow cells, and blood monocytes of the rat, mouse, guinea pig, and rabbit. It did not cross-react with macrophages of the lung, liver, spleen, lymph node, or thymus in any of those animals. In a followup study by Martinez and Montfort [66], specific antibody prepared against rat alveolar macrophages did not cross-react with peritoneal macrophages or blood monocytes. Results of this study are shown in Table 4. These differences have been confirmed by Dressler and Skornik [27] using antibodies prepared against rat alveolar and peritoneal macrophages and evaluated by cytotoxicity. Godleski et al. [39] have made similar observa-

TABLE 4 Frequency of Positive Fluorescent Staining of Rat Alveolar Macrophage Antigen(s) in Macrophages Taken from Other Rat Organs and in Other Animal Species [a,b]

	Animal species				
Source of macrophages	Rat	Mouse	Guinea pig	Rabbit	Chick
Fixed tissue macrophages					
Lung	90	28	5	3	0
Liver	90	5	0	2	8
Spleen	90	9	2	7	10
Thymus	85	2	0	0	18
Lymph node	80	10	12	7	8
Free macrophages					
Blood monocytes	0	0	0	0	0
Peritoneum	0	0	0	0	0
Undetermined [c]					
Bone marrow	20	4	2	12	16

[a](Adapted from Martinez and Montfort [66], by courtesy of the authors and publisher.)
[b]Percent of macrophages identified in a total of 300 cells using phase-contrast illumination.
[c]It was not established if these cells are bone marrow fixed macrophages or precursors.

tions in the mouse and hamster using natural antibody in normal rabbit serum. The differences between alveolar and peritoneal macrophages cited in the biochemical studies can probably be explained by adaptation to their locations, such as the very different P_{O_2}'s. However, the antigenic differences are difficult to explain on this basis. Studies of particle-stimulated animals could be used to determine whether increased numbers of macrophages remained antigenically the same. If the biochemical and antigenic changes result from maturation, the length of time and conditions needed for these adaptations need to be studied.

V. Fate of Pulmonary Macrophages

Having reviewed the origin and turnover of macrophages, let us now consider their fate. As before, differences exist among the varying classes of pulmonary macrophages and their fates will therefore be described separately.

A. Alveolar Macrophages

Although little concrete evidence regarding the latter stages of the life of the alveolar macrophages exists, the possibilities are finite and easily enumerated. They may be subject to alveolar-bronchiolar transport mechanisms; they may enter the lymphatics or connective tissue; or they may enter the circulation. Finally, some may never leave the alveolar surface; rather they may persist for long periods of time, die there, and then be ingested and digested by younger, more vigorous siblings.

B. Alveolar-Bronchiolar Transport

There is speculation about the mechanisms responsible for alveolar-bronchiolar transport, but little evidence exists to support the theories. We know that most particles deposited in alveoli are ingested by alveolar macrophages. Some of these cells find their way to the bronchioles, and are then carried to the pharynx by ciliary action. For example, Sorokin and Brain [87] found that following an iron oxide aerosol exposure, increasing numbers of alveolar macrophages, charged with particles, become concentrated near the openings of terminal bronchioles, and appear to be migrating toward the bronchiolar surface (see Plate 4a). One cannot exclude migration through alveolar pores, or other collateral pathways between adjacent bronchial paths. However, almost all of the macrophages are located unequivocally on the surfaces of alveolar bronchi. Thus, it seems unlikely that macrophages migrate to the bronchioles by penetrating between alveolar cells or by emerging from lymphatic pathways. Sorokin and Brain concluded that it is unlikely that more than a few of the particle-containing macrophages normally leave the respiratory zone by routes passing through the connective tissue compartments of the alveolar walls, a fate suggested by others [90]. Histochemical preparations reveal the presence of activated, stellate, or spindle-shaped macrophages in peribronchial and perivascular connective tissue, but these cells do not contain particles until the later phases of lung clearance.

Since some macrophages find their way to airways, we must ask how these cells move to the mucus escalator. It is possible that macrophages exhibit directed locomotion because of a concentration gradient of a chemotactic factor. The phenomenon of chemotaxis is well studied in vitro, particularly for neutrophils, much less so for macrophages [48,80,100]. Still less is known about the chemotactic behavior of alveolar macrophages [62,78] and no observations of alveolar macrophage movement in situ have been made. Ramsey and Grant [81] assert that, although alveolar macrophages can migrate in vitro, movement is less vigorous than that shown by neutrophils. Furthermore, Baum et al. [5] report that rabbit alveolar macrophages respond weakly to such chemotactic agents as a casein-complement mixture. The identities of possible chemotactic factors responsible for alveolar-bronchiolar transport in situ are unknown. There is also no evidence to suggest that other tropisms, such as geotropism, account for a purposeful migration of macrophages.

If macrophages do move in situ, it is possible that a purely random movement could account for some alveolar transport. If alveolar-airway distances and macrophage speeds were measured and then used in classic random walk calculations, the results might suggest that some macrophages can "blunder" toward ciliated airways and then be swept away. But, alveolar macrophages may reach the bronchial passages because they tend to passively follow the direction of alveolar fluid currents rather than because they are attracted to bronchial contents, or because of random movements.

There is little direct experimental evidence that the fluid lining of the alveolar region moves mouthward, but most investigators assume that it does [65]. It is possible that the continual production of surfactant and its tendency to remain as a monolayer might provide a moving surface for transport of macrophages. There may also be a surface-tension gradient which is important to the movement of the fluid surface. Kilburn [51] discussed the fluid dynamics of the surface and proposed mechanisms responsible for alveolar-bronchiolar transport. Staub [89] focused attention on the fluid currents that may sweep across alveolar surfaces; he described them as "liquid veins" resembling the drainage of soap bubbles and suggested that these "veins" might be involved in alveolar clearance. It seems likely that this flow, fed by transudation of pulmonary capillary fluid and cell secretion, may be influenced by shape and area changes associated with ventilation. Indeed, respiratory excursions seem to play a part in the movement of fluid, particles, and cells from the alveoli [42,44]. Klosterkotter [54] reported increased lung clearance in exercising animals, but Friedberg [34] could not confirm the result. Irmscher and Schulz [45] sectioned the left phrenic nerve of rats and examined the effect on clearance. The ventilatory excursions in the left lung were reduced, causing a reduction in clearance of dust in the left as compared to the right lung.

Although these reports taken in toto provide some support for the concept that the alveolar surface film may move toward the airways, this does not necessarily prove that macrophages are passive passengers on such a moving film. Observations regarding macrophage adhesion [17] suggest that alveolar macrophages are closely applied and strongly adherent to the alveolar surface. The alveolar lining film appears to cover the macrophages [37]; they do not rest on it. Thus, it is possible that a moving surface film might simply flow over adherent macrophages. Such a moving film might be responsible for the extracellular clearance of noningested particles and unwanted secretions, but not necessarily for the alveolar-bronchiolar transport of alveolar macrophages.

The direct entry of alveolar macrophages into lymphatic pathways and connective tissue has often been suggested but never proved. For many investigators, the presence of particle-containing macrophages in these compartments is compelling evidence. But the critical reader will observe that the entry of alveolar macrophages on the one hand and the entry of bare particles which are subsequently ingested by connective tissue macrophages already present on the other, cannot be readily distinguished. During alveolar clearance, some noningested particles may follow lymphatic or vascular channels from alveoli into the peribronchial, perivascular, or subpleural adventitiae and thus penetrate into the connective tissue of the lung. They are then stored by resident macrophages already present [87] (see Plate 3c). This route may be more pronounced when conditions favor increased lymphatic permeability (pulmonary edema). Then a greater number of particles might pass into these vessels through clefts between endothelial cells, and be carried along lymphatic drainage paths until filtered out by macrophages located farther along in lymphoid foci. In any event, although inhaled particles can be found in connective tissue macrophages, we are aware of no evidence that implicates movement of alveolar surface macrophages into connective tissue compartments. We cannot, however, totally exclude this possibility—although it must certainly be an uncommon event. Yet, it would be of consequence to immune mechanisms, since it provides a pathway for antigens in or on alveolar macrophages to meet reactive lymphocytes in the connective tissue.

Migration of alveolar macrophages into the circulation seems even less likely. To our knowledge, no investigator has presented evidence to support this possibility; furthermore, our knowledge of the nature of the air-blood barrier (see Chap. 18) makes this improbable. Also, in experiments with inhaled insoluble radioactive particles, essentially no activity appears in the blood despite alveolar macrophage ingestion of these particles.

Some alveolar macrophages might simply never leave the alveolar surface. Perhaps a few spend their entire mature lifespan there; once effete, they may be ingested and degraded by younger, more vigorous macrophages. This possibility must be considered in part by default. Since evidence for the kinetic importance of the other three pathways is incomplete, we are left with this option. It is consistent with the idea that the major biological function of the alveolar macrophage is to contend with pathogenic challenge. Microorganisms may be completely metabolized by phagocytes. Having killed and degraded pathogens, the economy of the body may dictate that the alveolar macrophage remains to serve again. Continuous confrontation with nondigestible, insoluble particles is probably a more recent evolutionary event, and the macrophages may not be designed for that challenge. Kilburn [53] expressed doubts regarding macrophage migration out of alveoli. He compared the known pool size of alveolar macrophages and estimated fluxes of macrophages exiting through the airways.

Studies using easily visualized particles of iron oxide [87] show that many particle-charged macrophages are resident on the alveolar surface for long periods of time. The number of particles per macrophage gradually decline with time. This suggests death and dissolution of some macrophages, followed by reingestion of particles by younger macrophages. Yet, if macrophages do not migrate from the alveoli, the younger cells should contain as many particles in their cytoplasm as the cells they replaced. Also relevant is the observation that particle-containing macrophages can be found on the airway surfaces many months after a single acute exposure to iron oxide particles [87]. It seems unlikely that such cells or their daughters have persisted in the airways for periods up to 13 months; more likely, they are the product of alveolar-bronchiolar transport.

C. Airway Macrophages

Before considering the fate of airway macrophages, the reader should be cautioned not to assume that the particle-containing mononuclear cells in the airways are necessarily the product of alveolar-bronchiolar transport. Some may be, but others may derive from blood monocytes which have migrated from the bronchial circulation directly to the airways. Alternatively, they may derive from local monocytic cell renewal systems (albeit undescribed) subjacent to the bronchial epithelium.

Some resident airway macrophages become enmeshed in the mucus and are propelled mouthward by the ciliary apparatus. Although, initially appearing as occasional islands of mucus, the moving mucus gradually becomes contiguous as airway diameter increases. Airway macrophages are ultimately swept past the larynx and into the oral pharynx. There respiratory tract fluid, macrophages, and debris mix with salivary secretions and are swallowed. Several investigators have attempted to monitor cleared cells as they exit the trachea of living animals. Spritzer et al. [88] used an esophageal cannula and plastic pouch attached to the flank to collect mucus and cells cleared via the trachea from unanesthetized rats. Of the cells collected, 82% were macrophages; 18% were polymorphonuclear leukocytes. The hourly clearance of pulmonary macrophages was estimated to be between 1.24 and 2.47 $\times 10^6$ cells. The effects of the surgical intervention and possible infection on these results is unknown.

Brain [13] studied the hourly output of cells from the tracheas of anesthetized cats. A glass collection tube was placed in the pharynx to collect the respiratory tract fluid (diluted with a retrograde saline infusion via the esophagus) coming from the trachea. Analysis of the cellular content showed that between 1.87 and 5.07 $\times 10^6$ large, mononuclear cells per hour (range of values for four cats) were removed from the lungs. He also counted the alveolar cells present in tracheal mucus washed from freshly excised tracheas. Acetylcysteine was used to dissolve any nonmiscible mucus. Based on the quantities of cells found in the tracheal mucus and on the assumption of a mucus transport rate of 1 cm/min, 2.05 $\pm$ 0.96 $\times 10^6$ cells/hr would be cleared from cat lungs.

These estimates of macrophage clearance from the airways do not necessarily prove that all airway macrophages are passive passengers on the mucus escalator and thus are hastily cleared. On the contrary, Sorokin and Brain [87] report that many macrophages appear to remain on the bronchial surface for extended periods of time and appear to go about their normal range of activities despite mucociliary currents. Macrophages were frequently found occupying niches bounded by the surfaces of ciliated cells and the adjacent sides of taller bronchiolar cells. Such macrophages tended to lie over several consecutive epithelial cells, extending protoplasmic processes over the surface and between neighboring cells. The mixed alveolar and bronchial secretions and rounded, detached cells float above these macrophages, while they remain bathed in the watery hypophase. Furthermore, in lungs of animals exposed to iron oxide, heavily particle-laden macrophages could often be seen aggregated above cells of the bronchial epithelium (see Plate 4b). The Prussian blue reaction revealed compounds which contained iron in the bronchial epithelial cells. Beneath, in the subjacent connective tissue, a number of connective tissue macrophages also exhibited Prussian blue granules. It seems reasonable that, at these points, macrophages pause and iron-containing material is transported into and not out of the connective tissue. This conclusion is supported by the appearance of iron-bearing cells on the bronchial surfaces long before the connective tissue macrophages became stainable. It is likely that transfers from adherent airway macrophages to the bronchial epithelium are fostered by cell damage and death causing release of ingested materials.

D. Connective Tissue Macrophages

Occasionally, investigators have suggested that connective tissue macrophages emerge from the airways and are cleared from the lungs. Brundelet [21], for example, stated that macrophages emerged from peribronchiolar lymphoid foci into the bronchiolar lumen. More recently, Tucker et al. [90] championed this view and suggested that interstitial macrophages may leave pulmonary connective tissue, cross the bronchial epithelium, and join the mucociliary escalator. This pathway appears most desirable since it provides a mechanism for the pulmonary connective tissue to cleanse itself of sequestered particle residues which are often toxic and cause disease. Unfortunately, the histological techniques used in these studies (sections $>5\ \mu m$) fail to give the needed resolution to prove this migration. Sorokin and Brain [87], using thick ($1\ \mu m$) and thin glycol methacrylate plastic sections, found no evidence for this pathway in mice. The importance of these tonsil-like lymphoid foci and this pathway may depend on the presence of considerable subepithelial lymphoid tissue (such as often occurs during chronic bronchial infection). Other pathological or pharmacological challenges such as that described by Kilburn [50] may make the lung rely to a greater extent on this pathway.

E. Significance of Macrophage Fate

Although the pulmonary macrophages are essential to host defense, the normal activity and movement of pulmonary macrophages may also cause harm. Because the macrophages avidly phagocytize, inhaled toxic, radioactive, or carcinogenic particles become concentrated within pulmonary macrophages. What begins as a diffuse and relatively even exposure becomes highly localized and nonuniform. If thresholds for certain effects exist, these hot spots of high dose may be of great significance. Localization is further enhanced by macrophage movement. In Plate 4c, for example, large iron-filled (black) alveolar macrophages can be seen lining the bronchial passages. To the extent that this nontoxic aerosol may serve as a model for highly toxic aerosols, the results suggest increased exposure of the bronchial epithelium to these aerosols.

Similarly, adherence of some airway macrophages to the airway epithelium may increase airway exposure to inhaled toxic materials. More important, perhaps, this close association with the bronchial epithelium may lead to transbronchial transport of inhaled particles and subsequent reingestion by subepithelial connective tissue macrophages. These cells, like their relatives in the alveolar and airway compartments, also segregate, retain, and perhaps metabolize carcinogenic and other toxic particles. It is intriguing to note that these final repositories of residual inhaled particles, the connective tissue macrophages, have a unique locus. Like fellow histiocytes through the body, they monitor the internal environment of the body through their contact with the systemic (bronchial) vascular circuit; however, they also receive particulate and antigenic matter from the peripheral lung, some of it unprocessed and the rest preprocessed either by alveolar or airway macrophages. Material from these divergent sources becomes concentrated in these relatively fixed cells. As the chronic phases of lung clearance continue, these cells and their contents become more prominent in the connective tissue of the larger airways, septa, and blood vessels. Unlike alveolar parenchyma, this region contains a great variety of the cells involved in immunological responses available for interaction with the macrophages. Sorokin and Brain [87] report close associations between these connective tissue macrophages and both lymphocytes and mast cells.

VI. Conclusions

Pulmonary macrophages have a central role in lung defense. It is essential that we formulate an accurate picture of the life of these cells and the pathways they follow while executing their clearing functions. Such a synthesis can yield new insight into the factors that predispose human populations to pulmonary disease. The control of disease lies in the recognition of factors important to the defense of the organism.

References

1. T. Alescio, Response to x-irradiation of mouse embryonic lung lung culture in vitro. Radiation effect on the epithelium growth rate, *Exp. Cell Res.*, **43**:459-473 (1966).
2. E. Agostoni, Mechanics of the pleural space, *Physiol. Rev.*, **52**:57-128 (1972).
3. H. Balner, Identification of peritoneal macrophages in mouse radiation chimeras, *Transplantation*, **1**:217-223 (1963).
4. H. Bartfield and T. Atoynatan, Cellular immunity. Activity and properties of human migration inhibitory factor, *Int. Arch. Allergy Appl. Immunol.*, **38**:549-553 (1970).
5. J. Baum, A. G. Mowat, and J. Kirk, A simplified method for the measurements of chemotaxis ofpolymorphonuclear leukocytes from human blood, *J. Lab. Clin. Med.*, **77**:501-509 (1971).
6. F. D. Bertalanffy, Respiratory tissue: Structure, histophysiology, cyto-

dynamics. II. New approaches and interpretations, *Int. Rev. Cytol.*, **17**: 213-297 (1964).

7. E. Bingham, E. A. Pfitzer, W. Barkley, and E. P. Radford, Alveolar macrophages: Reduced number in rat after prolonged inhalation of lead sesquioxide, *Science*, **162**:1297-1299 (1968).
8. D. H. Bowden, The alveolar macrophage, *Curr. Top. Pathol.*, **55**:1-36 (1973).
9. D. H. Bowden and I. Y. R. Adamson, The pulmonary interstitial cell as immediate precursor of the alveolar macrophage, *Am. J. Pathol.*, **68**:521-528 (1972).

9a. D. H. Bowden and I. Y. R. Adamson, The alveolar macrophage delivery system: Kinetic studies in cultured explants of murine lung, *Am. J. Pathol.*, **83**:123-134 (1976).

10. D. H. Bowden, I. Y. R. Adamson, G. Grantham, and J. P. Wyatt, Origin of the lung macrophage, *Arch. Pathol.*, **88**:540-546 (1969).
11. D. H. Bowden, E. Davies, and J. P. Wyatt, Cytodynamics of pulmonary alveolar cells in the mouse, *Arch. Pathol.*, **86**:667-670 (1968).
12. J. D. Brain, Clearance of particles from the lungs: Alveolar macrophages and mucus transport. Thesis, Harvard University School of Public Health, 1966.
13. J. D. Brain, Free cells in the lungs: Some aspects of their role, quantitation, and regulation, *Arch. Intern. Med.*, **126**:477-487 (1970).
14. J. D. Brain, The effects of increased particles on the number of alveolar macrophages. In *Inhaled Particles III.* Edited by W. H. Walton. London, Unwin, 1971, pp. 209-225.
15. J. D. Brain and N. R. Frank, Recovery of free cells from rat lungs by repeated washings, *J. Appl. Physiol.*, **25**:63-69 (1968).
16. J. D. Brain and N. R. Frank, The relation of age to the number of lung free cells, lung weight, and body weight in rats, *J. Gerontol.*, **23**:58-62 (1968).
17. J. D. Brain and N. R. Frank, Alveolar macrophage adhesion: Wash electrolyte composition and free cell yield, *J. Appl. Physiol.*, **34**:75-80 (1973).
18. A. R. Brody and J. E. Craighead, Pathogenesis of pulmonary cytomegalovirus infection in immunosuppressed mice, *J. Infect. Dis.*, **129**:677-689 (1974).
19. A. R. Brody, G. S. Davis, and J. E. Craighead, Intrapulmonary migration of mononuclear cells in human interstitial lung disease, *Am. J. Pathol.*, **78**:88 (1975).
20. J. S. Brody, A. Sun, A. D. Manalo, J. L. Nichol, and T. Rizzo, Oxygen toxicity: Pattern of injury revealed by lung washings, *Clin. Res.*, **21**:984 (1973) (Abstract).
21. J. P. Brundelet, Experimental study of the dust clearance mechanism of the lung. I. Histological study in rats of the intrapulmonary bronchial route of elimination. Academic Dissertation, *Acta Rathol. Microbiol. Scand.*, **175**, Suppl.:1-141 (1965).

22. M. Brunstetter, J. A. Hardie, R. Schiff, J. P. Lewis, and C. E. Cross, The origin of pulmonary alveolar macrophages, *Arch. Intern. Med.*, **127**:1064-1068 (1971).
23. H. M. Carleton, Studies on epithelial phagocytosis. II. A method for demonstrating the origin of dust cells, *Proc. R. Soc. Exp. Med. Biol. (Lond.)*, **114**:513-523 (1934).
24. R. L. Carter and J. D. B. Roberts, Macrophages and multinuclear giant cells in nitrosoquinoline-induced granulomata in rats: An autoradiographic study, *J. Pathol.*, **105**:285-288 (1971).
25. L. J. Casarett and P. S. Milley, Alveolar reactivity following inhalation of particles, *Health Phys.*, **10**:1003-1011 (1964).
26. A. M. Dannenberg, Jr., M. S. Burstone, P. C. Walter, and J. W. Kinsley, A histochemical study of phagocytic and enzymatic functions of rabbit mononuclear and polymorphonuclear enudate cells and alveolar macrophages. I. Survey and quantitation of enzymes and sites of cellular action, *J. Cell Biol.*, **17**:465-486 (1963).
27. D. P. Dressler and W. A. Skornik, Specificity of rat anti-alveolar macrophages serum, *J. Reticuloendothel. Soc.*, **15**:55a (1974) (Abstract).
28. P. Drinker and T. Hatch, *Industrial Dust.* New York, McGraw-Hill, 1954.
29. M. J. Evans, L. J. Cabral, R. J. Stephens, and G. Freeman, Cell division of alveolar macrophages in rat lung follwoing exposure to NO_2, *Am. J. Pathol.*, **70**:199-206 (1973).
30. J. Ferin, A. Vlckova, and G. Urbankova, Influence of trypan blue on the elimination of dust from the lungs, *Prac. Lek.*, **16**:202-205 (1964) (in Slovak).
31. J. Ferin, Elimination of dust from the lung and the influence of the reticuloendothelial system, *Ann. Occup. Hyg.*, **3**:1-5 (1960).
32. J. Ferin, Self-purification of the lungs from dust. V. Phagocytic capacity of the reticuloendothelial system on purification of the lungs from dust, *Prac. Lek.*, **12**:397-401 (1960) (in Slovak).
33. N. C. Foot, Studies on endothelial reactions. X. On the origin of the pulmonary "dust cell," *Am. J. Pathol.*, **3**:413-443 (1927).
34. K. D. Friedberg, Quantitative Untersuchungen über die Staubelimination in der Lunge und ihre Beeinflussbarkeit in Tierexperiment, *Beitr. Silikoseforsch.*, **69**:1-99 (1960).
35. L. U. Gardner and O. T. Smith, The origin of the alveolar phagocyte studied in paraffin sections of tissue stained supravitally with neutral red, *Am. J. Pathol.*, **3**:445-460 (1927).
36. R. Gersing and H. Schumacher, Experimentelle Untersuchungen über die Staubphagozytose, *Beitr. Silikoseforsch.*, **25**:31-34 (1955).
37. J. Gil and E. R. Weibel, Extracellular lining of bronchioles after perfusion-fixation of rat lungs for electron microscopy, *Anat. Rec.*, **169**:185-199 (1971).
38. J. J. Godleski and J. D. Brain, The origin of alveolar macrophages in mouse radiation chimeras, *J. Exp. Med.*, **136**:630-643 (1972).
39. J. J. Godleski, J. D. Brain, and D. L. Coffin, Relative toxicity of normal

serum to mouse and hamster alveolar and peritoneal macrophages, *J. Reticuloendothel. Soc.*, **15**:54a (1974).

40. D. W. Golde, T. N. Finley, and M. J. Cline, The pulmonary macrophage in acute leukemia, *N. Engl. J. Med.*, **290**:875-878 (1974).
41. J. W. Goodman, On the origin of peritoneal fluid cells, *Blood*, **23**:18-26 (1964).
42. P. Gross, The mechanisms of dust clearance from the lung: A theory, *Am. J. Clin. Pathol.*, **23**:116-120 (1953).
43. P. Gross, R. T. P. deTreville, E. B. Tolker, M. Kaschak, and M. A. Babyak, The pulmonary macrophage response to irritants, *Arch. Environ. Health*, **18**:174-185 (1969).
44. T. F. Hatch and P. Gross, *Pulmonary Deposition and Retention of Inhaled Particles.* New York, Academic Press, 1964.
45. G. Irmscher and G. Schulz, Experimentelle Silikose bei Ratten nach einseitiger Phrenicusexhairese, *Int. Arch. Arbeitsmed.*, **18**:422-441 (1961).
46. H. E. Karrer, The ultrastructure of the mouse lung, general architecture of capillary and alveolar walls, *J. Biophys. Biochem. Cytol.*, **2**:241-252 (1956).
47. H. E. Karrer, The ultrastructure of mouse lung: The alveolar macrophage, *J. Biophys. Biochem. Cytol.*, **4**:693-700 (1958).
48. H. V. Keller, M. W. Hess, and H. Cottier, Physiology of chemotaxis and random motility, *Semin. Hematol.*, **12**:47-57 (1975).
49. Y. Kikkawa and K. Koneda, The type II epithelial cell of the lung. I. Method of isolation, *Lab. Invest.*, **30**:76-84 (1974).
50. K. H. Kilburn, W. S. Lynn, L. L. Tres, and W. N. McKenzie, Leukocyte recruitment through airway walls by condensed vegetable tannins and quercitin, *Lab. Invest.*, **28**:55-59 (1973).
51. K. H. Kilburn, A hypothesis for pulmonary clearance and its implications, *Am. Rev. Respir. Dis.*, **98**:449-463 (1968).
52. K. H. Kilburn, Clearance zones in the distal lung, *Ann. NY Acad. Sci.*, **24**:276-281 (1974).
53. K. H. Kilburn, Functional morphology of the distal lung, *Int. Rev. Cytol.*, **37**:153-270 (1974).
54. W. Klosterkotter, Tierexperimentelle Untersuchungen über das Reinigungsvermögen der Lunge, *Arch. Hyg. Bakt.*, **141**:258-274 (1957).
55. J. Kouri and O. Ancheta, Transformation of macrophages into fibroblasts, *Exp. Cell Res.*, **71**:168-176 (1972).
56. C. W. LaBelle and H. Brieger, Synergistic effects of aerosols. II. Effects on rate of clearance from the lung, *Arch. Indust. Health*, **20**:100-105 (1959).
57. C. W. LaBelle and H. Brieger, The fate of inhaled particles in the early post-exposure period, **1**:432-437 (1960).
58. C. W. LaBelle and H. Brieger, Patterns and mechanisms in the elimination of dust from the lungs. In *Inhaled Particles and Vapours I.* Edited by C. N. Davis. London, Pergamon, 1961, pp. 356-368.
59. H. C. Langevoort, Z. A. Cohn, J. G. Hirsch, J. H. Humphrey, W. G. Spector,

and R. van Furth, The nomenclature of mononuclear phagocytic cells. Proposal for a new classification, In *Mononuclear Phagocytes.* Edited by R. van Furth. Philadelphia, Pa., F. A. Davis, 1970, pp. 1-6.

60. G. A. Laurenzi, R. T. Potter, and E. H. Kass, Bacteriological flora of the lower respiratory tract, *N. Engl. J. Med.*, **265**:173-178 (1961).
61. W. S. Lemon, The anatomic factors involved and mechanisms employed in removal of minute particles of foreign material from the lungs, *Trans. Assoc. Am. Phys.*, **52**:278-288 (1937).
62. R. W. Leu, A. Eddleston, R. Good, and J. Hadden, Paradoxical effects of ouabain on the migration of peritoneal and alveolar macrophages, *Exp. Cell Res.*, **76**:458-461 (1973).
63. R. W. Leu, A. L. Eddleston, J. W. Hadden, and R. A. Good, Mechanisms of action of migratory inhibitory factor (MIF). I. Evidence for a receptor for MIF present of the peritoneal macrophage but not on the alveolar macrophage, *J. Exp. Med.*, **136**:589-603 (1972).
64. F. N. Low, Electron microscopy of rat lung, *Anat. Rec.*, **113**:437-449 (1952).
65. C. C. Macklin, Pulmonary sumps, dust accumulations, alveolar fluid and lymph vessels, *Acta Anat.*, **23**:1-33 (1955).
66. R. D. Martinez and I. Montfort, A study of the specificity of alveolar macrophage antigen(s), *Immunology*, **25**:197-203 (1973).
67. G. Meuret and G. Hoffman, Monocyte kinetic studies in normal and disease states, *Br. J. Haematol.*, **24**:275-285 (1973).
68. I. Montfort and R. Perez-Tamayo, Two antigenically different types of macrophages, *Proc. Soc. Exp. Biol.*, **138**:204-207 (1971).
69. R. D. Moore and M. D. Schoenberg, Alveolar lining cells and pulmonary reticuloendothelial system of the rabbit, *Am. J. Pathol.*, **45**:991-1005 (1964).
70. P. E. Morrow, F. R. Gibb, and J. Leigh, Clearance of insoluble dust from the lower respiratory tract, *Health Phys.*, **10**:543-555 (1964).
71. G. P. Murphy, A. R. Brody, and J. E. Craighead, Monocyte migration across pulmonary membranes in mice infected with cytomegalovirus, *Exp. Mol. Pathol.*, **22**:35-44 (1975).
72. Q. N. Myrvik, E. S. Leake, and B. Fariss, Studies on pulmonary alveolar macrophages from the normal rabbit: A technique to procure them in a high state of purity, *J. Immunol.*, **86**:133-136 (1961).
73. Q. N. Myrvik, E. S. Leake, and B. Fariss, Lysozyme content of alveolar and peritoneal macrophages from the rabbit, *J. Immunol.*, **86**:133-136 (1961).
74. R. Oren, A. E. Farnham, K. Saito, E. Milofsky, and M. L. Karnovsky, Metabolic patterns in three types of phagocytizing cells, *J. Cell Biol.*, **17**: 487-500 (1963).
75. J. M. Papadimitriou and W. G. Spector, The origin properties and fate of epitheloid cells, *J. Pathol.*, **105**:187-203 (1971).
76. H. H. Permar, The development of the mononuclear phagocyte of the lung, *J. Med. Res.*, **42**:147-162 (1920).

77. M. O. Pinkett, C. R. Cowdrey, and P. C. Norwell, Mixed hematopoietic and pulmonary origin of "alveolar macrophages" as demonstrated by chromosome markers, *Am. J. Pathol.,* **48**:859-865 (1966).
78. E. M. Pollock, C. N. Pegram, and J. J. Vazquez, A comparison of the in vitro migration properties of alveolar and peritoneal macrophages, *J. Reticuloendothel. Soc.,* **9**:383-391 (1971).
79. S. A. Pratt, T. N. Finley, M. H. Smith, and A. J. Ladman, A comparison of alveolar macrophages and pulmonary surfactant obtained from the lung of human smokers and nonsmokers by endobronchial lavage, *Anat. Rec.,* **163**:497-507 (1969).
80. W. Ptak, Z. Porwit-Bobr, and Z. Chlap, Transformation of hamster macrophages into giant cells with antimacrophage serum, *Nature,* **225**:655-657 (1970).
81. W. S. Ramsey and L. Grant, Chemotaxis. In *Inflammatory Process,* Vol. I, 2nd ed. Edited by B. W. Zweifach, L. Grant, and R. T. McCluskey. New York, Academic Press, 1974, pp. 287-362.
82. M. A. Sackner, Bronchofiberscopy, *Am. Rev. Respir. Dis.,* **111**:62-88 (1975).
83. E. Schiller, Inhalation, retention and elimination of dusts from dogs' and rats' lungs with special reference to the alveolar phagocytes and bronchial epithelium. In *Inhaled Particles and Vapours,* Vol. I. Edited by C. N. Davis. London, Pergamon, 1961, pp. 342-347.
84. K. Shima, A. M. Dannenberg, M. Ando, S. Chandrasckhar, A. Seluzicki, and J. I. Fabrikant, Macrophage accumulation, division, maturation, and digestive and microbicidal capacities in tuberculous lesions. I. Studies involving their incorporation of tritiated thymidine and their content of lysosomal enzymes and bacilli, *Am. J. Pathol.,* **67**:159-174 (1972).
85. S. Sorokin, Recent work on developing lungs. In *Organogenesis.* Edited by R. L. DeHoan and H. Ursprung. New York, Holt, Rinehart, and Winston, 1965, pp. 467-491.
86. S. P. Sorokin and S. J. Adelstein, Failure of 1100 rads of x-radiation to affect ciliogenesis and centriole formation in cultured rat lungs, *Radiat. Res.,* **31**:748-759 (1967).
87. S. P. Sorokin and J. D. Brain, Pathways of clearance in mouse lungs exposed to iron oxide aerosols, *Anat. Rec.,* **181**:581-626 (1975).
88. A. A. Spritzer, J. A. Watson, J. A. Auld, and M. A. Guetthoff, Pulmonary macrophage clearance. The hourly rates of transfer of pulmonary macrophages to the oropharynx of the rat, *Arch. Environ. Health,* **17**:726-730 (1968).
89. N. C. Staub, The "liquid veins" of the lung, *Physiologist,* **9**:294 (1966).
90. A. D. Tucker, J. H. Wyatt, D. Undery, Clearance of inhaled particles from alveoli by normal interstitial drainage pathways, *J. Appl. Physiol.,* **35**: 719-732 (1973).
91. J. Ungar, Jr. and G. R. Wilson, Monocytes as a source of alveolar phagocytes, *Am. J. Pathol.,* **11**:681-691 (1935).

92. R. van Furth, The origin and turnover of promonocytes, monocytes, and macrophages in normal mice, In *Mononuclear Phagocytes.* Edited by R. van Furth. Philadelphia, Pa., F. A. Davis, 1970, pp. 151-165.
93. R. Van Furth and Z. A. Cohn, The origin and kinetics of mononuclear phagocytes, *J. Exp. Med.*, **128**:415-435 (1968).
94. G. P. Velo and W. G. Spector, The origin and turnover of alveolar macrophages in experimental pneumonia, *J. Pathol.*, **109**:7-19 (1973).
95. G. S. Vijeyaratnam and B. Corrin, Origin of the pulmonary alveolar macrophage studied in the iprindole-treated rat, *J. Pathol.*, **108**:115-118 (1972).
96. G. S. Vijeyaratnam and B. Corrin, Pulmonary histiocytosis simulating desquamative interstitial pneumonia in rats receiving oral iprindole, *J. Pathol.*, **108**:105-113 (1972).
97. M. Virolainen, Hematopoietic origin of macrophages as studied by chromosome markers in mice, *J. Exp. Med.*, **127**:943-952 (1968).
97a. A. Volkman, Disparity in origin of mononuclear phagocyte populations, *J. Reticuloendothel. Soc.*, **19**:249-268 (1976).
98. A. Volkman and J. L. Gowans, The origins of macrophages from bone marrow in the rat, *Br. J. Exp. Pathol.*, **46**:62-70 (1965).
99. Nai-sun Wang, The regional differences of pleural mesothelial cells in rabbits, *Am. Rev. Respir. Dis.*, **110**:623-633 (1974).
100. P. A. Ward, Leukotaxis and leucotactic disorders: A review, *Am. J. Pathol.*, **77**:520-538 (1974).
101. G. A. Warr and R. R. Martin, Response of human pulmonary macrophages to migration inhibition factor, *Am. Rev. Respir. Dis.*, **108**:371-373 (1973).
102. E. R. Weibel and R. P. Bolender, Stereological principles for morphometry in electron microscopic cytology. In *Principles and Techniques of Electron Microscopy*, Vol. 3. Edited by M. A. Hayat. New York, Van Nostrand-Reinhold, 1973, pp. 235-302.
103. D. M. Whitelaw, The intravascular lifespan of monocytes, *Blood*, **28**:455-464 (1966).
104. P. P. Yevich, Lung structure—relation to response to particulate, *Arch. Environ. Health*, **10**:37-43 (1965).

21

Metabolism of Alveolar Macrophages

ROBERT J. MASON

Cardiovascular Research Institute
University of California
San Francisco, California

I. Introduction

This chapter discusses the metabolism of alveolar macrophages and the alterations in metabolism that accompany several different physiologic states. The term "alveolar macrophage" is used to include all macrophages collected from the lung by any method. There are probably different subpopulations of macrophages within the lung, but they are not discussed separately because they have not been well characterized functionally, morphologically, or biochemically. Because experimental findings depend greatly on the source of macrophages and, perhaps, on the method of obtaining them, the source and method of collection is mentioned for many reports. Pertinent data obtained with peritoneal macrophages and polymorphonuclear leukocytes are used for illustrative purposes. Because of the author's past experience and relative knowledge of lipid metabolism, this subject is discussed in greater detail than other aspects.

The reader is encouraged to consult several reviews and collections of papers that discuss aspects of the metabolism of alveolar macrophages [12,30, 38,39,51,62,94,185], of cultured mouse peritoneal macrophages [72], and of other phagocytic cells [8,31,139,165,180,181].

II. The Importance of Alveolar Macrophages

Alveolar macrophages are the main cellular defense against inhaled organisms and other particulate material [73], and defects in this defense system can have serious consequences for the host. We inhale microorganisms and other particulate materials with every breath, and particles or aerosols 0.5-3.0 μm in diameter are likely to be deposited on the alveolar surface. It is surprising that the lungs and bronchi are sterile in normal individuals [98]. The importance of alveolar macrophages in handling inhaled bacteria has been recognized for many years [18,155], but only recently have quantitative studies been done by workers such as Green, Kass, Laurenzi, Huber, Goldstein, and their collaborators (see Chap. 23). There are a number of pathologic states, including uremia, alcoholism, immunosuppression, and oxygen toxicity, in which bacterial pneumonia frequently occurs. These altered states can be studied in rodents by measuring the removal and inactivation of radioactive live bacteria administered by aerosol [73]. Decreased bacterial clearance has been shown in these pathologic conditions, but studies of the biochemical or metabolic defects that account for the decreased clearance are just beginning. Prior coating of bacteria with pulmonary surface-active material may be an important adjunct for intracellular killing, and this process may be altered in certain pathologic states [96]; however, it is unlikely that this is the only defect, or that there is a single common defect, for the variety of abnormal states in which decreased bacterial clearance occurs.

Alveolar macrophages have been implicated also in the pathogenesis of several noninfectious diseases [134]. Human alveolar macrophages contain various acid and neutral proteases and elastases, some of which are inhibited by α_1-antitrypsin [26,150]. The hydrolytic enzymes of macrophages, as well as those of polymorphonuclear leukocytes, may be important in silent, chronic, degenerative diseases of the lungs such as emphysema, as well as in the more fulminant necrotizing types of pneumonitis [176]. Macrophages may also be involved in granulomatous diseases, such as sarcoidosis and Wegener's granulomatosis, which are likely to have an immunologic basis.

Another reason for interest in the metabolism of alveolar macrophages is that these are the only types of cells that can be obtained from the lung in large amounts and as a relatively homogeneous population. Alveolar macrophages can be used as indicators of how cells adapt to the lung and to the relatively high partial pressure of oxygen found in alveolar gas.

About 10^9 cells (2-4 ml of packed cells) can be collected by bronchopulmonary lavage from a rabbit several weeks after injection with BCG (bacillus Calmette-Guérin) or complete Freund's adjuvant [122,159]. This is at least 20 times the amount harvested from normal rabbits (4×10^7 cells per rabbit). In man, alveolar macrophages may be obtained by endobronchial lavage by means of balloon-tipped catheters under fluoroscopic control [58,68] or through a fiberoptic bronchoscope [147,195]. Similar cells can be obtained by lavage from resected surgical specimens [28]. Endobronchial lavage is probably the easiest means of obtaining members of the monocyte-macrophage series from man and is the only feasible method of isolating mature macrophages without the complexities of cell culture.

III. Problems in Studying Alveolar Macrophages

Cells obtained from lavage have been used for studies of such diverse areas as phagocytosis, synthesis of immunoglobulins [81,87], and release of histamine [137]. Although smears of alveolar macrophages may appear relatively homogeneous, cells obtained by lavage are not really homogeneous and may well represent one or more atypical and functionally distinct subpopulations of macrophages in the lung. The heterogeneity may be morphologic, functional, or both [184]. Cellular heterogeneity is an especially important problem in studies of specific biochemical functions in which individual cells are not examined. Giemsa-stained smears reveal great differences in cell size and appearance, especially in cells obtained from dogs and from humans who do not smoke [29,58,87,140, 144,147]. About 90% of cells obtained from normal rabbits by lavage with buffered saline and about 85% of cells from rabbits stimulated by Freund's adjuvant are macrophages as determined by light microscopy. As determined by electron microscopy up to 90% of cells lavaged from normal mice, rats, and rabbits appear to be alveolar macrophages (G. Huber, personal communication). Other investigators report lower percentages of macrophages in hamsters and guinea pigs [74,148,149,151].

In most studies, characterization of cells obtained by lavage is not carried further than examination of stained smears by light microscopy. More reports should include cell-specific means of characterization such as phagocytosis [197], adherence to glass, uptake of neutral red [153], content of nonspecific esterase [68], or presence of fc receptors. Unfortunately, even these types of tests are not totally specific. For example, some B lymphocytes adhere to glass surfaces, and nonspecific esterase activity and uptake of neutral red is found in type II alveolar epithelial cells (131; R. J. Mason, unpublished observations). Cellular heterogeneity is especially noticeable in animals exposed to high concentrations of toxic gases, such as ozone, in which circumstances up to 50% of cells recovered by lavage are polymorphonuclear leukocytes [25].

The functional state of alveolar macrophages used in various studies may differ, because the cells obtained depend on the host as well as on the method of obtaining cells. As mentioned above, the host may be a "normal" animal or a treated animal and, in man, a smoker or a nonsmoker. The number and, perhaps, the degree of activation of the cells may depend on the history of exposure of the host. It is well established that alveolar macrophages can be recruited by exposing the animals to a dust burden [15,74], but yield is also different in pathogen-free rodents [151]. The type and state of the cells may also depend on the age of the animal.

Early methods of obtaining alveolar macrophages used fluid for lavage that contained calcium and magnesium [126]. Brain and Frank [16] showed that the yield of cells could be doubled by omitting calcium and magnesium from buffer for lavage. It is not known if the cells obtained with different solutions are metabolically or functionally different. The exact source, age, and physiologic state of macrophages obtained by lavage is not known. There is also no information on the degree of similarity of the cells recovered by lavage to the majority of the macrophages that are left in the lung after lavage. It remains to be established whether cells obtained by lavage are representative of the cells that inactivate bacteria in the lung in situ. Kilburn [93,94] has suggested that cells harvested by endobronchial lavage come from small airways and not alveolar spaces or alveolar ducts.

Cells may be obtained by techniques other than bronchopulmonary lavage [132]. Oren and associates [132] conducted the most comprehensive study of the relative metabolic activities of different types of phagocytic cells; they isolated guinea pig alveolar macrophages by incubating minced pieces of lung tissue at 37°C and collecting the glass-adherent cells. Kikkawa and Yoneda [92] reported that the yield of macrophages could be increased 7-fold over techniques using lavage by mincing lung tissue and shaking the pieces vigorously. If this more recent technique were combined with glass adherence or rate sedimentation, a relatively pure population with a high yield might be obtained.

Some investigators use alveolar macrophages maintained in tissue culture, which presents other methodologic problems. There is a selection process for the cells that remain glass-adherent during the first 48 hr. The metabolic activity of mouse peritoneal macrophages maintained in culture can be altered by various conditions of incubation, especially the amount of serum present, and metabolism differs considerably from cells normally resident in the peritoneal cavity [32,33,35,158]. Consequently, extrapolation of data obtained from cultured cells to freshly obtained cells to cells in situ is difficult. The striking advantage of the tissue-culture system is, however, the ability to alter the environment in a controlled fashion and to measure alterations in metabolism over the course of days to weeks [69,158].

IV. General Metabolism

A. Energy Metabolism

This section begins with a discussion of the metabolism of different types of phagocytic cells. Later, I will explore the differences among alveolar macrophages obtained from lungs of different hosts. For comparative purposes, Table 1 shows representative values of oxygen consumption for the commonly studied phagocytic cells of rabbits and guinea pigs. I would like to stress two points. (a) In comparison to macrophages, polymorphonuclear leukocytes are a relatively homogeneous cell type. They are well differentiated cells when released from bone marrow, and they do not need to adapt to the local environments of different tissues. They contain glycogen as an endogenous energy supply, are able to process only one phagocytic load, and apparently do not have the ability to synthesize new granules or lysosomal enzymes. There are only two main populations of granules: the primary granules, which contain myeloperoxidase and most hydrolytic enzymes with an acidic pH optimum, and the secondary granules, which contain most of the lysozyme, lactoferrin, and alkaline phosphatase. No detailed biochemical or functional comparisons of polymorphonuclear leukocytes isolated from blood and from an exudate of the same species have been reported. (b) Macrophages, on the other hand, vary considerably in their metabolic activity depending on their location, and they differentiate in peripheral tissues after release from the bone marrow. They may depend on an exogenous

TABLE 1 Representative Values for Consumption of Oxygen by Phagocytic Cells

Cell	Species	Oxygen consumption ($\mu M\ O_2/10^8$ cells/hr)		Ref.
		Basal	During phagocytosis	
Polymorphonuclear leukocyte (exudate)	Guinea pig	2	4-13	132, 149
	Rabbit	2	8	149
Peritoneal macrophage (exudate)	Guinea pig	6	19	132, 149
	Rabbit	9	14	149
Alveolar macrophage	Guinea pig	9-32	14-41	132, 149
	Rabbit	8-10	12-16	56, 64, 149
Alveolar macrophage (exudate, stimulated by BCG)	Rabbit	12-17	–	56, 59

supply of energy for metabolism; they process many phagocytic loads, are capable of synthesizing new lysosomal and other enzymes, and have a complex array of primary and secondary lysosomes. There is no evidence that alveolar macrophages are dependent on external substrates for production of energy in short-term experiments, and the presence or absence of glucose has no effect on the rate of phagocytosis [113].

Available data do not allow comparison of metabolic variables within one species for different types of mononuclear phagocytes, i.e., monocytes, normal and exudative peritoneal macrophages, and normal and exudative alveolar macrophages. The major difficulty in interpreting studies using peritoneal macrophages and alveolar macrophages is simply that peritoneal macrophages usually come from an induced exudate and alveolar macrophages come from normal lungs. There are very little data on peritoneal macrophages from untreated animals, because few cells can be obtained from the peritoneal cavity under normal conditions [159].

Data for human cells are well characterized only for polymorphonuclear leukocytes isolated from peripheral blood. Other measurements, such as consumption of glucose and oxidation of 1-[^{14}C] glucose and 6-[^{14}C] glucose, were too variable to be collated. The reports by Romeo et al. [149] and Oren et al. [132] contain most of the comparative observations, but I have also included data from other laboratories in Table 1. Consequently, data are not strictly comparable because of differences in sources of cells, handling and incubating of cells, methods of measuring oxygen consumption, and phagocytic particles used. Oren and associates [132] used latex particles for phagocytosis, Warburg flasks for measurements of oxygen consumption during 1 hr of incubation, and alveolar macrophages in monolayers obtained from minced preparations of guinea pig lungs. Romeo et al. [149] used bacteria for phagocytosis, a polarographic measurement of consumption of oxygen during a short incubation, and alveolar macrophages obtained by lavage and incubated in suspension. The report by Romeo and associates indicates that the customary statement, that alveolar macrophages have a much higher level of oxygen consumption than peritoneal macrophages, may not be valid for all species. Other differences between alveolar and peritoneal macrophages are discussed in Sec. V.A.

The reason for belaboring differences among mononuclear phagocytes is that cells obtained by lavage are likely to be a mixture of many types. There are likely to be cells similar to monocytes, mature macrophages, and "activated" or exudative macrophages. Many studies have determined differences between monocytes and macrophages [10,31-33,35,69,106,159,160,181,182]. Structurally, monocytes are smaller and contain fewer lysosomes and mitochondria. Functionally, they have lower glycolytic and respiratory activity as measured by consumption of glucose and oxygen, and by content of pyruvate kinase and cytochrome oxidase. Monocytes have some peroxidase and can iodinate bacteria, but less well than polymorphonuclear leukocytes. Mature macrophages have very low levels of peroxidase and, apparently, cannot iodinate bacteria. The failure of iodination has caused much uncertainty and speculation about the predominant bactericidal mechanism in these cells [164]. Resident alveolar macrophages show high levels of consumption of glucose and oxygen with only slight changes during phagocytosis and very low peroxidase activity; they also lack the ability to iodinate bacteria.

Alveolar macrophages have been obtained from a variety of sources; these include cells obtained by lavage or from minced tissue of pathogen-free, germ-free, "normal," and stimulated hosts of several species (rat, rabbit, guinea pig, sheep, cow, and man). Cells are studied at once or after maintenance in culture. Therefore, evaluation of different studies requires information on the host (environmental history, age, sex, species) and on the methods of procurement, handling, performing the incubations, and measuring the biochemical or functional variables. Therefore, it is difficult to compare published data.

There are no biochemical data comparing cells obtained by lavage with buffered saline with those obtained by saline containing calcium and magnesium, or comparing cells obtained by lavage with those obtained from minces [132] or by the method of Kikkawa and Yoneda [92]. Cells adherent to plastic consume the same amount of oxygen but may incorporate more amino acids into proteins and phosphorus into lipids than similar cells in suspension [89,103,132]. Germ-free and pathogen-free animals yield fewer cells by lavage [151]. Stimulated hosts (BCG, dust loads, smoke) produce more cells than unstimulated animals. Although detailed comparative biochemical studies are not available, cells from stimulated hosts contain more mitochondria, rough endoplasmic reticulum, and lysosomes, and consume more glucose and oxygen than cells from unstimulated hosts [56,77,109,127].

Because macrophages are capable of synthesizing new enzymes, they can be affected by specific treatments of the host. For example, there are a series of microsomal enzymes that may be induced in macrophages in vivo or in vitro by exposing the lungs to specific substances, e.g., heme-oxygenase with methemoglobin or red cells [65,141], or aryl hydrocarbon hydroxylase with cigarette smoke [22]. It is probable that cells harvested from different types of hosts will be different, and they may also be affected by the manner of collection and handling for metabolic studies.

B. Metabolism of Carbohydrates

Alveolar macrophages can metabolize glucose by glycolysis, the pentose pathway, and Krebs cycle. The flux of glucose through these pathways and the proportion by which it is changed by phagocytosis is not precisely known. Unlike polymorphonuclear leukocytes, alveolar macrophages contain little glycogen and, therefore, may rely more on substrates from the circulation for their metabolism. Unlike other phagocytic cells, in which the rate of phagocytosis is affected only by glycolytic inhibitors [132], the rate of phagocytosis of alveolar macrophages is diminished by inhibitors of glycolysis and of the Krebs' cycle [27,113, 132]. Oren et al. [132] reported that guinea pig alveolar macrophages, unlike polymorphonuclear leukocytes and elicited peritoneal macrophages, lacked a Crabtree effect (depression of respiration by exogenous glucose). All three types of cells have a Pasteur effect (increased lactate production in the presence of glucose under anaerobic conditions) [132]. Lactate is readily produced by alveolar macrophages [59,132]. If these cells are incubated with a low concentration of glucose (0.4 mM) and a high concentration of lactate (1 mM), they will consume lactate, presumably as an alternative metabolic fuel [171]. As is pointed out in Sec. V.B, the control points for utilization of glucose in alveolar macrophages are not known. The pentose pathway uses 4% of available glucose in rabbit alveolar macrophages [59] and 6% in rat alveolar macrophages (R. J. Mason, unpublished observations). These data are similar to those for peritoneal macrophages from exudates in guinea pigs [192].

There are very little data on complex carbohydrates, such as glycoproteins or glycolipids, which may be useful as membrane markers, surface antigens, and binding sites for hormones or drugs. One sugar, α-L-fucose, is apparently required as part of the receptor for macrophage inhibitory factor (MIF) [146]. Although alveolar macrophages can respond to MIF, the response is not uniform [102,123,187]. Perhaps the variability is due to alterations in the complex carbohydrates on the cell surface. Little information has been reported on the composition of plasma membranes and receptors for physiologic regulators in these cells.

Alveolar macrophages can presumably digest the complex carbohydrates that are ingested. These cells contain a variety of hexosidases and hexosaminidases. Mouse peritoneal macrophages can digest most polysaccharides but they cannot degrade sucrose and β-glycosides [34]. When sucrose is pinocytosed and concentrated in the lysosomes, these organelles swell. They will return to normal size if yeast invertase or γ-glycosidase is pinocytosed and transported to the sucrose-laden inclusions. This observation is interesting by itself, and potentially important for the treatment of clinical storage diseases, as it shows that enzymes can get within cells and be transported to sites of storage of undigestible material, yet still function properly. A similar type of study was reported for the introduction of the enzyme uricase into alveolar macrophages [170]. The application of this principle to storage diseases of man is not yet practical but is certainly plausible [14].

C. Metabolism of Proteins

Alveolar macrophages readily synthesize protein, and this process can be studied in vitro [103,114-116,194]. There are little data about the synthesis of specific cellular proteins in the alveolar macrophage. The major proteins synthesized by BCG-stimulated and normal rabbit alveolar macrophages appear to be the same [103]. There is an increased content of lysosomal enzymes in alveolar macrophages from BCG-injected animals and from cigarette smokers; presumably, this is because of an increased rate of synthesis of these enzymes. There are, however, little data about the turnover of different enzymes or the contractile proteins in these cells. It has been reported that alveolar macrophages are able to synthesize certain circulating proteins and macromolecules including transferrin [163], components of the complement system (C3, C4, C1q) [82,163], immunoglobulins [81], interferon [2], endogenous pyrogen [4], and colony-stimulating factor [67]. Contamination of these preparations with lymphocytes and other cell types, however, must be considered.

Macrophages contain proteases that are important for the digestive functions of these cells, and that may also cause local injury to the lung. Most proteins ingested by macrophages are degraded to individual amino acids [44,95], but certain peptides with D-amino acids cannot be degraded [45,69]. There is a potential conflict; if macrophages digest proteins (antigens), how can they be effective on the afferent side of the immune response? The answer lies in incomplete digestion [193] and in the possibility of sequestration of some antigens on the cell surface or in RNA-antigen complexes. The actual role of the macrophage in processing antigen is still incompletely understood, and some of the evidence is contradictory [180]. A complete discussion of the processing of antigens is provided in Chap. 25.

D. Metabolism of Lipids

The major interest in metabolism of lipids within phagocytic cells is directed toward studying turnover and fusion of the cell membrane. During phagocytosis there is an extensive internalization and resealing of the plasma membrane, together with fusion of lysosomes with the phagocytic vesicle. The extent of the internalization is remarkable. It is estimated that up to 50% of the plasma membrane is internalized during phagocytosis [174]. What governs this reorganization of cellular membranes? How is the plasma membrane resynthesized? These are some of the questions that have prompted research during the past 15 years.

Reviews of metabolism of lipids in phagocytic cells are available that may be helpful to the reader [51,70].

1. Content and Synthesis of Lipids

The lipid composition of alveolar macrophages has not been examined in great detail, but there are some data for cells obtained from dogs [140], rabbits [111, 112], and rat [24]. Data on composition are difficult to evaluate because of the heterogeneity of cells obtained by lavage and because of the possibility of incomplete removal of surface-active material, which contains large amounts of phospholipid. The lipid composition of alveolar macrophages from newborn and adult animals is different (R. J. Mason and M. Williams, unpublished observations). Macrophages from newborn animals have a lipid composition consistent with the hypothesis, supported by their morphologic appearance, that they contain large amounts of ingested surface-active material. This is an example of the problems with compositional studies of phagocytic cells. Is ingested or absorbed material part of the cell?

Rabbit alveolar macrophages contain large amounts of lyso(bis)phosphatidic acid [112], but rat alveolar macrophages contain less than 2% of lyso(bis)-phosphatidic acid in their phospholipids [112]. This unusual lipid appears to be associated with lysosomal membranes, and it may serve as a stabilizing material that is resistant to most hydrolytic enzymes [20]. Analysis of macrophages from other species should include testing for this minor phospholipid.

Synthesis of lipids by alveolar macrophages has been investigated more extensively than has lipid composition of these cells. Components of complex lipids in macrophages can come from serum or be synthesized in situ. Precursors likely to come from serum include glucose, the various phospholipid bases, cholesterol, lysolecithin, and fatty acids. Intermediate compounds, cholesterol, and fatty acids are probably also synthesized by these cells. Alveolar macrophages can incorporate a variety of precursors (such as fatty acids, glycerol, choline, ethanolamine, and lysolecithin) into phospholipids and triglycerides [47-50,111]. These cells can readily synthesize the common phospholipids found in mammalian cells. Rabbit alveolar macrophages can synthesize disaturated phosphatidy-choline, the relatively unique phospholipid found in high concentrations in pulmonary surface-active material [111]. It is unlikely that macrophages contribute to the synthesis of surface-active material; it is more likely that they incorporate this phospholipid into their cellular membranes. The enzymes used in lipid synthesis have been only partially examined [48,186]. There is at least one enzyme, which is present in many cell types including polymorphonuclear leukocytes, that is apparently absent in alveolar macrophages. Rabbit alveolar macrophages are unable to convert lysolecithin to lecithin by the Erbland-Marinetti pathway (the transesterification pathway of lecithin biosynthesis) [48,54].

Synthesis of other lipids has not been thoroughly evaluated. Mixed human leukocytes lack acetyl CoA carboxylase, the first enzyme in the de novo synthesis of fatty acids and, therefore, cannot synthesize fatty acids, but they can elongate preexisting fatty acids [105]. Acetyl CoA carboxylase and fatty acid synthetase have not been studied in alveolar macrophages. Although the content of cholesterol in macrophages is quite high, the apparent rate of synthesis is quite low [189,190]. Cholesterol biosynthesis is, however, dependent on the activity of HMG CoA reductase (β-hydroxy-β-methylglutaryl coenzyme A reductase) which, in turn, is very dependent on the concentration of cholesterol in the medium. Some cells appear to have very low levels of synthesis of cholesterol in the presence of serum, but have higher rates of synthesis if deprived of serum. Alveolar macrophages can esterify cholesterol [175] and, under certain circumstances, store cholesterol as cholesterol esters [28]. There are no data on the composition or synthesis of complex glycolipids in these cells.

The possible role of lipid peroxides as part of the antimicrobial armamentarium of phagocytic cells has been suggested [168]. Lipid peroxides are known to be toxic to cells and destructive to subcellular organelles. Rancid oils have been reported to be bactericidal, and the products of lipid autoxidation have been shown to inhibit bacterial growth [75]. A major problem for this hypothesis is that polyunsaturated fatty acids are much more susceptible to lipid peroxidation than monoenic or saturated fatty acids, and bacteria and most fungi do not contain appreciable amounts of polyunsaturated fatty acids [90]. These fatty acids must, therefore, be in the phagocytic cells themselves. The amount of arachidonate (20:4) (the most likely source of lipid peroxides in phagocytic cells) varies greatly among different cell types and different species (Table 2). Information about the production of lipid peroxides is incomplete. Lipid peroxides have been found in cellular extracts and in the incubation medium during phagocytosis [112]. Malonyldialdehyde is a minor metabolite of the peroxidation of arachidonic acid and is bactericidal [168]. This compound was found in the incubation medium of phagocytosing human monocytes and alveolar macrophages from rabbits previously injected with Freund's adjuvant, but not in the medium of human polymorphonuclear leukocytes, guinea pig polymorphonuclear leukocytes, or unstimulated rabbit alveolar macrophages [112,168; R. J. Mason, unpublished observations]. The percentage of arachidonate found in total fatty acids (not shown in Table 2) and in fatty acids of phospholipids is significantly lower in normal alveolar macrophages as compared to its content in those from BCG-treated rabbits ($P < 0.05$, two-tailed t-test), but it is unlikely that this small difference in concentration of substrate is critical. It seems more plausible that the presence of detectable malonyldialdehyde in the medium is related to the efficiency of scavenging systems for degrading malonyldialdehyde. In other systems, where lipid peroxidation has been shown to be

TABLE 2 Fatty Acid Composition of Cellular Phospholipids[a]

Cell	Species	14:0[b]	16:0	16:1	18:0	18:1	18:2	20:1	20:4	20:5	22:4	22:5	22:6	24:1
Monocyte	Man	0.8	17.4	1.6	21.9	20.2	10.5	tr	20.2	tr	1.9	2.8	2.9	tr
Granulocyte	Man	0.9	20.8	0.9	17.9	29.2	11.5	tr	12.4	1.3	1.6	tr	tr	3.8
Alveolar macrophage	Rabbit	0.7	19.3	2.6	14.6	30.8	16.4	1.0	12.5	tr	0.8	tr	tr	1.4
Alveolar macrophage (BCG)	Rabbit	1.0	20.5	4.1	14.8	27.8	13.3	0.7	15.4	tr	1.1	tr	tr	1.3
Alveolar macrophage	Rat	3.6	47.4	4.8	12.6	8.6	6.5	tr	16.9	NA	NA	NA	NA	NA
Alveolar macrophage	Sheep	1.7	32.8	4.6	15.8	32.3	6.3	tr	6.0	NA	NA	NA	NA	NA
Alveolar macrophage	Dog	2.8	36.0	4.5	15.3	15.7[d]	3.1	tr	22.4	NA	NA	NA	NA	NA
Alveolar macrophage	Newborn sheep[c]	6.5	44.5	8.3	7.5	26.5	3.8	tr	2.2	NA	NA	NA	NA	NA
Alveolar macrophage	Newborn dog	4.0	46.3	5.8	10.1	8.5[d]	4.4	tr	20.9	NA	NA	NA	NA	NA

[a]The compositional data are expressed as mole percent. Methods for the analyses appear in report on human phagocytic cells [168]. All values are the mean of at least three different samples except values for newborn sheep, which are from a single sample. Methods for isolation of cells have been published [111,112,168]. Macrophages were isolated by bronchopulmonary lavage with buffered saline.

[b]The numbers represent the chain length and number of double bonds for the designated fatty acid. Trace (tr), $< 0.5\%$ of total; NA, not analyzed. Analysis of long-chain polyunsaturated fatty acids is performed with slightly different conditions than the routine method and is described [168]. There are some long-chain polyunsaturated fatty acids in the samples from dog and rat macrophages.

[c]Newborn animals are 1 week old.

[d]18:1 includes cis-5-18:1 as well as oleic acid.

important (such as in carbon tetrachloride poisoning of the liver), malonyldialdehyde does not accumulate in detectable amounts in whole tissues or slices, and is found only after incubation with subcellular organelles [145]. The mechanism of lipid peroxidation in phagocytic cells is not known. It may be enzymatic [118] or nonenzymatic, and is probably related to the hydrogen peroxide or free radicals of oxygen that are formed during phagocytosis. The physiologic importance of lipid peroxides in bacterial killing will have to be determined in future studies.

2. *Degradation of Lipids*

Alveolar macrophages, like other macrophages, must be able to digest what they ingest. They are capable of oxidizing fatty acids (R. J. Mason, unpublished observations) and hydrolyzing phospholipids [48,60,61], triglycerides [47], and cholesterol esters [40]. In the lung, these macrophages may also have the special function of removing surface-active material. During the respiratory cycle, surface-active material absorbs to the air-water interface at high lung volumes and then is compressed at low lung volumes. When the film is compressed to a low surface tension, the disaturated phosphatidylcholine that provides the low surface tension in the compressed film probably forms aggregates that will not readily resorb to the surface when the lung returns to high lung volumes. Hence, the physical state of surface-active material is probably changed during normal respiration, and new material must continually be brought to the surface to replace that which was converted to insoluble aggregates. Whereas this sequence of events is likely, there is little direct evidence to prove it.

The fate of these aggregates of disaturated phosphatidylcholine is unknown. One reasonable proposal is that the aggregates are ingested by alveolar macrophages and digested. Alveolar macrophages contain active phospholipases. These enzymes are usually assayed with phosphatidylethanolamine as the substrate [60,61], but similar hydrolysis and pH optima can also be obtained with a mixture of tritiated and hydrogenated egg phosphatidylcholine, perhaps more analogous to surface-active material (R. J. Mason, unpublished observations). In electron micrographs, occasional alveolar macrophages in normal adult animals are seen with myelinic swirls that may represent ingested surface-active material (G. Huber and M. Williams, personal communication). In newborn dogs, intracellular inclusions in macrophages stain as phospholipids by light microscopy, have an increased number of myelinic figures by electron microscopy, and an increased content of disaturated phosphatidylcholine by lipid analysis (R. J. Mason and M. Williams, unpublished observations).

This is circumstantial evidence that macrophages may be able to ingest and to digest surface-active material. It is very difficult to show significant ingestion of surface-active material by human alveolar macrophages in tissue culture, or by rabbit alveolar macrophages in suspension (A. B. Cohen and R. J. Mason, unpublished observations). Naimark [129] presented kinetic data that suggest that alveolar macrophages ingest disaturated phosphatidylcholine in vivo because of the time of appearance of labeled disaturated phosphatidylcholine onto the alveolar surface and into alveolar macrophages after the injection of [^{14}C] palmitate. Finley [57] found less extracellular surface-active material in lavage fluid from smokers than from nonsmokers. This suggests that macrophages from smokers may ingest more surface-active material than normal cells, and that this process might produce some of the pathologic lesions found in lungs of smokers. There are, however, alternative routes for the disposal of surface-active material, such as removal up the airway or transport across the alveolar epithelium.

E. Subcellular Fractionation

Isolation of subcellular organelles is important for localizing and studying the control of certain metabolic processes and for the initial purification of certain enzymes. This is especially important when the homogenate contains inhibitors of enzymatic reactions. The classic methods of subcellular fractionation, rate sedimentation and isopynic density centrifugation, have been applied to alveolar macrophages [36,37,61,124,161,162]. Because the intent of these studies was the purification of a single organelle or enzymatic activity, most studies have not included data on enzyme markers, balance sheets for calculations of recovery, or electron microscopic verification of the separated fractions. The separation of lysosomes from mitochondria is difficult [36,61,162]. Studies with isolated mitochondria from alveolar macrophages have not shown that the fraction was free of lysosomal contamination [124]. Similarly, isolated lysosomes have not been shown to be free of mitochondria [7,162]. An excellent study of the isolation and separation of acid phosphatase activity from alveolar macrophages was reported by Axline [7]. This paper shows the difficulties of solubilizing certain lysosomal enzymes and the advantages of using a nonionic detergent (Triton) in preference to serial freezing and thawing, vigorous homogenization with a Teflon pestle, and use of a French press. Measurement of different enzymatic activities in lysosomes of different densities has recently been reported, but definite resolution of various lysosomal enzymes into different populations of lysosomes has not been achieved [161,162]. In polymorphonuclear leukocytes, which are structurally less complex, different granule fractions with different enzymatic activities have been isolated and characterized [5,6,17,120, 188]. There have been two reports of isolation of plasma membrane fractions from alveolar macrophages [124,128], and one report of isolation of these fractions from mouse peritoneal macrophages in tissue culture [191]. Phagocytic vesicles, composed of plasma membrane, lysosomal membranes, lysosomal enzymes, and ingested particles, have been isolated by allowing cells to ingest particles and isolating the ingested particles and their cellular coat by buoyant density centrifugation [128,166,191].

V. Alterations in Metabolism

This section discusses changes in metabolism that accompany adaptation to the lung, phagocytosis, activation, and exposure to cigarette smoke. These changes are difficult to study in vivo because of turnover of cells (Chap. 20) and recruitment of new cells either from the blood or elsewhere in the lung when changes occur in the environment or in the host. Consequently, most studies examine freshly collected cells for short-term experiments in vitro. These studies are adequate for investigating phagocytosis and effects of some drugs, hormones, and toxic gases. However, processes that require cell division or new synthesis of enzymes cannot be studied in this manner; they must be investigated in vivo or in tissue culture where the environment can be partially regulated and the cells will survive for several days or weeks. Major questions are: How do these cells respond to changes in their environment? If most macrophages come from the bone marrow, how do these cells adjust to the lung? How do cells change in response to immunologic signals produced during viral infections or tuberculosis? Is it a failure in the "activation" of macrophages that allows primary tuberculosis or certain fungal diseases to disseminate in a few individuals? What is the role of transfer factor in the activation process caused by an immunologic challenge [23]? What is the role of the macrophage in surveillance for tumor cells? How are all these processes affected by the lung and by the dust burden we voluntarily or involuntarily give it?

A. Adaptation to the Lung

This section assumes that alveolar macrophages originate in the bone marrow, migrate to the lungs as monocytes, and develop into alveolar macrophages in the lung. This sequence of events has been demonstrated for the majority of alveolar macrophages lavaged from irradiated animals and from stimulated hosts [21,66,142,181]. Whether it is true in the normal animal is not known. There is, however, evidence that all alveolar macrophages do not originate in the bone marrow [13,43,68,110,158]. It is likely that alveolar macrophages have a very long lifetime (months) [31,69,181], but the exact duration is not known.

Very little is known about adaptation of macrophages to the lung. Differences between macrophages isolated from the peritoneum and those isolated from the lung suggest that there is some metabolic adaptation; for example, alveolar macrophages appear to have greater dependence on aerobic metabolism [27,132,133,149]. Some of the environmental differences that potentially affect the activity of macrophages in alveolar spaces are high oxygen tension, the presence of surface-active material, the possibility of a low pH and low concentrations of metabolic substrates in the hypophase, and the possibility of regional differences in types of lymphocytes in the lung [86]. The pH and composition of the fluid that lines the alveolar spaces in air-breathing animals is not known because of obvious sampling difficulties, but in the fetal lamb the pH of alveolar fluid is 6.3 [3]. In the adult it is likely that the fluid volume and the buffering capacity of the hypophase are very small. There are no reports on the concentrations of the substrates necessary for energy production, such as glucose, fatty acids, or lactate, in the hypophase or in liquid from fetal lung. Analysis of the types of lymphocytes obtained by endobronchial lavage has suggested there may be regional differences in lymphocytes within the lung. In healthy normal dogs only B cells are found in fluid obtained by lavage. After deposition of antigen or irritants through the airway, both B and T lymphocytes are recovered in the fluid from lavage [85-87]. It is probably the T lymphocytes that are important for activating or influencing behavior of macrophages by secreting various lymphokines [179].

Although the study of adaptation of macrophages to the lung is an intriguing subject, experimental approaches are difficult. Robin and coworkers have begun to examine this important problem. They measured the isoenzymes of lactate dehydrogenase in alveolar and exudative peritoneal macrophages of the rabbit [158]. The isoenzymes of lactate hydrogenase were markedly different in the two cell types, suggesting that there is enzymatic adaptation in the lung or that the cells arise from different precursors. This group of investigators have exposed mouse peritoneal macrophages in tissue culture to normal and low oxygen tensions, and followed changes in pyruvate kinase and cytochrome oxidase as indicators of glycolytic and oxidative metabolism [160]. There was an increase in pyruvate kinase and a decrease in cytochrome oxidase during hypoxia. In the normal adaptation to conditions of tissue culture in the presence of serum there is an increase in both cytochrome oxidase and pyruvate kinase [10,160]. To ascertain whether adaptation of macrophages to the lung is a physiologically important process will require greater knowledge of the source of these cells in the normal host, of the extent to which macrophages normally multiply in the interstitium of the lung, of the life span of alveolar macrophages in vivo, of the distribution and movement of macrophages within the lung, and of the location from which cells are obtained by lavage.

B. Phagocytosis

Metabolic alterations during phagocytosis are much easier to study. Phagocytosis includes two major sequential events. One is recognition and attachment of the particle—this step may not be energy-dependent and may occur at 4°C [177]; the other is the internalization of the particle—this step is energy-dependent. The second step includes fusion of the plasma membrane with the lysosomal membranes, and the concomitant release of lysosomal enzymes into the newly formed vesicle. Certain metabolic alterations are apparent only during the initial 10 min, when the uptake of most particles takes place; they may be missed if measurements are made only during prolonged periods [149]. Table 3 shows some of the metabolic alterations that have been reported to occur during phagocytosis by alveolar macrophages. No selection has been made for the type of particle ingested. The metabolic response may well depend on the nature of the particle [9,42,83,169] as well as on the basal activity of the cells. The only apparent discrepancy in the reports is the level of cyclic AMP in alveolar macrophages during phagocytosis. Manganiello and coworkers [107] found no changes in cyclic AMP in rabbit alveolar macrophages, and very large changes in mixed human leukocytes but not in purified phagocytic cells. Seyberth et al. [156] found a very small increase (note the values of the ordinate in their Fig. 3).

Energy for phagocytosis by alveolar macrophages is derived from the Krebs cycle, the pentose pathway, and glycolysis. This is the only phagocytic cell that uses the Krebs cycle for a major part of its energy production [28,132, 133,149]. The exact contribution of the different energy pathways has not been determined. The oxidation of glucose via the pentose pathway in human polymorphonuclear leukocytes is 1.3% during basal conditions and 30% during phagocytosis [164]. In guinea pig peritoneal macrophages from exudates, the pentose cycle accounts for 1% of glucose utilization during basal conditions and 3-6% during phagocytosis [192]. Increases in oxygen consumption and oxidation of 1-[^{14}C] glucose occur immediately at the start of ingestion [121,149, 167]. The initiation of the pentose pathway is likely to be caused by an increased concentration of $NADP^+$ [63,136], but the oxidases involved in the production of hydrogen peroxide and the ultimate formation of $NADP^+$ are still controversial [165]. There is evidence for a granule-associated cyanide-insensitive NADPH oxidase [83,136,138,164] and a cyanide-insensitive NADH oxidase in polymorphonuclear leukocytes [88]. In the alveolar macrophage there is a NADPH oxidase that is sensitive to cyanide [148,149]. Regardless of how hydrogen peroxide might be formed, it can generate $NADP^+$ by oxidizing reduced glutathione, and the oxidized glutathione can be reconverted to reduced glutathione by glutathione reductase with the resultant generation of $NADP^+$ [63,64].

Many of the metabolic concomitants of phagocytosis, such as increased oxygen consumption and activity of the pentose pathway, do not require uptake of particles. They can be produced by alterations in the plasma membrane by phospholipase C, endotoxin, digitonin, or detergents [71,152]. The mechanism

TABLE 3 Representative Values for Metabolic Changes During Phagocytosis by Alveolar Macrophages

Variable	Increase	No change	Decrease
Oxygen consumption	63, 64, 132, 56, 132, 149		
Glucose oxidation	64, 132, 152		
Pyruvate oxidation	63, 152		
Hydrogen peroxide production	63, 64		
Formate oxidation	64, 152		
Acetate oxidation		63, 152	
Succinate oxidation		152	
Lipid synthesis		132, 134, a	
Protein synthesis			117
Reduced glutathione level	152, 183		
NADPH oxidase activity[b]	148, 149		
Release of lysosomal enzymes	1, 152		
Cyclic AMP levels	156	107	
Uptake of amino acids and adenosine		174	

[a]R. J. Mason, unpublished observations.
[b]NADPH, reduced nicotinamide adenine dinucleotide phosphate.

of the coupling of changes in the plasma and lysosomal membranes to the metabolic processes in the cytosol is not known.

Because a great portion (~35-50%) of the plasma membrane may be internalized during phagocytosis, early attention was given to membrane synthesis, especially in terms of phospholipid synthesis [174]. There is no measurable net synthesis of membrane lipids during phagocytosis in mammalian cells or amoebae [46,132,133,178,191]. The most complete long-term studies are those by Werb and Cohn, who studied synthesis of membrane constituents in cultured mouse peritoneal macrophages [189-191]. New synthesis of plasma membrane was detectable 6 hr after ingestion as measured by incorporation of cholesterol, synthesis of phospholipids, and increase in the content of 5′-nucleotidase, an enzyme marker of the plasma membrane [191].

During phagocytosis in polymorphonuclear leukocytes, there is increased synthesis of two minor phospholipids, phosphatidic acid and phosphatidylinositol. This increased synthesis is not explained by changes in specific activity of adenosine triphosphate [154] and is, in part, caused by increased activity of diglyceride kinase [172]. In polymorphonuclear leukocytes, there is also increased incorporation of myo-[^{3}H] inositol, which has caused speculation about the turnover of cytidine diphosphate-diglyceride [172]. There is no increased synthesis of phosphatidylinositol or phosphatidic acid by alveolar macrophages during phagocytosis [132,133]. Elsbach has shown that, during phagocytosis, both alveolar macrophages and polymorphonuclear leukocytes incorporate more lysolecithin from the incubation medium into cellular lecithin [50]. The fatty acids used in the acylation of lysolecithin in polymorphonuclear leukocytes come predominantly from cellular triglycerides and not from fatty acids in the medium [52,157]. The lecithin that is formed is found in the plasma membrane and in the phagocytic vesicle [53]; there is, however, no change in the total content of cellular lecithin, so there must also be concomitant degradation equal to the new synthesis [46,51]. This rapid turnover of lysolecithin may be very important for fusion of the plasma membrane and the lysosomal membranes [104]. Thus, during phagocytosis there is a great rearrangement of parts of the plasma membrane associated with increased labeling of certain phospholipids, but no net synthesis of major membrane components.

C. Activation

Macrophages can be "activated," by which I mean macrophages can be treated so that functionally they have an increased ability to adhere to glass, oxidize a greater percentage of glucose via the pentose pathway (especially in response to a phagocytic load), have an increased content of lysosomal enzymes, and are probably better microbial killers. This process can be accomplished by a variety of means, including immunization with BCG, *Listeria,* or *Pertussis,* chronic exposure to noxious gases such as cigarette smoke, and maintenance in tissue culture in the presence of high concentrations of serum. These different processes have not been extensively studied in alveolar macrophages; the actual biochemical changes that lead to these functional and metabolic alterations are not known, and may be different for the different treatments. The effects of treatment of rabbits with BCG or Freund's adjuvant are discussed below, and the differences in alveolar macrophages obtained from smokers and nonsmokers are discussed in the following section.

The majority of the work on the effect of stimulation with BCG has been performed by Myrvik and his collaborators [56,99,125,127,162]. This treatment greatly increases the yield of cells obtained by bronchopulmonary lavage [127]. These cells differ morphologically from cells obtained from untreated rabbits in that they have more rough endoplasmic reticulum [11], increased numbers of microfilaments [99], increased numbers of dumbbell-shaped phagolysosomes [99,101], and increased numbers of mitochondria [125]. Biochemically these cells have increased oxygen consumption (Table 1), probably increased activity of the pentose pathway [56], increased creatine phosphokinase [41], and increased concentrations of lysosomal enzymes [36,78,127]. Conclusions about the pentose pathway from comparison of the oxidation of 1-[^{14}C]-glucose and 6-[^{14}] glucose without simultaneous measurement of glucose utilization are not justified [91].

Interestingly, the increase in lysosomal enzymes is not uniform, and there is a much greater increase in lysozyme and acid phosphatase than in β-glucuronidase or acid ribonuclease [162]. Depending on the particle or bacteria tested, these cells may or may not have increased rates of phagocytosis [113,169] and ability to kill organisms [55,100]; there is an increased rate of transfer of hydrolytic enzymes to the phagocytic vacuole [166]. "Toxic" polymorphonuclear leukocytes are somewhat similar in that they have increased numbers of dumbbell-shaped granules (increased β-glucuronidase but not acid phosphatase) and increased rough endoplasmic reticulum, as well as increased reduction of nitroblue tetrazolium (phagocytosis) [119].

Some "activation" of macrophages may be present (as a result of the previous exposure history of the host), which is apparently caused by subclinical infection. For example, Heise and associates reported a seasonal variation in the content of lysosomal enzymes of rabbit alveolar macrophages, presumably related to infection with *Bordetella bronchiseptica* [78]. Similarly, peripheral monocytes from patients with tuberculosis consume more oxygen and glucose than monocytes from control individuals [135]. One wonders about the metabolic state of monocytes from patients with other granulomatous diseases of the chest. Variations in hosts, in addition to cigarette smoking, may lead to considerable variation in the metabolic state of macrophages from human subjects. Whereas it is likely that alveolar macrophages do respond to challenges from inhaled material or from local pulmonary infections, it is less certain how systemic alterations caused by nonpulmonary disorders may affect alveolar macrophages. Truit et al. have indicated that it is difficult to activate pulmonary macrophages by systemic immunization [173].

D. Cigarette Smoke

There is an apparent paradox between the direct toxic effect of cigarette smoke on macrophages in vitro and the reduced bacterial clearance in vivo using rodent models in contrast with the very active, viable macrophages obtained from people who smoke cigarettes. The answer to the paradox is the difficulty in comparing the acute effects of very high doses of tobacco smoke with the chronic effects of low doses of tobacco smoke. Acute exposure to high concentrations of tobacco smoke causes decreased bacterial clearance in vivo [97]. However, there is no question that tobacco smoke is toxic to macrophages and other cell types in vitro [72,79,103]. Tobacco smoke and aqueous extracts of smoke produce decreased rates of phagocytosis [72], decreased oxygen consumption [196], and decreased protein synthesis in alveolar macrophages [80,103,194]. However, alveolar macrophages harvested by bronchopulmonary lavage from individuals who smoke cigarettes appear to be active, healthy cells. Smokers have increased numbers of alveolar macrophages in the small peripheral airways [130]. Pulmonary lavage produces more cells and a higher percentage of macrophages in smokers than in nonsmokers [68,77,143,147]. As contrasted to the appearance of cells from nonsmokers, the cells from smokers have many more pleomorphic cytoplasmic inclusions, a more extensive Golgi apparatus, more rough endoplasmic reticulum, and more microfilaments [19,77,109,143,144]. Metabolically, they oxidize more glucose and have a greater content of acid hydrolases, especially acid phosphatase, β-glucuronidase, and proteases [76,77, 109]. Functionally, they migrate more rapidly in vitro but do not respond to macrophage inhibitory factor [187]. There is no difference in the rate of phagocytosis of bacteria and yeasts by macrophages from these two different hosts [77,108].

These findings are quite similar to the differences in rabbit alveolar macrophages harvested from normal animals and from those stimulated with BCG. The explanation for the difference in findings of toxic effects of cigarette smoke on normal cells in vitro and the healthy cells from cigarette smokers is most likely related to the dose and duration of exposure. Holt and Keast showed that peritoneal macrophages in tissue culture actually have an increased rate of incorporation of amino acids into protein if they are given a low dose of smoke for 4 days [80]. There is still much to be learned about the effects of cigarette smoke on macrophages in vivo and in vitro, especially low-level chronic exposures.

VI. Future

The review of the literature for the preparation of this chapter suggested several areas of investigation that should be pursued in the near future. Are the cells recovered by endobronchial lavage the same cells that inactivate aerosolized bacteria in vivo? Because the percentage of macrophages that are recovered by lavage is low, one wonders if they are a peculiar and distinctive subpopulation of the total number of pulmonary macrophages. Answers to this problem will require a combination of biochemical, functional, and morphometric studies on intact lungs, and on cells harvested by lavage as well as from minced tissue [92, 132]. Another intriguing question is how do alveolar macrophages adapt to the lung? What makes some monocytes go to the spleen, peritoneum, liver, lymph nodes, or bone marrow and others go to the lung? Where do alveolar macrophages originate in the normal, nonirradiated animal? A final series of questions involves alveolar macrophages in man. Are there disease states in which the primary defect is in the pulmonary macrophage system? Are there disease states that could lead to understanding of chemotaxis and killing mechanisms, such as have been helpful in unraveling some of the metabolic processes in polymorphonuclear leukocytes [91,169]?

Acknowledgment

The author is an Established Investigator of the American Heart Association and a member of the Cardiovascular Research Institute, University of California, San Francisco, California.

This work was supported in part by the National Heart and Lung Institute (research grant HL-6285).

References

1. N. R. Ackerman and J. R. Beebe, Release of β glucuronidase and elastase from alveolar mononuclear cells, *Chest,* **66** [Suppl]: 21S-23S (1974).
2. J. D. Acton and Q. N. Myrvik, Production of interferon by alveolar macrophages, *J. Bacteriol.,* **91**:2300-2304 (1966).
3. T. M. Adamson, R. D. H. Boyd, H. S. Platt, and L. B. Strang, Composition of alveolar liquid in the foetal lamb, *J. Physiol.,* **204**:159-168 (1969).
4. E. Atkins, P. Bodel, and L. Francis, Release of an endogenous pyrogen in vitro from rabbit mononuclear cells, *J. Exp. Med.,* **126**:357-384 (1967).
5. J. L. Avila and J. Convit, Studies on human polymorphonuclear leukocyte enzymes. I. Assay of acid hydrolases and other enzymes, *Biochim. Biophys. Acta,* **293**:397-408 (1973).
6. J. L. Avila and J. Convit, Studies on human polymorphonuclear leukocyte enzymes. II. Comparative study of the physical properties of primary and specific granules, *Biochim. Biophys. Acta,* **293**:409-423 (1973).
7. S. G. Axline, Isozymes of acid phosphatase in normal and Calmette-Guérin bacillus-induced rabbit alveolar macrophages, *J. Exp. Med.,* **128**:1031-1048 (1968).
8. S. G. Axline, Functional biochemistry of the macrophage, *Semin. Hematol.,* **7**:142-160 (1970).
9. S. G. Axline and Z. A. Cohn, In vitro induction of lysosomal enzymes by phagocytosis, *J. Exp. Med.,* **131**:1239-1260 (1970).
10. W. E. Bennett and Z. A. Cohn, The isolation and selected properties of blood monocytes, *J. Exp. Med.,* **123**:145-160 (1966).
11. A. G. Bhagwat and P. E. Conen, Characterization of "free alveolar cells" in experimental adjuvant induced pneumonia, *Arch. Pathol.,* **88**:21-29 (1969).

12. D. H. Bowden, The alveolar macrophage, *Curr. Top. Pathol.*, **55**:1-36 (1971).
13. D. H. Bowden and I. Y. R. Adamson, The pulmonary interstitial cell as immediate precursor of the alveolar macrophage, *Am. J. Pathol.*, **68**:521-528 (1972).
14. R. O. Brady, A. E. Gal, and P. G. Pentchev, Evolution of enzyme replacement therapy for lipid storage diseases, *Life Sci.*, **15**:1235-1248 (1974).
15. J. D. Brain, The effects of increased particles on the number of alveolar macrophages. In *Inhaled Particles III*, Proceedings of an International Symposium Organized by the British Occupational Hygiene Society in London, 14-23 September 1970, Vol. 1. Edited by W. H. Walton. Surrey, England, Unwin, Gresham Press, Old Woking, 1971, pp. 209-225.
16. J. D. Brain and R. Frank, Alveolar macrophage adhesion; wash electrolyte composition and free cell yield, *J. Appl. Physiol.*, **34**:75-80 (1973).
17. U. Bretz and M. Baggiolini, Biochemical and morphological characterization of azurophil and specific granules of human neutrophilic polymorphonuclear leukocytes, *J. Cell Biol.*, **63**:251-269 (1974).
18. J. C. Briscoe, An experimental investigation of the phagocytic action of the alveolar cells of the lung, *J. Pathol. Bacteriol.*, **12**:66-96 (1908).
19. A. R. Brody and J. E. Craighead, Cytoplasmic inclusions in pulmonary macrophages of cigarette smokers, *Lab. Invest.*, **32**:125-132 (1975).
20. J. Brotherus, O. Renkonen, J. Herrmann, and W. Fischer, Novel stereoconfiguration in lyso-bis-phosphatidic acid of cultured BHK-cells, *Chem. Phys. Lipids*, **13**:178-182 (1974).
21. M. A. Brunstetter, J. A. Hardie, R. Schiff, J. P. Lewis, and C. E. Cross, The origin of pulmonary alveolar macrophages: Studies of stem cells using the Es-2 marker of mice, *Arch. Intern. Med.*, **127**:1064-1068 (1971).
22. E. T. Cantrell, G. A. Warr, D. L. Busbee, and R. R. Martin, Induction of aryl hydrocarbon hydroxylase in human pulmonary alveolar macrophages by cigarette smoking, *J. Clin. Invest.*, **52**:1881-1884 (1973).
23. A. Catanzaro, L. Spitler, and K. M. Moser, Immunotherapy of coccidiodomycosis, *J. Clin. Invest.*, **54**:690-701 (1974).
24. C. Champanet and G. Soula, Le phosphatidylglycérol des macrophages pulmonaires de rat: Composition en acides gras, *Biochimie*, **56**:1147-1150 (1974).
25. D. L. Coffin, D. E. Gardner, R. S. Holzman, and F. J. Wolock, Influence of ozone on pulmonary cells, *Arch. Environ. Health*, **16**:633-636 (1968).
26. A. B. Cohen, Interrelationships between the human alveolar macrophage and alpha-1-antitrypsin, *J. Clin. Invest.*, **52**:2793-2799 (1973).
27. A. B. Cohen and M. J. Cline, The human alveolar macrophage: Isolation, cultimation in vitro, and studies of morphologic and functional characteristics, *J. Clin. Invest.*, **50**:1390-1398 (1971).
28. A. B. Cohen and M. J. Cline, In vitro studies of the foamy macrophage of postobstructive endogenous lipoid pneumonia in man, *Am. Rev. Respir. Dis.*, **106**:69-78 (1972).
29. A. B. Cohen and D. Geczy, Purification of two populations of human

alveolar macrophages from surgical specimens, *Am. Rev. Respir. Dis.*, **108**: 972-975 (1973).

30. A. B. Cohen and W. M. Gold, Defense mechanisms of the lungs, *Annu. Rev. Physiol.*, **37**:325-350 (1975).
31. Z. A. Cohn, The structure and function of monocytes and macrophages, *Adv. Immunol.*, **9**:163-214 (1968).
32. Z. A. Cohn and B. Benson, The differentiation of mononuclear phagocytes: Morphology, cytochemistry, and biochemistry, *J. Exp. Med.*, **121**: 153-169 (1965).
33. Z. A. Cohn and B. Benson, The in vitro differentiation of mononuclear phagocytes. II. The influence of serum on granule formation, hydrolase production, and pinocytosis, *J. Exp. Med.*, **121**:835-848 (1965).
34. Z. A. Cohn and B. A. Ehrenreich, The uptake, storage, and intracellular hydrolysis of carbohydrates by macrophages, *J. Exp. Med.*, **129**:201-226 (1969).
35. Z. A. Cohn, J. G. Hirsch, and M. E. Fedorko, The in vitro differentiation of mononuclear phagocytes. IV. The ultrastructure of macrophage differentiation in the peritoneal cavity and in culture, *J. Exp. Med.*, **123**:747-756 (1966).
36. Z. A. Cohn and E. Wiener, The particulate hydrolases of macrophages. I. Comparative enzymology, isolation, and properties, *J. Exp. Med.*, **118**: 991-1008 (1963).
37. C. E. Cross, M. G. Mustafa, P. Peterson, and J. A. Hardie, Pulmonary alveolar macrophage: Membrane associated sodium ion, potassium ion, and magnesium ion adenosine triphosphatase system, *Arch. Intern. Med.*, **127**: 1069-1077 (1971).
38. C. N. Davies (ed.), *Inhaled Particles and Vapours,* Proceedings of an International Symposium Organized by the British Occupational Hygiene Society, Oxford, 29 March–1 April 1960. New York, Pergamon, 1961.
39. C. N. Davies (ed.), *Inhaled Particles and Vapours II,* Proceedings of an International Symposium Organized by the British Occupational Hygiene Society, Cambridge, 28 September–1 October 1965. New York, Pergamon, 1967.
40. A. J. Day, Lipid metabolism by macrophages and its relationship to atherosclerosis, *Adv. Lipid Res.*, **5**:185-207 (1967).
41. L. R. DeChatelet, C. E. McCall, and P. S. Shirley, Creatine phosphokinase activity in rabbit alveolar macrophages, *Infect. Immun.*, **7**:29-34 (1973).
42. L. R. DeChatelet, P. Wang, and C. E. McCall, Hexose monophosphate shunt activity and oxygen consumption during phagocytosis: Temporal sequence, *Proc. Soc. Exp. Biol. Med.*, **140**:1434-1436 (1972).
43. D. P. Dressler and W. A. Skornik, Specificity of rat anti-alveolar macrophage serum [abstract], *J. Reticuloendothel. Soc.*, **15**:55a (1974).
44. B. A. Ehrenreich and Z. A. Cohn, Fate of hemoglobin pinocytosed by macrophages in vitro, *J. Cell Biol.*, **38**:244-248 (1968).

45. B. A. Ehrenreich and Z. A. Cohn, The fate of peptides pinocytosed by macrophages in vitro, *J. Exp. Med.*, **129**:227-245 (1969).
46. P. Elsbach, Composition and synthesis of lipids in resting and phagocytizing leukocytes, *J. Exp. Med.*, **110**:969-980 (1959).
47. P. Elsbach, Uptake of fat by phagocytic cells. An examination of the role of phagocytosis. II. Rabbit alveolar macrophages, *Biochim. Biophys. Acta*, **98**:420-431 (1965).
48. P. Elsbach, Phospholipid metabolism by phagocytic cells. I. A comparison of conversion of [^{32}P]lysolecithin to lecithin and glycerylphosphorylcholine by homogenates of rabbit polymorphonuclear leukocytes and alveolar macrophages, *Biochim. Biophys. Acta*, **125**:510-524 (1966).
49. P. Elsbach, Metabolism of lysophosphatidyl ethanolamine and lysophosphatidyl choline by homogenates of rabbit polymorphonuclear leukocytes and alveolar macrophages, *J. Lipid Res.*, **8**:359-365 (1967).
50. P. Elsbach, Increased synthesis of phospholipids during phagocytosis, *J. Clin. Invest.*, **47**:2217-2229 (1968).
51. P. Elsbach, Lipid metabolism by phagocytes, *Semin. Hematol.*, **9**:227-239 (1972).
52. P. Elsbach and S. Farrow, Cellular triglyceride as a source of fatty acid for lecithin synthesis during phagocytosis, *Biochim. Biophys. Acta*, **176**:438-441 (1969).
53. P. Elsbach, P. Patriarca, P. Pettis, T. P. Stossel, R. J. Mason, and M. Vaughan, The appearance of lecithin-^{32}P, synthesized from lysolecithin-^{32}P, in phagosomes of polymorphonuclear leukocytes, *J. Clin. Invest.*, **51**:1910-1914 (1972).
54. J. F. Erbland and G. V. Marinetti, The enzymatic acylation and hydrolysis of lysolecithin, *Biochim. Biophys. Acta*, **106**:128-138 (1965).
55. D. G. Evans and Q. N. Myrvik, Increased phagocytic and bactericidal activities of alveolar macrophages after vaccination with killed BCG [abstract], *J. Reticuloendothel. Soc.*, **4**:428-429 (1967).
56. D. G. Evans and Q. N. Myrvik, Studies on glucose oxidation during the interaction of alveolar macrophages and bacteria, *Ann. NY Acad. Sci.*, **154**:167-176 (1968).
57. T. N. Finley and A. J. Ladman, Low yield of pulmonary surfactant in cigarette smokers, *N. Engl. J. Med.*, **286**:223-227 (1972).
58. T. N. Finley, E. W. Swenson, W. S. Curran, G. L. Huber, and A. J. Ladman, Bronchopulmonary lavage in normal subjects and patients with obstructive lung disease, *Ann. Intern. Med.*, **66**:651-658 (1967).
59. A. B. Fisher, S. Diamond, and S. Mellen, Effect of O_2 exposure on metabolism of the rabbit alveolar macrophage, *J. Appl. Physiol.*, **37**:341-345 (1974).
60. R. Franson, S. Beckerdite, P. Wang, M. Waite, and P. Elsbach, Some properties of phospholipases of alveolar macrophages, *Biochim. Biophys. Acta*, **296**:365-373 (1973).
61. R. C. Franson and M. Waite, Lysosomal phospholipases A_1 and A_2 of

normal and bacillus Calmette Guerin-induced alveolar macrophages, *J. Cell Biol.,* **56**:621-627 (1973).

62. J. B. L. Gee, The alveolar macrophage: Pulmonary frontiersman [editorial], *Am. J. Med. Sci.,* **260**:195-201 (1970).
63. J. B. L. Gee, C. L. Vassallo, P. Bell, J. Kaskin, R. E. Basford, and J. B. Field, Catalase-dependent peroxidative metabolism in the alveolar macrophage during phagocytosis, *J. Clin. Invest.,* **49**:1280-1287 (1970).
64. J. B. L. Gee, C. L. Vassallo, M. T. Vogt, C. Thomas, and R. E. Basford, Peroxidative metabolism in alveolar macrophages, *Arch. Intern. Med.,* **127**: 1046-1049 (1971).
65. D. Gemsa, H. H. Fudenberg, and R. Schmid, Steroid effect on erythrophagocytosis and heme oxygenase induction in macrophages in vitro, In *"Non-specific" Factors Influencing Host Resistance.* Edited by W. Braun and J. Ungar. Basel, S. Karger, 1973, pp. 129-136.
66. J. J. Godleski and J. D. Brain, The origin of alveolar macrophages in mouse radiation chimeras, *J. Exp. Med.,* **136**:630-643 (1972).
67. D. W. Golde, T. N. Finley, and M. J. Cline, Production of colony-stimulating factor by human macrophages, *Lancet,* **2**:1397-1399 (1972).
68. D. W. Golde, T. N. Finley, and M. J. Cline, The pulmonary macrophage in acute leukemia, *N. Engl. J. Med.,* **290**:875-878 (1974).
69. S. Gordon and Z. A. Cohn, The macrophage, *Int. Rev. Cytol.,* **36**:171-214 (1973).
70. E. L. Gottfried, Lipid patterns of leukocytes in health and disease, *Semin. Hematol.,* **9**:241-250 (1972).
71. R. C. Graham, Jr., M. J. Karnovsky, A. W. Shafer, E. A. Glass, and M. L. Karnovsky, Metabolic and morphological observations on the effect of surface-active agents on leukocytes, *J. Cell Biol.,* **32**:629-647 (1967).
72. G. M. Green and D. Carolin, The depressant effect of cigarette smoke on the in vitro antibacterial activity of alveolar macrophages, *N. Engl. J. Med.,* **276**:421-427 (1967).
73. G. M. Green and E. H. Kass, The role of the alveolar macrophage in the clearance of bacteria from the lung, *J. Exp. Med.,* **119**:167-176 (1964).
74. P. Gross, T. P. deTreville, E. B. Tolker, M. Kaschak, and M. A. Babyak, The pulmonary macrophage response to irritants: An attempt at quantitation, *Arch. Environ. Health,* **18**:174-185 (1969).
75. J. M. C. Gutteridge, P. Lamport, and T. L. Dormandy, Autoxidation as a cause of antibacterial activity in unsaturated fatty acids, *J. Med. Microbiol.,* **7**:387-389 (1974).
76. J. O. Harris, G. N. Olsen, J. R. Castle, and A. S. Maloney, Comparison of proteolytic enzyme activity in pulmonary alveolar macrophages and blood leukocytes in smokers and nonsmokers, *Am. Rev. Respir. Dis.,* **111**:579-586 (1975).
77. J. O. Harris, E. W. Swenson, and J. E. Johnson III, Human alveolar macrophages: Comparison of phagocytic ability, glucose utilization, and ultrastructure in smokers and nonsmokers, *J. Clin. Invest.,* **49**:2086-2096 (1970).

78. E. R. Heise, Q. N. Myrvik, and E. S. Leake, Effect of bacillus Calmette-Guérin on the levels of acid phosphatase, lysozyme and cathepsin in rabbit alveolar macrophages, *J. Immunol.*, **95**:125-130 (1965).
79. P. G. Holt and D. Keast, Route effects of cigarette smoke on murine macrophages, *Arch. Environ. Health,* **26**:300-304 (1973).
80. P. G. Holt and D. Keast, The effect of tobacco smoke on protein synthesis in macrophages, *Proc. Soc. Exp. Biol. Med.*, **142**:1243-1247 (1973).
81. M. Holub and R. E. Hauser, Lung alveolar histiocytes engaged in antibody production, *Immunology,* **17**:207-226 (1969).
82. C. L. Ilgen and P. M. Burkholder, Effect of anti-C_4 by guinea pig peritoneal macrophages, pulmonary macrophages, liver or spleen cells, *J. Reticuloendothel. Soc.*, **15**:185-192 (1974).
83. G. Y. N. Iyer, M. F. Islam, and J. H. Quastel, Biochemical aspects of phagocytosis, *Nature,* **192**:535-541 (1961).
84. T. C. Jones, Macrophages and intracellular parasitism, *J. Reticuloendothel. Soc.*, **15**:439-450 (1974).
85. H. B. Kaltreider, L. Kyselka, and S. E. Salmon, Immunology of the lower respiratory tract. II. The plaque-forming response of canine lymphoid tissues to sheep erythrocytes after intrapulmonary or intravenous immunization, *J. Clin. Invest.*, **54**:263-270 (1974).
86. H. B. Kaltreider and S. E. Salmon, Immunology of the lower respiratory tract: Functional properties of bronchoalveolar lymphocytes obtained from the normal canine lung, *J. Clin. Invest.*, **52**:2211-2217 (1973).
87. H. B. Kaltreider, F. N. Turner, and S. E. Salmon, A canine model for comparative study of respiratory and systemic immunologic reactions, *Am. Rev. Respir. Dis.*, **111**:257-265 (1975).
88. M. L. Karnovsky, Chronic granulomatous disease—pieces of a cellular and molecular puzzle, *Fed. Proc.*, **32**:1527-1533 (1973).
89. M. L. Karnovsky, S. Simmons, E. A. Glass, A. W. Shafer, and P. D. Hart, Metabolism of macrophages, in *Mononuclear Phagocytes.* Edited by R. van Furth. Philadelphia, Pa., F. A. Davis, 1970, pp. 103-120.
90. M. Kates, Bacterial lipids, *Adv. Lipid Res.*, **2**:17-90 (1964).
91. J. Katz and H. G. Wood, The use of $C^{14}O_2$ yields from glucose-1 and -6-C^{14} for the evaluation of the pathways of glucose metabolism, *J. Biol. Chem.*, **238**:517-523 (1963).
92. Y. Kikkawa and K. Yoneda, The type II epithelial cell of the lung. I. Method of isolation, *Lab. Invest.*, **30**:76-84 (1974).
93. K. H. Kilburn, Clearance zones in the distal lung, *Ann. NY Acad. Sci.*, **221**:276-281 (1974).
94. K. H. Kilburn, Functional morphology of the distal lung, *Int. Rev. Cytol.*, **37**:153-270 (1974).
95. R. E. Kirsch, L. O. Frith, and S. J. Saunders, Albumin catabolism in vitro by cultured peritoneal and pulmonary mononuclear phagocytes, *Biochim. Biophys. Acta,* **279**:87-91 (1972).
96. F. M. LaForce, W. J. Kelly, and G. L. Huber, Inactivation of staphylococci by alveolar macrophages with preliminary observations of the importance

of alveolar lining material, *Am. Rev. Respir. Dis.*, **108**:784-790 (1973).

97. G. A. Laurenzi, J. J. Guarneri, R. B. Endriga, and J. P. Carey, Clearance of bacteria by the lower respiratory tract, *Science*, **142**:1572-1573 (1963).

98. G. A. Laurenzi, R. T. Potter, and E. H. Kass, Bacteriologic flora of the lower respiratory tract, *N. Engl. J. Med.*, **265**:1273-1278 (1961).

99. E. S. Leake and Q. N. Myrvik, Changes in morphology and in lysozyme content of free alveolar cells after the intravenous injection of killed BCG in oil, *J. Reticuloendothel. Soc.*, **5**:33-53 (1968).

100. E. S. Leake and Q. N. Myrvik, Interaction of lysosome-like structures and phagosomes in normal and granulomatous alveolar macrophages, *J. Reticuloendothel. Soc.*, **8**:407-420 (1970).

101. E. S. Leake and Q. N. Myrvik, Rosette arrangement of electron-dense structures in granulomatous alveolar macrophages, *J. Reticuloendothel. Soc.*, **12**:305-313 (1972).

102. R. W. Leu, A. L. W. F. Eddleston, J. W. Hadden, and R. A. Good, Mechanism of action of migration inhibitory factor (MIF). I. Evidence for a receptor for MIF present on the peritoneal macrophage but not on the alveolar macrophage, *J. Exp. Med.*, **136**:589-603 (1972).

103. R. B. Low, Protein biosynthesis by the pulmonary alveolar macrophage: Conditions of assay and the effects of cigarette smoke extracts, *Am. Rev. Respir. Dis.*, **110**:466-477 (1974).

104. J. A. Lucy, Biochemistry of membrane interactions. In *Immunopathology of Inflammation*, Proceedings of a Symposium Sponsored by the International Inflammation Club at Brook Lodge, Augusta, Michigan, U. S. A., June 1, 2, and 3, 1970. *Excerpta Med. Int. Congr. Ser.*, **229**:98-106 (1971).

105. P. W. Majerus and R. R. Lastra, Fatty acid biosynthesis in human leukocytes, *J. Clin. Invest.*, **46**:1596-1602 (1967).

106. P. T. Major, A. S. Khandwala, and J. B. L. Gee, Human peripheral blood mononuclear cells: Biochemical features of phagocytosis [abstract], *J. Reticuloendothel. Soc.*, **15**:54a (1974).

107. V. Manganiello, W. H. Evans, T. P. Stossel, R. J. Mason, and M. Vaughan, The effect of polystyrene beads on cyclic 3′,5′-adenosine monophosphate concentration in leukocytes, *J. Clin. Invest.*, **50**:2741-2744 (1971).

108. P. E. G. Mann, A. B. Cohen, T. N. Finley, and A. J. Ladman, Alveolar macrophages: Structural and functional differences between nonsmokers and smokers of marijuana and tobacco, *Lab. Invest.*, **25**:111-120 (1971).

109. R. R. Martin, Altered morphology and increased acid hydrolase content of pulmonary macrophages from cigarette smokers, *Am. Rev. Respir. Dis.*, **107**:596-601 (1973).

110. R. D. Martinez and I. Montfort, A study of the specificity of alveolar macrophage antigen(s), *Immunology*, **25**:197-203 (1973).

111. R. J. Mason, G. Huber, and M. Vaughan, Synthesis of dipalmitoyl lecithin by alveolar macrophages, *J. Clin. Invest.*, **51**:68-73 (1972).

112. R. J. Mason, T. P. Stossel, and M. Vaughan, Lipids of alveolar macro-

phages, polymorphonuclear leukocytes, and their phagocytic vesicles, *J. Clin. Invest.*, **51**:2399-2407 (1972).

113. R. J. Mason, T. P. Stossel, and M. Vaughan, Quantitative studies of phagocytosis by alveolar macrophages, *Biochim. Biophys. Acta*, **304**:864-870 (1973).

114. D. Massaro, Alveolar cells: Incorporation of carbohydrate into protein and evidence for intracellular protein transport, *J. Clin. Invest.*, **47**:366-374 (1968).

115. D. Massaro, Alveolar macrophages: Cell-free protein synthesis, *Am. Rev. Respir. Dis.*, **100**:249-251 (1969).

116. D. Massaro, A. Handler, and L. Bottoms, Alveolar cells: Protein biosynthesis, *Am. Rev. Respir. Dis.*, **96**:957-961 (1967).

117. D. Massaro, K. Kelleher, G. Massaro, and H. Yeager, Jr., Alveolar macrophages: Depression of protein synthesis during phagocytosis, *Am. J. Physiol.*, **218**:1533-1539 (1970).

118. H. E. May and P. B. McCay, Reduced triphosphopyridine nucleotide oxidase-catalyzed alterations of membrane phospholipids: II. Enzymic properties and stoichiometry, *J. Biol. Chem.*, **243**:2296-2305 (1968).

119. C. E. McCall, I. Katayama, R. S. Cotran, and M. Finland, Lysosomal and ultrastructural changes in human "toxic" neutrophils during bacterial infection, *J. Exp. Med.*, **129**:267-293 (1969).

120. R. H. Mitchell, M. J. Karnovsky, and M. L. Karnovsky, The distributions of some granule-associated enzymes in guinea-pig polymorphonuclear leucocytes, *Biochem. J.*, **116**:207-216 (1970).

121. R. H. Mitchell, A. J. Pancake, J. Noseworthy, and M. L. Karnovsky, Measurement of rates of phagocytosis: The use of cellular monolayers, *J. Cell Biol.*, **40**:216-224 (1969).

122. R. D. Moore and M. D. Schoenberg, The response of the histiocytes and macrophages in the lungs of rabbits injected with Freund's adjuvant, *Br. J. Exp. Pathol.*, **45**:488-497 (1964).

123. V. L. Moore and Q. N. Myrvik, Inhibition of normal rabbit alveolar macrophages by factor(s) resembling migration inhibition factor, *J. Reticuloendothel. Soc.*, **16**:21-26 (1974).

124. M. G. Mustafa and C. E. Cross, Pulmonary alveolar macrophage: Oxidative metabolism of isolated cells and mitochondria and effect of cadmium ion on electron- and energy-transfer reactions, *Biochemistry*, **10**:4176-4185 (1971).

125. Q. N. Myrvik and D. G. Evans, Effect of bacillus Calmette Guerin on the metabolism of alveolar macrophages, *Adv. Exp. Med.*, **1**:203-213 (1967).

126. Q. N. Myrvik, E. S. Leake, and B. Farris, Studies on pulmonary alveolar macrophages from the normal rabbit: A technique to procure them in a high state of purity, *J. Immunol.*, **86**:128-132 (1961).

127. Q. N. Myrvik, E. S. Leake, and S. Oshima, A study of macrophages and epitheloid-like cells from granulomatous (BCG-induced) lungs of rabbits, *J. Immunol.*, **89**:745-751 (1962).

128. R. L. Nachman, B. Ferris, and J. G. Hirsch, Macrophage plasma membranes. I. Isolation and studies on protein components, *J. Exp. Med.*, **133**:785-806 (1971).
129. A. Naimark, Cellular dynamics and lipid metabolism in the lung, *Fed. Proc.*, **32**:1967-1971 (1973).
130. D. E. Niewoehner, J. Kleinerman, and D. B. Rice, Pathologic changes in the peripheral airways of young cigarette smokers, *N. Engl. J. Med.*, **291**: 755-758 (1974).
131. K. H. O'Hare, O. K. Reiss, and A. E. Vatter, Esterases in developing and adult rat lung. I. Biochemical and electron microscopic observations, *J. Histochem. Cytochem.*, **19**:97-115 (1971).
132. R. Oren, A. E. Farnham, K. Saito, E. Milofsky, and M. L. Karnovsky, Metabolic patterns in three types of phagocytizing cells, *J. Cell Biol.*, **17**:487-501 (1963).
133. E. Ouchi, R. J. Selvaraj, and A. J. Sbarra, The biochemical activities of rabbit alveolar macrophages during phagocytosis, *Exp. Cell Res.*, **40**: 456-468 (1965).
134. R. C. Page, P. Davies, and A. C. Allison, Participation of mononuclear phagocytes in chronic inflammatory diseases, *J. Reticuloendothel. Soc.*, **15**:413-438 (1974).
135. M. Para, A. Sagone, S. Balcerzak, and A. LoBuglio, Metabolism of normal and activated monocytes [abstract], *Clin. Res.*, **20**:742 (1972).
136. P. Patriarca, R. Cramer, S. Moncalvo, F. Rossi, and D. Romeo, Enzymatic basis of metabolic stimulation in leucocytes during phagocytosis: The role of activated NADPH oxidase, *Arch. Biochem. Biophys.*, **145**:255-262 (1971).
137. R. Patterson, Y. Tomita, S. Oh, I. M. Suszko, and J. J. Pruzansky, Immunoreactive respiratory basophil-like cells and mast cells, *Trans. Assoc. Am. Physicians*, **86**:95-100 (1973).
138. B. B. Paul, R. R. Strauss, A. A. Jacobs, and A. J. Sbarra, Direct involvement of NADPH oxidase with the stimulated respiratory and hexose monophosphate shunt activities in phagocytizing leukocytes, *Exp. Cell Res.*, **73**:456-462 (1972).
139. N. N. Pearsall and R. S. Weiser, *The Macrophage*. Philadelphia, Pa., Lea and Febiger, 1970.
140. R. C. Pfleger and H. G. Thomas, Beagle dog pulmonary surfactant lipids: Lipid composition of pulmonary tissue, exfoliated lining cells, and surfactant, *Arch. Intern. Med.*, **127**:863-872 (1971).
141. N. R. Pimstone, R. Tenhunen, P. T. Seitz, H. S. Marver, and R. Schmid, The enzymatic degradation of hemoglobin to bile pigments by macrophages, *J. Exp. Med.*, **133**:1264-1281 (1971).
142. M. O. Pinkett, C. R. Cowdrey, and P. C. Nowell, Mixed hematopoietic and pulmonary origin of 'alveolar macrophages,' as demonstrated by chromosome markers, *Am. J. Pathol.*, **48**:859-867 (1966).
143. S. A. Pratt, T. N. Finley, M. H. Smith, and A. J. Ladman, A comparison of alveolar macrophages and pulmonary surfactant(?) obtained from the

lungs of human smokers and nonsmokers by endobronchial lavage, *Anat. Rec.*, **163**:497-507 (1969).

144. S. A. Pratt, M. H. Smith, A. J. Ladman, and T. N. Finley, The ultrastructure of alveolar macrophages from human cigarette smokers and nonsmokers, *Lab. Invest.*, **24**:331-338 (1971).
145. R. O. Recknagel and A. K. Ghoshal, Lipoperoxidation as a vector in carbon tetrachloride hepatotoxicity, *Lab. Invest.*, **15**:132-146 (1966).
146. H. G. Remold, Requirement for α-L-fucose on the macrophage membrane receptor for M. I. F., *J. Exp. Med.*, **138**:1065-1076 (1973).
147. H. Y. Reynolds and H. H. Newball, Analysis of proteins and respiratory cells obtained from human lungs by bronchial lavage, *J. Lab. Clin. Med.*, **84**:559-573 (1974).
148. D. Romeo, G. Zabucchi, M. R. Soranzo, and F. Rossi, Macrophage metabolism: Activation of NADPH oxidation by phagocytosis, *Biochem. Biophys. Res. Commun.*, **45**:1056-1062 (1971).
149. D. Romeo, G. Zabucchi, T. Marzi, and F. Rossi, Kinetic and enzymatic features of metabolic stimulation of alveolar and peritoneal macrophages challenged with bacteria, *Exp. Cell Res.*, **78**:423-432 (1973).
150. R. Rosenberg, R. Sandhaus, and A. Janoff, Further studies of human alveolar macrophage alanine-P-nitrophenyl esterase: Evidence of resistance to endogenous antiproteases, *Am. Rev. Respir. Dis.*, **106**:114-115 (1972).
151. R. Rylander, Influence of infection on pulmonary defense mechanisms, *Ann. NY Acad, Sci.*, **221**:282-289 (1974).
152. F. L. Sachs and J. B. L. Gee, Comparison of the effects of phagocytosis and phospholipase C on metabolism and lysozyme release in rabbit alveolar macrophages, *J. Reticuloendothel. Soc.*, **14**:52-58 (1973).
153. J. A. Sandler, R. I. Clyman, V. C. Manganiello, and M. Vaughan, The effect of serotonin (5-hydroxytryptamine) and derivatives on guanosine 3′,5′-monophosphate in human monocytes, *J. Clin. Invest.*, **55**:431-435 (1975).
154. P. S. Sastry and L. E. Hokin, Studies on the role of phospholipids in phagocytosis, *J. Biol. Chem.*, **241**:3354-3361 (1966).
155. W. T. Sewell, The phagocytic properties of the alveolar cells of the lung, *J. Pathol. Bacteriol.*, **22**:40-55 (1918-1919).
156. H. W. Seyberth, H. Schmidt-Gayk, K. H. Jakobs, and E. Hackenthal, Cyclic adenosine monophosphate in phagocytizing granulocytes and alveolar macrophages, *J. Cell Biol.*, **57**:567-571 (1973).
157. S. B. Shohet, Changes in fatty acid metabolism in human leukemic granulocytes during phagocytosis, *J. Lab. Clin. Med.*, **75**:659-672 (1970).
158. L. H. S. Sieger, M. Altman, and E. D. Robin, Lactate dehydrogenase characteristics of rabbit alveolar and peritoneal macrophages, *J. Lab. Clin. Med.*, **75**:721-728 (1970).
159. S. R. Simmons and M. L. Karnovsky, Iodinating ability of various leukocytes and their bactericidal activity, *J. Exp. Med.*, **138**:44-63 (1973).

160. L. M. Simon, S. G. Axline, B. R. Horn, and E. D. Robin, Adaptations of energy metabolism in the cultivated macrophage, *J. Exp. Med.*, **138**:1413-1425 (1973).

161. W. A. Sorber, E. S. Leake, and Q. N. Myrvik, Comparative densities of hydrolase-containing granules from normal and BCG-induced alveolar macrophages, *Infect. Immun.*, **7**:86-92 (1973).

162. W. A. Sorber, E. S. Leake, and Q. N. Myrvik, Isolation and characterization of hydrolase-containing granules from rabbit lung macrophages, *J. Reticuloendothel. Soc.*, **16**:184-192 (1974).

163. V. J. Stecher, Synthesis of proteins by mononuclear phagocytes. In *Mononuclear Phagocytes.* Edited by R. van Furth. Philadelphia, Pa., F. A. Davis, 1970, pp. 133-150.

164. R. L. Stjernholm and R. C. Manak, Carbohydrate metabolism in leukocytes. XIV. Regulation of pentose cycle activity and glycogen metabolism during phagocytosis, *J. Reticuloendothel. Soc.*, **8**:550-560 (1970).

165. T. P. Stossel, Phagocytosis, *N. Engl. J. Med.*, **290**:717-723; 774-780; 833-839 (1974).

166. T. P. Stossel, R. J. Mason, T. D. Pollard, and M. Vaughan, Isolation and properties of phagocytic vesicles. II. Alveolar macrophages, *J. Clin. Invest.*, **51**:604-614 (1972).

167. T. P. Stossel, R. J. Mason, J. Hartwig, and M. Vaughan, Quantitative studies of phagocytosis by polymorphonuclear leukocytes: Use of emulsions to measure the initial rate of phagocytosis, *J. Clin. Invest.*, **51**:615-624 (1972).

168. T. P. Stossel, R. J. Mason, and A. L. Smith, Lipid peroxidation by human blood phagocytes, *J. Clin. Invest.*, **54**:638-645 (1974).

169. M. Stubbs, A. V. Kühner, E. A. Glass, J. R. David, and M. L. Karnovsky, Metabolic and functional studies on activated mouse macrophages, *J. Exp. Med.*, **137**:537-542 (1973).

170. J. Theodore, J. C. Acevedo, and E. D. Robin, Implantation of exogenous enzymatic activity in isolated alveolar macrophages, *Science*, **178**:1302-1304 (1972).

171. D. F. Tierney, Lactate metabolism in rat lung tissue, *Arch. Intern. Med.*, **127**:858-860 (1971).

172. J.-S. Tou and R. L. Stjernholm, Stimulation of the incorporation of $^{32}P_i$ and *myo*-[2-^{3}H] inositol into the phosphoinositides in polymorphonuclear leukocytes during phagocytosis, *Arch. Biochem. Biophys.*, **160**:487-494 (1974).

173. G. L. Truitt and G. B. Mackaness, Cell-mediated resistance to aerogenic infection of the lung, *Am. Rev. Respir. Dis.*, **104**:829-843 (1971).

174. M. F. Tsan and R. D. Berlin, Effect of phagocytosis on membrane transport of nonelectrolytes, *J. Exp. Med.*, **134**:1016-1035 (1971).

175. R. K. Tume and A. J. Day, Cholesterol esterifying activity of rabbit alveolar macrophages, *J. Reticuloendothel. Soc.*, **7**:338-354 (1970).

176. G. M. Turino, R. J. Rodriguez, L. M. Greenbaum, and I. Mandl, Mechanisms of pulmonary injury, *Am. J. Med.*, **57**:493-505 (1974).

177. F. Ulrich and D. B. Zilversmit, Release from alveolar macrophages of an inhibitor of phagocytosis, *Am. J. Physiol.,* **218**:1118-1127 (1970).
178. A. G. Ulsamer, F. R. Smith, and E. D. Korn, Lipids of *Acanthamoeba castellani:* Composition and effects of phagocytosis on incorporation of radioactive precursors, *J. Cell Biol.,* **43**:105-114 (1969).
179. F. T. Valentine, Soluble factors produced by lymphocytes, *Ann. NY Acad. Sci.,* **221**:317-323 (1974).
180. R. van Furth (ed.), *Mononuclear Phagocytes.* Philadelphia, Pa., F. A. Davis, 1970.
181. R. van Furth, Origins and kinetics of monocytes and macrophages, *Semin. Hematol.,* **7**:125-141 (1970).
182. R. van Furth, J. G. Hirsch, and M. E. Fedorko, Morphology and peroxidase cytochemistry of mouse promonocytes, monocytes, and macrophages, *J. Exp. Med.,* **132**:794-812 (1970).
183. M. T. Vogt, C. Thomas, C. L. Vassallo, R. E. Basford, and J. B. L. Gee, Glutathione-dependent peroxidative metabolism in the alveolar macrophage, *J. Clin. Invest.,* **50**:401-410 (1971).
184. W. S. Walker, Functional heterogeneity of macrophages: Subclasses of peritoneal macrophages with different antigen-binding activities and immune complex receptors, *Immunology,* **26**:1025-1037 (1974).
185. W. H. Walton (ed.), *Inhaled Particles III,* Proceedings of an International Symposium Organized by the British Occupational Hygiene Society in London, 14-23 September, 1970, Vols. 1 and 2. Surrey, England, Unwin, Gresham Press, Old Woking, 1971.
186. P. Wang, L. R. DeChatelet, M. Waite, and C. E. McCall, Phospholipid synthesis in rabbit alveolar macrophages and neutrophils [abstract], *Clin. Res.,* **21**:65 (1973).
187. G. A. Warr and R. R. Martin, In vitro migration of human alveolar macrophages: Effects of cigarette smoking, *Infect. Immun.,* **8**:222-227 (1973).
188. I. R. H. Welsh and J. K. Spitznagel, Distribution of lysosomal enzymes, cationic proteins, and bactericidal substances in subcellular fractions of human polymorphonuclear leukocytes, *Infect. Immun.,* **4**:97-102 (1971).
189. Z. Werb and Z. A. Cohn, Cholesterol metabolism in the macrophage. I. The regulation of cholesterol exchange, *J. Exp. Med.,* **134**:1545-1569 (1971).
190. Z. Werb and Z. A. Cohn, Cholesterol metabolism in the macrophage. II. Alteration of subcellular exchangeable cholesterol compartments and exchange in other cell types, *J. Exp. Med.,* **134**:1570-1590 (1971).
191. Z. Werb and Z. A. Cohn, Plasma membrane synthesis in the macrophage following phagocytosis of polystyrene latex particles, *J. Biol. Chem.,* **247**:2439-2446 (1972).
192. J. West, D. J. Morton, V. Esmann, and R. L. Stjernholm, Carbohydrate metabolism in leukocytes. VIII. Metabolic activities of the macrophage, *Arch. Biochem. Biophys.,* **124**:85-90 (1968).
193. E. Wiener and Z. Curelaru, The incomplete digestion of proteins taken up by macrophages, *J. Reticuloendothel. Soc.,* **13**:210-220 (1973).

194. H. Yeager, Jr., Alveolar cells: Depression effect of cigarette smoke on protein synthesis, *Proc. Soc. Exp. Biol. Med.*, **131**:247-250 (1969).

195. H. Yeager, Jr., S. M. Zimmet, and S. L. Schwartz, Pinocytosis by human alveolar macrophages: Comparison of smokers and nonsmokers, *J. Clin. Invest.*, **54**:247-251 (1974).

196. G. K. York, C. Arth, J. A. Stumbo, C. E. Cross, and M. G. Mustafa, Pulmonary macrophage respiration as affected by cigarette smoke and tobacco extract, *Arch. Environ. Health*, **27**:96-98 (1973).

197. D. Zucker-Franklin, The percentage of monocytes among "mononuclear" cell fractions obtained from normal human blood, *J. Immunol.*, **122**: 234-240 (1974).

22

Motility, Transport, and Endocytosis in Lung Defense Cells

J. BERNARD L. GEE

Yale University School of Medicine and
Yale-New Haven Hospital
New Haven, Connecticut

ATUL S. KHANDWALA

Yale University Lung Research Center
New Haven, Connecticut

I. Introduction

Cellular lung defense mechanisms depend on two phagocytes, blood phagocytes, mainly polymorphonuclear leukocytes (PMN), and the alveolar macrophages (AM). In general terms, PMN respond rapidly to acute inflammatory challenges, whereas AM accumulate more slowly following low grade inflammatory challenges. Further, the AM are the major resident cellular mechanism which maintains the normal lung sterility. AM are also of major importance in that they exhibit adaptive biochemical features. Such adaptations vary with the nature and immunogenicity of the inhaled materials.

The defense systems require cellular mobilization, particle ingestion and metabolic processes which nullify some of the noxious hazards associated with inhaled particles. Our account will therefore largely deal with cellular motility and phagocytosis. Brief reference to general transport physiology and pinocytosis will be included. We will describe these mechanisms in both PMN and AM in some detail. Emphasis on these two cells is appropriate since both are lung defense cells and many studies of PMN have laid the foundation for the subsequent study of AM. Brief references to other phagocytic cells such as protozoa and peritoneal macrophages (PM) will be made occasionally where studies of

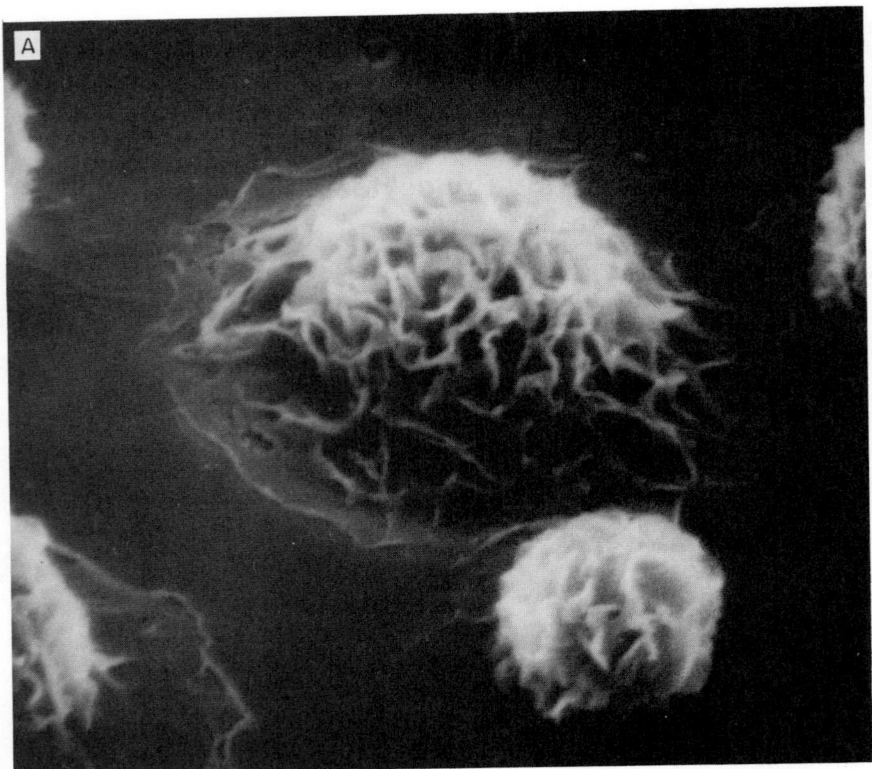

FIGURE 1 Scanning electron micrographs of normal rabbit alveolar macrophages adhered to a glass coverslip. Note the ruffled surfaces and the flattening at the periphery of some of the cells. The macrophages are very similar in size. X7800. (From Leake et al. [105a].)

specific aspects of phagocytosis have been particularly well documented in these cells. It will become apparent that there is a considerable variation between the characteristics of PMN and AM phagocytes. No attempt will be made to analyze the species variations which are much smaller than variations associated with the cell types. Further, there are some variations in the homogeneity of the AM obtained by the now classic procedure of pulmonary lavage. In rabbits, the cells obtained by lavage are apparently of uniform type; in man this is probably not the case, at least two populations having been described [34].

The reader is referred to general reviews of the subject [19,22,23,69,168, 202] and to specific accounts of the antimicrobial defense systems [99,101]. A complete review of defective cellular defense mechanisms is beyond the scope of this review but a number of instances of such defects will be indicated while describing the relevant mechanisms.

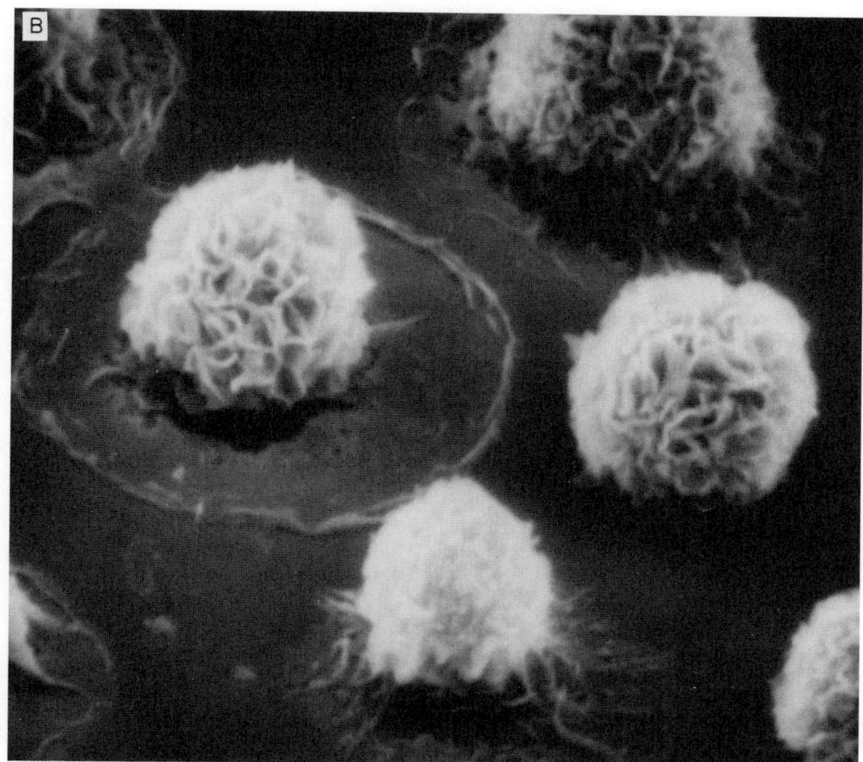

FIGURE 1 (continued)

II. Cellular Motility

Some features of the motility of AM are shown in Fig. 1. These include the long tentacle-like pseudopodia of AM. Cell motility may be taken to include both movement in the extracellular environment and the internal movement of subcellular structures, such as lysosomes and the nucleus. Phagocytosis involves both types of movement. Particles, initially adherent to the plasma membrane, are engulfed by pseudopodia. The resulting phagocytic vacuole (PV) is ingested in association with lysosomal counterflow from the centriolar region of the cell. Directional movement in the extracellular environment is usually associated with ruffling movements of the plasma membrane at the leading edge of the cell. All these forms of cell motility appear to depend mainly on some contractile mechanisms operating on intracellular materials possessing intrinsic rigidity.

In the last decade, extensive biochemical work has demonstrated that many cell types [145], including phagocytes, possess groups of proteins which serve these functions. Electron-microscopic studies have also shown two types of subcellular structures which are now known to provide a basis for cell motility. They are microfilaments and microtubules. The simplest hypothesis for their functions is that microfilaments serve a primary contractile function, whereas microtubules provide both mechanical support and flow orientation.

In addition to these contractile elements, the plasma membrane requires consideration. Aside from providing sites which trigger motile and other responses, this membrane also provides sites of insertion for the contractile proteins. Further, lateral mobility of proteins within the fluid lipids of cell membranes can also occur. This is exemplified by the variable distribution of surface immunoglobulins following reaction with antiimmunoglobulin sera. For instance, such bivalent antibodies bind diffusely at 0-4°C to the plasma membrane of lymphocytes and other cell types but at 37°C become redistributed into patches or "caps." The latter are then found at the trailing edge of these cells when they are in motion [178]. The regulation of the mobility of such receptors within the membrane per se depends on the contractile proteins and cyclic nucleotides, notably, cGMP (guanosine 3′,5′-cyclic monophosphate) [129].

We will first describe the microfilaments and microtubules. Their role in organized cell motility and the broader aspects of cellular motility in the pulmonary defenses will be indicated subsequently.

A. Microfilaments

In the briefest terms, contraction in skeletal muscle involves a number of steps which include the binding of actin to myosin with activation of an ATPase activity, the dissociation of the products of ATP hydrolysis, contraction generation and the dissociation of the actin-myosin complex. The process is regulated by other proteins and divalent cations. Many features of this contractile process have been identified in the cytoplasm of a wide range of cells including phagocytes. The present state of this area of molecular biology has been recently reviewed [144,145] and our comments will be confined to general remarks and to reports specifically concerned with the AM.

Cytoplasmic actins have been identified in a number of cells. They consist of a single globular polypeptide chain with a double helical conformation of molecular weight of about 45,000 daltons. The physical properties are similar to those of muscle actin. A characteristic amino acid, 3-methylhistidine, is consistently present. In general, such actins appear to bind single molecules of ATP which undergo hydrolysis to ADP and inorganic phosphate, a process associated with polymerization of the actin chain. The actins so far identified in a wide range of biological systems (ameba, slime molds, granulocytes, and macrophages, etc.) have a similar helical configuration and orientation of binding sites, since they can react with heavy meromyosin, a portion of rabbit muscle myosin obtained by trypsinization. This interaction with myosin leads to a characteristic electron-microscopic configuration, namely, an electron-dense arrowhead shape. This feature is particularly useful since it may be employed in the intact cell suspended in glycerine to identify actin filaments.

Myosins have now been described in many cell types. As a class, myosins are characterized as enzymes possessing actin-activated Mg^{2+}-dependent ATPase activity. Thus they all presumably serve to transduce chemical energy from ATP into contractile force. At present, most is known about striated muscle myosin which comprises two large heavy polypeptide chains and two or more light polypeptide chains. Myosin Mg^{2+}-ATPase activity is activated by the binding to actin which appears to promote the dissociation of the ATP hydrolysates and in some unknown way may cause both the sliding contractile motion and the dissociation of the actin-myosin complex. Subsequent rebinding of ATP to free myosin permits the process to recycle. Cytoplasmic myosins have been biochemically identified in leukocytes, platelets, and rabbit AM. Immunofluorescent techniques with myosin antibodies have shown myosin to be present in mouse peritoneal macrophages [7]. The latter method is particularly useful, since there are no presently available morphologic mechanisms for demonstrating the presence of myosin. Formation of decorated actin filaments and bipolar myosin filaments, in the presence of divalent cations from purified guinea pig PMN myosin, has been demonstrated [174].

In the AM, there is one important biochemical study of contractile proteins. This study is of interest since it directly concerns the AM and since it permits a comparison of both cytoplasmic and muscle contractile protein in the same species, the rabbit. Stossell and Hartwig [171] have shown the presence of peptides in AM cytoplasm with the electrophoretic mobilities of muscle actin and myosin. They constitute, respectively, 0.7% and 7% of the total cellular protein. Further characterization of these materials [171] has shown that AM myosin consists of a single polypeptide chain which has a molecular weight of 200,000 daltons and has the same electrophoretic mobility as the heavy chain of rabbit muscle myosin. In addition, two light chains of rabbit AM myosin with molecular weight of ~20,000 daltons comigrate with the light chains of muscle myosin. Under certain conditions, AM myosin exhibits an ATPase activity. This activity is maximal in the presence of 0.6 M KCl and EDTA, and is approximately 1200 times the activity of AM homogenates. AM myosin in the presence of 0.1 M KCl and either Mg^{2+} or Ca^{2+} forms bipolar filaments identifiable in uranyl acetate stains (Fig. 3). AM myosin also binds rabbit muscle F actin. This actin-myosin complex is dissociable by $MgCl_2$ and ATP and may be visualized electron microscopically by the formation of "arrowhead" complexes. As pointed out earlier, activation of the Mg-ATPase activity is generally regarded as important for contraction and hence cell mobility. This important step appears to require a protein cofactor which does not possess independent ATPase activity nor directly increase the ATPase activity of either muscle or AM myosin unless these are already complexed with actin. These three components, actin, myosin, and cofactor, appear to confer Ca^{2+} sensitivity to the Mg^{2+} ATPase activity. In some, at present obscure way, this system may provide a molecular basis for contractility in the AM.

Microfilaments have been identified morphologically in macrophages. Detailed electron-microscopic studies of the subplasmalemmal location of microfilaments of various sizes and their involvement in pseudopodia formation have been performed in cultured mouse peritoneal macrophages [148]. Employing guinea pig peritoneal macrophages, treated with glycerine and rabbit muscle myosin, Allison demonstrated networks of actin filaments, many of which were in close apposition to the plasma membrane [7]. However, direct biochemical evidence equating actin with all forms of these microfilaments is lacking. It is clearly necessary to provide further details on the distribution of myosin within the cell if a fuller understanding of microfilament function is to emerge. Myosin antibody techniques are currently being employed to define this distribution. These studies [80,194,203] indicate that myosin can be found at cell surfaces and also in linear parallel strands with defined periodicity. The latter features evoke the image of striated muscle.

Microfilaments (Fig. 2) have also been described in rabbit AM [111]. Indirect evidence that microfilaments are involved in phagocytosis by the AM has been obtained employing the mold metabolite, cytochalasin B [111]. This drug reversibly inhibits the uptake of bacteria by rabbit AM. It also diminishes the number of microfilaments observed by electron microscopy. In contrast, microtubules were unaffected by cytochalasin B (Fig. 3). It is a reasonable presumption that these two effects are causally related. There are, to date, no studies of effects of this drug on other aspects of cell motion in the AM. However, cytochalasin B does inhibit ruffled membrane movement in other macrophages [7, 10], and in leukocytes at high cytochalasin B concentrations, chemotaxis is sharply diminished. Additional morphologic effects of cytochalasin B on AM include a flattening, an unusually wide spread on glass surfaces and nuclear displacement (Fig. 4). While these effects of cytochalasin B on phagocytosis and cell morphology presumably depend on some action on microfilaments, this interpretation remains unproved. Indeed, there is considerable disagreement concerning the mode of action of cytochalasin B (for discussion see Refs. 51 and 199). There are claims that cytochalasin B reacts stoichiometrically with rabbit striated muscle actin and acts by preventing actin-myosin binding [166]. However, the concentrations of cytochalasin B in these experiments were much higher than those usually employed in most studies of phagocytic cells.

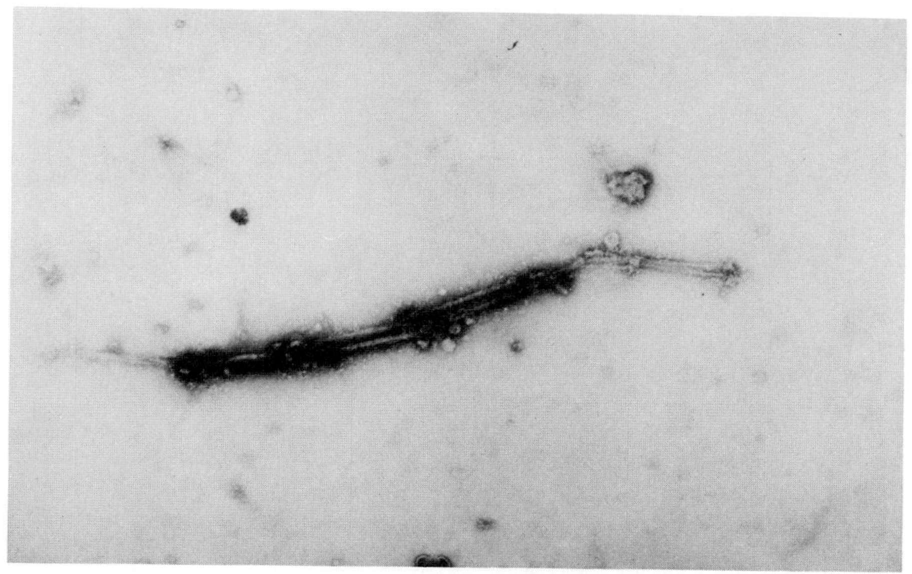

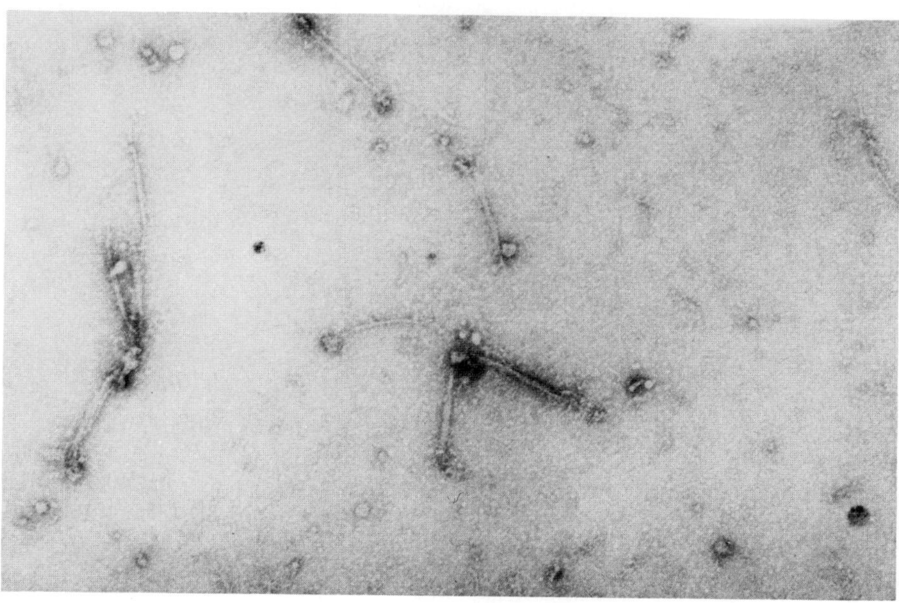

FIGURE 2 AM myosin bipolar filament in uranyl acetate stain. (From Stossel et al. [171].)

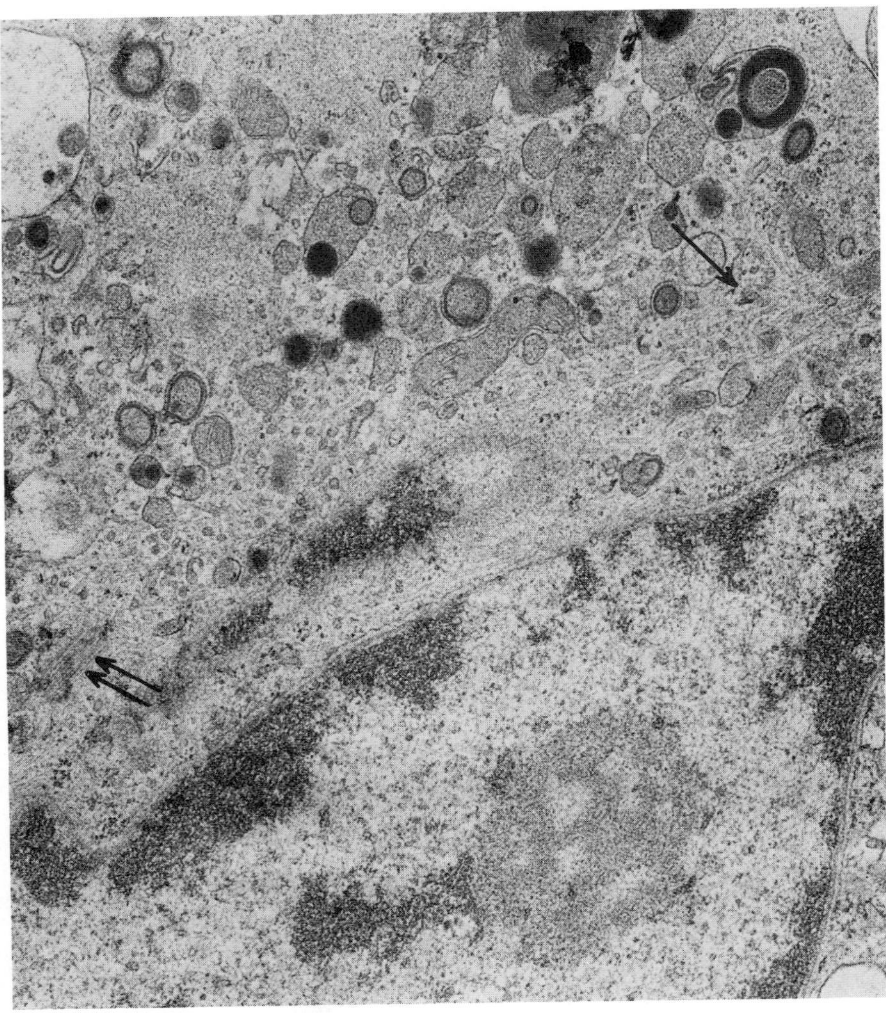

FIGURE 3 Part of a macrophage exposed to 5 μg/ml cytochalasin B (20-min preincubation) and incubated with bacteria for 60 min is seen. Microfilaments are not observable, but microtubules are prominent (arrow); a centriole is present on the left margin of the photograph (double arrow). ×35,000. (From Malawista et al. [111].)

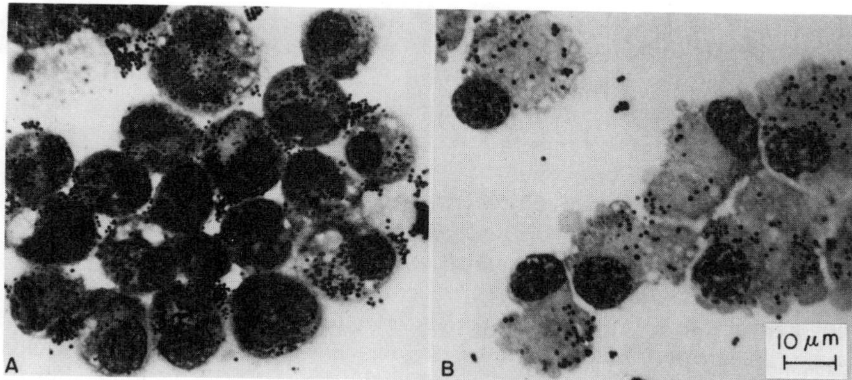

FIGURE 4 The effect of cytochalasin B on rabbit alveolar macrophages incubated with bacteria for 60 min is seen in cells centrifuged on to glass slides. (A) No drug. Many bacteria per cell are seen. The cells have depth, bacteria are in different planes. (B) Cytochalasin B, 5 μg/ml, 10-min preincubation. Fewer bacteria per cell are seen, and the cells appear flatter and more spread out than in (A). Wright's stain. (From Malawista et al. [111].)

Further, cytochalasin B sharply impairs the uptake of glucose analogs and other small molecules in many cell lines [208] including the AM [60]. A related drug, cytochalasin D, does not affect such small molecule uptake but produces in many cell lines an appearance under phase microscopy that includes microvilli withdrawal, inhibition of ruffled membrane movement, sustained cytoplasmal contraction, and nuclear herniation [122,123]. Some of these effects have been shown in the AM exposed to cytochalasin B [111].

A single case of neutrophil actin dysfunction causing diminished migration, bacterial uptake, and degranulation has been described. This infant was subject to recurrent staphylococcal infections [25].

B. Microtubules

These subcellular structures have been widely recognized in many biologic systems since the use of glutaraldehyde as a fixative for electron-microscopic studies. This subject has been recently reviewed [132]. Their length varies from elongated microtubules of flagellae and neuronal cells to shorter ones observed in endocytic cells including leukocytes and macrophages. Their diameter, ~240 nm, is substantially larger than those of microfilaments, and in section comprises an outer core of electron-dense material and an inner electron-lucent core. Further, they tend to be arranged along the long axis of cellular extensions. This orientation implies a role in both preserving cellular morphology and channeling intracellular movement. The microtubules are of two general types: the stable form, characteristic of flagellae and the labile forms which are found in neural cells, the mitotic apparatus and the cytosol of many cells, including the mammalian phagocyte. The labile microtubules are in dynamic equilibrium with preformed subunits present in the cytosol. Microtubular function is therefore understandably unaffected by inhibitors of protein synthesis. These subunits, tubulins, are specific dimeric proteins whose molecular weight is 120,000 daltons and which appear to comprise two somewhat dissimilar monomeric polypeptides. Their amino acid sequence has been partially characterized in material from two such diverse sources as chicken brain and sea urchin sperm. It appears that the microtubule is composed of 13 tubulin units, sometimes termed protofilaments, and that cross bridges link the individual microtubules. An ATPase activity has been described in some microtubules (e.g., flagella) but there is no current evidence for such activity in mammalian phagocytes.

The function and assembly mechanism of microtubules has been investigated by pharmacologic agents which, at appropriate concentrations, act largely on the microtubular apparatus. These drugs are generally known as "spindle-poisons" since they cause metaphase arrest. They include colchicine and colchemid which irreversibly bind to tubulin dimers and cause microtubular disappearance by preventing their reassembly from these tubulin units. Colchicine does not attack organized microtubules. Similar effects occur with mechanical pressure and many inhalation anesthetics [8,9]. Stabilization of microtubular structure occurs with high concentrations of heavy water (D_2O). Vinblastine and other related vinca alkaloids cause an irreversible precipitation of microtubules into a paracrystalline form. Griseofulvin also modifies microtubule function in a similar manner to colchicine but acts at a different site [132].

The factors regulating in vivo assembly and disassembly of the microtubules are unknown. Ca^{2+} combines with microtubular protein and probably plays an important role in microtubule assembly. Repolymerization of tubulin appears to proceed best in the presence of guanosine triphosphate and Mg^{2+}, at low concentrations of Ca^{2+}. Nucleotide triphosphates, notably guanosine triphosphate, are required for assembly in vitro. In some systems, it has been suggested that tubulin acts as an acceptor for phosphate in cAMP mediated protein kinase reactions [68]. Further, cGMP itself and two agents which elevate intracellular cGMP (carbachol and phorbol myristate acetate) have been shown to regulate surface capping, a phenomenon believed to be regulated by microtubules [129]. This suggests that microtubular function is also regulated by cGMP levels.

Some examples of the effects of spindle-poisons on cell function may be given. First, colchicine affects both chemotaxis in PMN [118] and directional movement in a number of other cell types, including peritoneal macrophages. Usually ruffled membrane movement is confined to limited areas of the cell membrane and thus confers a specific direction to the cell motion. Colchicine diminishes these localized ruffling movements and transforms directional motion into random pseudopodial formation, so-called ameboid movement [7]. Second, colchicine affects both the distribution and motion of intracellular particles. Freed and Lebowitz studied HeLa cells and fibroblasts in tissue culture and showed that the radial pericentriolar distribution of acid-phosphatase rich particles, presumably lysosomes, became randomized within the cytosol following treatment with spindle-poisons. Further, they demonstrated that such particles were capable of discrete jumping motions, the long saltatory movements [53, 149]. These movements were virtually abolished by colchicine, podophyllin, and vinblastine. These treated cells also showed random pseudopodial formation. Third, Malawista and Bodel [110] showed that colchicine (1×10^{-4} M) caused a diminution of the extracellular release of lysosomal enzymes from the PMN during phagocytosis without affecting either bacterial uptake or the metabolic changes associated with such uptake. This dissociation of lysosomal enzyme release from particle entry and accompanying metabolic changes was associated with the disappearance of microtubules. It was therefore suggested that microtubules directed the flow of phagocytic vacuoles toward lysosomes. Fusion of these two organelles is then required for external lysosomal enzyme release. While there is little question that low concentrations of colchicine (10^{-6}-10^{-5} M) affect microtubular function, the proposed explanation of the site of action of colchicine has been questioned. Employing cultured mouse PM, 10^{-6} M colchicine sharply diminished the induction of the lysosomal enzyme acid phosphatase following a phagocytic pulse [141]. Since the degradation of endocytosed materials was unaffected by colchicine, it has been proposed that the microtubules do not influence phagolysosome formation but act elsewhere to influence lysosomal enzyme formation. This alternative site is uncertain, but it has been suggested that the egress of lysosomes from the Golgi apparatus might be microtubule-dependent and therefore colchicine-sensitive. It should be noted that these effects of colchicine may depend on either the cell type or the experimental conditions or both. Finally, there is an interesting effect of colchicine on the transport of the amino acid lysine during phagocytosis by PMN. Neither low concentrations of colchicine nor phagocytosis per se have an effect on lysine transport which is mediated by a membrane "carrier" mechanism (Sec. III.B). However, the combination of phagocytosis and colchicine does produce a sharp drop in lysine transport rate [185]. This observation, also noted with vinblastine, has been interpreted to mean that the micro-

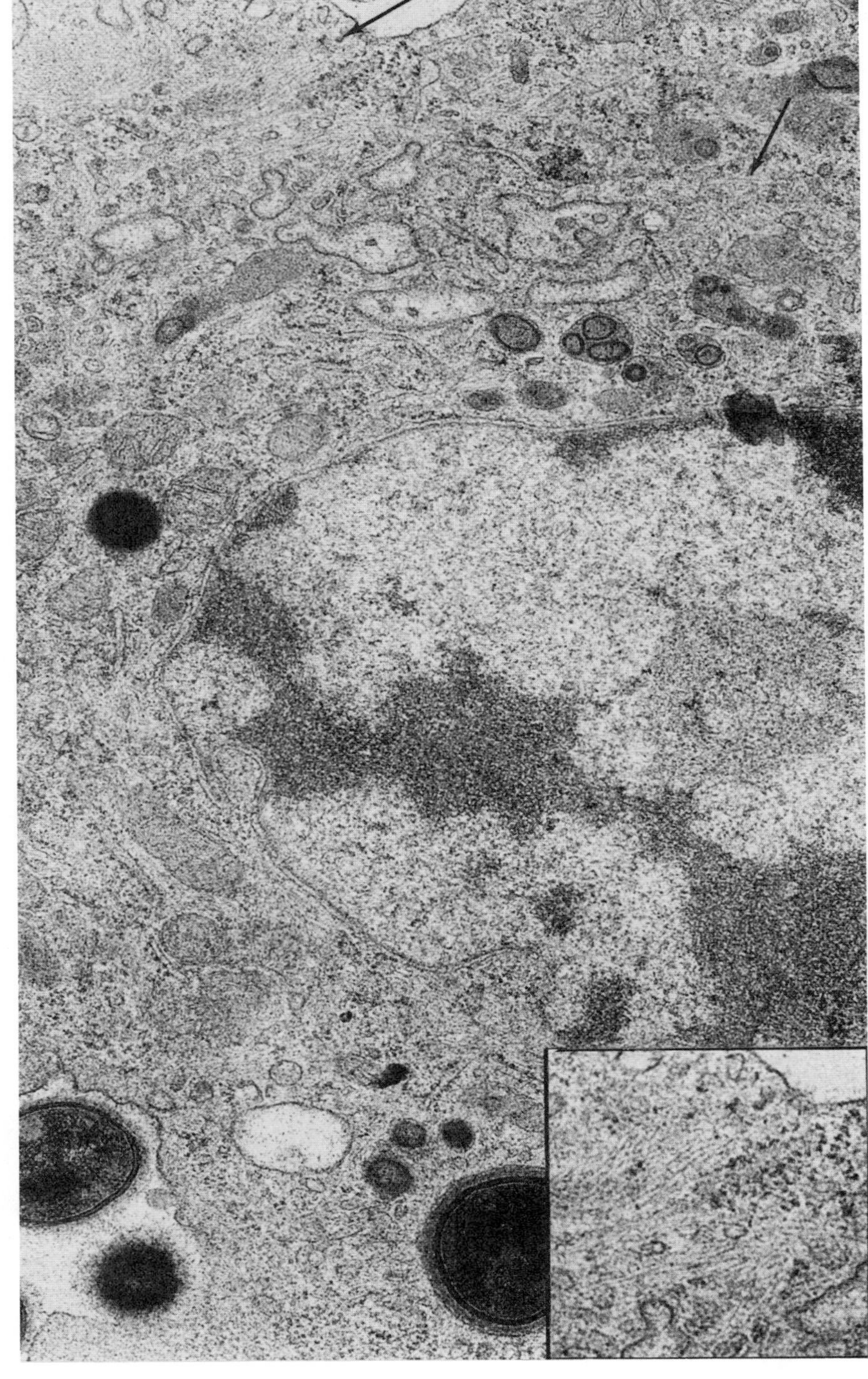

tubules maintain a topographical separation of different membrane receptors involved in the two separate types of transport, namely, lysine transport and particle uptake [20,185].

While there is no doubt that these spindle-poisons do affect microtubule function, it would be unwise to ascribe all their actions on cell function to alteration in microtubular activity. For instance, there is evidence that colchicine can react with cell membrane proteins [167,205].

Microtubules are predictably present in the AM (Fig. 5) but there are few studies of their role in this cell type. Colchicine (10^{-3} M) diminishes glucose conversion to CO_2 with a small effect on bacterial uptake (Gee and Khandwala, unpublished observation) and also produces a small decrement in the uptake of oil droplets by AM [172]. The effects, however, require colchicine concentrations about two orders of magnitude higher than those usually required to prevent tubule reassembly. It is therefore unlikely that the metabolic effects of colchicine depend on microtubule function. Colchicine does not affect regulatory enzymes involved in glucose metabolism but does impair the uptake of glucose analogs. Thus, the metabolic effects may reflect diminished glucose transport [181].

C. Regulation of Cell Motility

The three previously described components, membranes, microfilaments, and microtubules, are important in many aspects of cell motility. The manner in which the contractile proteins and microtubules are integrated in order to perform any specific type of cell motion is at present obscure. Involvement of changing localized concentrations of Ca^{2+} at various subcellular sites is suggested by analogy with muscular contraction, the ability of Ca^{2+} both to activate ATPases, including actin-myosin complexes, and also to bind to microtubule subunits. It is supported by changes in Ca^{2+} stimulated ATPase at different phases of cell division [7]. An additional regulatory factor may well be the intracellular concentrations of cyclic nucleotides. These are discussed further in relation to lysosomal activation (Sec. IV.F), but there are two lines of evidence that cAMP may play such a regulatory role in cell motility. cAMP diminishes the PM migration from capillary tubes. Further, the chemotactic responses of

---

FIGURE 5 Part of a control macrophage, incubated with bacteria for 60 min, shows ingested microorganisms (lower margin of illustration). Note the abundant microtubules (arrow) and microfilaments (insert) which are particularly prominent in the upper one-third of the illustration. ×30,000. Insert: ×50,000. (From Malawista et al. [111].)

PMN are diminished by caffeine and theophylline, an action that may be associated with the elevated levels of cAMP resulting from phosphodiesterase inhibition.

Whatever the mechanism(s) involved in the distribution and activity of microtubules and microfilaments may be, it is clear that both these structures are "organized" within such phagocytes as the PM. Reaven and Axline showed both structures to be concentrated in the subplasmalemmal area of the attached cell surface and also in regions of the cell participating in the attempted ingestion of large polystyrene particles. In contrast, the free aspects of the cells only contained a filamentous network.

Several aspects of cellular motility deserve separate comments.

1. Energetics

It is clear that cellular motility is an energy-requiring process. The cytosol actin-myosin system is an ATPase. External ATP in the presence of divalent cations causes rounding contraction of PM suspended in glycerine [7]. Further external ATP promotes the uptake of latex particles by guinea pig PM. If large particles ($>1.3\ \mu m$) are employed, more particles are ingested in a given time period in the presence of external ATP [58]. While the energy cost of cell locomotion is not known, an estimate of the energy cost of particle uptake by PMN can be calculated from measurements of the increased lactate formation occurring in anerobically phagocytosing PMN. These calculations indicate that 1×10^{-15} mol ATP are required for the ingestion of a single $1.17\ \mu m$ diam particle. In the AM, particle ingestion is inhibited by inhibitors of oxidative phosphorylation [134] and by low O_2 tensions [33]. This is in sharp contrast to the PMN, where anaerobic glycolysis can sustain phagocytosis. AM increase O_2 consumption ($^{Q}O_2$) by 0.9 nM/min-10^6 AM during phagocytosis. Assuming similar ATP expenditures during phagocytosis in AM and PMN, approximately 1% of this increased $^{Q}O_2$ would be required for movement and ingestion by AM. The majority of the increase in $^{Q}O_2$ associated with phagocytosis by AM is therefore utilized for other functions. These presumably include the production of microbicidal O_2 metabolites, such as H_2O_2 (Sec. IV.C.1).

Cigarette smoke [74,76,146] and aqueous extracts therefrom [24] impair bacterial uptake by the AM in vitro. The complete smoke acts on glyceraldehyde 3-phosphate dehydrogenase and its effects are reversed by SH-containing antioxidants. By contrast, aqueous extracts of smoke impair ATP formation by some unidentified effect on mitochondrial function. This is not prevented by antioxidants. Both appear to act on energy metabolism at substrate or mitochondrial levels.

2. Surface Interaction

Studies of cell motility and phagocytosis are frequently performed on solid surfaces such as glass or polystyrene. The cells adhere to this substructure. This adherence in the AM occurs in the cold at 4°C, and is prevented by lethal concentrations of KCN (10^{-2} M), but neither KCN nor cytochalasin B causes detachment from the surface once it has occurred [120; P. E. McKeever and J. B. L. Gee, unpublished observations]. Established adherence therefore may depend on physicochemical, non-energy-requiring forces. There is evidence that ionic forces are involved in adherence to artificial surfaces [142]. An additional attempt to define the physicochemical forces has been made employing the concept of "contact-angle." This parameter, which may reflect the surface energy of a cell monolayer, requires a measurement of the angle between the suspending fluid and the cell monolayer [186]. This angle is lowered by migration inhibitory factor [180]. The significance and importance of this approach needs further study.

3. Chemotaxis

Directional movement of phagocytic cells is clearly an important component of the inflammatory response in which there is a rapid influx of PMN and a slow influx of mononuclear phagocytes. Substances causing such movements, i.e., chemotaxins, are important. Those inducing PMN chemotaxis include: bacterial products, components derived from the classical complement pathway, notably C_{3a}, C_{5a} and $C_{\overline{567}}$ [201] and materials derived from the alternate properdin pathway [156]. They also result from Hageman factor activation [168]. Further, products of PMN lysis are chemotactic for mononuclear cells and also for the PMN themselves. Thus, PMN exhibit "autochemotaxis," a feature which sustains and may even amplify the inflammatory response [92].

Becker has emphasized the role of serine esterases in neutrophil chemotaxis [17,18]. He proposes that these enzymes, which are probably microsomal, exist in an inactive proesterase form. The chemotactic components of complement and bacterial chemotaxins activate the proesterase, an effect blocked by the contemporaneous presence of certain serine esterase inhibitors. While neutrophil chemotaxis requires Ca^{2+} and Mg^{2+}, these ions are not required for the esterase activation. Little is known about the natural substrate of these particular esterases or how their activation promotes the vectorial motion characteristic of chemotaxis.

Transfer factor is also chemotactic for PMN and at least nonalveolar macrophages. This material, originally obtained from disrupted leukocytes by Lawrence has been recently studied [56]. Transfer factor has been used in the immunotherapy of two pulmonary disorders, tuberculosis [200] and coccidiomycosis [30].

While the foregoing chemotaxins are characterized by their effects on cell motility, it must be emphasized that many of them produce important internal structural and metabolic responses. These responses include microtubule assembly, lysosomal enzyme release and metabolic perturbations. For instance, Goldstein and colleagues have shown that chemotaxis in human PMN is enhanced by a factor in human serum. This factor appears to be the C_{5a} component of complement [67]. They provide evidence that in addition to its chemotactic and lysosomal enzyme releasing effect (Sec. IV.F), it transiently promotes the assembly of microtubules. This effect is associated with changes in Ca^{2+} distribution [57]. These latter are also features of phagocytosis. These effects operate by alterations in the cell membrane in both chemotaxis and phagocytosis. It is an example of physiologic economy that the processes which attract phagocytes to an ingestate are also part of the process of ingestion [64].

In human monocytes, IgG receptors have also been implicated in chemotaxis [112].

The action of chemotaxins is opposed by certain inhibitory factors notably described by Ward and colleagues [189]. These factors are of clinical importance in several disorders including hepatic cirrhosis [109], systemic infections [165], and in lymphoproliferative disorders.

The in vivo movement of PMN and monocytes into lung tissue from pulmonary capillaries is poorly understood in spite of its obvious importance in defense mechanisms. The phenomenon of margination of PMN in the capillary circulation has long been recognized [28]. It is presumed that such margination is a prerequisite for migration into the lung and is thus a component of general chemotactic mechanisms. The subject is poorly understood and forms part of the general subject of migration of cells on biologic as opposed to artificial surfaces. A number of clinical observations are relevant to this discussion. First, epinephrine diminishes neutrophil margination and shifts the cells into the circulating pool, particularly from the pulmonary circulation [104]. By contrast, early in hemodialysis, the reverse occurs [84]. Second, vascular endothelial injury provokes local neutrophil adhesion. Third, shock causes pulmonary leukocyte deposition [204]. Fourth, it is obvious that diapedesis of neutrophils must precede the local leukocytosis characteristic of pneumonias. Fifth, margination appears to depend on "stickiness," an ill-defined but measurable phenomenon [108]. This stickiness is diminished by ethanol [27] and prednisone [108]. These features were largely observed in clinical situations and have potential clinical relevance in defense mechanisms; one may speculate that they bear on such disorders as asthma and shock lung. Is the diminished neutrophil margination by epinephrine and prednisone at least partly responsible for a diminution of the inflammation which, along with bronchial smooth muscle contraction, is a component of asthma? Are the neutrophil accumulations seen in shock lung a source of lysosomal enzymes which may be partly responsible for the edema of this entity?

The in vivo mobilization of AM following inhalation of a wide range of particles including microbes, dusts, and cigarette smoke indicates that some stimulatory mechanism must operate. However, there is little information on their nature. Further, there are very few in vitro studies of AM chemotaxins. Ward [188] demonstrated a very weak chemotactic effect with factors derived from pneumococci and no effect with agents that are chemotactic for peritoneal macrophages, such as rabbit serum treated with either immune complexes or streptokinase or plasminogen. Likewise, PMN lysates were chemotactic for PM but not for AM. Another and somewhat mysterious difference between PM and AM has been reported. Employing capillary tube migration techniques, ouabain appears to enhance AM migration but diminishes PM migration. This strange difference occurs in spite of a similar effect of ouabain on ion transport in the two cell types. Ethanol has been shown to minimize AM migration into the alveoli [79] and to selectively affect antimicrobial defense mechanisms [75,77]. The mechanism is obscure since there are no major effects of ethanol on AM metabolism [59].

4. Lymphokines

The last decade has witnessed a major development in the area of cellular "cross-talk," particularly lymphocyte factors which regulate macrophage behavior. This subject has been recently reviewed [42]. Both lymphocytes and polypeptides derived therefrom have been shown to exert effects on macrophages. These effects include increases in surface adherence, ruffling movement, surface spreading, phagocytic activity and glucose oxidation via the pentose shunt. Increases or decreases in lysosomal enzyme specific activities have been variously reported. In general these responses appear to enhance microbicidal activity. There will be major advances in the chemical structure, mechanisms, and specificities of these factors in the next few years. For instance, it is already clear that PM reactivity to MIF depends on a receptor containing a sugar, α-L-fucose [150]. At present these factors include migration inhibitory [102] macrophage enhancement factors [196] and chemotactic factors [191]. Most of these studies concern nonalveolar macrophages. Studies of the AM are relatively few and are limited by two factors, namely, even "normal" AM are frequently activated by occult infections and the frequent use of BCG and Freund's adjuvant to increase the AM yield obtained by pulmonary lavage. The response of human AM to migration inhibitory factor is variable [193] but is strikingly reduced in AM obtained from smokers [192].

There is some substantial evidence that delayed hypersensitivity (i.e., cell-mediated immunologic activation) mechanisms may operate via blood monocytes recruited to the lung rather than by activation of the normally resident AM. Specifically, thymidine-labeled peripheral blood monocytes accumulate in experimental bacterial infections in mice [182]. While these important experiments seem to argue that recruitment is more important than local intrapulmonary activation, there is also evidence that intrapulmonary exposure to *M. tuberculosis* confers a greater immunity than nonpulmonary tuberculosis challenge [16]. Whatever their immediate origin, cells lavaged from lungs made granulomatous by intracheal instillation of BCG into previously immunized rabbits are morphologically similar to other AM and show marked increases in the lysosomal enzyme specific activities [55]. Further work is required to determine whether pulmonary challenge works via chemotactic substances causing monocyte recruitment or local AM activation.

III. General Features of Transport

The entry of materials into cells depends on many factors, including molecular size. Small molecules may enter without major structural deformation of the cell membrane. They enter by simple or carrier-mediated facilitated diffusion along activity or concentration gradients and also by active transport against such gradients. Larger molecules are selectively admitted by mechanisms which specifically require overt morphologic changes in the cell membrane, namely, endocytosis. This mechanism, also termed bulk transport, includes both pinocytosis and phagocytosis. Pinocytosis and phagocytosis are appropriately regarded as transport mechanisms since they permit cells to take up materials required for biosynthetic and other purposes. However, in view of their specific host defense function, they will be treated separately. At this point, brief comments on active and carrier transport in the AM are appropriate.

A. Active Transport

Most mammalian cells maintain internal ionic concentrations different to those of the extracellular fluid. AM intracellular ion concentrations measured in the presence of normal serum electrolytes were: Na^+, 83 ± 7.1; K^+, 75 ± 13.2; and Cl^-, 59 ± 4.1 meq/kg cell water [152]. It is probable that Cl^- is in thermodynamic equilibrium with extracellular fluid. An active sodium pump must exist in view of the $[Na^+]$ gradient and the ouabain sensitivity of Na^+ efflux. This pump is some 10 times more active than that of the rabbit erythrocyte and its energy requirements exceed the energy available from purely glycolytic pathways. The AM therefore depend on oxidative phosphorylation for internal ionic homeostasis. The external surface of the AM plasma membrane contains Na^+-K^+-dependent ATPase [41]. This is activated by Mg^{2+}. It is inhibited by certain divalent cations notably Cd^{2+} [124]. This ATPase has been demonstrated histochemically and appears conspicuously in pseudopodia [120]. Ouabain, an inhibitor of this ATPase, has no effect on particle ingestion by AM in short-term in vitro experiments employing shaking cell suspensions (J. B. L. Gee and A. S. Khandwala, unpublished observation). This contrasts with the effects of ouabain on macrophage migration from capillary tubes [106] and the inhibition of chemotaxis in PMN by ouabain [190]. The explanation for these differences is unclear but may relate to experimental conditions in that migration and chemotaxis were studied on solid surfaces as opposed to liquid suspensions.

B. Carrier Transport

Glucose is both a substrate for energy production and a source of reducing equivalents. The entry of glucose into the AM is therefore important. In most mammalian cells, intracellular glucose is largely present as glucose 6-phosphate but is transported by a carrier mechanism as free glucose. Glucose transport is most easily approached experimentally employing glucose analogs such as ^3H-labeled 2-deoxy-D-glucose (2DG) which is phosphorylated at the 6 position but not further metabolized. This description will largely be confined to studies with the AM [96,122].

Carrier-mediated facilitated diffusion transport systems exhibit certain characteristics. First, unlike simple diffusion, the initial uptake rates are an alinear function of the external solute concentration and exhibit saturation kinetics, i.e., an external solute concentration above which no further increases in uptake rate occur. This reflects saturation of the carrier. 2DG transport shows these characteristics with maximal uptake at an external 2DG concentration of approximately 8 mM (K_m; 0.66 mM). Second, transport should not be against a concentration gradient. Over a wide range of external 2DG concentrations, free intracellular 2DG is always less than the external concentration. However, since over 80% of intracellular 2DG normally exists as 2DG 6-phosphate, the total 2DG, free and phosphorylated, does exceed the external 2DG concentration. Third, such carrier mediated transport systems show competitive inhibition by substrate analogs; 2DG transport is inhibited by increasing external glucose concentrations.

A number of drugs exert important effects on 2DG transport. Inhibition of oxidative phosphorylation by cyanide, antimycin A and dinitrophenol causes a sharp drop in 2DG uptake and inversion of the ratio of the free to phosphorylated 2DG. This effect presumably depends on decreased availability of ATP for 2DG phosphorylation. The drug, cytochalasin B [60], sharply diminishes 2DG uptake but does not affect phosphorylation. In the narrow concentration range of 0.05 to 2.0 μg/ml, cytochalasin B appears to act as a competitive inhibitor of 2DG transport. One molecule of cytochalasin B blocks a single transport site. This effect is probably not related to microfilament disruption, since, in other cell types, the related mold metabolite, cytochalasin A, disrupts microfilaments without affecting hexose transport. The influence of drugs usually associated with elevations of cAMP are of interest [96]. While PGE_1, $PGF_{2\alpha}$, and dibutyryl cAMP have no effect on 2DG transport, three presumed inhibitors of phosphodiesterases (theophylline, caffeine, and papaverine) depress 2DG uptake without affecting the ratio of free to phosphorylated 2DG. The mechanism is uncertain. Colchicine (10^{-5} M) also inhibits glucose transport. Finally, in short-term in vitro experiments, insulin does not affect 2DG transport by AM from normal rabbits [98].

Other important compounds are transported in a similar manner, e.g., adenosine and amino acids, notably lysine [182,183]. Lysine transport is inhibited by serum and by agents which bind to external membrane SH groups [176,177,182].

These aspects of transport physiology bear on the endocytic defense mechanisms of the PMN and AM in several ways. First, ionic homeostasis is required for normal cell function. Second, pharmacologic effects on metabolism may depend on how the drug affects transport mechanisms. Third, both endocytosis and the two forms of transport previously discussed depend on cell membrane function. Transport sites, receptors for chemotaxins and opsonins and such membrane bound enzymes as the transport ATPases are viewed as a dynamically changing mosaic in the normal fluid cell membrane. The role of microtubules in maintaining this mosaic has been discussed. Two further examples of this mosaicism may now be mentioned. Employing PMN, phagocytosis diminished the number of binding sites for a mitogen, concanavalin A [131], and also diminished the transport of potassium [48].

IV. Phagocytosis

Phagocytosis is often described as occurring in several sequential steps. The initial contact between the phagocyte and particle leads to adherence which depends on physicochemical forces. This step is also a discriminatory one in which an important selection of the ingestate occurs. In this step, immunologic factors are of great importance. The selection of one particle over another frequently depends on such factors. Macrophages also show sharp, immunologically determined, increases in their phagocytic activity and mobility. The second step is the formation of the phagocytic vacuole (PV) by the formation of plasma membrane lined vacuoles. These are then transported within the cell and fused with lysosomes whose enzymes are released from a latent form into an active state. This step may render the PV a discrete subcellular microenvironment in which a variety of chemical processes can occur. These processes serve a microbicidal or degradative function. Phagocytosis is associated with a number of metabolic changes involved with energy production, membrane resynthesis and the generation of vigorous oxidizing substances such as H_2O_2 and the superoxide anion ($O_2^{-}\cdot$). The latter are microbicidal. While these steps may be described separately, the process of biochemical changes including lysosomal enzyme release can occur without the active ingestion of a particle and are therefore thought to follow some, as yet uncharacterized, change in the plasma membrane. This process, in which lysosomal enzymes are released without actual particle ingestion, is similar to the process whereby latent particle-bound substances are released from certain cells, e.g., histamine release from the mast cell. This process is often termed reverse endocytosis or exocytosis. The external release of degradative lysosomal hydrolases and other enzymes can be a particularly disruptive component of the inflammatory response. It is evident therefore that endocytosis can be either defensive or injurious, depending on the degree to which the lysosomal system remains within the PV.

It should be noted that, while studies of PMN show relatively consistent results, considerable variation in the features of phagocytosis by AM occurs. This presumably reflects the exposure and immunologic history of the rabbits from which the AM were obtained.

A. Adherence

Information on the forces whereby particles adhere to phagocytes is limited particularly with respect to the AM. A few general statements may be made. First, attachment of particles to phagocytes frequently occurs at low temperature suggesting that physicochemical forces are involved. Second, there are factors derived from the particle which promote attachment but not ingestion. Capsulated organisms and mycoplasma pneumonia adhere but are not ingested without immune serum. Third, there is an important group of adherence and ingestion promoting materials termed opsonins. For example, low concentrations of heat stable opsonins are found in normal serum and are greatly elevated by hyperimmunization. They require both F_c and F_{ab} fragments of the IgG_1 and IgG_3 molecules. In addition, there are opsonins which are destabilized by heating to 60°C. These derive from the complement system. There is a recent report that IgE can also bind to certain macrophages [29].

Studies on the surface receptors of macrophages have been reviewed by Rabinovitch [147], Cohn [35,69], and Pearsall and Weiser [139]. Very little is known about the chemical nature of the F_c receptor in macrophages. The receptor is resistant to proteolytic enzymes and neuraminidase but is destroyed by crude phospholipases. The receptor persists in prolonged tissue culture. It is present in all macrophages including AM [143]. Binding of IgG to AM appeared to be enhanced by the presence of polyvalent and divalent haptens both at equivalence and in moderate antigen excess. Further, antigen-antibody complexes bind more tightly than antibody alone. Saturation studies indicate that each AM has approximately 2×10^6 binding sites [143]. These receptors play a role in the selection of the ingestate. Particulate antigens coated with such antibodies bind to macrophage receptors. This selective "recognition" process also serves to enhance the intensity of the phagocytic process. The F_c component is critical in enhancing the uptake of immunoglobulin coated particles [87]. The C_3 component of complement can promote attachment but only IgG promotes ingestion of immune complexes by macrophages [114]. On the other hand, the C_3 component of the complement promotes both attachment and ingestion of microorganisms by PMN leukocytes [170]. Inert particles added to macrophages in the presence of immunologically adherent red cells do not promote red cell ingestion whereas anti-red cell IgG will stimulate red cell uptake [78]. Thus, there is a selectivity in the ingestive as well as the adherence process.

B. Ingestion

The role of microfilaments and microtubules in particle uptake has been discussed in relation to cell motility. The use of albumin stabilized oil droplets [116,172] is a major advance in the methodology of phagocytosis, since it permits precise quantitation without the problem of distinguishing adherent from ingested particles. The technique is particularly valuable, since initial uptake rates can be measured and so employed in kinetic studies. A number of factors modify uptake rates. These include extracellular fluid osmolality and pH [134]. In addition, divalent cations are probably essential for ingestion, notably Ca^{2+} and Mg^{2+} [168,169]. The absence of Ca^{2+} or presence of EDTA suppresses ingestion by AM completely (J. B. L. Gee and A. S. Khandwala, unpublished observation). A number of agents diminish ingestion by PMN. These include exogenous cyclic nucleotides, prostaglandins, and theophylline [38]. Attempts to alter cell surfaces by enzymatic tools and SH binding agents have not lead to any understanding of the biochemistry of ingestion. One potentially fruitful approach derives from the use of specific peptide fragments derived from the constant portions of the IgG molecule. For instance, "tuftsin" [36,126], a tetrapeptide [Thr-Lys-Pro-Arg], has been offered as a phagocytosis stimulator but this work needs confirmation and a broader study of such components of the IgG molecule.

The mechanism(s) initiating ingestion are unknown. Speculations include the role of the particle induced intracellular leak of Na^+ causing membrane depolarization [7]. This in turn may evoke Ca^{2+} exchange and activation of the microfilament system.

The AM operates in a different milieu than that of other macrophages at least while within the alveolar spaces. It has been suggested that IgA represents an important opsonin for AM [21]. There is also evidence that cystic fibrosis serum inhibits both the particle uptake and killing of pseudomonas aeruginosa by rabbit AM [26].

C. Oxygen Metabolism

This important area of biochemistry of phagocytosis will be reviewed with special reference to antimicrobial function of three oxygen metabolites, namely, hydrogen peroxide, superoxide anion, and singlet excited oxygen.

1. Hydrogen Peroxide

O_2 consumption in the phagocyte serves an important function as the source of active oxidizing products capable of microbicidal action [95,99,101]. This role was suggested by several key studies in the PMN. First, PMN will ingest bacteria anaerobically but require O_2 for maximal killing. Second, PMN show characteristic metabolic responses to phagocytosis. These responses include increases in O_2 consumption (${}^{Q}O_2$) and H_2O_2 formation. In the PMN, this increase in ${}^{Q}O_2$ is cyanide insensitive suggesting that hemeproteins are not involved in the O_2 utilization pathway. These two features are associated with a stimulation of glucose conversion to CO_2 via the hexose monophosphate shunt (HMP), as judged by the preferential oxidation of glucose labeled in the 1 position as opposed to the 6 position. These observations are summarized in Table 1, right-hand two columns. There are a number of uncertainties in the precise mechanisms responsible for these effects. For instance, at least three enzymes have been proposed as H_2O_2 generating oxidases, NADH oxidase, NADPH oxidase, and d-amino acid oxidase. There are two well-established pathways which remove excess H_2O_2, namely, catalase and the glutathione system linked to the HMP by a NADPH-specific glutathione reductase (Fig. 6). The HMP provides reducing equivalents both for the formation of reduced glutathione in the H_2O_2 disposal pathway and also for the regeneration of NADPH from $NADP^+$ generated by the NADPH oxidase systems.

TABLE 1 Metabolic Features of Phagocytosis for AM and PMN

	AM[a]		PMN[b]	
	Rest	Phagocytosis	Rest	Phagocytosis
Q_{O_2}	1.70	2.60	0.29	0.80
$^{14}CO_2$ from 1-[^{14}C] glucose[d]	9.60	40.00	1.35	21.30
$^{14}CO_2$ from 6-[^{14}C] glucose[d]	1.80	7.00	0.34	0.70
$^{14}CO_2$ from [^{14}C] formate[d]	0.30	0.56	0.60	2.90
H_2O_2 production[e]	0.16	0.24	0.59	1.02

[a]Data from Refs. 59 and 64.
[b]Data from Refs. 137 and 160.
[c]nmol O_2/min-10^6 cells.
[d]pmol CO_2/min-10^6 cells.
[e]nmol/10^6 cells.

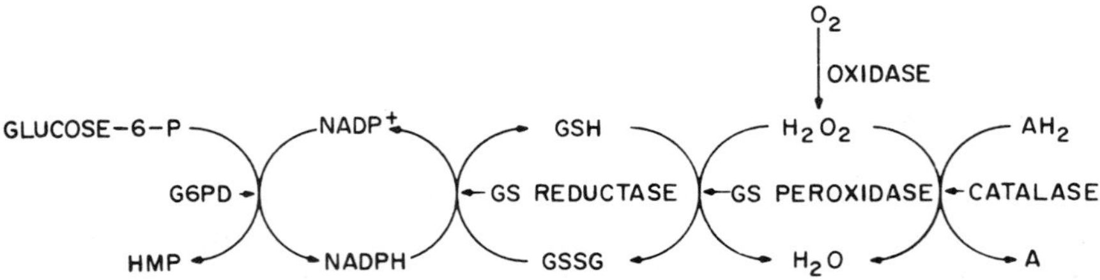

FIGURE 6 Peroxidative metabolic pathways. GSH = reduced glutathione; GSSG = oxidized glutathione; G6PD = glucose 6-phosphate dehydrogenase; HMP = hexose monophosphate shunt; AH_2 represents unknown hydrogen donors for catalase. GS reductase and GS perioxidase refer to glutathione enzymes. (From Vogt et al. [187].)

This biochemical pathway has been shown in the PMN to be part of an important microbicidal system comprising myeloperoxidase, H_2O_2 and an halide. In addition, d-amino acid oxidase has a bactericidal activity in its own right since it can attack the d-alaninine present in the teichoic acids of certain bacteria. The action of this system on bacteria may be exerted by one of three mechanisms, directly on the microbes, halide fixation to bacterial protein, or the formation of toxic aldehydes from amino acids. This system has been extensively reviewed [99,101,159]. The importance of this system is highlighted in the hereditary disorder of PMN function, chronic granulomatous disease [94]. In this disorder, there is a striking absence of the metabolic response to bacterial ingestion. The bacterial uptake rates are normal, but there are no associated changes in Q_{O_2},

H_2O_2 formation or glucose oxidation. In chronic granulomatous disease, the bactericidal activity against organisms which do not produce H_2O_2 is severely impaired. The precise primary defect is obscure, but there is no doubt that PMN from these patients show diminished H_2O_2 formation. The defect in the X-linked form of this disease has been variously ascribed to a deficiency of either NADH or NADPH oxidase and in the recessive form to deficient glutathione peroxidase [85,94]. There are two other disorders involving this aspect of PMN antimicrobial ability. Certain PMN with less than 5% of normal glucose 6-phosphate dehydrogenase (G6PD) activity kill bacteria poorly. G6PD plays a dual role, first in the glutathione H_2O_2 disposal pathway and second, in regenerating reduced pyridine nucleotides oxidized during the reduction of O_2 to H_2O_2 [13, 37]. This defect is rare but clinical infections occur in such patients. Second, a rare deficiency of PMN myeloperoxidase has been reported. In these patients, there is little evidence of major susceptibility to infections even though their PMN kill *Candida* and some bacteria more slowly than normal PMN. Peroxide formation and glucose oxidation appear normal in these PMN. This suggests that myeloperoxidase is not the only mechanism whereby peroxidative killing can occur and, more importantly, indicates that this enzyme is not the major one responsible for H_2O_2 formation as has been proposed by some workers [99].

In the AM, some of the features observed in the PMN also occur (Table 1, left-hand columns, and Ref. 63). There is a smaller but definite increase in H_2O_2 formation and also increased $^{Q}O_2$ and glucose conversion to CO_2. However, the increased oxidation of both forms of labeled glucose is similar and specific stimulation of the HMP shunt probably does not occur at least during normal phagocytosis. Since it is known that, in the AM, H_2O_2 formation is increased during phagocytosis [62], and since the glutathione H_2O_2 disposal pathway contains a NADPH specific glutathione reductase [187], it is likely that the HMP pathway is activated concurrently with glycolytic pathway. The two glucose oxidation pathways may be linked by a transhydrogenase or lactic acid dehydrogenase. Alternatively separate stimulation may also occur.

There are two possible sources for the generation of H_2O_2 in AM. First, there is an NADPH oxidase described by Rossi and colleagues which is detergent activated, requires MN^{2+} as a cofactor and has optimum activity at pH 5.5 [153]. Alternatively, H_2O_2 can be generated by d-amino acid oxidase present in AM cytosol [187].

One important unanswered question concerning the AM is the mechanism whereby H_2O_2 is bactericidal. Histochemical and a number of biochemical assays failed to detect myeloperoxidase activity [62] in the AM. However, two later groups used somewhat different assay conditions, particularly H_2O_2 concentrations, and reported peroxidase activity with guaiacol as the substrate [153, 138]. Sbarra and colleagues have shown that I^-, H_2O_2 and a granular fraction of homogenized AM (200,000 g pellet) exert significant antimicrobial activity [138]. They have not defined the precise mechanism but, in contrast to PMN, amino acids are not converted to bactericidal aldehydes by the material present in this fraction of AM. The "peroxidase" activity of AM also differs from PMN myeloperoxidase in that it will only kill with I^- and not Cl^-. In PMN, myeloperoxidase activity is greater with I^- but still present with Cl^-. Further evidence that this activity is "peroxidase-like" is its sensitivity to aminotriazole. This peroxidase-like enzyme or catalase or both, together with I^- and H_2O_2, may therefore serve an antimicrobial role. It should be noted that variation in H_2O_2 utilizing peroxidases has been previously appreciated; eosinophil leukocyte peroxidase has different biochemical features to PMN myeloperoxidase.

2. *Superoxide Anion*

The preceding discussion describes the state of the art until the last few years. It has recently become clear that other highly reactive products of O_2 metabolism are involved in bactericidal activity. Fridovich and coworkers [54] described the biologic importance of the superoxide anion ($O_2^{-}\cdot$), which is a one electron reduction of O_2 and is a free radical, i.e., a variety of O_2 in which there is an unpaired electron. This and other reduction products are highly reactive in their own right and capable of vigorous direct oxidation of many substances. The $O_2^{-}\cdot$ may undergo spontaneous dismutation to H_2O_2 and O_2 and this process is also catalyzed by an enzyme, superoxide dismutase (SOD). The precise product of O_2 reduction varies with different oxidases. For instance, d-amino oxidase generates H_2O_2 and xanthine oxidase generates superoxide anion [11]. Odajima and colleagues have reported that leukocytic myeloperoxidase can act as an NADH oxidase which generates superoxide anion [127,128]. The exact product(s) of the NADH or NADPH oxidases in either PMN or AM are not presently known even though H_2O_2 is clearly generated at some point during the reduction of O_2. Thus, more work on the intermediates of O_2 reduction by phagocytic cell oxidases is required to establish the quantitative formation of various O_2 moieties.

Babior and colleagues have now shown that PMN release $O_2^{-}\cdot$ in low concentrations into the medium [12]. Further, bacterial ingestion increases $O_2^{-}\cdot$ release with a time course paralleling that of the $^{Q}O_2$ increase [195]. $O_2^{-}\cdot$ production during phagocytosis is enhanced by the inclusion of serum in the system [39]. Since PMN of patients with chronic granulomatous disease produce little $O_2^{-}\cdot$, this anion may also be a bactericidal agent [40]. Klebanoff has suggested that myeloperoxidase system utilizes H_2O_2 generated by dismutation from $O_2^{-}\cdot$ for bacterial killing [100]. However, an important series of experiments by Johnston and colleagues on PMN provided some evidence that $O_2^{-}\cdot$

might be bactericidal [93]. Latex particles were coated with SOD. PMN were allowed to ingest these particles and live bacteria *(E. coli* or *S. aureus).* The normal increase in $^{Q}O_2$ as well as glucose oxidation occurred but bactericidal activity was sharply decreased by the ingestion of SOD. This experiment suggests that, provided normal $O_2^{-}\cdot$ production occurs, the presence of excess ingestate-bound SOD within the PV prevents the $O_2^{-}\cdot$-mediated bacterial killing. A similar experiment was performed using catalase bound to latex. This, presumably decomposed H_2O_2 and again killing was diminished. This is anomalous, since excess SOD should increase H_2O_2 formation by the dismutation reaction from $O_2^{-}\cdot$. Yet, excess SOD diminished killing. Likewise, while catalase decomposes H_2O_2 and also is not normally found in PMN PV, ingestate bound catalase impairs killing. One possibility is that both $O_2^{-}\cdot$ and H_2O_2 cooperate in their individual bactericidal mechanisms. Alternatively, $O_2^{-}\cdot$ and H_2O_2 react together to form the highly unstable and reactive hydroxy free radical (OH·):

$$O_2^{-}\cdot + H_2O_2 \rightarrow OH\cdot + OH^{-} + {}^{1}O_2^{*} \qquad (1)$$

In the AM, cytoplasmic SOD activity is present and $O_2^{-}\cdot$ generation occurs at rest and is increased in phagocytosing cells [45,47]. Studies of the bactericidal roles of $O_2^{-}\cdot$ in the AM are lacking. However, they are important since, apart from catalyzed reactions, these O_2 moieties are highly reactive in their own right and AM from some species form large amounts of $O_2^{-}\cdot$ during phagocytosis [47].

3. *Singlet Excited Oxygen*

An additional species of the O_2 molecules has to be considered, namely singlet excited oxygen, ${}^{1}O_2^{*}$. This is a form of O_2 in which one electron has been shifted from a ground state orbital to an orbit of higher energy [117]. ${}^{1}O_2^{*}$ may be formed by three distinct mechanisms. They are indicated in reactions (1)-(4). One of these pathways may be associated with the halide bactericidal system:

$$H_2O_2 + Cl^{-} \xrightarrow{\text{myeloperoxidase}} H_2O + OCl^{-} \qquad (2)$$

$$OCl^{-} + H_2O_2 \rightarrow H_2O_2 + Cl^{-} + {}^{1}O_2^{*} \qquad (3)$$

An alternative mechanism for ${}^{1}O_2^{*}$ formation is spontaneous or enzymatic dismutation of superoxide anions [4,5]:

$$2O_2^{-}\cdot + 2H^{+} \rightarrow H_2O_2 + {}^{1}O_2^{*} \qquad (4)$$

The $^1O_2$*, so produced, may be an additional antimicrobial agent. This possibility is suggested by comparative studies employing two variants of *S. lutea* [103]. One variant, containing a carotenoid pigment, is not killed by human PMN. The other variant, lacking this pigment, is killed normally. Carotenoids are efficient scavengers of $^1O_2$*. There are no studies of $^1O_2$* in the AM.

There are also a number of very "simple" artificial systems in which oxidizing free radicals are bactericidal. For example, ascorbic acid and low concentrations of H_2O_2 are together antimicrobial. The effectiveness of this "simple" system is prevented by thiosulfate, a free radical scavenger [121]. At this point, it appears clear that various products of O_2 reduction are heavily implicated in antimicrobial activities in the PMN, but their relative importance is uncertain.

4. Activation and Localization

The activation mechanisms of these O_2 reducing systems are poorly understood. It is believed that some mechanism similar to the lysosomal releasing systems may well operate. Plasma membrane "trigger mechanisms" have been proposed in both PMN and AM on the basis of experiments utilizing detergents [73,207], phospholipase C [136,158], concanavalin A [150] and Ca^{2+} ionophores (J. B. L. Gee and A. S. Khandwala, unpublished observation; 161). Involvement of adrenergic receptors in the regulation of O_2 metabolism and hence, glucose metabolism, has been suggested by experiments on the PMN [168] but are not a feature of the AM [61]. The suggestion that the oxidases are plasma membrane bound is unproved but possible [168]. However, 60% of the nucleotide oxidases found in both the PMN and AM are granular and are detergent activated. D-amino acid oxidase is a soluble cytoplasmic enzyme in the AM [187].

It is clear that there is a complex interaction between the variation in the antioxidant capabilities of bacterial species and the oxidant activities of the particular phagocytes. For instance, in addition to the variable susceptibility of strains of *S. lutea* to leukocytic killing, virulent and avirulent forms of *S. typhi* show differing resistance to killing by PMN. The avirulent strains evoke increased $^{Q}O_2$ in PMN but the virulent strains do not. A further consideration may be of crucial importance, namely, the balance between the subcellular localization and extracellular release of the O_2 metabolites. If these products are so biologically active as to kill microbes, toxic effects on the host cell may be expected. The notion that these materials are largely generated within the microenvironment of the phagocytic vacuole is therefore appealing. Under certain conditions, this may be the case. However, there is no doubt that $O_2^{-}\cdot$ and H_2O_2 can be released extracellularly. During this process the antioxidant functions of SOD on $O_2^{-}\cdot$, of catalase and glutathione peroxidase on H_2O_2 and the latter enzymes on lipid peroxides [97,115,187] presumably protect the phagocyte cytosol from auto-oxidation. It is intriguing to realize that in the AM, O_2 reduction in one location, the mitochondria, is the main source of energy, while in another location, the PV, O_2 reduction serves the cell's primary function of host defense [54].

The preceding emphasis on O_2 metabolism as an antimicrobial defense should not obscure recent exciting developments which indicate that O_2 metabolites can also exert important cytolytic effects [31,32,49]. The immunologic surveillance of tumor cells by phagocytes may depend on O_2 metabolites.

D. Phagocytic Vacuole

Identification of the PV by morphologic and histochemical techniques was an early development in the study of phagocytosis. The fusion of the PV with cytoplasmic granules which suddenly "degranulated" on contact with the PV was strikingly documented by Hirsch and colleagues. However, the actual isolation of the vacuole and documentation of the transfer of latent granule associated enzymes into the PV has only recently been accomplished. The first approach, in protozoa, employed latex particles and transfer of lysosomal enzymes into the PV was successfully shown. Stossel, Mason, Vaughan, and colleagues provided a more stringent separation of the PV by using a "soft diet" of albumin stabilized paraffin oil droplets containing a lipid-soluble red dye [175]. This technique permitted the quantification and isolation of PV by sucrose density centrifugation. This technique is particularly valuable in that the PV could be isolated with minimal damage to its membrane. This technique provokes little release during phagocytosis of the lysosomal enzymes into either the cytosol or into the external medium.

The PV of two particular cells were studied, the PMN [175] and AM [173]. In both cells, approximately 25% of the total cellular lysosomal enzyme activities were exchanged from the cell pellets into the PV. These included the lysosomal phosphatases and β-glucuronidase. There was a striking absence from the PV of such marker materials as succinic dehydrogenase (mitochondria) DNA, RNA (nuclei), and glucose 6-phosphatase (microsome). There were several important differences between the contents of the PV in the two cell types. For instance, the enzymes associated with peroxidative killing mechanisms were found in PMN PV. These include NADH oxidase and myeloperoxidase. Little or no catalase enters the PV of PMN. In contrast, while the AM PV contained lysosomal hydrolases, about 50% of the total cellular catalase activity was found within the PV. Further, the AM vacuoles contained considerable quantities of lipid hydroperoxides which may be bactericidal. These biochemical data provide direct evidence that agents derived from cellular organelles can be selectively concentrated within the PV. They indicate the crucial importance of the PV as a subcellular chemical microenvironment providing a powerful localized antimicrobial system within the cell. Variations in the composition of PV from AM depend upon the exposure history of rabbits from which they are obtained.

These studies are in contrast with earlier studies in which there were either considerable increases in lysosomal enzyme activity in the cell "sap" or frank exocytosis of such solubilized enzymes after phagocytosis by the intact cell. The studies with oil droplets indicate that lysosomal enzyme release into the soluble phase of cell homogenates is not an obligatory concomitant of ingestion. The release of hydrolases into the cytosol and extracellular fluid may depend on the nature of the ingestate and immunologic factors. They confirm earlier studies with sheep red cells which likewise do not induce lysosomal enzyme leak into the medium [197]. It appears likely that disruption of the PV depends on the physical characteristics of the ingestate, the associated presence on the ingestate inflammatory mediators (e.g., complement) and perhaps on the particle load. This flexibility in the localization of the microbicidal agents derived from either lysosomes or O_2 reduction perhaps represents an autoregulation of the defense mechanism.

In addition to the usefulness of oil droplets in measuring the kinetics of particle uptake (Sec. IV.C), the kinetics of the transfer of lysosomal enzymes can also be observed with this technique. The transfer process is intimately related to ingestion [175]. It varies with the individual lysosomal and peroxidative enzymes, possibly because they are initially sequestered in different granules [15,46]. The transfer process into the PV ceases in the absence of ingestate. This suggests that either there is some regulation of the PV content of hydrolases or, more likely, that the formation and movement of the PV is intimately associated with lysosomal flow and degranulation. Such a mechanistic association of these processes may depend upon a plasma membrane trigger and intracellular messenger system. The potential role of cyclic nucleotides in this system is discussed below.

E. Membrane Resynthesis

During the processes of ingestion and PV formation, a significant amount of plasma membrane is interiorized. This raises the question whether phagocytes can sufficiently rapidly synthesize the new plasma membrane necessary for the continuation of phagocytosis. Studies from several laboratories have clearly shown that phagocytosis increases the rate of incorporation of labeled precursors into various lipids in all three phagocytes, namely, PMN, PM, and AM. It was, however, difficult to assess whether this increased incorporation of precursors represented increased turnover of lipids as a general consequence of increased metabolic activity during phagocytosis or a net increase in lipid biosynthesis to replace the lost plasma membrane.

Cohn [198] capitalized on the inability of isolated PM to synthesize cholesterol, an important structural component of cell membranes and employed the ectoenzyme 5′-nucleotidase as a marker for plasma membrane. His studies showed: the amount of 5′-nucleotidase found in PV following ingestion of latex particles is proportional to the amount of plasma membrane interiorized as judged by the amount of plasma membrane cholesterol found in PV; 5′-nucleotidase activity in PV decreases reaching a minimum at 6 hr; the residual plasma membrane 5′-nucleotidase associated with the noninternalized plasma membrane remains constant for 6 hr after phagocytosis and then increases and reaches prephagocytosis levels at 10-12 hr; an increase in lysosomal cholesterol and concomitant decrease in plasma membrane cholesterol occurs immediately after phagocytosis; plasma membrane cholesterol returns to prephagocytosis levels after 12 hr. These studies and measurements of protein synthesis indicate that new plasma membrane synthesis occurs after a lag of 6 hr and is essentially complete in 12 hr. This time table for biosynthetic activity in PM was further confirmed by Lutton using concavalin A binding sites as markers for plasma membrane. In still another phagocyte, namely, human blood monocytes, Schmidt et al. [163] have shown that IgE receptor sites disappear immediately following phagocytosis but are restored in about 6-8 hr. In contrast, PMN, which are short lived and contain a nonrenewable population of granules show only an increased turnover of lipids which may be due to increased metabolism during phagocytosis. Detailed studies of the AM are lacking.

In summary, ephemeral phagocytes such as PMN have little endoplasmic reticulum and synthesize little new plasma membrane. In contrast, macrophages, which live longer and are capable of synthesizing lysosomal enzymes, require new plasma membrane synthesis in order to maintain their endocytic function.

F. Regulation of Lysosomal Enzyme Release

Lysosomal enzymes are stored in granular inactive forms. Phagocytosis causes the lysosomes to fuse with the PV and the enzymes are solubilized and activated. Some of the features of the transfer of these enzymes to the PV have already been discussed. It is generally thought that the PV milieu is highly acid (pH ~ 5.0), so permitting the maximum activity of the lysosomal acid proteases. These and other lysosomal enzymes are also released into the extracellular fluid. The relative contributions of various lysosomal enzymes in tissue fluids then depend on their activities and the local pH which may range from pH 7.45 to acid values in severe inflammatory reactions where anaerobiosis is enforced by local O_2 depletion.

The release of the enzymes can be considered from four separate viewpoints. First, what are the mechanisms involved in fusion and degranulation?

Second, what factors regulate the secretion of lysosomal enzymes? Third, since there are several types of granules, is there a sequence of release? Fourth, are any lysosomal enzymes secreted independently of a phagocytic stimulation? In addition, it should be noted that lysosomal enzyme content in the macrophage group, as opposed to PMN, can be induced de novo or increased further by both phagocytosis and the pinocytosis of certain materials. This induction process will be described in relation to pinocytosis.

1. Degranulation

One approach regards contact between the PV and lysosome as the crucial factor. This view is certainly consistent with the morphologic evidence of contact degranulation. Hawiger and colleagues [83] have devised models for this system in which PMN granules are lysed by contact with artificial liposomes. The studies demonstrated that liposomes made with phosphatidyl inositol, a plasma membrane component, induced both degranulation and lysosomal enzyme activation in direct proportion to the liposome concentrations. This effect by some types of liposomes has pH optimum of 5.0 and incorporation of cortisol into the liposomes diminishes the lysosomal activation by liposomes. These effects of liposomes are diminished by basic proteins. This view speculates that phagocytosis induces changes in the plasma membrane during PV formation. The altered membrane might then trigger lysosomal degranulation. This view is compatible with a role for microtubules in directing PV motion towards the lysosome. Poor degranulation is a feature of Chediak-Higashi PMN [155].

2. Regulation of Secretion

This has been extensively studied employing a pharmacologic analysis of the process of lysosomal release. The analysis focuses on the "messenger" roles of cyclic nucleotides similar to those which regulate secretory phenomena. Indeed, this view regards lysosomal extrusion as a form of "exocytosis." The evidence for this view is strong in the PMN and PM but limited in the AM.

Before describing the effects of particle uptake on lysosomal enzyme release, it is useful to remind the reader that this release can occur without the ingestion of particles (Sec. IV.F.3). This has been demonstrated with two activating systems, antigen-antibody complexes bound to nonphagocytosable surfaces such as millipore filters [197,209] and a component of serum released by zymosan granules [89]. This component has many characteristics of the C_{5a} component of complement. In addition, it is possible, at least in the PMN, to dissociate ingestion from the adhesion of particles to the plasma membrane by the use of cytochalasin B which selectively depresses ingestion. In all these systems, lysosomal enzymes such as β-glucuronidase show about 25% release into the extracellular fluid. This release is not associated with the loss of a soluble cytosol enzyme, lactic acid dehydrogenase. This indicates that the process is indeed selective and that cytosol leakage cannot explain the lysosomal enzyme release. In such systems, it is possible to examine the roles of cyclic nucleotides and microtubules. For instance, employing surface bound antigen-antibody complexes and agents which presumably increase intracellular cAMP, β-glucuronidase release is diminished. These agents include cAMP, its dibutyryl analog, PGE_1, and theophylline. While cAMP levels were not measured, the similar effects of the above drugs is most economically explained by their common action in raising cAMP levels within the cells. Further, colchicine (10^{-5} M) causes a 27% diminution of β-glucuronidase release in the same system, suggesting that β-glucuronidase release depends on intact microtubular function. Similarly cytochalasin B treated PMN [210] and AM [3] all release lysosomal enzymes following exposure to particles. In the PMN and PM but not AM, the release in the presence of cytochalasin B is diminished by the above agents which presumably elevate cAMP. Further, employing PMN and zymosan induced release of the C_{5a} component of complement from serum in the presence of cytochalasin B; there were similar inhibitory effects of cAMP, theophylline, PGE_1, and colchicine on β-glucuronidase release [210]. This C_{5a} like material transiently increased the numbers of microtubules. In addition, cGMP enhanced the β-glucuronidase release. These observations support the hypothesis that lysosomal release is regulated by levels of cAMP and cGMP via their effects on the polymerization of tubulin to form organized microtubules.

A comment on the mechanism whereby cytochalasin B promotes lysosomal release without ingestion is germane. Cytochalasin B may disrupt a subplasmalemmal microfilament network which maintains subcellular organelles within the cell. Alternatively, incomplete fusion of pseudopodia around the particle may result in incomplete PV formation and lysosomal enzyme leakage.

Somewhat similar studies have been reported in association with particle ingestion. Ignarro [88,90,91] also employed human PMN. Heat aggregated human IgG complexes were used as the test particles. These caused release of neutral proteases and β-glucuronidase. In addition to showing a decrease of this release by cAMP and theophylline, and an increase in release with cGMP, they were able to show that effects could be obtained by certain neurohormones. For instance, cholinergic drugs stimulated release but were blocked by atropine. Studies with adrenergic drugs and appropriate blocking agents showed that lysosomal enzyme release was depressed by stimulation of the β-receptor. The additional observation that neurohumoral antagonists do not block the effects of either cyclic nucleotide suggests that the neurohormones act via their "second messenger," the appropriate cyclic nucleotide.

Further evidence that neurohumoral factors regulate lysosomal behavior comes from observation on fibroblasts and PMN in Chediak-Higashi syndrome. In this disorder, macrolysosomes are observed. They can be disaggregated by the cholinergic agonist, carbamyl choline [130].

Confirmation of the role of cyclic nucleotides in the modulation of lysosomal responses during phagocytosis requires a number of steps. First, detailed information on the concentrations and turnover rates of intracellular cyclic nucleotides during phagocytosis is required. At present the data on PMN are conflicting. Two reports claim increased cAMP levels and six failed to detect any change during phagocytosis. The increased cAMP level during phagocytosis is somewhat unexpected since it depressed lysosomal enzyme release which is usually promoted by phagocytosis. Second, measurements of cGMP during phagocytosis are not presently available. Third, detailed information on the behavior of adenylate and guanylate cyclases and phosphodiesterases are also lacking. Finally, the present evidence implicating these cyclic nucleotides with in vivo microtubule organization is incomplete.

Turning to the AM, phagocytic release of lysosomal enzymes has been less well studied. Variable extracellular release of lysosomal enzymes during phagocytosis has been reported [1,2,44,207]. Possible factors in this variability include the necessity for maintaining high O_2 tensions to achieve lysosomal release and species variations. Ackerman (personal communication) failed to obtain any effects of cholinergic or adrenergic agents on lysosomal release during phagocytosis. Similarly, prostaglandins E_1, E_2, F_{2a} and theophylline had no effect on lysosomal release [3]. This contrasts with the ability of these agents to diminish glucose conversion to CO_2 in both resting and phagocytosing AM [61] and with their ability to increase intracellular cAMP levels [162]. Cytochalasin B and zymosan caused comparable release of β-glucuronidase and these effects were colchicine-sensitive [2]. One study of cAMP levels during phagocytosis showed similar levels to those in resting AM [113]; another reported transient rises in cAMP occurring during the first 2-5 min of particle exposure [162,164].

3. *Release Sequence*

It is clear that PMN contain at least two types of granules, the azurophil and the so-called specific granule. These granules contain different enzymes. Peroxidase and proteases, notably elastase, characterize azurophils. Alkaline phosphatase and collagenase characterize specific granules which also contain most of the lysozyme [46,151]. Bainton [15] has shown, using some of the above enzymes as markers, that the specific granules discharge their enzymes in the first minute of phagocytosis. The azurophil granules discharge their enzymes into PV somewhat later. By 10 min, PV contain enzymes from both granules. The mechanisms responsible for this sequence are not known but may depend on the differences in the phospholipid composition of the granule membranes [81].

There is less information on the distribution of enzymes in macrophage granules. Indeed there are no overt morphologic and little cytochemical differences between the lysosomes within any given macrophage type. However, it is clear that developing monocytes, a macrophage precursor, acquire two types of granules. The promonocyte contains granules with peroxidase and arylsulfatase activities. During maturation, peroxidase negative granules appear. Their biochemical features are unknown [125].

There are no studies of AM granule variations; to the extent AM derive from monocytes, such variations appear likely.

4. Phagocytosis Independent Lysosomal Enzyme Release

Certain lysosomal enzymes are secreted independently of phagocytosis. The best example of this is lysozyme (muramidase) which has been extensively studied [133]. It hydrolyzes N-acetyl muramic β-1,4 N-acetyl glucosamine linkages. It is a weak antimicrobial agent attacking bacterial cell wall peptidoglycans. It potentiates the antimicrobial effects of one peroxidative system [121]. In PMN, lysozyme is found largely but not exclusively in the specific granules. It is present in high specific activity in rabbit and human AM [55,82]. Human monocytes, mouse PM and rabbit AM secrete lysozyme in tissue culture [70]. The secretion rate is little influenced by massive phagocytic pulses.

This enzyme can be used as a marker of the PMN and/or macrophage pool in disease states. Serum lysozyme levels reflect the activities and/or pool size of these phagocytes. For instance, Finch developed this marker in myeloid and monocytic leukemias. Serum lysozyme levels may be also used to define activity in such granulomatous lung diseases as tuberculosis [140] and sarcoidosis [135]. In the latter, lysozyme levels fall rapidly with steroid administration.

5. Lysosomal Enzymes and Lung Disease

Lung diseases may arise either from the failure of these defense mechanisms or their inappropriate use. This failure leads to opportunistic infections. The effects of corticosteroids on AM lysosomal release is well documented [50] and has obvious reference to lung defense mechanisms. Clinical aspects of cellular lung defense failure in the compromised host and the effects of drugs on lysosomal function and other aspects of phagocytosis have been recently reviewed [43,107].

Lysosomal enzymes may be released inappropriately and induce inflammatory, degradative or fibrogenic responses in the lung. Chemotaxis of PMN and lysosomal release will follow immune-complex deposition in diseases associated with biologic dust inhalation, e.g., farmer's lung. Since both PMN and AM contain collagenases and elastases, these may account for the degradative loss of structural proteins when the enzymes are not subject to circulating antiprotesase as in familial α_1-antitrypsin deficiency. Green's group has recently studied the effects of inhaled materials on human AM in tissue culture [44]. They find that some materials, e.g. bacteria and zymosan, evoke selective lysosomal enzyme release. Others, e.g. silica and asbestos, cause cytoxicity (LDH and lysosomal enzyme release). Of considerable interest is their observation that Kaolinite, a nonbiodegradable material present in both cigarette smoke and human AM from smoking subjects, also provokes a cytotoxic lysosomal enzyme release.

Thus, it is already apparent that the effects of a given particle type on the defense cells, particularly the AM, will depend on their ability to induce or enhance specific lysosomal enzyme activities and on the state of activation present in the macrophage. For instance, repeated bacterial challenge may cause activation; inert particles may then induce persistent release of preformed lysosomal enzymes. A good example of the interaction between activation and phagocytosis producing vigorous secretion of the neutral protease, plasminogen activator, is seen in PM. Such cells, "primed" with endotoxin, persistently secrete the activator following a phagocytic pulse of latex particles, but show transient secretion when digestible materials are phagocytosed [71]. It is tempting to analyze the course of obstructive lung disease as a consequence of repeated infections causing AM activation which in turn sets the stage for inert kaolinite particles to evoke the persistent release of neutral proteases such as collagenase. A detailed analysis of such interactions in the AM may well be most rewarding.

Finally, a study of the interaction between fibroblasts and macrophages will also help elucidate the fibrosis associated with granulomatous and other infiltrative lung diseases.

V. Pinocytosis

Pinocytosis was originally thought to be the process of "drinking" or uptake of fluid by cells. It more properly concerns the uptake of solutes or colloids. As opposed to phagocytosis in which macrophages take up insoluble or particulate material, pinocytosis refers to the uptake of soluble materials which cannot penetrate the intact cell membrane but enter the cell by the formation of vacuoles.

Pinocytosis may be divided into two types, depending upon the molecular weight of the solute and the type of deformation of the membrane. The term micropinocytosis refers to pinocytosis of solutes of low molecular weight, e.g., sucrose (MW 340) which results in small undulations of the membrane. On the other hand in macropinocytosis solutes of large molecular weight are interiorized by the formation of a vacuole by fusion, e.g., DNA (MW 2×10^6). The pinocytic vacuole migrates within the cell and usually fuses with the lysosomes. Since there are so few studies of pinocytosis by the AM and since PMN exhibit little or no pinocytosis, we will only sketch a few studies by Cohn of pinocytosis in the PM [35], and refer the reader to general reviews [72,86,157]. The process is energy requiring. In tissue culture, protein synthesis inhibitors diminish pinocytosis presumably by interference with cell membrane renewal. Certain materials are readily pinocytosed, e.g., sucrose, dextran and colloidal gold. Other materials induce pinosome formation; these include anionic proteins, nucleoside phosphates, and a number of proteins often used in tissue culture media, e.g., bovine sera. There are several important consequences of pinocytosis. For instance, the uptake of nondegradable substances, e.g., sucrose, causes lysosomal swelling and sequestration of the substance in the pinolysosomes. Certain enzymes can be pinocytosed and thereby alter the degradability of materials present in pinolysosomes, e.g., invertase which can thereby degrade preingested sucrose. Further, certain materials evoke lysosomal enzyme synthesis. Originally it was thought that lysosomal enzyme induction only occurred if the materials being pinocytosed were degradable. This is probably not the case and detailed studies of the relationship between the effects of pinocytosed materials and the synthetic and other cellular responses are required.

In the AM, sucrose can be taken up [206]. The enzyme uricase can be introduced into the cell [179]. While these studies indicate that the AM exhibit pinocytosis, the behavior of AM following ingestion of biologically important materials is an open field for investigation.

VI. Cell Function in the Intact Lung

The major thrust of the foregoing discussion has been based on in vitro studies of lung defense cells. These studies have provided intimate mechanistic details of their behavior. They have begun to elucidate the immunologic and biochemical features which serve their defensive function. In vitro studies permit a discrete analysis of these specific cellular mechanisms. They further demonstrate the multiple antimicrobial defensive potentialities and the amplification of these responses particularly by inflammatory and immunologic response mediators. While it is clear that we have much more mechanistic information about PMN

TABLE 2 Possible Defects in Alveolar Macrophage Function

Condition	Defect
Acidosis	Mobilization
Anesthesia	Microtubule
Cigarette smoke	Energy
Cold	?
Epinephrine	?
Ethanol	Mobilization
Hypoxia	Energy, H_2O_2 formation
Immuno suppression	Activation mechanism
Oxidants (NO_2, O_3, O_2)	Uptake
Renal failure	? and acidosis
Steroids	Lysosome hyperstability
Theophylline	Chemotaxis, lysosome release
Viruses	Particle blockade of uptake

than AM, the efficiency of the AM is demonstrated by the sterility of the healthy lung. This sterility is achieved without any inflammatory response and little or no PMN mobilization both of which would affect the lung gas exchange function. The absence of this inflammatory response indicates that AM as opposed to PMN are the major resident defense cells. The AM or their precursors can be regulated immunologically by intrapulmonary cellular and humoral amplification mechanisms since serum and secretory immunoglobulins and also lymphocytes can be identified in lung washes from animals and man.

Important approaches to the function of the AM in the intact lung derives from the extensive studies from the laboratories of Kass, Green [75], Goldstein [66], and Huber. The technique involves inhalation challenge with ^{32}P-labeled bacteria and measuring the viability of the organisms which are retained within the lung. The intrapulmonary microbicidal activity can thus be measured under various experimental conditions. A summary of the possible defects in AM function accounting for experimental impairment of intrapulmonary killing is presented in Table 2.

The interrelation between components of the lung lining fluid and AM should be emphasized. These components, so far unidentified, potentiate AM microbicidal activity [105].

Limited space precludes a full discussion of neutrophil dysfunction syndromes [99] which frequently but not universally predispose to pulmonary infections.

VII. Prospects

Basic and applied research on endocytosis has developed rapidly in the last decade. Areas of importance for the future may be highlighted. From the standpoint of cell biology the following questions seem important. What are the mechanisms of excitation coupling whereby plasma membrane binding sites evoke vectorial motion? What is the chemical nature of these binding sites? How do materials entering endolysosomes cause changes in protein synthesis and to what extent are the enzymes produced specific for specific ingestates?

From the applied and clinical standpoint, certain problems are unique to the lung. Since AM chemotaxins are hard to define, does this mean that the activated AM obtained by lavage are activated by local humoral mechanisms or are the AM derived from monocytes? If it is the latter, are there specific monocyte chemotaxins? Are monocytes becoming activated in the peripheral blood in some diseases, e.g., sarcoid?

Intraalveolar phagocytosis occurs in a unique biologic fluid with high lipid content and a low surface tension. How does this milieu affect the phagocytic mechanism of AM? In this connection it is known that lung lipids include polyunsaturated fatty acids which form lipid peroxides following the inhalation of oxidants. Such lipid peroxides diminish bacterial uptake in vitro [97]. Are there other interactions between lung lining fluids and AM function?

If neutral protease release is important in lung tissue degradation, can we develop new methods for diminishing the release? Finally, can industrially important, cytotoxic respirable particles be "coated" in such a manner as to minimize their toxicity while preserving their value in modern industrial society?

Recent Developments

In the past two years, several important developments have occurred.

1. Chemotaxis and Opsonization

A number of small peptides, e.g., formyl-methionine-leucine-phenylalanine, have been shown to act both as chemotaxins and metabolic stimulants in PMN [225, 226]. It seems very likely that similar effects will occur with AM.

Further evidence indicating the amplification of the inflammatory response derived from the observation that AM can release materials which are chemotactic from PMN [218].

Reynolds has provided direct evidence that human AM contain receptors for both IgG and the C_{3b} fragment of complement [220]. In addition, the opsonic antibody for *P. aeruginosa* is largely found in IgG class [221], an immunoglobulin found in the lavage fluid from the human lung.

2. Oxygen Metabolism

While there is considerable species variation, further evidence for the formation of $O_2^{-}\cdot$ and H_2O_2 in phagocytosing AM has now been obtained [213,214, and G. Bolen and R. K. Root, unpublished observation]. The precise quantities and metabolic sequences of these O_2 metabolites remains to be defined; however, their potential role in microbicidal mechanisms is further suggested by the recent demonstration that human AM contain a "peroxidase" which can be assayed with o-dianisidine as opposed to guaiacol as a substrate [212]. This peroxidase is found in the 20,000 g fraction and has characteristics consistent with an antimicrobial function.

The system generating the O_2 reduction products has been reexamined in the PMN. There now seems little doubt that the major pathway involves NADPH as opposed to NADH, possibly by a chain reaction involving NADP· [219]. Evidence for a cell membrane localization of the NADPH oxidase now exists [223, 228].

The "cost-benefit ratio" of these reduction products of O_2 requires comment. As suggested earlier, the extracellular release of these products can play both defensive and destructive roles within the host. For instance, during phagocytosis, cultured human PMN self-destruct, a process preventable by the antioxidants SOD, catalase, and manitol [224]. By contrast, AM can adapt to increased O_2 tensions by increasing the levels of superoxide dismutase. Two examples of this adaptive antioxidant response may be given. First, in tissue cultures, AM adapt to changes to O_2 tension [227]. Second, the AM are the major source of increased SOD activity in the fetal lung undergoing adaptation to hyperoxia [211].

3. Neutral Proteases

The presence, in PMN, of proteases which attack native insoluble elastin and collagen at the neutral pH of extracellular fluid has been known for some time. Similar enzymes have now been identified in macrophages obtained from various sites and species. While there is some storage of these enzymes, under certain circumstances, including phagocytosis, they are continuously secreted. Crystal's group has demonstrated a collagenase in AM [216]. This enzyme is activated by another AM enzyme, a neutral protease [217]. In addition, an elastase has been identified in human AM, particularly in cigarette smokers [222]. This enzyme has a different inhibitor profile from the elastase present human PMN (L. Hinman and J. B. L. Gee, unpublished observation). Further, the release of this enzyme by mouse AM is temporarily diminished by tetracycline [229].

4. *Recent Review*

Further details of lung defense cells may be found in a recent publication [215].

Acknowledgment

This work was supported in part by the National Heart and Lung Institute Grant (USPHS HL 14179, SCOR Program).

References

1. N. R. Ackerman and J. R. Beebe, Release of β-glucuronidase and elastase from alveolar mononuclear cells, *Chest,* **66**:21S-23S (1974).
2. N. R. Ackerman and J. R. Beebe, Release of lysosomal enzymes by alveolar mononuclear cells, *Nature,* **247**:475-477 (1974).
3. N. R. Ackerman and J. R. Beebe, Effects of pharmacologic agents on the release of lysosomal enzymes from alveolar mononuclear cells, *J. Pharmacol. Exp. Ther.,* **193**:603-613 (1975).
4. R. C. Allen, R. L. Stjernholm, and R. H. Steele, Evidence for the generation of an electronic excitation state(s) in human polymorphonuclear leukocytes and its participation in bactericidal activity, *Biochem. Biophys. Res. Commun.,* **47**:679-684 (1972).
5. R. C. Allen, S. J. Yevich, R. W. Orth, and R. H. Steele, The superoxide anion and singlet molecular oxygen: Their role in the microbicidal activity of the polymorphonuclear leukocyte, *Biochem. Biophys. Res. Commun.,* **60**:909-917 (1974).
6. A. C. Allison, The role of lysosomes in the action of drugs and hormones, *Adv. Chemother.,* **3**:253-302 (1968).
7. A. C. Allison, The role of microfilaments and microtubules in cell movement, endocytosis and exocytosis, *Ciba Found. Symp.,* **14**:109-148 (1973).
8. A. C. Allison, G. H. Hulands, J. F. Nunn, J. A. Kitching, and A. C. MacDonald, The effect of inhalational anaesthetics on the microtubular system in actinosphaerium nucleofilum, *J. Cell. Sci.,* **7**:483-499 (1970).
9. A. C. Allison and J. F. Nunn, Effects of general anaesthetics on microtubules, *Lancet,* **36**:1326-1329 (1968).
10. S. G. Axline and E. P. Reaven, Inhibition of phagocytosis and plasma membrane mobility of the cultivated macrophage by cytochalasin B. Role of subplasmalemmal microfilaments, *J. Cell. Biol.,* **62**:647-659 (1974).

11. B. M. Babior, J. T. Curnutte, and R. S. Kipnes, Biological defense mechanisms. Evidence for the participation of superoxide in bacterial killing by xanthine oxidase, *J. Lab. Clin. Med.*, **85**:235-244 (1975).
12. B. M. Babior, R. S. Kipnes, and J. T. Curnutte, Biological defense mechanisms. The production by leukocytes of superoxide, a potential bactericidal agent, *J. Clin. Invest.*, **52**:593-597 (1974).
13. R. L. Baehner, R. B. Johnston, Jr., and D. G. Nathan, Reduced pyridine nucleotide (RPN) content in G6PD-deficient granulocytes (PMN): An explanation for their defective bactericidal function, *J. Clin. Invest.*, **50**: 4a (1971).
14. D. F. Bainton, The origin, content and fate of polymorphonuclear leukocyte granules. In *Phagocytic Mechanisms in Health and Disease.* Edited by R. C. Williams and H. H. Fundenberg. New York, Intercontinental Medical Book, 1972, pp. 123-150.
15. D. F. Bainton, Sequential degranulation of two types of polymorphonuclear leukocytes granules during phagocytosis of microorganisms, *J. Cell. Biol.*, **58**:249-264 (1973).
16. W. R. Barclay, W. M. Bussey, D. W. Dalgard, R. C. Good, B. W. Janicki, J. E. Kasik, E. Ribi, C. E. Ulrich, and E. Wolinsky, Protection of monkeys against airborne tuberculosis by aerosol vaccination with Bacillus Calmette-Guerin, *Am. Rev. Respir. Dis.*, **107**:351-366 (1973).
17. E. L. Becker, Enzyme activation and the mechanism of polymorphonuclear leukocytes chemotaxis. In *Phagocytic Cell in Host Resistance.* Edited by J. A. Bellanti and D. H. Dayton. New York, Raven Press, 1975, pp. 1-14.
18. E. L. Becker, The relationship of the chemotactic behavior of the complement derived factors, C3a, C5a, and $C\overline{567}$, and a bacterial chemotactic factor to their ability to activate the proesterase 1 of rabbit polymorphonuclear leukocytes, *J. Exp. Med.*, **135**:376-387 (1972).
19. J. A. Bellanti and D. H. Dayton, *Phagocytic Cell in Host Resistance.* New York, Raven Press, 1975.
20. R. D. Berlin, J. M. Oliver, T. E. Ukena, and H. H. Yin, Control of cell surface topography, *Nature*, **247**:45-46 (1974).
21. W. D. Biggar, B. Holmes, and R. A. Good, Opsonic defect in patients with cystic fibrosis of the pancreas, *Proc. Natl. Acad. Sci. USA*, **68**:1716-1721 (1971).
22. D. H. Bowden, The alveolar macrophage, *Curr. Top. Pathol.*, **55**:1-36 (1971).
23. D. H. Bowden, The alveolar macrophage and its role in toxicology, *CRC Crit. Rev. Toxicol.*, pp. 95-124 (1973).
24. B. R. Boynton, A. S. Khandwala, and J. B. L. Gee, Effect of aqueous extract of cigarette smoke on the metabolism of alveolar macrophages, *Clin. Res.*, **23**:345A (1975).
25. L. A. Boxer, E. T. Hedley-Whyte, and T. P. Stossel, Neutrophil actin dysfunction and abnormal neutrophil behavior, *N. Engl. J. Med.*, **291**:1093-1100 (1974).
26. B. Boxerbaum, M. Kagremba, and L. W. Matthew, Selective inhibition of

phagocytic activity of rabbit alveolar macrophages by cystic fibrosis serum, *Am. Rev. Respir. Dis.*, **108**:777-783 (1973).

27. R. G. Brayton, P. E. Stokes, M. S. Schwartz, and D. B. Louria, Effect of alcohol and various diseases on leukocyte mobilization, phagocytosis and intracellular bacterial killing, *N. Engl. J. Med.*, **282**:123-128 (1970).
28. L. H. Burbaker, Unsticky neutrophils, *N. Engl. J. Med.*, **291**:674-675 (1974).
29. A. Capron, J. P. Dessaint, M. Capron, and H. Bazin, Specific IgE antibodies in immune adherence of normal macrophages to schistosoma mansoni schistosomules, *Nature*, **253**:474-476 (1975).
30. A. Catanzaro, L. Spitler, and K. M. Moser, Immunotherapy of coccidiomycosis, *J. Clin. Invest.*, **54**:690-701 (1974).
31. R. A. Clark and S. J. Klebanoff, Neutrophil mediated tumor cell cytotoxicity: Role of the peroxidase system, *J. Exp. Med.*, **141**:1442-1447 (1975).
32. R. A. Clark, S. J. Klebanoff, A. B. Einstein, and A. Fefer, Peroxidase H_2O_2-halide system: Cytotoxic effect on mammalian tumor cells, *Blood*, **45**:161-170 (1975).
33. A. B. Cohen and M. J. Cline, The human alveolar macrophage: Isolation, cultivation in vitro, and studies of morphologic and functional characteristics, *J. Clin. Invest.*, **50**:1390-1398 (1971).
34. A. B. Cohen and D. Geczy, Purification of two populations of human alveolar macrophages from surgical specimens, *Am. Rev. Respir. Dis.*, **108**:972-975 (1973).
35. Z. A. Cohn, The structure and function of monocytes and macrophages, *Adv. Immunol.*, **9**:163-214 (1968).
36. A. Constantopoulous and V. A. Najjar, Tuftsin, a natural and general phagocytosis stimulating peptide affecting macrophages and polymorphonuclear granulocytes, *Cytobiosis*, **6**:97-100 (1972).
37. M. R. Cooper, L. R. DeChatelet, C. E. McCall, M. F. Lavia, C. L. Spurr, and R. L. Baehner, Complete deficiency of leukocyte G6PD with defective bactericidal activity, *J. Clin. Invest.*, **49**:21a (1970).
38. J. P. Cox and M. L. Karnovsky, The depression of phagocytosis by exogenous cyclic nucleotides, prostaglandins and theophylline, *J. Cell. Biol.*, **59**:480-490 (1973).
39. J. T. Curnutte and B. M. Babior, Biologic defense mechanisms: The effect of bacteria and serum on superoxide production by granulocytes, *J. Clin. Invest.*, **53**:1662-1672 (1974).
40. J. T. Curnutte, D. M. Whitten, and B. M. Babior, Defective superoxide production by granulocytes from patients with chronic granulomatous disease, *N. Engl. J. Med.*, **290**:593-597 (1974).
41. C. E. Cross, A. B. Ibrahim, M. Ahmed, and M. G. Mustafa, Effect of cadmium ion on respiration and ATPase activity of the pulmonary alveolar macrophage: A model for the study of environmental interference with pulmonary cell function, *Environ. Res.*, **3**:512-520 (1970).
42. J. R. David, A brief review of macrophage activation by lymphocyte medi-

ators. In *The Phagocytic Cell in Host Resistance.* Edited by J. A. Bellanti and D. H. Dayton. New York, Raven Press, 1975, pp. 143-153.

43. P. Davies, Drugs effecting the golgi apparatus and lysosomes. In *Fundamentals of Cell Pharmacology.* Edited by S. Dikstein. Springfield, Ill., Charles C Thomas, 1973, pp. 231-250.
44. G. S. Davis, M. Mortara, and G. M. Green, Lysosomal enzyme release from human and guinea pig alveolar macrophages, during phagocytosis, *J. Clin. Res.,* **23**:346A (1975).
45. L. R. DeChatelet, C. E. McCall, L. C. McPhail, and R. B. Johnston, Jr., Superoxide dismutase activity in leukocytes, *J. Clin. Invest.,* **53**:1197-1201 (1974).
46. B. Dewald, R. Rindler-Ludwig, U. Bretz, and M. Baggiolini, Subcellular localization and heterogeneity of neutral proteases in neutrophilic polymorphonuclear leukocytes. *J. Exp. Med.,* **141**:709-723 (1975).
47. D. B. Drath and M. L. Karnovsky, Superoxide production by phagocytic leukocytes, *J. Exp. Med.,* **141**:257-262 (1975).
48. P. B. Dunham, I. M. Goldstein, and G. Weissmann, Potassium and amino acid transport in human leukocytes exposed to phagocytic stimuli, *J. Cell Biol.,* **63**:215-226 (1974).
49. P. J. Edelson and Z. A. Cohn, Peroxidative-mediated mammalian cell cytotoxicity, *J. Exp. Med.,* **138**:318-323 (1973).
50. S. M. Epstein, E. Verney, T. D. Miale, and M. Sidaransky, Studies on the pathogenesis of experimental pulmonary aspergillosis, *Am. J. Pathol.,* **51**: 769-781 (1967).
51. R. D. Estensen, M. Rosenberg, and J. D. Sheridan, Cytochalasin B: Microfilaments and "contractile" processes, *Science,* **173**:356-357 (1971).
52. A. Finazzi Agro, P. De Sole, G. Rotilio, and B. Mondovi, Influence of catalase and superoxide dismutase on side oxidations involving singlet oxygen, *Ital. J. Biochem.,* **22**:217-231 (1973).
53. J. J. Freed and M. M. Lebowitz, The association of a class of saltatory movements with microtubules in cultures cells, *J. Cell Biol.,* **45**:334-354 (1970).
54. I. Fridovich, Oxygen: Boon and bane, *Am. Sci.,* **63**:54-59 (1975).
55. B. Galindo and Q. N. Myrvik, Migratory response of granulomatous alveolar cells from BCG sensitized rabbits, *J. Immunol.,* **105**:227-237 (1970).
56. J. I. Gallin and C. H. Kirkpatrick, Chemotactic activity in dialyzable transfer factor, *Proc. Natl. Acad. Sci.,* **71**:498-502 (1974).
57. J. I. Gallin and A. S. Rosenthal, The regulatory role of davalent cations in human granulocyte chemotaxis. Evidence for an association between calcium exchanges and microtubule assembly, *J. Cell Biol.,* **62**:594-609 (1974).
58. J. B. L. Gee and C. E. Cross, Drugs affecting phagocytosis and pinocytosis. In *Fundamentals of Cell Pharmacology.* Edited by S. Dikstein. Springfield, Ill., Charles C Thomas, 1973, pp. 349-372.
59. J. B. L. Gee, J. Kaskin, M. P. Duncombe, and C. L. Vassallo, The effects of ethanol on some metabolic features of phagocytosis in the alveolar macrophage, *J. Reticuloendothel. Soc.,* **15**:61-68 (1974).

60. J. B. L. Gee, A. S. Khandwala, and R. W. Bell, Hexose transport in the alveolar macrophage: Kinetics and pharmacologic features, *J. Reticuloendothel. Soc.*, **15**:394-405 (1974).
61. J. B. L. Gee, A. S. Khandwala, P. E. McKeever, and S. E. Malawista, Glucose oxidation in alveolar macrophages: Pharmacologic features, *J. Reticuloendothel. Soc.*, **15**:387-393 (1974).
62. J. B. L. Gee, C. L. Vassallo, P. Bell, J. Kaskin, R. E. Basford, and J. B. Field, Catalase dependent peroxidative metabolism in the alveolar macrophage during phagocytosis, *J. Clin. Invest.*, **50**:1280-1287 (1970).
63. J. B. L. Gee, C. L. Vassallo, M. L. Vogt, C. Thomas, and R. E. Basford, Peroxidative metabolism in alveolar macrophages, *Arch. Intern. Med.*, **127**: 1046-1049 (1971).
64. E. J. Goetzl and K. F. Austen, Simulation of human neutrophil leukocyte aerobic glucose metabolism by purified chemotactic factors, *J. Clin. Invest.*, **53**:591-599 (1974).
65. D. W. Golde, T. N. Finley, and M. J. Cline, The pulmonary macrophage in acute leukemia, *N. Engl. J. Med.*, **290**:875-878 (1974).
66. E. Goldstein, W. Lippert, D. Warshauer, Pulmonary alveolar macrophage (defender against bacterial infection of the lung), *J. Clin. Invest.*, **54**:519-528 (1974).
67. I. Goldstein, S. Hoffstein, J. Gallin, and G. Weissmann, Mechanisms of lysosomal enzyme release from human leukocytes: Microtubule assembly and membrane fusion induced by a component complement, *Proc. Natl. Acad. Sci. USA*, **70**:2916-2920 (1973).
68. D. B. P. Goodman, H. Rasmussen, F. DiBella, and C. E. Guthrow, Jr., Cyclic adenosine 3′:5′-monophosphate-stimulated phosphorylation of isolated neurotubule subunits, *Proc. Natl. Acad. Sci. USA*, **67**:652-659 (1970).
69. S. Gordon and Z. A. Cohn, The macrophage, *Int. Rev. Cytol.*, **36**:171-214 (1973).
70. S. Gordon, J. Todd, and Z. A. Cohn, In vitro synthesis and secretion of lysozyme by mononuclear phagocytes, *J. Exp. Med.*, **139**:1228-1248 (1974).
71. S. Gordon, J. C. Unkeless, and Z. A. Cohn, Induction of macrophage plasminogen activator by endotoxin stimulation and phagocytosis, *J. Exp. Med.*, **140**:995-1010 (1974).
72. R. E. Gosselin, Kinetics of pinocytosis, *Fed. Proc.*, **29**:687-691 (1967).
73. R. C. Graham, Jr., M. J. Karnovsky, A. W. Shafer, E. A. Glass, and M. L. Karnovsky, Metabolic and morphological observations on the effect of surface active agents on leukocytes, *J. Cell Biol.*, **32**:629-639 (1967).
74. G. M. Green, Cigarette smoke: Protection of alveolar macrophages by glutathione and cysteine, *Science*, **162**:810-811 (1968).
75. G. M. Green, Pulmonary clearance of infectious agents, *Annu. Rev. Med.*, **19**:315-336 (1968).
76. G. M. Green and D. Carolin, The depressant effect of cigarette smoke on the in vitro antibacterial activity of alveolar macrophages, *N. Engl. J. Med.*, **276**:421-428 (1967).

77. L. H. Green and G. M. Green, Differential suppression of pulmonary antibacterial activity as the mechanism of selection of a pathogen in mixed bacterial infection of the lung, *Am. Rev. Respir. Dis.*, **98**:819-824 (1968).
78. F. M. Griffin, Jr., and S. C. Silverstein, Segmental response of the macrophage plasma membrane to a phagocytic stimulus, *J. Exp. Med.*, **139**:323-336 (1974).
79. J. J. Guarneri and G. A. Laurenzi, Effect of alcohol on the mobilization of alveolar macrophages, *J. Lab. Clin. Med.*, **72**:40-51 (1968).
80. I. Gwynn, R. B. Kemp, B. M. Jones, and U. Groschell-Stewart, Ultrastructural evidence for myosin of the smooth muscle type at the surface of trypsin-dissociated embryonic chick cells, *J. Cell Sci.*, **15**:279-290 (1974).
81. R. Hachman, J. G. Hirsch, and M. Baggiolini, Studies on isolated membranes of azurophil and specific granules from rabbit polymorphonuclear leukocytes, *J. Cell Biol.*, **54**:133-140 (1972).
82. J. O. Harris, G. N. Olsen, J. R. Castle, and A. S. Maloney, Comparison of proteolytic enzyme activity in pulmonary alveolar macrophages and blood leukocytes in smokers and nonsmokers, *Am. Rev. Respir. Dis.*, **111**:579-586 (1975).
83. J. Hawiger, R. Horn, M. Koenig, and R. Collins, Activation and release of lysosomal enzymes from isolated leukocytic granules by liposomes. A. Proposed model for degranulation in polymorphonuclear leukocytes, *Yale J. Biol. Med.*, **42**:57-70 (1969).
84. L. W. Henderson, M. E. Miller, R. W. Hamilton, and M. E. Norman, Hemodialysis leukopenia and polymorph random mobility—a possible correlation, *J. Lab. Clin. Med.*, **85**:191-197 (1975).
85. D. C. Hohn and R. I. Lehrer, NADPH oxidase deficiency in X-linked chronic granulomatous disease, *J. Clin. Invest.*, **55**:707-713 (1975).
86. M. Holter, Pinocytosis, *Int. Rev. Cytol.*, **8**:481-504 (1959).
87. H. Huber and H. H. Fudenberg, Receptor sites of human monocytes for IgG, *Int. Arch. Allergy Appl. Immunol.*, **34**:18-31 (1968).
88. L. J. Ignarro, Neutral protease release from human leukocytes regulated by neurohormones and cyclic nucleotides, *Nature [New Biol.]*, **245**:151-154 (1973).
89. L. J. Ignarro, Nonphagocytic release of neutral protease and β-glucuronidase from human neutrophils, *Arthritis Rheum.*, **17**:25-36 (1974).
90. L. J. Ignarro and W. J. George, Hormonal control of lysosomal enzyme release from human neutrophils: Elevation of cyclic nucleotide levels by autonomic neurohormones, *Proc. Natl. Acad. Sci. USA*, **71**:2027-2031 (1974).
91. L. J. Ignarro, R. J. Paddock, and W. J. George, Hormonal control of neutrophil lysosomal enzyme release: Effect of epinephrine on adenosine 3′,5′-monophosphate, *Science*, **183**:855-857 (1974).
92. A. Janoff, Neutrophil proteases in inflammation, *Annu. Rev. Med.*, **23**:177-190 (1972).
93. R. B. Johnston, Jr., B. R. Keele, H. P. Misra, L. S. Webb, J. E. Lehmeyer, and K. V. Rajagopalan, Superoxide anion generation and phagocytic bac-

tericidal activity. In *The Phagocytic Cell in Host Resistance.* Edited by J. A. Bellanti and D. H. Dayton. New York, Raven Press, 1975, pp. 61-75.

94. M. L. Karnovsky, Chronic granulomatous disease–pieces of a cellular and molecular puzzle, *Fed. Proc.,* **32**:1527-1533 (1973).

95. M. L. Karnovsky, Metabolic basis of phagocytic activity, *Physiol. Rev.,* **42**:143-167 (1962).

96. A. S. Khandwala and J. B. L. Gee, Inhibition of 2-deoxy-D-glucose transport by theophylline, caffeine and papaverine in alveolar macrophages, *Biochem. Pharmacol.,* **23**:1781-1786 (1974).

97. A. S. Khandwala and J. B. L. Gee, Linoleic acid hydroperoxide: Impaired bacterial uptake by alveolar macrophages, a mechanism of oxidant lung injury, *Science,* **182**:1364-1365 (1973).

98. A. S. Khandwala and J. B. L. Gee, Factors in glucose oxidation by alveolar macrophages: Glucose transport and glycogenolysis, *Chest,* **67**:60S-63S (1975).

99. S. J. Klebanoff, Antimicrobial mechanisms in neutrophilic polymorphonuclear leukocytes, *Semin. Hematol.,* **12**:117-142 (1975).

100. S. J. Klebanoff, Role of the superoxide anion in the myeloperoxidase-mediated antimicrobial system, *J. Biol. Chem.,* **249**:3724-3728 (1974).

101. S. J. Klebanoff and C. B. Hamon, Antimicrobial systems of mononuclear phagocytes. In *Mononuclear Phagocytes in Immunity, Infection and Pathology.* Edited by R. van Furth. Oxford, Blackwell, 1975.

102. W. J. Koopman and J. R. David, Pharmacologic modulation of the biologic activity of MIF. In *Inflamation-Mechanisms and Control.* Edited by I. H. Lepow and P. A. Ward. New York, Academic Press, 1972, pp. 151-161.

103. N. I. Krinsky, Singlet excited oxygen as a mediator of the antibacterial action of leukocytes, *Science,* **186**:363-365 (1974).

104. C. Kuhn, Fine structure of bronchiolo-alveolar cell carcinoma, *Cancer,* **30**:1107-1118 (1972).

105. M. F. LaForce, W. J. Kelly, and G. L. Huber, Inactivation of staphylococci by alveolar macrophages with preliminary observations on the importance of alveolar lining material, *Am. Rev. Respir. Dis.,* **108**:784-794 (1973).

105a. E. S. Leake, M. J. Wright, and Q. N. Myrvik, *J. Reticuloendothel. Soc.,* **17**:370-379 (1975).

106. R. W. Leu, A. W. L. F. Eddleston, R. A. Good, and J. W. Hadden, Paradoxical effects of ouabain on the migration of peritoneal and alveolar macrophages, *Exp. Cell Res.,* **76**:458-461 (1973).

107. A. S. Levine, S. C. Schmpiff, D. G. Graw, Jr., and R. C. Young, Hematologic malignancies and other marrow failure states: Progress in the management of complicating infections, *Semin. Hematol.,* **11**:141-202 (1974).

108. R. R. MacGregor, P. J. Spagnuolo, and A. L. Lentnek, Inhibition of granulocyte adherence by ethanol, prednisone and aspirin measured with an assay system, *N. Engl. J. Med.,* **291**:642-646 (1974).

109. E. G. Maderazo, P. A. Ward, and R. Quintiliani, Defective regulation of chemotaxis in cirrhosis, *J. Lab. Clin. Med.,* **85**:621-630 (1975).

110. S. E. Malawista and P. T. Bodel, The dissociation by colchicine of phagocytosis from increased oxygen consumption in human leukocytes, *J. Clin. Invest.*, **46**:786-796 (1967).
111. S. E. Malawista, J. B. L. Gee, and K. G. Bensch, Cytochalasin B reversibly inhibits phagocytosis: Functional, metabolic, and ultrastructural effects in human blood leukocytes and rabbit alveolar macrophages, *Yale J. Biol. Med.*, **44**:286-300 (1971).
112. H. L. Malech, A. D. Schreiber, and R. K. Root, Changes in mononuclear leukocyte IgG receptors by chemotactic stimulus, Proceedings of the 14th Interscience Conference on Antimicrobial Agents and Chemotherapy, Abstract 10, American Society of Microbiology, San Francisco, California, Sept. 1974.
113. V. Manganiello, W. H. Evans, T. P. Stossel, R. J. Mason, and M. Vaughan, The effect of polystyrene beads on cyclic 3′,5′-adenosine monophosphate concentration in leukocytes, *J. Clin. Invest.*, **50**:2741-2744 (1971).
114. B. Mantovani, M. Rabinovitch, and V. Nussenzweig, Phagocytosis of immune complexes by macrophages, *J. Exp. Med.*, **135**:780-792 (1972).
115. R. J. Mason, T. P. Stossel, and M. Vaughan, Lipids of alveolar macrophages, polymorphonuclear leukocytes and their phagocytic vesicles, *J. Clin. Invest.*, **51**:2399-2407 (1972).
116. R. J. Mason, T. P. Stossel, and M. Vaughan, Quantitative studies of phagocytosis by alveolar macrophages, *Biochim. Biophys. Acta,* **304**:864-870 (1973).
117. T. H. Maugh II, Singlet oxygen: A unique microbicidal agent in cells, *Science,* **182**:44-45 (1973).
118. D. J. McCarty, Urate crystal phagocytosis by polymorphonuclear leukocytes and the effects of colchicine. In *Phagocytic Mechanism on Health and Disease.* Edited by R. C. Williams, Jr. and H. H. Fudenberg. New York, Intercontinental Medical Book, 1972, pp. 107-122.
119. P. E. McKeever, Methods to study pulmonary alveolar macrophage adherence, micromanipulation and quantitation, *J. Reticuloendothel Soc.*, **16**:313-317 (1974).
120. C. Meban, The localization of adenosine triphosphatase activity in the alveolar macrophages of hamster lung, *Experientia,* **15**:473-474 (1974).
121. T. E. Miller, Killing and lysis of gram-negative bacteria through the synergistic effect of hydrogen peroxide, ascorbic acid, and lysozyme, *J. Bacteriol.*, **98**:949-959 (1969).
122. A. F. Miranda, G. C. Godman, A. D. Deitch, and S. W. Tanenbaum, Action of cytochalasin D on cells of established lines. I. Early events, *J. Cell Biol.*, **61**:481-500 (1974).
123. A. F. Miranda, G. C. Godman and S. W. Tanenbaum, Action of cytochalasin D on cells of established lines. II. Cortex and microfilaments, *J. Cell Biol.*, **62**:406-423 (1974).
124. M. G. Mustafa, C. E. Cross, R. J. Munn, and J. A. Hardie, Effects of divalent metal ions on alveolar macrophage membrane adenosine triphosphatase activity, *J. Lab. Clin. Med.*, **77**:563-571 (1971).

125. B. A. Nichols and D. F. Bainton, Differentiation of human monocytes in bone marrow and blood. Sequential formation of two granule populations, *Lab. Invest.*, **29**:27-31 (1973).
126. K. A. Nishioka, A. Constantopoulous, P. S. Satoh, and V. A. Najjar, The characteristics, isolation and synthesis of the phagocytosis stimulating peptide tuftsin, *Biochem. Biophys. Res. Commun.*, **47**:172-179 (1972).
127. T. Odajima, Myeloperoxidase of the leukocyte of normal blood. II. The oxidation-reduction reaction mechanism of the myeloperoxidase system, *Biochim. Biophys. Acta*, **235**:52-60 (1971).
128. T. Odajima and I. Yamazaki, Myeloperoxidase of the leukocyte of normal blood. III. The reaction of ferric myeloperoxidase with superoxide anion, *Biochim. Biophys. Acta*, **284**:355-359 (1972).
129. J. M. Oliver and R. D. Berlin, Macrophage membrane. In *Immunobiology of the Macrophages*. Edited by D. S. Nelson. New York, Academic Press, 1975.
130. J. M. Oliver, J. A. Krawice, and R. D. Berlin, Carbamylcholine prevents giant granule formation in cultured fibroblasts from beige (Chediak-Higashi) mice, *J. Cell Biol.*, **69**:205-210 (1976).
131. J. M. Oliver, T. E. Ukena, and R. D. Berlin, Effects of phagocytosis and colchicine on the distribution of lectin-binding sites on cell surfaces, *Proc. Natl. Acad. Sci.*, **71**:394-398 (1974).
132. J. B. Olmsted and G. G. Borisy, Microtubules, *Annu. Rev. Biochem.*, **42**:507-540 (1973).
133. E. Ossermann, R. Canfield, and S. Beychok, *Lysozyme*, New York, Academic Press, 1974.
134. E. Ouchi, R. J. Selvaraj, J. Sbarra, The biochemical activities of rabbit alveolar macrophages during phagocytosis, *Exp. Cell Res.*, **40**:456-468 (1965).
135. R. S. Pascual, J. B. L. Gee, and S. C. Finch, Usefulness of serum lysozyme measurement in diagnosis and evaluation of sarcoidosis, *N. Engl. J. Med.*, **289**:1074-1076 (1973).
136. P. Patriarca, R. Cramer, M. Marossi, S. Moncalvo, and R. Rossi, Phospholipid splitting and metabolic stimulation in polymorphonuclear leukocytes, *J. Reticuloendothel. Soc.*, **10**:251-268 (1971).
137. B. Paul and A. J. Sbarra, The role of phagocyte in host-parasite interactions. XII. The direct quantitative estimation of H_2O_2 in phagocytosing cells, *Biochem. Biophys. Acta*, **156**:168-178 (1968).
138. B. B. Paul, R. R. Strauss, R. J. Selvaraj, and A. J. Sbarra, Peroxidative mediated antimicrobial activities of alveolar macrophage granules, *Science*, **181**:849-850 (1973).
139. N. N. Pearsall and R. S. Weiser, *The Macrophage*. Philadelphia, Pa., Lea and Febiger, 1970.
140. P. E. Perillie, K. Khan, and S. C. Finch, Serum lysozyme in pulmonary tuberculosis, *Am. J. Med. Sci.*, **265**:297-302 (1973).
141. E. L. Pesanti and S. G. Axline, Colchicine effects on lysosomal enzyme induction and intracellular degradation in the cultivated macrophage, *J. Exp. Med.*, **141**:1030-1046 (1975).

142. B. A. Pethica, The physical chemistry of cell adhesion, *Exp. Cell Res. [Suppl.]*, **8**:123-125 (1961).
143. J. M. Phillips-Qualiata, B. B. Levine, F. Qualiata, and J. W. Uhr, Mechanisms underlying binding of immune complexes to macrophages, *J. Exp. Med.*, **133**:589-601 (1971).
144. T. D. Pollard and R. R. Weihing, Actin and myosin and cell movement, *CRC Crit. Rev. Biochem.*, pp. 1-65 (1974).
145. R. Porter and D. W. Fitzsimons, Locomotion of tissue cell, *Ciba Found. Symp.* **14**. New York, American Elsevier Publishing Company, 1973.
146. G. M. Powell and G. M. Green, Cigarette smoke–A proposed metabolic lesion in alveolar macrophages, *Biochem. Pharmacol.*, **21**:1785-1798 (1972).
147. M. Rabinovitch, Phagocytosis: The engulfment stage, *Semin. Hematol.*, **5**:134-155 (1968).
148. E. P. Reaven and S. G. Axline, Subplasmalemmal microfilaments and microtubules in resting and phagocytozing cultivated macrophages, *J. Cell Biol.*, **59**:12-27 (1973).
149. L. I. Rebhun, Polarized intracellular particle transport: Saltatory movements and cytoplasmic streaming, *Int. Rev. Cytol.*, **32**:93-137 (1972).
150. H. G. Remold, Requirement for α-L-fucose on the macrophage membrane receptor for migration inhibitory factor, *J. Exp. Med.*, **138**:1065-1076 (1973).
151. P. B. Robertson, R. B. Ryel, R. E. Taylor, K. W. Shyv, and H. M. Fullmer, Collagenase: Localization in polymorphonuclear leukocyte granules in the rabbit, *Science*, **177**:64-65 (1972).
152. E. D. Robin, J. D. Smith, A. R. Tanser, J. S. Adamson, J. E. Millen, and B. Packer, Ion and macromolecular transport in the alveolar macrophage, *Biochim. Biophys. Acta*, **241**:117-128 (1971).
153. D. Romeo, R. Cramer, T. Marzi, N. R. Soranno, G. Zabucchi, and F. Rossi, Peroxidase activity of alveolar and peritoneal macrophages, *J. Reticuloendothel. Soc.*, **13**:399-409 (1973).
154. D. Romeo, G. Zabucchi, and F. Rossi, Reversible metabolic stimulation of polymorphonuclear leukocytes and macrophages by concanavalin A, *Nature [New Biol.]*, **243**:111-112 (1973).
155. R. K. Root, A. S. Rosenthal, and D. J. Balestra, Abnormal bactericidal, metabolic and lysosomal functions of Chediak-Higashi syndrome leukocytes, *J. Clin. Invest.*, **51**:649-665 (1972).
156. S. Ruddy, K. F. Austen, and E. J. Goetzl, Chemotactic activity derived from interaction of factors $\overline{D}$ and B of the properdin pathway with cobra venom factor of C3b, *J. Clin. Invest.*, **55**:587-592 (1975).
157. H. J. P. Ryser, Uptake of protein by mammalian cells: An underdeveloped area. The penetration of foreign proteins into mammalian cells can be measured and their functions explored, *Science*, **159**:390-398 (1968).
158. F. L. Sachs and J. B. L. Gee, Comparison of the effects of phagocytosis and phospholipase C on metabolism and lysozyme release in rabbit alveolar macrophages, *J. Reticuloendothel. Soc.*, **14**:52-58 (1973).

159. A. J. Sbarra, B. B. Paul, R. R. Strauss, and G. W. Mitchell, Jr., Metabolic and bactericidal activities of phagocytosing leukocytes. In *Regulation of Hematopoiesis,* Vol. 2. Edited by A. S. Gordon. New York, Appleton-Century-Crofts, 1970, pp. 1081-1108.
160. A. J. Sbarra and R. J. Selvaraj, Relationship of glycolytic and oxidative metabolism to particle entry and destruction in phagocytosing cells, *Nature,* **211**:1272-1276 (1966).
161. E. Schell-Frederick, Stimulation of the oxidative metabolism of polymorphonuclear leukocytes by the calcium ionophore A23187, *FEBS Lett.,* **48**:37-40 (1974).
162. H. E. Schmidt-Gayk, K. H. Jakobs, and E. Hackenthal, Cyclic AMP and phagocytosis in alveolar macrophages: Influence of hormones and dibutyryl cyclic AMP, *J. Reticuloendothel. Soc.,* **17**:251-261 (1975).
163. M. E. Schmidt and S. D. Douglas, Disappearance and recovery of human monocyte IgG receptor activity after phagocytosis, *J. Immunol.,* **109**: 914-917 (1972).
164. H. W. Seyberth, H. Schmidt-Gayk, K. H. Jakobs, and E. Hackenthal, Cyclic adenosine monophosphate in phagocytizing granulocytes and alveolar macrophages, *J. Cell Biol.,* **57**:567-571 (1973).
165. R. Snyderman, L. C. Altman, A. Frankel, and R. M. Blaese, Defective mononuclear leukocyte chemotaxis: A previously unrecognized immune dysfunction, *Ann. Intern. Med.,* **78**:509-513 (1973).
166. J. A. Spudich and S. Lin, Cytochalasin B, its interaction with actin and actomyosin from muscle. (Cell movement/microfilaments/rabbit striated muscle), *Proc. Natl. Acad. Sci. USA,* **69**:442-446 (1972).
167. J. Stadler and W. W. Franke, Characterization of the colchicine binding of membrane fractions from rat and mouse liver, *J. Cell Biol.,* **60**:297-303 (1974).
168. T. P. Stossel, Phagocytosis, *N. Engl. J. Med.,* **290**:717-723; 774-780; 833-839 (1974).
169. T. P. Stossel, Quantitative studies of phagocytosis: Kinetic effects of cations and heat-labile opsonin, *J. Cell Biol.,* **58**:346-356 (1973).
170. T. P. Stossel, R. J. Field, J. D. Gitlin, C. A. Alper, and F. S. Rosen, The opsonic fragment of the third component of human complement, *J. Exp. Med.,* **141**:1329-1347 (1975).
171. T. P. Stossel and J. H. Hartwig, Phagosomes in macrophages: Formation and structure. Interaction of actin, myosin and a new actin binding protein of rabbit pulmonary macrophages, *J. Biol. Chem.,* **250**:5706-5712 (1975).
172. T. P. Stossel, R. J. Mason, J. Hartwig, and M. Vaughn, Quantitative studies of phagocytosis by polymorphonuclear leukocytes: Use of emulsions to measure the initial rate of phagocytosis, *J. Clin. Invest.,* **51**:615-624 (1972).
173. T. P. Stossel, R. J. Mason, T. D. Pollard, and M. Maughn, Isolation and properties of phagocytic vesicles. II. Alveolar macrophages, *J. Clin. Invest.,* **51**:604-614 (1972).

174. T. P. Stossel and T. D. Pollard, Myosin in polymorphonuclear leukocytes, *J. Biol. Chem.*, **248**:8288-8294 (1973).
175. T. P. Stossel, T. D. Pollard, R. J. Mason, and M. Vaughn, Isolation and properties of phagocytic vesicles from polymorphonuclear leukocytes, *J. Clin. Invest.*, **50**:1745-1757 (1971).
176. P. R. Strauss, Effects of serum on membrane transport. II. Serum and the stimulation of adenosine transport, a possible mechanism, *J. Cell Biol.*, **60**:571-585 (1974).
177. P. R. Strauss and R. D. Berlin, Effects of serum on membrane transport. I. Separation and preliminary characterization of factors which depress lysine or stimulate adenosine transport in rabbit alveolar macrophages, *J. Exp. Med.*, **137**:359-368 (1973).
178. R. B. Taylor, P. H. Duffus, M. C. Raff, and S. de Petris, Redistribution and pinocytosis of lymphocyte surface immunoglobulin molecules induced by anti-immunoglobulin antibody, *Nature [New Biol.]*, **233**:225-229 (1971).
179. J. Theodore, J. C. Acevedo, and E. D. Robin, Implantation of exogenous enzymatic activity in isolated alveolar macrophages, *Science*, **178**:1302-1304 (1972).
180. S. G. Thrasher, T. Yoshida, C. J. van Oss, S. Cohen, and N. R. Rose, Alteration of macrophage interfacial tension by supernatants of antigen-activated lymphocyte cultures, *J. Immunol.*, **110**:321-326 (1973).
181. G. L. Truitt and G. B. Mackaness, Cell mediated resistance to aerogenic infection of the lung, *Am. Rev. Respir. Dis.*, **104**:829-843 (1971).
182. M. F. Tsan and R. D. Berlin, Effect of phagocytosis on membrane transport on nonelectrolytes, *J. Exp. Med.*, **134**:1016-1035 (1971).
183. M. F. Tsan and R. D. Berlin, Membrane transport in the rabbit alveolar macrophage. The specificity and characteristics of amino acid transport systems, *Biochim. Biophys. Acta*, **241**:155-169 (1971).
184. M. Tsan, R. A. Taube, and R. D. Berlin, The effect of trypsin on membrane transport of non-electrolytes, *J. Cell Physiol.*, **81**:251-256 (1973).
185. T. E. Ukena and R. D. Berlin, Effect of colchicine and vinblastine on the topographical separation of membrane functions, *J. Exp. Med.*, **36**:1-7 (1972).
186. C. J. van Oss and C. F. Gillman, Phagocytosis as a surface phenomenon. I. Contact angles and phagocytosis of non-opsonized bacteria, *J. Reticuloendothel. Soc.*, **12**:283-292 (1972).
187. M. T. Vogt, C. Thomas, C. L. Vassallo, R. E. Basford, and J. B. L. Gee, Glutathione-dependent peroxidative metabolism in the alveolar macrophage, *J. Clin. Invest.*, **50**:401-410 (1971).
188. P. A. Ward, Chemotaxis of mononuclear cells, *J. Exp. Med.*, **128**:1201-1219 (1968).
189. P. A. Ward, Natural and synthetic inhibitors of leukotaxis. In *Inflammation Mechanisms and Control.* Edited by I. H. Lepow and P. A. Ward. New York, Academic Press, 1972, pp. 301-310.
190. P. A. Ward and E. L. Becker, Potassium reversible inhibition of leukotaxis by ouabain, *Life Sci.*, **9**:355-360 (1970).

191. P. A. Ward, H. G. Remold, and J. R. David, Leukotactic factor produced by sensitized lymphocytes, *Science,* **163**:1079-1081 (1969).
192. G. A. Warr and R. Russell Martin, In vitro migration of human alveolar macrophages: Effects of cigarette smoking, *Infect. Immun.,* **8**:222-227 (1973).
193. G. A. Warr and R. Russell Martin, Response of human pulmonary macrophage to migration inhibition factor, *Am. Rev. Respir. Dis.,* **108**:371-373 (1973).
194. K. Weber and U. Groeschel-Stewart, Antibody to myosin: The specific visualization of myosin containing filaments in non-muscle cells, *Proc. Natl. Acad. Sci. USA,* **71**:4561-4564 (1974).
195. R. S. Weening, R. Wever, and D. Roos, Quantitative aspects of the production of superoxide radicals by phagocytizing human granulocytes, *J. Lab. Clin. Med.,* **85**:245-252 (1975).
196. R. H. Weisbart, R. Bluestone, L. S. Goldberg, and C. M. Pearson, Migration enhancement factor: A new lymphokine, *Proc. Natl. Acad. Sci. USA,* **71**:875-879 (1974).
197. G. Weissman, P. Dukor, and R. Zurier, Effect of cyclic AMP release of lysosomal enzymes from phagocytes, *Nature [New Biol.],* **231**:131-135 (1971).
198. Z. Werb and Z. Cohn, Plasma membrane synthesis in the macrophage following phagocytosis of polystyrene latex particles, *J. Biol. Chem.,* **247**: 2439-2446 (1972).
199. N. K. Wessells, B. S. Spooner, J. F. Ash, M. O. Bradley, M. A. Luduena, E. L. Taylor, J. T. Wrenn, and K. M. Yamada, Microfilaments in cellular and developmental processes. Contractile microfilament machinery of many cell types is reversibly inhibited by cytochalasin B, *Science,* **171**: 135-143 (1971).
200. M. E. Whitcomb and R. E. Rocklin, Transfer factor therapy in a patient with progressive primary tuberculosis, *Ann. Intern. Med.,* **79**:161-166 (1963).
201. P. C. Wilkinson, J. F. Borel, V. J. Stecher-Levin, and E. Sorkin, Macrophage and neutrophil specific chemotactic factors in serum, *Nature,* **222**: 244-247 (1969).
202. R. C. Williams and H. H. Fudenberg, *Phagocytic Mechanisms in Health and Disease.* New York, Intercontinental Medical Book, 1972.
203. M. C. Willingham, R. E. Ostlund, and I. Pastan, Myosin is a component of the cell surface of cultural cells, *Proc. Natl. Acad. Sci. USA,* **71**:4144-4148 (1974).
204. J. W. Wilson, Treatment or prevention of pulmonary cellular damage with pharmacologic doses of corticosteroid, *Surg. Gynecol. Obstet.,* **134**:675-681 (1972).
205. F. Wunderlich, R. Muller, and V. Speth, Direct evidence for a colchicine-induced impairment in the mobility of membrane components, *Science,* **182**:1136-1138 (1973).
206. H. Yeager, Jr., S. M. Zimmet, and S. L. Schwartz, Pinocytosis by human alveolar macrophages, *J. Clin. Invest.,* **54**:247-251 (1974).

207. M. Zatti and F. Rossi, Relationship between glycolysis and respiration in surfactant-treated leukocytes, *Biochim, Biophys. Acta,* **148**:553-563 (1967).

208. S. H. Zigmond and J. G. Hirsch, Cytochalasin B: Inhibition of D-2-deoxy-glucose transport into leukocytes and fibroblasts, *Science,* **176**:1432-1434 (1972).

209. R. B. Zurier, S. Hoffstein, and G. Weissmann, Mechanisms of lysosomal enzyme release from human leukocytes, *J. Cell Biol.,* **58**:27-41 (1973).

210. R. B. Zurier, G. Weissmann, S. Hoffstein, S. Kammerman, and H. H. Tai, Mechanisms of lysosomal enzyme release, *J. Clin. Invest.,* **53**:297-309 (1974).

211. A. P. Autor and J. B. Stevens, Biochemical changes in alveolar macrophages of neonatal rat lungs: Association with pulmonary development, *Am. Rev. Resp. Dis.,* **115** (Abstr.):302 (1977).

212. G. S. Davis, M. Mortara, L. M. Pfeiffer, and G. M. Green, Bactericidal and biochemical peroxidase activity in human alveolar macrophages, *Am. Rev. Resp. Dis.,* **115** (Abstr.):210 (1977).

213. D. B. Drath and M. L. Karnovsky, Superoxide production by phagocytic leukocytes, *J. Exp. Med.,* **141**:257-262 (1975).

214. J. B. L. Gee and A. S. Khandwala, Oxygen metabolism in the alveolar macrophage: Friend or foe? *J. Reticuloendoth. Soc.,* **19**:229-236 (1976).

215. G. M. Green, G. J. Jakab, R. B. Low, and G. S. Davis, Defense mechanisms of the respiratory membrane, *Am. Rev. Resp. Dis.,* **115**:479-514 (1977).

216. A. L. Horwitz and R. G. Crystal, Collagenase from rabbit pulmonary alveolar macrophages, *Biochem. Biophys. Res. Commun.,* **69**:296-303 (1976).

217. A. L. Horwitz, J. A. Kelman, and R. G. Crystal, Activation of alveolar macrophage collagenase by a neutral protease secreted by the same cell, *Nature,* **264**:772-774 (1976).

218. J. A. Kazmierowski, J. I. Gallin, and H. Y. Reynolds, Mechanism for the inflammatory response in primate lungs: Demonstration and partial characterization of an alveolar macrophage-derived chemotactic factor with preferential activity for polymorphonuclear leukocytes, *J. Clin. Invest.,* **59**:273-281 (1977).

219. P. Patriarca, P. Dri, K. Kakinuma, F. Tedesco, and F. Rossi, Studies on the mechanism of metabolic stimulation in polymorphonuclear leukocytes during phagocytosis. I. Evidence for superoxide anion involvement in the oxidation of $NADPH_2$, *Biochim. Biophys. Acta,* **385**:380-386 (1975).

220. H. Y. Reynolds, J. P. Atkinson, H. H. Newball, and M. M. Frank, Receptors for immunoglobulin and complement on human alveolar macrophages, *J. Immunol.,* **114**:1813-1819 (1975).

221. H. Y. Reynolds, J. A. Kazmierowski, and H. H. Newball, Specificity of opsonic antibodies to enhance phagocytosis of *Pseudomonas aeruginosa* by human alveolar macrophages, *J. Clin. Invest.,* **56**:376-385 (1975).

222. R. J. Rodriguez, R. R. White, R. M. Senior, and E. A. Levine, Elastase secretion by human alveolar macrophages, *Am. Rev. Resp. Dis.*, **115** (Abstr.):371 (1977).
223. R. K. Root and J. Metcalf, Initiation of granulocyte (PMN) $O_2^{-}\cdot$ and H_2O_2 formation by stimulation of membrane phagocytic receptors (PR), *Clin. Res.*, **24**:352A (1976).
224. M. L. Salin and J. M. McCord, Free radicals and inflammation. Protection of phagocytosing leukocytes by superoxide dismutase, *J. Clin. Invest.*, **56**:1319-1323 (1975).
225. E. Schiffmann, B. A. Corcoran, and S. M. Wahl, N-Formylmethionyl peptides as chemoattractants for leukocytes, *Proc. Natl. Acad. Sci. USA*, **72**:1059-1062 (1975).
226. H. J. Showell, R. J. Freer, S. H. Zigmond, E. Schiffmann, S. Aswanikumar, B. Corcoran, and E. L. Becker, The structure-activity relations of synthetic peptides as chemotactic factors and inducers of lysosomal enzyme secretion for neutrophils, *J. Exp. Med.*, **143**:1154-1169 (1976).
227. L. M. Simon, J. Liu, J. Theodore, and E. D. Robin, Effect of hyperoxia, hypoxia, and maturation on superoxide dismutase activity in isolated alveolar macrophages, *Am. Rev. Resp. Dis.*, **115**:279-284 (1977).
228. K. Takanaka and P. J. O'Brien, Mechanism of H_2O_2 formation by leukocytes. Evidence for a plasma membrane location, *Arch. Biochem. Biophys.*, **169**:428-435 (1975).
229. R. R. White and C. Kuhn, The effect of tetracycline on elastase secretion by mouse peritoneal exudative and alveolar macrophages, *Am. Rev. Resp. Dis.*, **115** (Abstr.):387 (1977).

23

Experimental Models and Pulmonary Antimicrobial Defenses

GARY L. HUBER

Harvard Medical School
Boston, Massachusetts

F. MARC LaFORCE

Veterans Administration Hospital
Denver, Colorado

W. G. JOHANSON, JR.

University of Texas
San Antonio, Texas

I. Introduction

A. Historical Contributions

Advances in understanding of antimicrobial defenses of the lung have occurred in several cycles over the past century. The initial cycle followed the mid-nineteenth century discoveries of Pasteur, Tyndall, and others suggesting airborne transmission of infectious agents might be important in human disease. A number of investigators employed experimental animals to study the deposition of aerosolized bacteria within the respiratory tract [1,2]. That bacteria could be recovered from the lungs following such airborne inoculations was clearly shown. However, primarily due to a lack of understanding of aerobiology and aerosol physics, evidence to support the airborne transmission of infectious agents was not immediately forthcoming. In contrast, bacterial transmission by direct contact was more readily demonstrable and the concept that the lung might be a major organ of host defense remained obscure. Bloomfield reviewed this work in light of the remarkable observations that the respiratory tract distal to the trachea or major bronchi is normally sterile [3]. He concluded that such sterility was due primarily to the efficiency of the filtering and cleansing actions of the upper respiratory passages and that only a rare bacterium penetrated deep into the lung, a concept no longer held valid. Bacteria deposited infrequently in the lung were disposed of by the protective mechanisms of the lung, which at the time were thought to include mucociliary activity, drainage by lymphatics and bacterial death in situ due to "environmental influences." This deemphasis of lung defense mechanisms was due in part to the concept that pneumonia resulted from bacteremia produced by penetration of the upper respiratory tract epithelium, a hypothesis that was not put to rest until the mid-1930s, when it was shown that bacteria deposited in the upper respiratory tract of experimental animals appeared virtually immediately in the lung and that bacteremia rarely occurred subsequently, if at all [4,5].

It was clearly evident during these early investigations, however, that phagocytosis of inhaled or injected material occurred within the lung. The nature and source of the pulmonary phagocytic cells were less clear. At the turn of the century, Briscoe summarized the existing theories of his day and on the basis of his own observations concluded that: (a) alveoli were lined by nucleated epithelium consisting of several types of cells; (b) only the large mononuclear cells were actively phagocytic; (c) new mononuclear cells were recruited from the alveolar walls in response to the alveolar deposition of bacteria or other foreign particulate matter; and (d) under most conditions the phagocytic activity of the mononuclear cells was by itself sufficient and circulating leukocytes became involved only if and when the mononuclear cells were unable to contain the challenge[6]. Thus, the concept of an antibacterial defense mechanism intrinsic to the lung that inherently depended on phagocytosis by macrophages was established by the turn of the century.

B. Development of Animal Models

A second cycle of interest in lung antibacterial defenses occurred during the first several decades of this century as a consequence of numerous investigations into the pathogenesis of bacterial pneumonia. These studies included investigations with a variety of bacteria and manipulations of the host but, in general, only the development of pneumonia histologically or the death of the animal were used as the endpoint. Thus, little was learned about the role of intrapulmonary antimicrobial defenses. For example, Stillman studied the persistence of various bacterial species in the lungs of mice following aerosol exposure [7]. Pneumococci were rapidly eliminated and did not produce generalized infection. On the other hand, hemolytic streptococci persisted in the lungs and led to fatal septicemia. Staphylococci were slowly cleared from the lungs but did not produce septicemia and *Hemophilus* were handled irregularly. These observations were important in that they indicated that the efficiency of the pulmonary defenses varied for different bacterial species. However, the mechanism of these defenses was not characterized. Rather, in a further series of studies Stillman showed that the administration of alcohol to the test animals prior to exposure led to the persistence of pneumococci in the lungs [8] and subsequently to the development of pneumonia [9]. Thus, it was demonstrated that the outcome of an interaction between bacteria and the lung depended on a balance of two basic factors: (a) the apparent virulence of the organism differed with bacterial species, and (b) the resistance of the host could be experimentally altered. Wadsworth had earlier emphasized the interplay between these variables but his observations were concerned primarily with the factors which determined whether a local or systemic infection could result from a given bacterial challenge [10]. Experimental models of pneumonia provided a means of testing the integrated defenses of the host but tended to obscure the intrinsic defenses of the lung. Extensive studies by Robertson of experimental pneumonia led him to conclude that the primary defense of the lung against invading bacteria was phagocytosis by circulating polymorphonuclear cells [11], a concept also subsequently shown to be incorrect.

The development of a theory for airborne transmission of infectious agents and the accompanying technology emerged in the 1930s largely due to the work of Wells and his associates[12]. With quantitative bacteriologic methods it became possible to estimate more precisely the number of bacteria deposited in the respiratory tract during aerosol exposure and to follow changes in this bacterial population with time [13]. The use of radioactively labeled bacteria to facilitate the determination of the distribution of inhaled bacteria was introduced in 1950 by Goldberg and Leif [14].

On this background, Kass, Laurenzi, Green, and coworkers performed a series of experiments in the early 1960s which focused specifically on the antimicrobial defenses of the lung [15-17]. These investigators combined advances in aerosol technology, as pioneered by First [17], quantitative bacteriologic methods and isotopic and immunologic techniques with the use of nonpathogenic and pathogenic bacterial species to elucidate for the first time the quantitative aspects of the pulmonary antibacterial defenses. In so doing, the alveolar macrophage was identified as the principal cellular component in this system. These series of experiments conducted by several different investigators working in the laboratories of Kass, to be summarized below, have provided most of the basis of our current understanding of pulmonary antibacterial defenses.

II. Theoretical Considerations of Aerosol Challenge with Bacteria

A. Theoretical Considerations

As described in other chapters of this series, the physical fate of an inhaled particle depends on its site of deposition within the respiratory system. Viable and nonviable particles are presumably handled similarly, although little data exist to confirm that assumption. In the case of viable particles, however, the rate at which the organisms are inactivated and the rate at which they multiply in the lungs must both be considered, as each may be the dominant determinant of the interaction. The exposure systems, an example of which is depicted schematically in Fig. 1, used in current studies of lung defense mechanisms provide aerosols in which over 85-90% of viable particles are less than 2 μm mass median diameter. Thus, deposition distally at the alveolar level in the lung and a slow rate of physical removal by mucociliary transport mechanisms of the airways from the lung would be expected. By providing an inoculation of aerosol of this size, a physiologic analog to droplet infection in humans is achieved in these model systems. Although data are incomplete on the probable size of droplet nuclei carrying human infections, most infections appear to spread by particles of these relative dimensions. Bacteria labeled with radioactive isotopes, thus providing labeled particles with aerodynamic properties essentially identical to those of the viable bacteria, have been used to evaluate the rate of physical removal of inhaled organisms from the lung. The published data on the rate of removal of bacteria labeled with radioactive phosphorous (^{32}P) [18], sulfur (^{35}S) [19,20], pertechnetate (^{99}Tc) [21], or selenium (^{75}Se) [22] appear to indicate somewhat different rates of clearance of these isotopes. The reasons for such differences have not been established and possibly could include differences in particle size due to labeling or aerosolizing procedures, differing rates of dissociation of isotopes from bacteria or varying affinity of dissociated isotopes for pulmonary tissue. However, the rate of transport or physical clearance of each isotope is small compared to the decline in the number of viable bacteria in the lungs of normal animals. Therefore, it is reasonable to believe that following an aerosol exposure to most bacterial species the physical removal of bacteria plays a relatively minor role in the defense of the lung and that mechanisms which are bactericidal in situ are quantitatively far more important. Rylander has emphasized that physical removal of bacteria may be quantitatively important in the reduction of viable bacteria essentially only during the first 30 min following aerosol exposure [19].

In that the airways are lined with a mucous blanket that contains antimicrobial factors, such as bactericidal enzymes and antimicrobial immunoglobulins, killing of bacteria by contact with the respiratory tract and its secre-

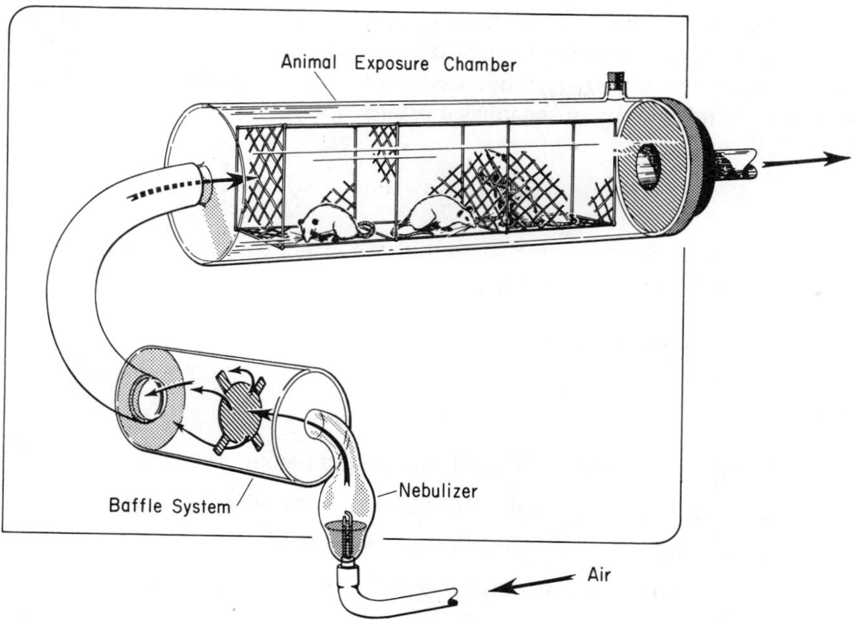

FIGURE 1 Schematic representation of an aerosol generator inoculating apparatus, with bacterial nebulizer, baffle-dehydrating aerosol conditioner and animal exposure chamber.

tions, excluding the role of actively phagocytizing cells, could also contribute to the immediate bactericidal activity of the lung in vivo. For example, the ratio of viable organisms to radioactive particles in the lungs of animals sacrificed shortly after exposure begins to decrease immediately relative to the ratio of the bacteria to the isotope in the aerosol [18]. It has been established that this decrease is not due to killing of the organisms by or during the aerosolization process. Considering that inoculating exposure periods are usually 30 min or more in duration, the observed decrease, amounting to only 15-30% or more of the initial challenge at most, is likely due to slower bactericidal mechanisms than killing on contact. Whether or not the importance of this mechanism differs among various bacterial species is poorly appreciated.

Most of the pulmonary antibacterial activity for organisms deposited by aerosol inhalation can be attributed to the alveolar macrophage system and its associated alveolar lining material. Both in vivo and in vitro studies have demonstrated the phagocytic potential of these cells. Bacteria in the lung are engulfed by macrophages and, at least for many bacterial species, neither specific antibody, serum factors nor other cell types or products of other cell types are required for phagocytosis or bacterial killing. Thus the differences observed in bactericidal activity between bacterial species, and the changes in this activity produced by various manipulations of the host, reside in large part in the physical interaction of the alveolar macrophage system with the inhaled microorganism, as well as in the capacity of the inhaled organism to multiply in the lungs.

B. Microbial Replication vs. Inactivation

The opposing activities of bacterial multiplication and bacterial inactivation can be represented by the relationship:

$$C_t = C_o \exp(k_g - k_i)t \tag{1}$$

where

C_t = the concentration of viable bacteria in the lungs at time t

C_o = the concentration of viable bacteria in the lungs at time 0

k_g = a constant representing the rate of bacterial multiplication

k_i = a constant representing the rate of bacterial inactivation

t = time

If nonpathogenic bacteria are unable to multiply in the lung in vivo, then $k_g = 0$ and the decrease in the number of viable bacteria in the lung should follow a single exponential function, the slope of which is k_i. Published "lung clearance" curves for *Staphylococcus albus* are generally single exponential curves in agreement with this hypothesis [23]. Since k_i represents the combined effect of both physical removal and the in vivo killing of bacteria, this observation suggests that each of the processes is a single exponential function over the short time periods usually employed in these studies.

In the case of pathogenic bacterial strains, bacterial multiplication in vivo may be retarded or prevented by the administration of a bacteriostatic antibiotic, such as tetracycline for one illustrative example. If $k_g = 0$, Eq. (1) can be rewritten

$$C_{tet_t} = C_{tet_o} e^{-k_i t} \tag{2}$$

where C_{tet_t} = the concentration of viable bacteria in the lungs of antibiotic-treated animals at time t; and C_{tet_o} = the concentration of viable bacteria in the lungs of tetracycline-treated animals at time 0.

An estimate of the rate of bacterial multiplication in vivo can be obtained by dividing (1) by (2):

$$\frac{C_t}{C_{tet_t}} = e^{k_g t} \tag{3}$$

These relationships are shown in Fig. 2.

Using this approach, it has been demonstrated, as summarized in Fig. 3, that marked impairment in apparent bactericidal activity of the hemorrhagic rat lung following acid instillation, as one specific example, is due to the combined effects of a decreased k_i and a markedly increased k_g [24]. The mechanisms of the change in k_i in this situation, or in other circumstances which are known to decrease the bactericidal activity of the lungs, remain speculative. Such a decrease could be due to an impairment in phagocytosis, due to an impairment in intracellular bacterial killing or due to both. For example, the rate of bacterial multiplication in vivo could increase if the alveolar environment becomes more favorable for multiplication. However, if only extracellular bac-

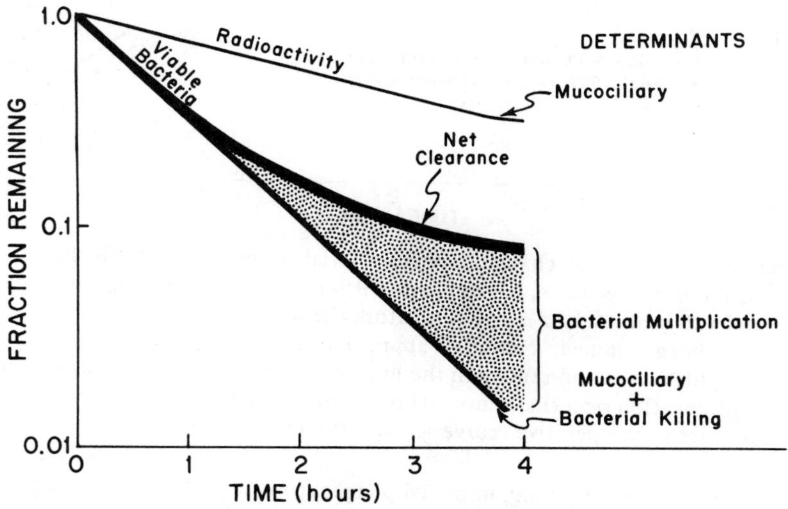

FIGURE 2 The determinants of lung bacterial clearance are plotted as the fraction of original counts (radioactive or viable bacteria) remaining in the lung against time postexposure. The decrease in radioactive counts is due primarily to mucociliary activity. The lowermost line represents the change in viable bacteria counts in the lungs of animals in which bacterial multiplication is prevented by the administration of tetracycline; the slope of this line represents the combined effects of mucociliary activity and bacterial killing in situ (k_i). "Net clearance" or "net inactivation" represents the change in viable bacteria in the lungs of control animals; the difference between this line and k_i is due to bacterial multiplication. In this example, bacterial multiplication begins between 1 and 2 hr postexposure. Such lag periods have been observed with some, but not all, bacterial strains.

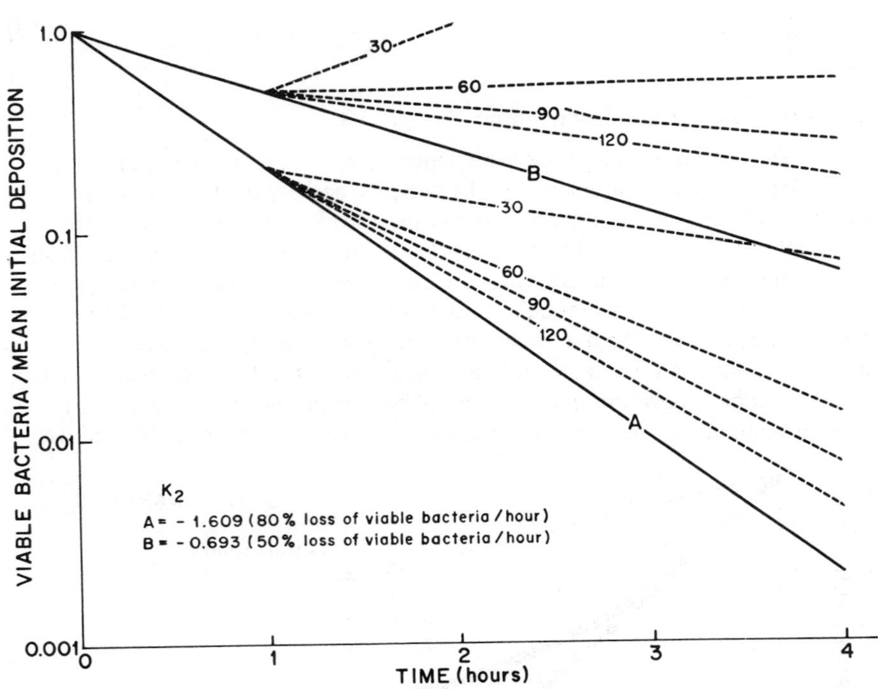

FIGURE 3 The predicted change in lung bacterial counts with time is shown for two different values for k_i (curves A and B) and bacterial doubling times of 30, 60, and 120 min. A 1-hr lag period before the initiation of bacterial multiplication has been assumed. Note that approximately 10% of the original bacterial population would remain in the lung at 4 hr if either slow inactivation but no multiplication occurred (curve B) or if rapid inactivation and rapid multiplication were both operative (curve A plus 30-min doubling time).

teria are capable of multiplying, impaired phagocytosis would result in an apparent increase in k_g without an actual shortening of the doubling time of individual bacterial cells. Or, alternatively, the alveolar lining material could have been altered by the experimental effect and result in impaired intracellular killing in the presence of normal phagocytosis.

An alternative attempt to increase the power of this type of experiment through modeling has been presented [25,26]. This alternative approach was developed using data obtained with staphylococcal inoculations and assumed that bacteria in the lung were subjected to a uniform death rate and that multiplication did not occur. That assumption remains to be confirmed by experimental data and, indeed, recent studies using antibiotic administration partially support this conclusion in the case of the staphylococci but indicate that other species of bacteria do multiply in the lungs of normal animals [27]. Therefore, considerable care should be exercised in using this simplistic approach.

The fundamental difficulty in developing adequate statistical models to describe the activity of the pulmonary antibacterial mechanisms is the variability of the data obtained. Despite the multiplicity of possible sources of such variability between different experiments, including slurry concentrations, uncontrolled chamber conditions, the level of ventilation of individual animals and the errors introduced by the sampling techniques used, it seems clear that the source of the largest variance resides in the varying capacity of individual animals to inactivate inhaled bacteria. In other words, animals vary in their intrapulmonary inactivation rates from one to the next and sometimes this variation is quite significant. No adequate explanation for these individual differences has been advanced, nor has this problem been systematically investigated. However, a means of either reducing the variability of experimental results, or a statistical method for dealing with data which frequently is neither distributed normally or Poisson, is needed to refine current models and therefore improve the ability to resolve the many remaining questions about the antibacterial defenses of the lung.

III. In Vivo Models of Intrapulmonary Antibacterial Defenses

A. Background and Clinical Relevance

Careful medical histories obtained from patients with pneumonia usually reveal specific predisposing factors that may have led to bacterial infection in the respiratory tract. Such clinical associations providing a link between altered resistance of the host and pulmonary infection have been delineated further by a limited number of epidemiologic investigations, the scope of which is beyond review here. It is not surprising, then, that a proliferation of contributions utilizing models to study experimental animal analogs of human disease states would occur following the introduction by Kass and his coworkers [17] of physiologic and readily applicable quantitative techniques capable of precisely defining the antibacterial action of the lung. Before the advent of the aerosol generator system introduced by First [17], most studies of the interaction of bacteria with host defenses of the lung involved evaluations of tissue reactions on a qualitative basis or mortality rates secondary to overwhelming infection. Contributions utilizing the aerosol generator system are summarized in Table 1 [15-21,23,24,27-145].

TABLE 1 Models of Intrapulmonary Antibacterial Defenses

Category	Animal Species	Response	Ref.
Environmental oxidants and pollutants			
Carbon black particulate loading	Mice	No effect	28
Cigar smoke	Rats	Impaired	a
Marijuana smoke	Rats	Impaired	29-31
Nitrogen dioxide	Mice	Impaired	32
Ozone	Mice, rats	Impaired	33-40
and silicosis	Mice	Impaired	41
and nitrogen dioxide	Mice	Impaired	42
and vitamin E deficiency	Mice	Impaired	37
Epoxy paint fumes	Mice	Impaired	43
Quartz pneumonitis	Mice	Enhanced	44
Silicosis	Mice	Impaired	45
Tobacco smoke	Mice, rats	Impaired	46, 28
Synthetic tobacco substitutes	Rats	Impaired	a
Therapeutic agents			
Aminophylline	Mice	Impaired	50
Anesthetics			
Cyclopropane	Mice	Impaired	47, 48
Halothane	Mice	No effect	47, 48
Methoxyflurane	Mice	Impaired	47, 48
Pentobarbital	Mice	No effect	47-49
Barbiturates	Mice	Impaired	28
Topical cold remedies	Mice	Impaired	51, 52
Corticosteroids	Mice, rats	Impaired	53-58, 28

Epinephrine	Mice	Impaired	50, 15
Immunosuppressants			
Azathioprine	Mice	Impaired	57, 85
Antilymphocytic serum	Mice	Impaired	57, 85, 86
Oxygen	Mice	Impaired	59-82
X-Irradiation	Mice	Impaired	83, 84
Infectious agents			
Candida pyelonephritis	Mice	Impaired	88
Streptococcal abscess	Mice	Impaired	87
Virus infection			
Encephalomyocarditis virus			
Columbia SK virus	Mice	Impaired	89
Mengo 37A virus	Mice	Impaired	89
Influenza	Mice	Impaired, no effect	90, 91, b, c
Parainfluenza (Sendai virus)	Mice	Impaired	92-94
Reovirus	Mice	Impaired, No effect	147, 148, g, c
General disease analogs			
Acidosis	Mice	Impaired	95-97
Bone fracture	Rats	No effect	98
Dehydration	Mice	Impaired	99-102
Diabetes	Mice	Impaired	104
Ethanol	Mice	Impaired	105, 15, 23, 91, 58, 106, 62, 28, 107
Endotoxin	Mice	Impaired	28
Hemorrhage	Rats	Impaired	108-112
Hypoxia	Mice	Impaired	95, 23, 58, 28
Hydrocarbon ingestion	Mice	Impaired	118, 56, 119, 120, 121
Interstitial fibrosis	Mice	Impaired	44
Liver disease	Rats	Impaired	122-129

TABLE 1 (continued)

Category	Animal Species	Response	Ref.
Therapeutic agents			
Renal failure	Mice	Impaired	97, 44, 113, 88, 91
Starvation	Mice	Impaired	87, 58, 15
Stress			
Cold exposure	Mice	Impaired	23
General stress	Rats	Impaired	114-117, 103
Thyroidism			
Hypothyroidism	Rats	Impaired	130, 66, 74
Hyperthyroidism	Rats	Enhanced	130, 66, 74
Cardiopulmonary disease analogs			
Acidosis	Rats	Impaired	136
Aspiration	Rats	Impaired	24, 131-135
Congestive heart failure	Rats	Impaired	137-140
Consolidation	Mice, rats	Impaired	141
Fat embolism	Rats	Impaired	98
Hypercapnia	Mice	Impaired	95
Hypersensitivity pneumonitis	Guinea pig	Enhanced	142
Mechanical ventilation	Rats	Impaired	49
Positive end expiratory pressure	Rats	Impaired	49
Pulmonary edema	Mice, rats	Impaired	102, 143-145

[a]G. L. Huber, personal communication of work in progress.
[b]G. L. Huber and N. Young, personal communication of work in progress.
[c]G. L. Huber and F. M. LaForce, personal communication of work in progress.

B. Animal Model Analogs to Human Infection

This list of animal experiments is extensive and the numerous contributions cannot be reviewed individually in detail here. They are listed in summary in Table 1. It is our intent to confine our discussion of these contributions to broader perspectives of their application, including identification of specific problems and limitations of their use. Many of these studies have been the subject of general reviews of pulmonary host defenses in man and the experimental animal [148-152,209-212]. The vast majority of conditions and models utilized have demonstrated an impairment, not an enhancement, in host intrapulmonary antibacterial defenses. Exceptions to this include experimental hypersensitivity pneumonitis [141], quartz pneumonitis [44], ethanol intoxication [62], oxygen toxicity [62], hyperthyroidism [68,74,130], hyperglucosemia in the absence of ketoacidosis or significant hyperosmolarity [106; G. L. Huber, personal communication of work in progress] and moderate and low dosage exposure to tobacco smoke (Huber, personal communication), all of which have been associated, under selected circumstances, with enhanced or improved intrapulmonary inactivation rates.

C. Experimental Design of Animal Models

The first few models developed [15-17,28] carefully controlled all parameters of aerosol inoculation and reported initial bacterial deposition data, exposure conditions and rates of inactivation at various intervals after inoculation. This practice soon gave way, somewhat unfortunately, to expression of simple statistical comparisons of arithmetic mean inactivation values, usually obtained only at one time interval after bacterial exposure and computed by a t-test for unpaired data, between experimental and control groups. The term "clearance" was initially introduced to describe the rapid decrease in viable bacteria recovered from the lung at various periods after inoculation. This has led to some confusion, however, in that it is now generally held that "clearance" might better be used in reference to the physical removal or transport of organisms from the lung and "intrapulmonary bacterial killing" employed to denote inactivation of the microbes in situ. With the introduction of alternative methods for computing inactivation [18], emphasis on "zero hour animals" and quantitation of initial bacterial deposition was replaced by the study of larger numbers of animals at the arbitrary point chosen for comparative analyses during the inactivation process. Comparisons thus computed were usually obtained from data on animals sacrificed at 4 or 6 hr after bacterial aerosolization, points probably chosen more for their convenience to the usual working day of the laboratory technical staff than for any other reason. That these analytical time intervals represent the most sensitive or reliable points for quantitative comparisons for each of the many experimental conditions employed to date has not been adequately evaluated. By increasing the numbers of animals so analyzed at only one specific point in the inactivation process, the varying capacity of individual animals to inactivate inhaled bacteria, and the source of largest variance, can be better contained statistically. However, in that the exposure capacity of most aerosol inoculation units is limited, this "improvement" in statistical comparative analysis unfortunately has been obtained at a loss of information on other potential sources of variability, including the variable inoculating concentrations, chamber conditions, and altered levels of ventilation of individual animals. Also, rates of intrapulmonary bacterial growth, as well as an assessment of phagocytic uptake versus intracellular killing, cannot be adequately evaluated independently under conditions limited primarily to a comparative analysis of one point. The term "intrapulmonary bacterial inactivation" was coined, as a by-product of the isotope-ratio method for quantitating host defense activity in individual animals [18], in an attempt to denote the overall result or sum effect of these individual variables. Historically, the net result of this methodologic approach has been the production of a large number of descriptive studies, which by themselves are useful in providing quantitative assessments of the host-microbe interaction under conditions of altered intrapulmonary antibacterial defenses. At the same time, however, these studies are limited in providing a comprehensive understanding of the mechanism of the observed impairments.

Measurement of intrapulmonary bacterial inactivation rates with radiotracer labeled bacteria has permitted the determination of bacterial viability by relating that parameter of quantitation of the physical presence of the organisms [18]. This method has been extensively well characterized for the use of ^{32}P-labeled *Staphylococcus aureus,* somewhat less well evaluated for ^{32}P- or ^{35}S-labeled *Proteus mirabilis* and inadequately studied in experiments using other radiotracers. Radioactive phosphorus (^{32}P) appears to bind tightly to the DNA of the test-microbe over a significantly long period and is more than satisfactory for evaluations by this method, but other radiotracers are less tightly retained by the bacteria and thus present wider variability and perhaps somewhat less reliability in results. The use of radiolabeled bacteria has strengthened the concept that the decay in viable bacteria following the initial deposition is an intrapulmonary phenomenon, closely linked to pulmonary alveolar macrophage phagocytic function and not related to physical transport of the inoculating aerosol from the lung. Once the initial ratio of bacterial to isotope activity is determined, a subsequent decrease in this ratio within the lung represents a decline in the number of viable organisms, since there is no internal source of additional radioactivity. An expression of intrapulmonary bacterial inactivation by this method, then, represents primarily in situ bacterial killing at the alveolar level in that radiolabeled bacteria depositing on the mucociliary stream would be physically cleared, for the most part, over conventional periods of study commonly utilized [18].

Although not extensively studied per se, it would appear from information incorporated in other studies that the antibacterial defense system of the lung cannot be overwhelmed by increasing numerically the deposition of bacteria. For example, the majority of studies published reported initial deposition values of 10^3 to 10^5 bacteria, ranging from a low of 10^2 in several studies to a high of 10^6 to 10^9 [37,153]. The magnitude of initial bacterial deposition in the pathogenesis of pulmonary infection in man is not known, but it is likely that it is considerably less than the bacterial challenge used in these studies. It is unlikely that inocula of a higher magnitude can be readily achieved by aerosol deposition techniques. Using another approach, Green has evaluated intrapulmonary bacterial inactivation rates during 8 hr of continuous aerosol inoculation [154]. The bacterial inactivation rates for all organisms studied to date appear to be essentially identical within a given bacterial species and independent of the initial magnitude of the inoculum.

A major problem, accentuated by the use of very small numbers of experimental and control animals under conditions of a single bacterial exposure, has been the day-to-day reproducibility of "normal" inactivation rates for a given animal strain and bacterial species within any one laboratory or between laboratories. Systematic comparisons of species and strain variations have apparently never been undertaken. In one of the earliest contributions [28], Laurenzi and coworkers avoided these problems by utilizing the concept of a "relative retention ratio" to compare differences between animal groups. Unfortunately, this practice has been employed little, if at all, since then and data are now generally reported as the arithmetic mean of bacterial inactivation values in individual "runs" or bacterial exposures for control and experimental groups. In almost all publications, data from all experimental and all control animals are then processed further by pooling, without restriction, into what has commonly been called a "grand mean" for each group. No investigator to date has reported firm criteria for pooling data in this manner, nor alternative criteria for rejecting a single set of experiments in which the mean control values differ significantly from one bacterial inoculation to the next. For example, the degree of variation of intrapulmonary bacterial inactivation reported for control animals in a set of experiments often has been very large, sometimes differing in magnitude by as much as two- to threefold and occasionally as high as fivefold. In many instances, the differences between "normal" or control animals from one day to another are much greater than the differences between experimental and control groups in one given day.

Several refinements have been made on basic methodology. It appears that the magnitude of the initial deposition within the lung is proportional, on a lobar basis, to the size of the lobe [20,141]. It also appears that inactivation rates are uniform on a regional basis [20,141]. Thus, the lung of a single animal can be partitioned for comparative evaluations, allowing correlation of intrapulmonary bacterial inactivation with fluid accumulation (wet-dry lung weights), light- or electron-microscopic structure, phagocytosis or other parameters. Experimental models of intrapulmonary bacterial inactivation should, in future studies, include an analysis of as many of the factors that can potentially affect lung structure and function. The availability of additional tissue through partitional analyses should provide this opportunity. It appears that under certain conditions of consolidation [93], intrapulmonary bacterial inactivation may be progressively more impaired in extensively consolidated areas than in the more aerated portions.

Another important advancement in the understanding of the defenses of the lung against bacterial infection was made by Goldstein and coworkers [37]. By using a large aerosol inoculum of 10^8 bacteria/ft^3 air, an initial intrapulmonary bacterial inactivation could be determined on the left lung of animals and rates of phagocytosis determined within the right lung by examining microscopically the percentage of organisms engulfed by alveolar macrophages. These data indicate that phagocytic uptake of the bacterial challenge occurs very rapidly within the alveolar spaces. This method of investigation provides one means of distinguishing between impaired phagocytosis versus impaired intracellular killing, and should be employed more extensively in future studies.

Probably because of its small size and the feasibility of exposing relatively large numbers of animals within the aerosol generator, the mouse has been the most widely studied host species. Pathogen-free vs. pathogen-bearing differences in inactivation rates have been demonstrated [28]. Larger animals, including various strains of rats, as well as guinea pigs and hamsters, have been less completely evaluated. Clearly, animal species and even animal strain differences in intrapulmonary inactivation rates exist. In this context, changes in the ability of the lung to kill bacteria as a function of age, and thus size, have not been adequately controlled, making it often impossible to compare results from one laboratory to another.

D. Application of Animal Models

Use of animal models employed to study factors responsible for impaired host defenses may require a redefinition of the concept of pathogens. The complex interaction between the microorganism and the host that results in infection and disease has been the subject of many extensive studies. It is now well established that bacteria of different species or even different strains of the same species vary widely in their capacity to produce disease, and that different hosts are not equally susceptible to disease caused by a given infecting agent. Unlike nonliving agents toxic to the lung, infectious microbes can replicate and, in the presence of impaired defenses, could lead to the demise of the host through overwhelming infection of the lung. Thus, the concept of "pathogen" must be defined in terms of both the host and the potential infecting agent, not in terms of the microbe alone. From the standpoint of the host, antimicrobial defenses can be achieved by destruction of the viability of the infecting organism, by limitation of replication of the organism within the lung, by structural breakdown or alteration of the microbe in the lung or by physical removal of the agent from the pulmonary tissue. The net response—that is, whether bacterial infection, through intrapulmonary replication exceeding inactivation, develops, or pulmonary sterility, through intrapulmonary inactivation exceeding replication—is the quantitative outcome of the infectious challenge. In other words, proliferation of bacteria within the lung at a rate sufficient to cause infectious disease is in competition with the defense mechanisms of the host attempting to inactivate the challenge. As demonstrated in Table 1, a variety of agents, ranging from inert inorganic to organic materials or viable organisms, may impair the host defense system of the lung. This impairment may be direct, or indirect through responses within the host or within the lung other than directly affecting the host defense system itself.

As might be expected in phagocytic systems, different bacterial species are killed at different rates within the lung. Bacteria pathogenic and nonpathogenic to man, including *Staphylococcus albus* and *aureus, Diplococcus pneumoniae, Proteus mirabilis, Klebsiella pneumoniae, Pseudomonas aeruginosa,* as well as the murine pathogen *Pastuerella pneumotropica,* have been studied in animals with the aerosol generator system. From a limited number of studies, it would appear that when multiple bacterial species are inoculated as a mixed aerosol infection, each organism is killed at the same rate as in a monoinoculation of the individual microbes [23,93,107,108,155]. The implication that selection of one bacterial species out of a mixed inoculum during impairment of host antibacterial defenses, induced by an agent such as ethanol [23], is selective may not be valid in that studies reported to date have not considered intrapulmonary bacterial growth rates or alterations in the surrounding pulmonary milieu that might enhance or alter these growth rates [24]. Further work is thus needed to clarify this concept.

Although there have been attempts to the contrary, radiolabeling bacteria has not provided a precisely accurate method of quantifying physical clearance or transport by the mucociliary stream during study with the aerosol generator system, except to say that it is not very significant over the primary period of intrapulmonary bacterial inactivation (note Fig. 2). Recent experience with noninvasive techniques, introduced by Sackner and his coworkers [156-158], may provide the most physiologic alternative to answering this difficult problem.

Studies with electron microscopy [153], fluorescent antibodies [16] and radiolabeled bacteria [16,18] have indicated that the alveolar macrophage is the key cellular element in the intrapulmonary antibacterial host defense network. The role of other cells recoverable from the alveolar surface, such as polymorphonuclear leukocytes, plasma cells, and lymphocytes, all of which comprise less than 1-5% of the recoverable cells in most animal species, has not been adequately determined. Stereologic investigations, using techniques that permit quantitation of anatomic structures within cells on a three-dimensional basis, have demonstrated that the mononuclear cell recoverable by bronchopulmonary lavage is morphologically or morphometrically identical to the alveolar macrophage responsible for in situ phagocytosis [159]. The role of alveolar lining materials in the killing of phagocytized bacteria appears to be of crucial importance, both in the experimental animals and in man [77,114-117, 160-163]. Studies with "alveolar lining material" refer to the noncellular fractions recoverable by bronchopulmonary lavage of the respiratory tree. Although the components apparently essential for intracellular killing by phagocytes of some bacterial species are recovered in the "surfactant fraction" of lung washings, it remains to be determined if the active antimicrobial component is the surfactant per se. In that these lining materials can be recovered and isolated by differential centrifugation of lavage fluid, further clarification of their role can be elucidated through in vitro techniques.

IV. In Vitro Models of Microbial Inactivation by Cellular and Acellular Fractions of the Lung

A. Introduction and Historical Perspectives

As has been amply demonstrated in the in vivo studies listed in Table 1, the alveolar macrophage defense network is a key factor in the maintenance of pulmonary sterility. For the purposes of the discussion to follow it is important to consider this cellular network as a system complex, consisting not only of macrophages but of important local factors such as surfactant and locally produced immunoglobulins as well.

Over the past 10-15 years, a great deal of attention has been focused on the functional, biochemical, ultrastructural and immunologic capabilities of this cell system. Much of this work has been and will be summarized in other chapters of this monograph. The following discussion will focus on (a) methods used to assess in vitro bactericidal activity of alveolar macrophages; (b) a resume of reported results using alveolar macrophages harvested from experimental animals; (c) studies using acellular lung fractions; (d) correlations with disease states, and, lastly, (e) a critique of the limitations of in vitro studies. For all practical purposes, virtually all functional measurements of in vitro bactericidal activity of alveolar macrophages seek to answer two questions: (a) how well is the test organism ingested (phagocytosis), and (b) what is the effect of intracellular residence on viability of the phagocytized organism (intracellular bactericidal activity).

B. Methods of in Vitro Bactericidal Bioassay Systems

Several techniques have been used to quantitate phagocytosis. Perhaps the most widely used is a calculation of the phagocytic index. Using this technique, bacteria and phagocytes are incubated, usually with added serum, and at various time intervals smears are prepared, stained and examined microscopically. The percent cells that have phagocytized organisms are then counted [166]. Other refinements include the calculation of the mean number of phagocytized organisms per phagocytic cell. These studies can easily be done in conjunction with quantitative bacterial or fungal counts to determine the overall "static" or "cidal" activity of the system [165]. Microorganisms can also be radiolabeled and macrophage uptake of bacteria or fungi may be quantitated by isotopic measurements [166,167].

The measurement of intracellular bactericidal activity of alveolar macrophages required the isolation of those bacteria located intracellularly. A commonly used technique in macrophage suspensions is that of differential centrifugation whereby cell-associated bacteria are isolated, the cells ruptured and intracellular bacteria counted [168]. When monolayers of macrophages are used, extracellular bacteria can be rinsed from the cells [170]. Another method of isolating phagocytized bacteria involved the introduction of an antibiotic which does not penetrate cells into the macrophage-bacterial system after phagocytosis has taken place. Thus, extracellular bacteria are killed and accurate counts of intracellular organisms can subsequently be made [170,171].

Yet another but less commonly employed method used to study the interaction of microorganisms and alveolar macrophages involves the effect of intracellular residence of phagocytized organisms on overall viability of alveolar macrophages. In brief, alveolar macrophage monolayers are challenged with a specific microorganism, and macrophage death, as a result of this interaction, is determined by dye exclusion studies [172,173].

C. Resume of in Vitro Bactericidal Studies

Numerous studies defining the interaction of alveolar macrophages with various microorganisms have been published and a summary of these studies is presented in Table 2.

TABLE 2 Summary of in Vitro Phagocytic Studies Using Alveolar Macrophages from Experimental Animals

Species	Otganism	Summary of results	Ref.
Calf	*Staphylococcus aureus*	Bovine alveolar macrophage easily grown in tissue culture and demonstrated good phagocytosis against staphylococci	174
Rabbit	*Bacillus anthracis*	Excellent phagocytosis with germination of spores and destruction of alveolar macrophages	175
	Mycobacterium tuberculosis	Enhanced phagocytosis by alveolar macrophages from a strain of rabbits relatively resistant to inhaled challenges of *M. tuberculosis;* with bacteria to phagocytic ratio of greater than 100:1 significant degree of alveolar macrophage death	176
	Francisella tularensis	Bactericidal activity decreased with increased strain virulence. Alveolar macrophage from immune animals had better bactericidal activity	177
		Marked degree of alveolar macrophage death with bacteria to phagocyte ratio of 10:1 and virulent strain	173
	Listeria monocytogenes	Activated macrophages have enhanced listericidal activity	178

	Fungal spores	Enhanced phagocytosis of fungal spores when compared to polystyrene particles of equal size	179
	Staphylococcus aureus	Excellent phagocytosis with 97% of bacterial inoculum inactivated in 90 min	180
	Staphylococcus albus	About 80% of initial inoculum inactivated in 2 hr	164
	Pseudomonas aeruginosa	Greater bactericidal activity with increased macrophage to bacteria ratios	181
		Good bactericidal activity; phagocytosis enhanced with immune IgG and IgA	180, 182
	Escherichia coli	Excellent bactericidal activity	180, 183
Guinea pig	*Staphylococcus aureus*	Very poor intracellular bactericidal activity	169
	Salmonella typhymurium	Limited bactericidal activity	169
Rat	*Staphylococcus aureus*	Limited intracellular bactericidal activity	160, 184
	Staphylococcus albus	Good intracellular bactericidal activity	160
Mouse	*Hemophilus influenza*	Excellent bactericidal activity with about 75% of inoculum inactivated at 1 hr	185

Allowing for differences in experimental protocols, several important points can be noted from a review of these studies. These include:

1. Alveolar macrophages from all species tested are avidly phagocytic.
2. Marked species differences occur in bactericidal activity of alveolar macrophages. For example, rat alveolar macrophages readily ingest but kill very poorly *S. aureus,* whereas rabbit alveolar macrophages ingest and kill *S. aureus* quite well [160, 161,180,184].
3. Rather pronounced intraspecies variations in intracellular bactericidal activity are seen for different organisms. Rabbit alveolar macrophages kill *S. aureus* and *P. aeruginosa* well but cannot inactivate *Bacillus anthracis* [175,180].

In an effort to mimic in vivo conditions as closely as possible, some investigators have quantitated in vitro bactericidal activity of alveolar macrophages after phagocytosis has occurred in vivo. For example, when rat alveolar macrophages are harvested and challenged with *S. aureus* in vitro, these cells are unable to kill *S. aureus.* However, if rats are allowed to inhale *S. aureus,* their lungs lavaged and intracellular bactericidal activity of alveolar macrophages then determined in vitro after in vivo phagocytosis, efficient bactericidal activity is demonstrable [161]. These data suggest that purely in vitro studies may not reflect macrophage bactericidal activity in vivo. This phenomenon may be species-specific since similar studies in guinea pigs in which *S. aureus* was delivered by intratracheal injection failed to show any enhanced bactericidal activity [169].

In vivo response of rabbit alveolar macrophages to intratracheal *Mycobacterium smegmatis* has also been examined [186]. In these studies, rabbit alveolar macrophages were lavaged and studied with electron microscopy at intervals following challenge. These studies demonstrated little change in intracellular morphology of phagocytized organisms but a progressive decrease in viability such that 10 days after challenge, no viable organisms could be recovered from alveolar macrophages. Similarly, mice have been challenged by aerosol techniques with *Aspergillus* spores, their lungs lavaged, and alveolar macrophages studied ultrastructurally. Phagocytosis with progressive disintegration of spores was demonstrated in normal animals [187].

D. The Role of Acellular Lung Lining Materials

Little work has been done on direct antibacterial activity of pulmonary secretions or the interaction that these secretions may have with alveolar macrophages.

Lysozyme has bactericidal activity and is known to be present in tracheobronchial secretions. However, its role in the maintenance of bronchopulmonary sterility is unclear [188]. Jalowayski and Giamonna have measured the rate of growth of *Escherichia coli* and *Streptococcus viridans* incubated in surfactant harvested from dog lungs [189]. Enhanced growth was noted in surfactant incubation when compared to controls. Similarly, no inhibition of growth was noted when surfactant fraction from rats was incubated with *S. aureus* [160,161]. It would appear that at least the phospholipid-protein moieties in bronchopulmonary secretions from unstimulated animals do not have important bactericidal activity alone, at least against the bacterial strains tested to date.

Recently, Reynolds and Thompson have described inhibition of growth of *P. aeruginosa* with IgA from bronchopulmonary lavage fluid obtained from animals immunized by the nasal route [190]. This inhibition was strain-specific and was not enhanced with the addition of either complement or lysozyme. It was postulated that this effect was due to agglutinative properties of immune IgA. Of interest, immune IgG which was also shown to agglutinate *P. aeruginosa* did not inhibit growth of lag phase bacteria. These studies suggest an agglutinative role for immune secretory IgA in local antibacterial defenses of the lung.

Alveolar lining material has been shown to enhance intracellular bactericidal activity of alveolar macrophages [77,114-117,160-163]. For example, rat alveolar macrophages kill phagocytized *S. aureus* poorly in a standard in vitro test system. However, if *S. aureus* are preincubated in and thus coated by alveolar lining material prior to inoculation into the phagocyte system, intracellular bactericidal activity can be demonstrated [160-163]. Similar results using rat alveolar macrophages have been demonstrated when the challenge organism was *P. aeruginosa,* [191,192] and this phenomenon has also been observed in man [162,163]. These studies suggest that local factors may play a far more important role in macrophage function than has been previously suspected. In fact, depressed bactericidal activity of rat lung in the initial phase of experimental oxygen toxicity and restraint-induced stress is due to a failure of surfactant enhancement of alveolar macrophage bactericidal activity [77,114].

The most comprehensive studies of the influence of respiratory antibodies on the functional activity of alveolar macrophages has recently been published by Reynolds and Thompson [182,190]. These investigators carefully evaluated the immunoglobulin composition of respiratory secretions in rabbits before and after local and systemic immunization with *P. aeruginosa.* IgG antibody was found in lung washings after systemic immunization whereas both IgA and IgG antibodies were demonstrable after nasal immunization. IgM and complement were absent from bronchial secretions. Careful phagocytic studies using IgA and IgG antibodies revealed that, while both IgG and IgA antibodies enhanced phagocytosis, IgG was more active. Intracellular killing of *P. aeruginosa* was unrelated to the immune status of the animal. These studies emphasized the importance of local acellular factors which may modify alveolar macrophage function as determined by in vitro studies.

E. Correlation of Bioassay Systems with Disease States of Man

Functional and ultrastructural studies have been done using alveolar macrophages from experimental animals with pathophysiologic conditions felt to be associated with increased risk of bronchopulmonary infection in man. Lockard et al. [193] have demonstrated decreased in vitro bactericidal activity of alveolar macrophages harvested from rabbits subjected to tumbling stress. Electron microscopy studies suggested that this inhibition may be due to a primary failure in phagocyte killing activity. Studies from our laboratory, however, have indicated this impairment may be due solely to an alteration in the alveolar lining material and does not involve phagocytic or bactericidal function of alveolar macrophages per se [114]. Alveolar macrophages from rats with chemically induced pulmonary edema have decreased bactericidal activity against *S. albus* [143,145]. Degre has demonstrated impaired phagocytosis in alveolar macrophages from animals previously infected with Sendai virus [194]. Prior viral infection did not affect bactericidal activity.

Immunosuppressed animals have also been studied. Alveolar macrophages from cyclophosphamide-treated rats were unable to degrade ingested bacteria [195] and cortisone-treated rats after challenge with *Aspergillus flavus* spores failed to form phagolysosomes presumably because of stabilization of lysosomes by steroids [187].

Ozone, sulfur dioxide, and oxides of nitrogen have all been shown to be toxic for alveolar macrophages recoverable from treated animals [196,197]. Depressed staphylococcidal activity of both rabbit and rat alveolar macrophage has been demonstrated when these cells are exposed in vitro to freshly drawn cigarette smoke [30,31,165,198-208]. Related studies have demonstrated similar effects following the addition of cigar [206-208], marijuana [30,31,201-203, 208], or smoke from synthetic tobacco substitutes [204,207,208]. This effect can be blocked by the addition of glutathione or cysteine to the culture medium [198-200].

Conversely, heightened alveolar macrophage bactericidal activity against *Listeria monocytogenes* has been documented in macrophages harvested from animals previously given BCG [178]. Reynolds and Thompson have also demonstrated enhanced phagocytosis of *P. aeruginosa* by rabbit alveolar macrophages with immune IgG and IgA from bronchopulmonary lavage fluid [183].

F. Limitations of in Vitro Studies

Working with relatively pure cell fractions of alveolar macrophages has obvious advantages. Experimental conditions can be carefully defined and specific variables may be more easily controlled. However, phagocytic and bactericidal results from in vitro studies using alveolar macrophages from experimental animals may not be entirely applicable to a similar in vivo animal experiment or disease as it occurs in man.

First, there are rather pronounced species variations in in vitro bactericidal studies. Thus, it may be erroneous to extrapolate results using macrophages from experimental animals directly to man. Second, alveolar macrophages in the lung exist in a highly complex environment. They are bathed in a highly surface active material, as well as locally produced immunoglobulins and other proteins. What effect these local factors have in terms of alveolar macrophage function is largely unknown. Nevertheless, if appropriate conclusions are to be drawn from in vitro functional studies, efforts in this field will have to be expanded greatly. Similarly, it would appear crucial that all in vitro observations be confirmed using more physiologic in vivo studies.

V. Other Antimicrobial Models

The review of antimicrobial models, presented above [148-152], indicates that reasonable methods have been developed for quantitating antibacterial defenses, both in vivo and in vitro. Similar approaches still are needed for the study of infections by viruses, mycoplasma, fungi, and parasites. To date, there has been a paucity of information generated for these agents. The direct effect of virus agents on the alveolar macrophage directly or on other components of the pulmonary defense system are poorly appreciated [148,213]. Limited data imply that virus particles can be taken up by pulmonary alveolar macrophages after inhalation inoculation [214], wherein they potentially can (a) multiply, (b) be digested and inactivated, (c) be passively transferred to underlying pulmonary parenchyma, or (d) spread systemically via the circulatory or lymphatic systems. Other investigators have confirmed that influenza A (G. L. Huber and N. Young, personal communication) and influenza B [215] particles are rapidly phagocytized and viral antigen can be demonstrated in the macrophages of infected lung [216]. It also appears that influenza A virus, at least, can replicate within the alveolar macrophage during the first 48 to 72 hr after inoculation (Huber and Young, personal communication). Fungi are also phagocytized very rapidly [217] and the clearance or inactivation of mycoplasma is less well appreciated [148].

It is generally accepted that in experimental animal models viral infection impairs antibacterial defenses [89-94,146,147]. Although there are many clinical observations that would support this hypothesis [93,218,219], the mechanism of viral-induced impairment deserves further clarification. Experimental results reported have been somewhat confusing and complicated by the demonstration of "mouse cytopathic agent," apparently representing unidentified endogenous viral infecting agents inherently present in many animal species [146,147]. Several attempts to repeat these investigations in experiments controlling for "mouse cytopathic agent" have not been able to reproduce the initial studies (Huber and Young, personal communication; G. L. Huber and F. M. LaForce, personal communication). It is probable that the development of bacterial pneumonia under these circumstances is dependent on the virus-induced inflammatory lesion, and perhaps not due directly to the virus itself, in that hard data to the contrary have not yet surfaced. An alternative hypothesis has been a direct viral-induced impairment of macrophage function per se that is not mediated indirectly through the viral-induced inflammatory response of the underlying parenchyma [92-94]. Part of the basis for this proposal is the alleged lack of edema in the presence of impaired inactivation rates for *S. aureus* in reovirus-infected lungs, although quantitative data for fluid accumulation or lack thereof have not been presented [146,147]. Use of light microscopic histology alone to evaluate fluid accumulation within the lung is no longer acceptable, as significant interstitial edema can occur without detectable morphologic changes on histologic examination [137-140]. A further alternative proposal has been that of "overloading" macrophages in aerated portions of virus-infected lungs through selective shunting of the aerosolized bacterial challenge from consolidated areas [92,191]. This, too, seems a most unlikely explanation in that this intact system appears to be inexhaustible at considerably higher levels of bacterial inoculation [153,154]. Clearly, more work is needed to understand not only the pulmonary defenses against viral infection alone but the interaction between viral infection and impaired antibacterial defenses.

VI. Conclusion and Extrapolations

The past century of investigation has most dramatically increased our understanding of the host defense mechanisms of the lung. The growth of knowledge relative to intrapulmonary antibacterial activity has far exceeded our insight into other antimicrobial defenses of the lung, as models for the study of virus, fungal, mycoplasma, and parasitic infections are now at best only in their infancy, if even conceived at all. The state-of-the-art of physiologic delivery of bacterial aerosols to experimental animals has reached a point of high sophistication and precise techniques for the quantification of intrapulmonary bacterial inactivation have been refined. Experimental animal models, developed almost exclusively with few exceptions by Kass or his disciples, for the study of antibacterial defenses now are almost a hundred in number (Table 1) and continue to grow in both quantity and complexity. Most contributions have been descriptive in nature and clearly more studies in greater depth to carefully identify pathophysiologic mechanisms of impaired antimicrobial function are needed. Statistical analyses performed on data gathered to date have been almost entirely restricted to simple comparisons of intrapulmonary bacterial inactivation values at a given point after inoculation, with the subsequent interpretations very much oversimplified. Better understanding perhaps could be derived from calculation of inactivation rates on a log-normal basis with specific attention given to each individual factor, as well as the combined effect of experimental variables. Almost all attention has been focused on the pulmonary alveolar macrophage as the key defender of the lung, at the exclusion of the inherent growth characteristics of the microorganism, at the exclusion of the effect on the lung or lung injury on these bacterial growth characteristics, at the exclusion of evaluating alterations in lung parenchyma and pulmonary metabolism and, perhaps most importantly of all, at the exclusion of an understanding of the noncellular components of an integrated macrophage-humoral pulmonary defense network. These "exclusions" should be carefully considered in further investigations with animal models.

Essentially all in vivo studies with antimicrobial animal models to date have been performed on rodents, apparently the smaller the size the better from the standpoint of both host and convenience of large-scale inoculations. A mouse, however, is not a man. Studies with larger animals, including primates, are feasible from the current knowledge of aerosol physics and microbial delivery systems. Cells and humoral components harvested by bronchopulmonary lavage appear to be representative of those active at the airway and alveolar surfaces. In that both these cells and these noncellular factors can be recovered from both the human and the animal lung, in vitro bioassays, then, may provide the bridge for linking, at a limited number of points at least, extensive investigations on experimental animals to limited studies in man and a better understanding of the pathogenesis of infection in humans.

References

1. N. Tchistovitch, Des phenomenes de phagocytose dans les poumons, *Ann. Inst. Pasteur,* **3**:337-361 (1889).
2. L. Paul, Ueber die Bedingungen des Eindringens der Bakterien der Inspiration Sluff in die Lungen, *S. Hyg.,* **40**:468-504 (1902).
3. A. L. Bloomfield, The mechanism of elimination of bacteria from the respiratory tract, *Am. J. Med. Sci.,* **164**:854-867 (1922).

4. G. Rake, Pathogenesis of pneumococcus infections in mice, *J. Exp. Med.*, **63**:191-208 (1936).
5. P. R. Cannon and T. E. Walsh, Studies on the fate of living bacteria introduced into the upper respiratory tract of normal and intranasally vaccinated rabbits, *J. Immunol.*, **32**:49-62 (1937).
6. J. C. Briscoe, An experimental investigation of the phagocytic action of the alveolar cells of the lung, *J. Pathol. Bacteriol.*, **12**:66-100 (1908).
7. E. G. Stillman, The presence of bacteria in the lungs of mice following inhalation, *J. Exp. Med.*, **38**:117-126 (1923).
8. E. G. Stillman, Persistence of inspired bacteria in the lungs of alcoholized mice, *J. Exp. Med.*, **40**:353-361 (1924).
9. E. G. Stillman and A. Branch, Experimental production of pneumococcus pneumonia in mice by the inhalation method, *J. Exp. Med.*, **40**:733-742 (1924).
10. A. Wadsworth, Experimental studies on the etiology of acute pneumonitis, *Am. J. Med. Sci.*, **127**:851-877 (1904).
11. O. H. Robertson, Phagocytosis of foreign material in the lung, *Physiol. Rev.*, **21**:112-139 (1941).
12. W. F. Wells, *Airborne Contagion and Air Hygiene.* Cambridge, Mass., Harvard University Press, 1955.
13. A. M. Ames and W. J. Nugester, The initial distribution of airborne bacteria in the host, *J. Infect. Dis.*, **84**:56-63 (1949).
14. L. J. Goldberg and W. R. Leif, The use of a radioactive isotope in determining the retention and initial distribution of airborne bacteria in the mouse, *Science*, **112**:299-300 (1950).
15. G. M. Green and E. H. Kass, Factors influencing the clearance of bacteria by the lung, *J. Clin. Invest.*, **43**:769-776 (1964).
16. G. M. Green and E. H. Kass, The role of the alveolar macrophage in the clearance of bacteria by the lung, *J. Exp. Med.*, **119**:167-176 (1964).
17. G. A. Laurenzi, L. Berman, M. First, and E. H. Kass, A quantitative study of the deposition and clearance of bacteria in the murine lung, *J. Clin. Invest.*, **43**:759-768 (1964).
18. G. M. Green and E. Goldstein, A method for quantitating intrapulmonary bacterial inactivation in individual animals, *J. Lab. Clin. Med.*, **68**:669-677 (1966).
19. R. Rylander, Pulmonary defense mechanisms to airborne bacteria, *Acta Physiol. Scand. [Suppl.]*, **306**:1-89 (1968).
20. G. J. Jakab and G. M. Green, Regional defense mechanisms of the guinea pig lung, *Am. Rev. Respir. Dis.*, **107**:776-783 (1973).
21. W. G. Johanson, M. G. Kennedy, and F. J. Bonte, Use of technetium (^{99m}Tc) as a bacterial label in lung clearance studies, *Appl. Microbiol.*, **25**:592-594 (1973).
22. J. A. Watson, J. A. Auld, and G. C. Meyer, Clearance and inactivation of the vegetative and spore forms of *Bacillus subtilis* var.Niger in rat lungs, *Am. Rev. Respir. Dis.*, **107**:975-984 (1973).
23. G. M. Green and E. H. Kass, The influence of bacterial species on pulmon-

ary resistance to infection in mice subjected to hypoxia, cold stress and ethanolic intoxication, *Br. J. Exp. Pathol.*, **46**:360-366 (1965).

24. W. G. Johanson, S. J. Jay, and A. K. Pierce, An important determinant of the pulmonary clearance of *Diplococcus pneumoniae* in rats, *J. Clin. Invest.*, **53**:1320-1325 (1974).
25. P. S. Levy and G. M. Green, A use of Fieller's theorem in a pulmonary clearance problem, *Biometrics*, **23**:382-383 (1967).
26. P. S. Levy and G. M. Green, A stochastic model of the bactericidal activity of the lung, *J. Theor. Biol.*, **21**:103-112 (1968).
27. S. J. Jay, W. G. Johanson, and A. K. Pierce, Interaction of three parameters in lung bacterial clearance, *Am. Rev. Respir. Dis.*, **107**:1116 (1973).
28. G. Laurenzi, J. J. Guarneri, and R. B. Endriga, Important determinants in pulmonary resistance to bacterial infection, *Med. Thorac.*, **22**:48 (1965).
29. W. Pereira, T. McLaughlin, M. T. Baranano, S. Dudley, D. O'Connell, M. Cutting, and G. Huber, The acute effect of marijuana smoke on antibacterial defense mechanisms of the lung, *Clin. Res.*, **23**:351A (1975).
30. C. McCarthy, M. E. Cutting, G. A. Simmons, W. Pereira, R. Laguarda, and G. L. Huber, The effect of marijuana on the in vitro function of pulmonary alveolar macrophages. In *Pharmacology of Marijuana.* Edited by M. C. Braude and S. Szara. New York, Raven Press, 1976, pp. 211-216.
31. G. L. Huber, M. E. Cutting, C. R. McCarthy, G. A. Simmons, R. Laguarda, and W. Pereira, The depressant effect of marijuana smoke on the antibacterial activity of pulmonary alveolar macrophages, *Chest*, **68**:769-773 (1975).
32. E. Goldstein, M. C. Eagle, and P. D. Hoeprich, Effect of nitrogen dioxide on pulmonary bacterial defense mechanisms, *Arch. Environ. Health*, **26**: 202-204 (1973).
33. G. L. Huber and F. M. LaForce, Comparative effects of ozone and oxygen on pulmonary antibacterial defense mechanisms, *Antimicrob. Agents Chemother.*, **10**:129-136 (1970).
34. G. L. Huber and N. J. Spencer, Alterations in pulmonary antibacterial defense mechanisms following exposure to ozone, *Am. Rev. Respir. Dis.*, **101**:1016-1017 (1970).
35. F. E. Speizer and G. L. Huber, Some physiologic biochemical and cellular responses of the lung to air pollutants, *Milbank Mem. Fund. Q.*, **41**:256-268 (1969).
36. E. Goldstein, W. Lippert, and D. Warshauer, Pulmonary alveolar macrophage: Defender against bacterial infection of the lung, *J. Clin. Invest.*, **54**:519-528 (1974).
37. D. Warshauer, E. Goldstein, P. D. Hoeprich, and W. Lippert, Effect of vitamin E and ozone on the pulmonary antibacterial defense mechanisms, *J. Lab. Clin. Med.*, **83**:228-240 (1974).
38. G. L. Huber, R. J. Mason, F. M. LaForce, D. E. Gardner, and D. L. Coffin, Alterations in the lung following the administration of ozone, *Arch. Intern. Med.*, **128**:81-87 (1971).
39. E. Goldstein, W. S. Tyler, P. D. Hoeprich, and M. C. Eagle, The effect of

ozone on the anti-bacterial defense mechanisms of the murine lung, *Arch. Intern. Med.,* **127**:1099-1102 (1971).

40. E. Goldstein, W. S. Tyler, P. D. Hoeprich, and M. C. Eagle, Adverse influence of ozone on pulmonary bactericidal activity of the murine lung, *Nature,* **229**:262-263 (1971).
41. E. Goldstein, M. C. Eagle, and P. D. Hoeprich, Influence of ozone on pulmonary defense mechanisms of silicotic mice, *Arch. Environ. Health,* **24**: 444-448 (1972).
42. E. Goldstein, D. Warshauer, W. Lippert, and B. Tarkington, Effect of ozone and nitrogen dioxide on murine pulmonary defense mechanisms, *Arch. Environ. Health,* **28**:85-90 (1974).
43. G. L. Huber, S. W. Burley, N. J. Spencer, and F. M. LaForce, Impairment of intrapulmonary antibacterial defense mechanisms by exposure to a freshly painted room, *Clin. Res.,* **19**:729 (1971).
44. G. M. Green and E. Goldstein, Non-specific resistance to bacterial infection in laboratory models of chronic pulmonary disease, *Am. Rev. Respir. Dis.,* **94**:491-492 (1966).
45. E. Goldstein, G. M. Green, and C. Seamans, The effect of silicosis on the antibacterial defense mechanisms of the murine lung, *J. Infect. Dis.,* **120**: 210-216 (1969).
46. G. A. Laurenzi, J. J. Guarneri, R. B. Endriga, and J. P. Carey, Clearance of bacteria by the lower respiratory tract, *Science,* **142**:1572-1573 (1963).
47. E. Goldstein, E. S. Munson, C. Eagle, R. W. Martucci, and P. D. Hoeprich, Influence of anesthetic agents on murine pulmonary bactericidal activity, *Antimicrob. Agents Chemother.,* **10**:231-235 (1971).
48. E. Goldstein, E. S. Munson, C. Eagle, R. W. Martucci, and P. D. Hoeprich, The effects of anesthetic agents on murine pulmonary bactericidal activity, *Anesthesiology,* **34**:344-352 (1971).
49. R. Laguarda, M. Calihan, S. Nyman, G. Simmons, T. Dempsey, C. McCarthy, and G. Huber, Pulmonary infection during the use of mechanical ventilation, *Clin. Res.,* **22**:508 (1974).
50. G. S. Davis, D. S. Newcombe, and G. M. Green, Inhibition of bacterial killing in epinephrine and aminophylline in the murine lungs: Possible role of cyclic AMP, *Clin. Res.,* **21**:659 (1973).
51. A. Broderick, E. Finder, G. Simmons, D. O'Connell, and G. Huber, The effect of a commonly used cold remedy on host antibacterial defense mechanisms of the lung, *Clin. Res.,* **21**:593 (1973).
52. G. Huber, A. Broderick, E. Finder, G. Simmons, and D. O'Connell, Impairment of intrapulmonary bacterial inactivation following administration of a commonly used cold remedy, *Chest,* **64**:397 (1973).
53. G. Huber, C. McCarthy, J. Mullane, R. Laguarda, and W. Pereira, Variability in impairment of host intrapulmonary antibacterial defenses as a function of steroid turnover, *Clin. Res.,* **23**:221A (1975).
54. R. Laguarda, C. McCarthy, D. Redder, S. Goodenough, G. Simmons, D. O'Connell, and G. Huber, Impairment of in vivo bactericidal activity and in vitro phagocytic ability of pulmonary alveolar macrophages by systemic steroids, *Clin. Res.,* **22**:320 (1974).

55. D. Redder, C. McCarthy, S. Goodenough, G. Simmons, D.O'Connell, R. Laguarda, and G. Huber, The effect of experimental steroid administration on the rate of in vitro phagocytosis by alveolar macrophages, *Clin. Res.,* **21**:957 (1973).
56. D. O'Connell, E. Lewin, and G. Huber, Effects of steroids and oxygen in experimental kerosene ingestion, *Pediatr. Res.,* **7**:430 (1973).
57. G. L. Huber, F. M. LaForce, R. J. Mason, and A. P. Monaco, Acute and chronic effects of immunosuppressive agents on intrapulmonary defense mechanisms, *Clin. Res.,* **18**:485 (1970).
58. G. A. Laurenzi, G. M. Green, L. Berman, and E. H. Kass, Antibacterial activity of the bronchopulmonary tree, *Clin. Res.,* **9**:173 (1961).
59. C. McCarthy, D. O'Connell, E. Finder, G. Simmons, and G. Huber, The effect of prolonged exposure to 100% oxygen on the intrapulmonary inactivation of various bacterial pathogens, *Clin. Res.,* **21**:607 (1973).
60. G. L. Huber, S. L. Porter, S. W. Burley, F. M. LaForce, and R. J. Mason, The effect of oxygen toxicity on the inactivation of bacteria by the lung, *Chest,* **61**:66s (1972).
61. G. L. Huber, S. W. Burley, L. Porter, R. J. Mason, and F. M. LaForce, Pulmonary oxygen toxicity, *J. Clin. Invest.,* **50**:46a (1971).
62. P. A. Sturin, S. Permutt, and R. L. Riley, Pulmonary antibacterial defenses with pure oxygen breathing, *Proc. Soc. Exp. Biol. Med.,* **137**:1202-1208 (1971).
63. G. L. Huber and F. M. LaForce, Progressive impairment of pulmonary antibacterial defense mechanisms associated with prolonged oxygen administration, *Ann. Intern. Med.,* **72**:808 (1970).
64. G. L. Huber, F. M. LaForce, and R. J. Mason, Impairment and recovery of pulmonary antibacterial defense mechanisms after oxygen administration, *J. Clin. Invest.,* **49**:47a (1970).
65. C. McCarthy and G. Simmons, The effect of supplemental oxygenation on the antibacterial host defense networks of the lung, *Aerospace Med.,* **1**:71 (1974).
66. C. McCarthy, H. Nicholas, C. Pollack, G. Simmons, R. Laguarda, and G. Huber, The effect of experimentally altered thyroid activity on alveolar macrophage function and pulmonary oxygen toxicity, *Clin. Res.,* **22**:509 (1974).
67. E. Finder, G. Simmons, M. LaForce, and G. Huber, The role of edema in the development of adaptive tolerance to pulmonary oxygen toxicity, *Clin. Res.,* **21**:985 (1973).
68. C. McCarthy and G. Huber, The dose-dependent nature of pulmonary oxygen toxicity, *Chest,* **64**:402 (1973).
69. E. Finder, M. LaForce, and G. Huber, Prevention of pulmonary oxygen toxicity, *Clin. Res.,* **20**:577 (1972).
70. E. Finder, M. LaForce, and G. Huber, Prevention of oxygen toxicity of the lung, *Chest,* **62**:365 (1972).
71. C. McCarthy, J. Slade, D. O'Connell, G. Simmons, E. Fincer, M. LaForce, and G. Huber, Comparative resistance to pulmonary inactivation of bacterial species by the lung in oxygen toxicity, *Clin. Res.,* **20**:879 (1972).

72. S. Johnson, L. Harris, D. Malik, D. O'Connell, G. Simmons, E. Finder, M. LaForce, and G. Huber, Recovery of lung injury and host antibacterial defenses following experimental oxygen toxicity, *Clin. Res.,* **20**:888 (1972).
73. D. Levens, G. Simmons, and G. Huber, Basic physiologic changes and antibacterial defenses in mice exposed to 100% oxygen, *Clin. Res.,* **20**:888 (1972).
74. H. Nicholas, C. McCarthy, C. Pollack, G. Simmons, J. Mullane, R. Laguarda, W. Pereira, and G. Huber, Thyroid activity, alveolar macrophage function and pulmonary oxygen toxicity, *Clin. Res.,* **22**:718A (1974).
75. S. Couzens, M. Calihan, R. Laguarda, and G. Huber, Additive, potentiating and protecting effects of oxygen administration on acute lung injury, *Chest,* **66**:321 (1974).
76. G. Huber, C. McCarthy, G. Simmons, E. Finder, J. Mullane, R. Laguarda, and M. LaForce, Oxygen toxicity and bacterial infection in the lung, *Chest,* **65**(5):589-590 (1974).
77. G. Huber, S. Goodenough, and D. O'Connell, Oxygen toxicity and bacterial infection in the lung: Impairment of alveolar lining materials versus alveolar macrophage bactericidal activity, *Clin. Res.,* **22**:506 (1974).
78. F. Segal, G. Simmons, A. Watson, D. Levens, E. Finder, R. Laguarda, and G. Huber, Evaluation of nutritional factors in the development of tolerance to oxygen toxicity, *Clin. Res.,* **21**:981 (1973).
79. E. Finder, G. Simmons, and G. Huber, Adaptive tolerance to pulmonary oxygen toxicity following hypoxia or intermittent hyperoxia, *Ann. Intern. Med.,* **78**:832 (1973).
80. E. Finder, G. Simmons, and G. Huber, Pulmonary adaptive tolerance, *Fed. Proc.,* **32**:341 Abs. (1973).
81. C. McCarthy, D. O'Connell, M. LaForce, and G. Huber, How much oxygen is toxic? *Clin. Res.,* **21**:666 (1973).
82. M. Dodd, S. Johnson, L. Harris, D. O'Connell, E. Finder, M. LaForce, and G. Huber, Recovery and adaptation of the lung to injury induced by prolonged exposure to 100% oxygen, *Clin. Res.,* **21**:659 (1973).
83. F. F. Hahn, E. Goldstein, and D. L. Dungworth, Effect of whole body x-irradiation on pulmonary bactericidal function, *Radiat. Res.,* **47**:461-471 (1971).
84. H. A. Nicholas, F. M. LaForce, and G. L. Huber, The effect of experimental irradiation on the antibacterial defense system of the lung, *Clin. Res.,* **19**:739 (1971).
85. G. L. Huber, F. M. LaForce, R. J. Mason, and A. P. Monaco, Impairment of pulmonary bacterial defense mechanisms by immunosuppressive agents, *Surg. Forum,* **21**:285-286 (1970).
86. G. L. Huber, S. W. Burley, M. Wood, F. M. LaForce, and A. P. Monaco, The effect of antilymphocytic serum on alveolar macrophages, *Clin. Res.,* **19**:443 (1971).
87. F. M. LaForce and G. L. Huber, Effect of a sub-acute extrapulmonary infection on the antibacterial mechanisms of the lung, *Antimicrob. Agents Chemother.,* **10**:332-334 (1970).

88. E. Goldstein and G. M. Green, Inhibition of pulmonary bacterial clearance during acute renal failure, *Antimicrob. Agents Chemother.*, **5**:22-25 (1965).
89. E. Goldstein, T. Akers, and C. Prato, Role of immunity in viral induced bacterial super infections of the lung, *Infect. Immun.*, **8**:757-761 (1973).
90. G. M. Green, Patterns of bacterial clearance in murine influenza, *Antimicrob. Agents Chemother.*, **6**:26-29 (1966).
91. G. M. Green, Current research in chronic obstructive lung disease, USPHS publication 1787, Washington, D.C., 1967.
92. G. J. Jakab and G. M. Green, Pulmonary defense mechanisms in nonconsolidated and consolidated regions of sendai virus infected lungs, *J. Infect. Dis.*, **129**:263 (1974).
93. G. J. Jakab and G. M. Green, Effects of pneumonia on intrapulmonary distribution of inhaled particles, *Am. Rev. Respir. Dis.*, **107**:675-678 (1973).
94. G. J. Jakab and G. M. Green, The effect of sendai virus infection on bactericidal and transport mechanisms of the murine lung, *J. Clin. Invest.*, **51**:1989 (1973).
95. G. M. Green, Resistance to bacterial infection in experimental simulated respiratory insufficiency, *Clin. Res.*, **15**:345 (1967).
96. E. Goldstein, G. M. Green, and C. Seamans, The effect of acidosis on pulmonary clearance of inhaled bacteria, *Clin. Res.*, **14**:339 (1966).
97. E. Goldstein, G. M. Green, and C. Seamans, The effect of acidosis on pulmonary bacterial function, *J. Lab. Clin. Med.*, **75**:912 (1970).
98. E. Glucksman, M. LaForce, and G. Huber, Susceptibility to pulmonary infection following bone trauma and experimental fat embolism, *Clin. Res.*, **20**:881 (1972).
99. J. F. Mullane, R. G. Wilfong, T. O. Phelps, and G. L. Huber, Dehydration and factors affecting pulmonary antibacterial defenses, *J. Surg. Res.*, **16**:44-49 (1974).
100. F. M. LaForce and G. L. Huber, Impaired inactivation of inhaled staphylococci following experimental dehydration, *Clin. Res.*, **19**:731 (1971).
101. J. F. Mullane, R. G. Wilfong, T. O. Phelps, D. M. O'Connell, and G. L. Huber, Dehydration and pulmonary host defense mechanisms, *Clin. Res.*, **21**:669 (1973).
102. J. F. Mullane, F. M. LaForce, and G. L. Huber, Variations in lung water and pulmonary host defenses, *Am. Surg.*, **39**:630-636 (1973).
103. J. F. Mullane, R. G. Wilfong, J. C. Smith, T. O. Phelps, and G. L. Huber, Lung injury, hypoxia, stress, and gastric lesions in the rat, *Clin. Res.*, **21**:963 (1973).
104. G. L. Huber, D. O'Connell, L. Chen, J. Mullane, and M. LaForce, Experimental diabetes mellitus and pulmonary antibacterial host mechanisms, *Clin. Res.*, **20**:530 (1972).
105. L. H. Green and G. M. Green, Differential suppression of pulmonary antibacterial activity as the mechanism of selection of a pathogen in mixed bacterial infection of the lung, *Am. Rev. Respir. Dis.*, **98**:819 (1968).

106. L. H. Green and G. M. Green, Selective multiplication of single bacterial species in a mixed infection of the lung, *Antimicrob. Agents Chemother.*, **7**:67-69 (1967).
107. J. J. Guarneri and G. A. Laurenzi, Effect of alcohol on the mobilization of alveolar macrophages, *J. Lab. Clin. Med.*, **72**:40-51 (1968).
108. R. R. Roth, J. F. Mullane, G. L. Huber, T. O. Phelps, and R. G. Wilfong, Blood loss and factors affecting pulmonary antibacterial defenses, *J. Surg. Res.*, **17**:36-42 (1974).
109. J. F. Mullane, F. M. LaForce, and G. L. Huber, Intrapulmonary bacterial inactivation following acute blood loss, *Chest*, **62**:372-373 (1972).
110. R. R. Roth, J. F. Mullane, F. M. LaForce, R. G. Wilfong, T. O. Phelps, and G. L. Huber, Pulmonary host defense mechanisms in the rat after blood loss, *Clin. Res.*, **21**:610 (1973).
111. J. F. Mullane, F. M. LaForce, D. M. O'Connell, and G. L. Huber, Acute blood loss and pulmonary host defense mechanisms in the rat, *J. Surg. Res.*, **14**:228-234 (1973).
112. J. F. Mullane, F. M. LaForce, R. G. Wilfong, D. M. O'Connell, and G. L. Huber, Intra-alveolar blood and pulmonary antibacterial defense, *Am. Rev. Respir. Dis.*, **107**:1093 (1973).
113. E. Goldstein and G. M. Green, Alteration of the pathogenicity of pasteruella pneumotropica for the murine lung caused by changes in pulmonary antibacterial activity, *J. Bacteriol.*, **93**:1651-1656 (1967).
114. J. Mullane, S. Goodenough, C. McCarthy, G. Simmons, D. O'Connell, M. LaForce, R. Laguarda, and G. Huber, Alterations in alveolar lining material as the key factor in depression of interpulmonary antibacterial defenses following stress, *Chest*, **66**:333 (1974).
115. S. Goodenough, G. Simmons, J. Mullane, N. Feldman, and G. Huber, Impairment of pulmonary antibacterial defenses by experimental stress, *Clin. Res.*, **22**:442 (1974).
116. J. F. Mullane, R. G. Wilfong, F. M. LaForce, and G. L. Huber, Effect of acute stress on pulmonary host defenses, *Clin. Res.*, **20**:580 (1972).
117. P. Overson, D. O'Connell, G. Simmons, E. Finder, M. LaForce, and G. Huber, The effect of experimental stress on pulmonary alveolar macrophage function, *Clin. Res.*, **20**:879 (1972).
118. S. Goodenough, D. O'Connell, M. LaForce, and G. Huber, Aspiration versus systemic absorption as a mechanism of lung injury in experimental kerosene pneumonitis, *Clin. Res.*, **22**:442 (1974).
119. S. W. Burley, D. M. O'Connell, F. M. LaForce, and G. L. Huber, The effect of kerosene ingestion on pulmonary antibacterial defense mechanisms, *Clin. Res.*, **18**:696 (1970).
120. S. W. Burley and G. L. Huber, The effect of toxic agents commonly ingested by children on antibacterial defenses in the lung, *Pediatr. RFs.*, **5**:405 (1971).
121. C. McCarthy, L. Holmes, S. Goodenough, G. Simmons, J. Mullane, R. Laguarda, W. Pereira, and G. Huber, A problem of the fuel shortage: Aspiration pneumonitis and impaired antibacterial defenses after ingestion of gasoline and kerosene, *Clin. Res.*, **22**:717A (1974).

122. D. O'Connell, J. Libertoff, L. Chen, J. Mullane, M. LaForce, and G. Huber, The effect of partial hepatectomy on alveolar macrophage structure and function, *Clin. Res.,* **20**:462 (1972).
123. G. Huber, D. O'Connell, J. Libertoff, L. Chen, J. Mullane, and M. LaForce, Impairment of pulmonary alveolar macrophage function following experimental liver injury, *Gastroenterology,* **62**:871 (1972).
124. J. F. Mullane, F. M. LaForce, and G. L. Huber, The effect of experimental liver injury on pulmonary antibacterial defenses, *Clin. Res.,* **19**:723 (1971).
125. G. L. Huber, F. M. LaForce, and J. F. Mullane, The effect of liver impairment on lung function and pulmonary antibacterial defenses, *Ann. Intern. Med.,* **76**:879-880 (1972).
126. D. O'Connell, J. Libertoff, L. Chen, J. Mullane, M. LaForce, and G. Huber, Alterations in the pulmonary alveolar macrophage defense system with chronic biliary obstruction, *Clin. Res.,* **20**:496 (1972).
127. J. F. Mullane, N. A. Popovic, F. M. LaForce, and G. L. Huber, Influence of liver damage on the lung, *Chest,* **62**:372 (1972).
128. D. O'Connell, J. Libertoff, S. Couzens, G. Simmons, R. Birns, J. Mullane, and G. Huber, Recovery of antibacterial defense mechanisms in the lung following partial hepatectomy, *Clin. Res.,* **20**:871 (1972).
129. J. Mullane, N. Popovic, J. Liang, D. O'Connell, M. LaForce, and G. Huber, Experimental biliary obstruction and the lung, *Gastroenterology,* **64**:188 (1973).
130. H. Nicholas, C. Pollack, C. McCarthy, D. O'Connell, R. Laguarda, and G. Huber, The effect of experimentally altered thyroid activity on alveolar macrophage function, *Clin. Res.,* **21**:973 (1973).
131. J. F. Mullane, G. L. Huber, N. A. Popovic, R. G. Wilfong, S. R. Bielke, D. M. O'Connell, and F. M. LaForce, Aspiration of blood and pulmonary bost defense mechanisms, *Ann. Surg.,* **180-2**:236-242 (1974).
132. C. McCarthy, R. Laguarda, K. Sobel, H. Nicholas, C. Pollack, G. Simmons, J. Mullane, and G. Huber, An experimental evaluation of therapeutic measures used in the treatment of aspiration pneumonitis, *Clin. Res.,* **22**: 450 (1974).
133. K. Sobel, C. McCarthy, G. Simmons, H. Nicholas, R. Laguarda, J. Mullane, and G. Huber, Aspiration of blood, *Clin. Res.,* **21**:968 (1973).
134. J. Mullane, M. LaForce, R. Wilfong, D. O'Connell, and G. Huber, Aspiration of blood and pulmonary host defense mechanisms in the rat, *Clin. Res.,* **20**:889 (1972).
135. G. Huber, D. O'Connell, C. McCarthy, R. Birns, and J. Mullane, The effect of oxygen administration on aspiration pneumonitis, *Clin. Res.,* **21**:662 (1973).
136. D. O'Connell, G. Huber, G. Simmons, I. Barrett, M. LaForce, and J. Mullane, Chest strapping, bacterial infection and the lung: A model for experimental respiratory acidosis, *Clin. Res.,* **21**:670 (1973).
137. J. Mullane, G. Huber, and F. M. LaForce, Congestive heart failure and pulmonary host defense mechanisms, *Circulation,* **50**:111-122 (1974).

138. G. Huber, D. O'Connell, C. McCarthy, R. Birns, M. LaForce, and J. Mullane, Oxygen administration and antibacterial defenses of the lung in experimental congestive heart failure, *Clin. Res.*, **21**:426 (1973).
139. J. F. Mullane, F. M. LaForce, R. G. Wilfong, and G. L. Huber, Effect of suprahepatic caval constriction and congestive heart failure on stress ulcer formation, *Clin. Res.*, **20**:462 (1972).
140. D. O'Connell, M. LaForce, J. Mullane, and G. Huber, Hepatic versus pulmonary congestion in the impairment of pulmonary antibacterial defenses with congestive heart failure, *Clin. Res.*, **20**:859 (1972).
141. G. L. Huber, C. A. Vater, A. J. Huber, S. W. Burley, and F. M. LaForce, An experimental model for correlative quantification of bacterial inactivation with consolidation and fluid accumulation in the lung, *Clin. Res.*, **19**:741 (1971).
142. G. J. Jakab and G. M. Green, The effect of hypersensitivity pneumonitis on the pulmonary defense mechanisms of the guinea pig lung, *Infect. Immun.*, **7**:39-45 (1973).
143. F. M. LaForce, J. F. Mullane, R. F. Boehme, W. J. Kelly, and G. L. Huber, The effect of pulmonary edema on antibacterial defenses of the lung, *J. Lab. Clin. Med.*, **82**:634-638 (1973).
144. F. M. LaForce, R. F. Boehme, and G. L. Huber, The effect of pulmonary edema on antibacterial defenses of the lung, *Ann. Intern. Med.*, **74**:840 (1971).
145. F. M. LaForce, R. F. Boehme, and G. L. Huber, Impaired pulmonary bactericidal activity in pulmonary edema, *Clin. Res.*, **19**:324 (1971).
146. J. O. Klein, G. M. Green, J. G. Tilles, E. H. Kass, and M. Finland, Bactericidal activity of mouse lung in reovirus infection, *Antimicrob. Agents Chemother.*, **8**:164-167 (1968).
147. J. O. Kelin, G. M. Tilles, E. H. Kass, and M. Finland, Effect of intranasal reovirus infection on antibaxterial activity of the mouse lung, *J. Infect. Dis.*, **119**:43-50 (1969).
148. G. M. Green, Pulmonary clearance of infectious agents, *Annu. Rev. Med.*, **19**:315-336 (1968).
149. G. M. Green, Defenses of the lung, *Clin. Notes Respir. Dis.*, **11**:3-12 (1972).
150. G. M. Green, Lung Defense mechanisms, *Med. Clin. N. Am.*, **57**:547-562 (1973).
151. G. M. Green, In defense of the lung, *Am. Rev. Respir. Dis.*, **102**:691-703 (1970).
152. G. M. Green, The study of integrated defense mechanisms in models of chronic pulmonary disease, *Arch. Intern. Med.*, **126**:500-503 (1970).
153. J. Libertoff and G. Huber, The in situ inactivation of inhaled bacteria by the pulmonary alveolar macrophage, *J. Cell Biol.*, **59**:194A (1973).
154. G. M. Green, Quoted in Ref. 149.
155. L. H. Green and G. M. Green, A direct method for determining the viability of a freshly generated mixed bacterial aerosol, *Appl. Microbiol.*, **16**: 78-81 (1968).

156. M. A. Sackner, J. Landa, J. Hirsch, and A. Zapata, Pulmonary effects of oxygen breathing; a 6-hr study in normal men, *Ann. Intern. Med.*, **82**: 40-43 (1975).
157. M. A. Sackner, M. J. Rosen, and A. Wanner, Effects of oxygen breathing and endotracheal intubation on tracheal mucus velocity of anesthetized dogs, *Bull. Physiopathol. Respir. (Nancy)*, **9**:403-413 (1973).
158. M. A. Sackner, M. J. Rosen, and A. Wanner, Estimation of tracheal mucous volocity by bronchofiberoscopy, *J. Appl. Physiol.*, **34**:495-499 (1973).
159. G. Huber, H. Schauffler, C. McCarthy, and M. Hayashi, Comparative morphometric analysis of recoverable and in situ pulmonary alveolar macrophages, *J. Cell Biol.*, **63**:148A (1974).
160. M. LaForce, W. Kelly, and G. Huber, The role of recoverable alveolar macrophages in pulmonary bacterial activity, *Clin. Res.*, **20**:532 (1972).
161. F. M. LaForce, W. J. Kelly, and G. L. Huber, Inactivation of staphylococci by alveolar macrophages with preliminary observations on the importance of alveolar lining material, *Am. Res. Respir. Dis.*, **108**:784-790 (1973).
162. R. M. Rogers, J. Juers, and J. B. McCurdy, Influence of rat and human alveolar lining material on bactericidal capacity of alveolar macrophages, *Fed. Proc.*, **34**:269 (1975).
163. J. Juers, R. M. Rogers, and J. B. McCurdy, Enhancement of bactericidal capacity of alveolar macrophages by human "alveolar lining material," *Clin. Res.*, **23**:348A (1975).
164. L. J. Berry and T. D. Spies, Phagocytosis, *Medicine*, **28**:239-300 (1949).
165. G. M. Green and D. Carolin, The depressant effect of cigarette smoke on the in vitro antibacterial activity of the alveolar macrophages, *N. Engl. J. Med.*, **276**:421-427 (1967).
166. R. H. Michell, S. J. Pancake, J. Noseworthy, and M. L. Karnovsky, Measurement of rates of phagocytosis, *J. Cell Biol.*, **40**:216-224 (1969).
167. F. Ulrich, Phagocytosis of *E. coli* by enzyme-treated alveolar macrophages, *Am. J. Physiol.*, **220**:958-966 (1971).
168. G. B. Mackaness, The phagocytosis and inactivation of staphylococci by macrophages of normal rabbits, *J. Exp. Med.*, **112**:35-53 (1960).
169. I. Auzins and D. Rowley, Factors involved in the adherence of *S. typhimurium* C5 and mouse peritoneal macrophages, *Aust. J. Exp. Biol.*, **41**: 539-546 (1963).
170. W. Brumfitt, A. A. Glynn, and A. Percival, Factors influencing the phagocytosis of *Escherichia coli*, *Br. J. Exp. Pathol.*, **46**:215-226 (1965).
171. J. S. Tan, C. Watanakakunakorn, and J. P. Phair, A modified assay of neutrophil function: Use of lysostaphin to differentiate defective phagocytosis from impaired intracellular killing, *J. Lab. Clin. Med.*, **78**:316-322 (1971).
172. M. Nakashima, Studies on the resistance of rabbit alveolar macrophages to the toxicity of tubercule bacilli in tissue culture, *Acta Tuberc. Jpn.*, **14**:75-88 (1965).
173. J. E. Nutter and Q. N. Myrvik, In vitro interactions between rabbit alveolar macrophages and *Pasteurella tularensis*, *J. Bacteriol.*, **92**:645-651 (1966).

174. M. L. Fox, The bovine alveolar macrophage: Isolation, in vitro cultivation, ultrastructure and phagocytosis, *Can. J. Microbiol.*, **19**:1207-1212 (1973).
175. F. Shafa, B. J. Moberly, and P. Gerhardt, Cytological features of anthrax spores phagocytized in vitro by rabbit alveolar macrophages, *J. Infect. Dis.*, **116**:401-413 (1966).
176. H. J. Henderson, A. M. Dannenberg, and M. B. Lurie, Phagocytosis of tubercle bacilli by rabbit pulmonary alveolar macrophages and its relation to native resistance to tuberculosis, *J. Immunol.*, **91**:553-556 (1963).
177. B. D. Thorpe and S. Marcus, Phagocytosis and intracellular fate of *Pasturella tularensis*, *J. Immunol.*, **93**:558-565 (1964).
178. Q. N. Myrvik, Function of the alveolar macrophage in immunity, *J. Reticuloendothel. Soc.*, **11**:459-468 (1972).
179. M. Lundborg and B. Holma, In vitro phagocytosis of fungal spores by rabbit lung macrophages, *Sabouraudia*, **10**:152-156 (1972).
180. E. Ouchi, R. J. Selvaraj, and A. J. Sbarra, The biochemical activity of rabbit alveolar macrophages during phagocytosis, *Exp. Cell. Res.*, **40**:456-468 (1966).
181. J. B. Grogan and V. Lockard, Acute alterations in the bactericidal capacity of rabbit alveolar macrophages following stress, *J. Trauma*, **13**:877-883 (1973).
182. H. Y. Reynolds and R. E. Thompson, Pulmonary host defenses: Interaction of respiratory antibodies with *Pseudomonas aeruginosa* and alveolar macrophages, *J. Immunol.*, **111**:369-380 (1973).
183. B. B. Paul, R. R. Strauss, and R. J. Selvaraj, Peroxidase-mediated antimicrobial activities of alveolar macrophage granules, *Science*, **181**:849-850 (1973).
184. E. J. Pavillard, In vitro phagocytic and bactericidal ability of alveolar and peritoneal macrophages of normal rats, *Aust. J. Exp. Biol.*, **41**:265-274 (1963).
185. M. Degre, Phagocytic and bactericidal activities of peritoneal and alveolar macrophages from mice, *J. Med. Microbiol.*, **2**:353-357 (1969).
186. E. S. Leake and Q. N. Myrvik, Digestive vacuole formation in alveolar macrophages after phagocytosis of *Mycobacterium smegmatis* in vivo, *J. Reticuloendothel. Soc.*, **3**:83-100 (1966).
187. L. P. Merkow, S. M. Epstein, and H. Sidransky, The pathogenesis of experimental pulmonary aspergillosis: An ultrastructural study of alveolar macrophages after phagocytosis of aflavus spores in vivo, *Am. J. Pathol.*, **62**:57-74 (1971).
188. H. Yeager, Tracheobronchial secretions, *Am. J. Med.*, **50**:493-509 (1971).
189. A. A. Jalowayski and S. T. Gramniona, The interaction of bacteria with pulmonary surfactant, *Am. Rev. Respir. Dis.*, **105**:236-241 (1972).
190. H. Y. Reynolds and K. E. Thompson, Pulmonary host defenses: Analysis of protein and lipids in bronchial secretions and antibody responses after vaccination with *Pseudomonas aeruginosa*, *J. Immunol.*, **111**:358-368 (1973).
191. W. A. Skornik, D. P. Dressler, and P. Nathan, Intracellular killing of

Ps. aeruginosa by rat alveolar macrophages stimulated by normal lung lavage fluid, *Physiologist,* **16**:456 (1973).

192. W. A. Skornik, D. P. Dressler, and P. Nathan, Identification of a humoral alveolar-macrophage enhancement factor, *Physiologist,* **17**:332 (1974).
193. V. G. Lockard, J. B. Grogan, and J. G. Brunson, Alterations in the bactericidal ability of rabbit alveolar macrophages as a result of tumbling stress, *Ann. J. Pathol.,* **70**:57-68 (1973).
194. M. Degre, Synergistic effect in viral-bacterial infection: Influence of viral infection in the phagocytic ability of alveolar macrophages, *Acta Pathol. Microbiol. Scand.,* **78**:41-50 (1970).
195. V. G. Lockard, R. J. Rharbawgh, R. B. Arhelger, and J. B. Grogan, Ultrastructural alterations in phagocytic functions of alveolar macrophages after cyclophosphamide administration, *J. Reticuloendothel. Soc.,* **9**: 97-107 (1971).
196. L. Weissbecker, R. D. Carpenter, P. C. Luchsinger, and T. S. Osdene, In vitro alveolar macrophage viability, *Arch. Environ. Health,* **18**:756-759 (1969).
197. J. D. Acton and Q. N. Myrvik, Nitrogen dioxide effects on alveolar macrophages, *Arch. Environ. Health,* **24**:48-52 (1972).
198. G. M. Green, Cigarette smoke: Protection of alveolar macrophages by blutathione and cysteine, *Science,* **162**:810-811 (1968).
199. G. M. Powell and G. M. Green, Cigarette smoke: A proposed metabolic lesion in alveolar macrophages, *Biochem. Pharmacol.,* **21**:1785-1787 (1972).
200. G. M. Green, Protection of the alveolar macrophage from the cytotoxic activity of cigarette smoke by glutathione and cysteine, *J. Clin. Invest.,* **47**:42a-43a (1968).
201. M. Cutting, A. Watson, S. Goodenough, G. Simmons, R. Laguarda, and G. Huber, The effect of exposure to marijuana smoke on the bactericidal activity of pulmonary alveolar macrophages, *Clin. Res.,* **22**:501 (1974).
202. M. Cutting, A. Watson, S. Goodenough, G. Simmons, R. Laguarda, and G. Huber, Impairment of bactericidal activity of pulmonary alveolar macrophages by exposure to marijuana smoke, *Proc. Int. Union Physiol. Sci.,* **21**:361 (1974).
203. M. Cutting, S. Goodenough, G. Simmons, A. Watson, R. Laguarda, and G. Huber, Marijuana and pulmonary antibacterial defenses: Depression of alveolar macrophage function following experimental exposure to marijuana smoke, *Chest,* **66**:321-322 (1974).
204. M. Cutting, A. Watson, S. Goodenough, G. Simmons, R. Laguarda, and G. Huber, Impairment of alveolar macrophage bactericidal activity by synthetic tobacco substitutes, *Am. Rev. Respir. Dis.,* **109**:726-727 (1974).
205. M. Cutting, R. Laguarda, W. Pereira, and G. Huber, The effect of in vitro exposure to cigar smoke on alveolar macrophage bactericidal function, *Clin. Res.,* **22**:716A (1974).
206. M. Cutting, R. Laguarda, W. Pereira, J. Mullane, and G. Huber, In vitro impairment of murine alveolar macrophage bactericidal activity by tobacco smoke, *Clin. Res.,* **22**:717A (1974).

207. M. Cutting, W. Pereira, R. Laguarda, and G. Huber, Comparable impairment of alveolar macrophage (AM) bactericidal activity by commonly consumed smoking materials, *Clin. Res.*, **23**:302A (1975).
208. M. Cutting, G. Huber, G. Simmons, W. Pereira, and R. Laguarda, A comparative evaluation of impaired antibacterial defenses of the lung by products commonly smoked by man, *Chest*, **68**:407 (1975).
209. D. W. Gump and G. M. Green, Bacterial pneumonia, *Curr. Diagnosis*, **3**: 164-167 (1971).
210. G. M. Green, The response of the alveolar macrophage system to host and environmental changes, *Arch. Environ. Health*, **18**:548-550 (1969).
211. G. M. Green, Alveolo-bronchiolar transport; observations and hypothesis of a pathway, *Chest*, **59**:1S-2S (1971).
212. G. M. Green, Cell dysfunction as a pathogenetic determinant in chronic broncho pulmonary disease, *Arch. Environ. Health*, **21**:481-482 (1970).
213. J. Guillaume, F. Wattell, and C. Macke-Van-Moorleghem, Etude de la phagocytose du virus grippal par les macrophages alveolaires de cobaye: Effets de la phagocytose du virus grippal dur le metabolisme cellulaire, *Ann. Inst. Pasteur*, **16**:17-20 (1965).
214. C. A. Mims, Aspects of the pathogenesis of virus diseases, *Bacteriol. Rev.*, **28**:30-71 (1964).
215. C. Voisin, C. Vivier, and C. Aerts, Etude de la phagocytose du virus grippal par les macrophages alveolaries du cobaye: Aspects morphologiques et cinetiques en microscopie electronique et en microcinematographie en contraste de phase, *Ann. Inst. Pasteur*, **16**:1-10 (1965).
216. J. A. Roberts, Histopathogenesis of mouse pox, *Br. J. Exp. Pathol.*, **43**: 451-461 (1962).
217. Y. C. Kong, H. B. Levine, and S. H. Madin, Fungal multiplication and histopathologic changes in vaccinated mice infected with *Coccidiodes immitis*, *J. Immunol.*, **92**:779-790 (1964).
218. C. G. Loosli, Synergism between viruses and bacteria, *Yale J. Biol. Med.*, **40**:522-540 (1968).
219. C. G. Hartford, V. Leidler, and M. Hara, Effects of the lesion due to influenza virus on the resistance of mice to inhaled pneumococci, *J. Exp. Med.*, **89**:53-68 (1949).

24

Antimicrobial Activities
Intracellular Mechanisms and Extracellular Influences

QUENTIN N. MYRVIK and JEAN D. ACTON

The Bowman Gray School of Medicine
Wake Forest University
Winston-Salem, North Carolina

I. Introduction

There is ample evidence to support the conclusion that normal alveolar macrophages have the capability to ingest and kill many types of microorganisms that gain entrance to the respiratory tract [27,30,37,42,47-49]. It has also been recognized that some microorganisms, particularly the virulent intracellular parasites, have characteristics which allow them to survive in normal macrophages [5,24,40]; it is apparent that this latter class of parasite can be controlled only when the forces of acquired immunity orchestrate the macrophage system into more potent antimicrobial action, both qualitatively and quantitatively [79].

On the basis of hydrolase content, rate of O_2 consumption, and gluconic shunt activity [51,61], the steady-state normal alveolar macrophage is relatively mature, as compared to the peritoneal macrophage; thus, the pathways of differentiation produced by an immunologic stimulus may produce qualitatively different lines of macrophages. In other words, an immune alveolar macrophage (as observed in a cellular immune reaction) in all likelihood is mobilized and derived from immature monocytes and not from existing "steady state" alveolar macrophages present in the normal lung. This possibility would allow variable pathways of differentiation and, accordingly, the epithelioid cell in the immune granuloma may differ physiologically from the normal alveolar macrophage. It would be advantageous for an epitheliloid cell not to be a preferential aerobe like the normal alveolar macrophage because of the nature of the organized structure of the granuloma. Since most studies have been carried out on free alveolar cells, it is still uncertain as to the physiologic status or comparative antimicrobial capabilities of "interstitial" macrophages or epithelioid cells in situ in an immune structure like the granuloma or tubercle.

The above considerations prompt a brief examination of terminology. The term "lung macrophage," which is commonly used, is a collective term that refers to macrophages located anywhere in the lung. The term "alveolar macrophage" or "pulmonary macrophage" refers to macrophages obtained by lung lavage; however, these preparations may also contain "airway macrophages" which may or may not have had an alveolar entrance. Nevertheless, the term alveolar macrophage is a descriptive and convenient term and, in spite of this uncertainty, will be used throughout this chapter in accordance with the above definition.

It is important to emphasize that the alveolar macrophage system is part of a highly integrated pulmonary defense system which includes (a) the acute inflammatory phagocytic (neutrophil) system, (b) the mucociliary escalator apparatus, (c) humoral immune mechanisms, including specific Ab and nonspecific antibacterial factors, and (d) cellular immune mechanisms. Normal lungs contain a resident population of alveolar macrophages, which function as the first line of phagocytic defense in the lower airways. Accordingly, it is of obvious importance to understand the capabilities and limitations of this unique phagocytic system which functions so efficiently in this special location under circumstances of continuing insult.

II. Antibacterial Functions of Normal Alveolar Macrophages

A. Conditions Necessary for the Phagocytic Event

Alveolar macrophages appear to have the same requirements for phagocytosis that macrophages at other anatomical sites demand. In the case of normal flora and the common airborne bacteria (*Bacillus subtilus,* staphylococci, micrococci), there is an adequate supply of "natural" opsonins available and these organisms are readily phagocytized. The major functional opsonins in the normal lung are probably small quantities of IgG and even lesser quantities of IgM. In this regard, some gram-positive bacteria (*Listeria monocytogenes*) as well as acid-fast and alcohol-fast mycobacteria can be readily phagocytized in vitro without the presence of opsonins; presumably this also could occur in vivo. Robbins et al. [68] observed that the opsonizing power of purified IgM antisalmonella Abs was 500 to 1,000 times more effective than purified IgG. Rowley et al. [70] reported that approximately 10 molecules of IgM per bacterium were sufficient for opsonization. With respect to secretory IgA (sIgA), observations to date indicate that it is a poor opsonin, compared to IgG or IgM [67,81]. Since the IgM levels in the respiratory tract are very low or absent, it appears that IgG is the major opsonin in the airways [66].

Since the level of complement components in normal lung secretions is extremely low [66], its exact role as an amplification mechanism of the opsonins present is yet undefined. In a study on alveolar macrophages Mason et al. [54] observed that active component(s) in serum (nondialyzable and heat-labile) more than doubled the uptake of paraffin oil emulsions stabilized with albumin. Since zymosan removed serum-containing opsonic activity, they suggested that the properdin system (complement-bypass system) might involve those complement components. However, the presence of low levels of natural opsonins could have accounted for their results, a point that was not ruled out. If the appropriate complement components are available, a synergistic effect with natural or immune opsonins would be a likely expectation, particularly if the opsonin concentration is limiting. This issue is unduly complex because transient, local inflammatory reactions in the lung could cause sufficient transudation to bring in plasma Ab (both IgG and IgM) and necessary complement components. This undoubtedly occurs during clinically apparent pulmonary infections.

The absence of specific opsonins directed against surface components of certain pathogenic bacteria may prevent phagocytosis. Surface moieties may be capsules (*Streptococcus pneumoniae*) or surface chains of polysaccharides (*Salmonella typhi*) that are highly specialized components exhibiting antiphagocytic properties. These surface Ags do not usually show cross-reactivity with natural opsonins against related nonvirulent bacteria.

A case in point is *S. typhi.* Rabbit alveolar macrophages will not phagocytose these organisms unless specific opsonins are supplied and such opsonins are not present in normal rabbit serum. In contrast, *Escherichia coli,* a normal flora organism, also requires opsonins, but an abundant supply exists in normal rabbit serum because of natural immunization from the *E. coli* present in the gastrointestinal tract. It is of interest that, during the course of incubation (6-24 hr) of rabbit macrophages, *S. typhi* adheres to the surface of the macrophages, but no phagocytosis is detectable [50]. When specific opsonins are added, the adherent organisms are rapidly phagocytosed. This observation illustrates that adherence, which is opsonin independent in this case, does not trigger phagocytosis; it also establishes that phagocytosis is at least a two-step process.

Other examples of bacteria that resist phagocytosis, unless specific opsonins are present, include *Hemophilus influenzae, Pseudomonas aeruginosa, Neisseria meningitidis,* and *Streptococcus pyogenes.* Essentially all classical extracellular parasites possess some attribute which interferes with their being phagocytosed. However, once these organisms are phagocytosed, normal macrophages as well as polymorphonuclear cells are quite capable of killing them. This naturally raises the question as to how might opsonins or Ab against surface moieties influence the intracellular fate of ingested microorganisms. Jenkin [38] approached this problem in a novel way by using phage adsorbed to bacteria and Ab to phage as opsonin and compared the intracellular fate of *Salmonella typhimurium* phagocytosed by this means with this organism opsonized with specific opsonin. He observed that specific Ab against *S. typhimurium* facilitated intracellular killing of this organism, whereas Ab against phage attached to *S. typhimurium* promoted phagocytosis but failed to promote equivalent killing. This principal has not been tested with gram-positive or other gram-negative organisms.

B. Mechanisms of Intracellular Killing

Particle contact with the surface membrane of the phagocyte appears to stimulate metabolic activation. Once phagocytosis has occurred, the bacterium encased in a phagosomal membrane, contributed by the cytoplasmic membrane of the phagocyte, usually interacts with primary and secondary lysosomes to form a phagolysosome. Under some circumstances, fusion of two or more phagosomes or phagolysosomes probably occurs. Lysosome-phagosome fusion brings about the environmental changes which make the phagolysosome the prime compartment for effecting killing and digestion of the engulfed bacterium. With the exception of virulent intracellular parasites, normal alveolar macrophages are effective if opsonins are available, assuming they are not overwhelmed by excessive numbers of such bacteria.

Whereas we have a working concept on the requirements for phagocytosis, we are deficient in our knowledge as to what happens to the bacterium after the phagocytic event. It is likely that killing in the phagosome is related to some product of metabolism. The myeloperoxidase-H_2O_2-halide system in neutrophils [43] has been examined rather thoroughly in alveolar macrophages. The first problem encountered was the difficulty in demonstrating significant peroxidase activity in macrophages. Recently, Paul et al. [62] have reported on peroxidase-mediated killing by alveolar macrophage preparations. However, since the peroxidase activity was only 10% of that found in neutrophils, there is a question as to the relative importance of this system in alveolar macrophages; the peroxidase activity demonstrated in this case could be due to contamination from other cell types.

Hydrolases undoubtedly play an important role in the breakdown of the microbial carcass but the direct role of hydrolases in bactericidal events is questionable. Lysozyme is an exception; when bacteria with large amounts of murein

(*Sarcina lutea*) are exposed to lysozyme, rapid hydrolysis, and killing results. Another example involves a synergism between antibody plus complement and lysozyme in the case of some gram negative bacteria. Also it is possible that lysozyme could facilitate metabolic-mediated killing events by creating breaks in the murein layer and further exposing the cell membrane to peroxidation or the action of other hydrolases.

The studies of Zeya and Spitznagel [83] have revealed a spectrum of interesting antibacterial cationic proteins in neutrophils. However, this system could not be identified in alveolar macrophages.

Another point of consideration relates to the possibility that "old" multilamellar phagosomes may exert some degree of nutrient deprivation. Accordingly, "slow death" could be produced when resistant or refractory parasites are ingested. Multilamellar phagosomes are relatively common in normal alveolar macrophages (Fig. 1). However, little is known about the process of forming multiple membranous layers. Presumably this is the result of an endophagic process involving refractory residues in a long-lived macrophage.

III. Antibacterial Functions of Alveolar Macrophages in Acquired Cellular Immunity

The expression of acquired cellular immunity in the lung is similar to its expression in other organ systems. Accordingly, sensitive T lymphocytes circulating through the small vessels can be triggered by the corresponding Ag to undergo a blastogenic response and sequester on the vascular endothelium with subsequent migration through the tight junctions of small vessels into the interstitium of the lung. Blasting T lymphocytes then secrete a series of mediators which attract, mobilize and activate bloodborne mononuclear phagocytic cells to the focus of Ag deposition. The mononuclear phagocytes become activated and transform into mature macrophages and ultimately into epithelioid cells and occasional giant cells which have enhanced killing potential [22,44,46,60]. The differentiated mononuclear phagocytes aggregate and form the classical allergic granuloma which is cuffed by lymphocytes.

The available evidence strongly supports the concept that cellular immunity provides mechanisms to mobilize a large number of activated macrophages to a focus of infection. Some of the macrophages ultimately move into the alveolar space. However, if the cellular immune reaction is intense, the tendency toward aggregation of macrophages in the interstitium is strong and few free cells accumulate in the alveoli (Fig. 2).

If alveolar cell populations derived from allergic granulomatous (BCG-induced) lungs are procured and studied in vitro, three general observations can

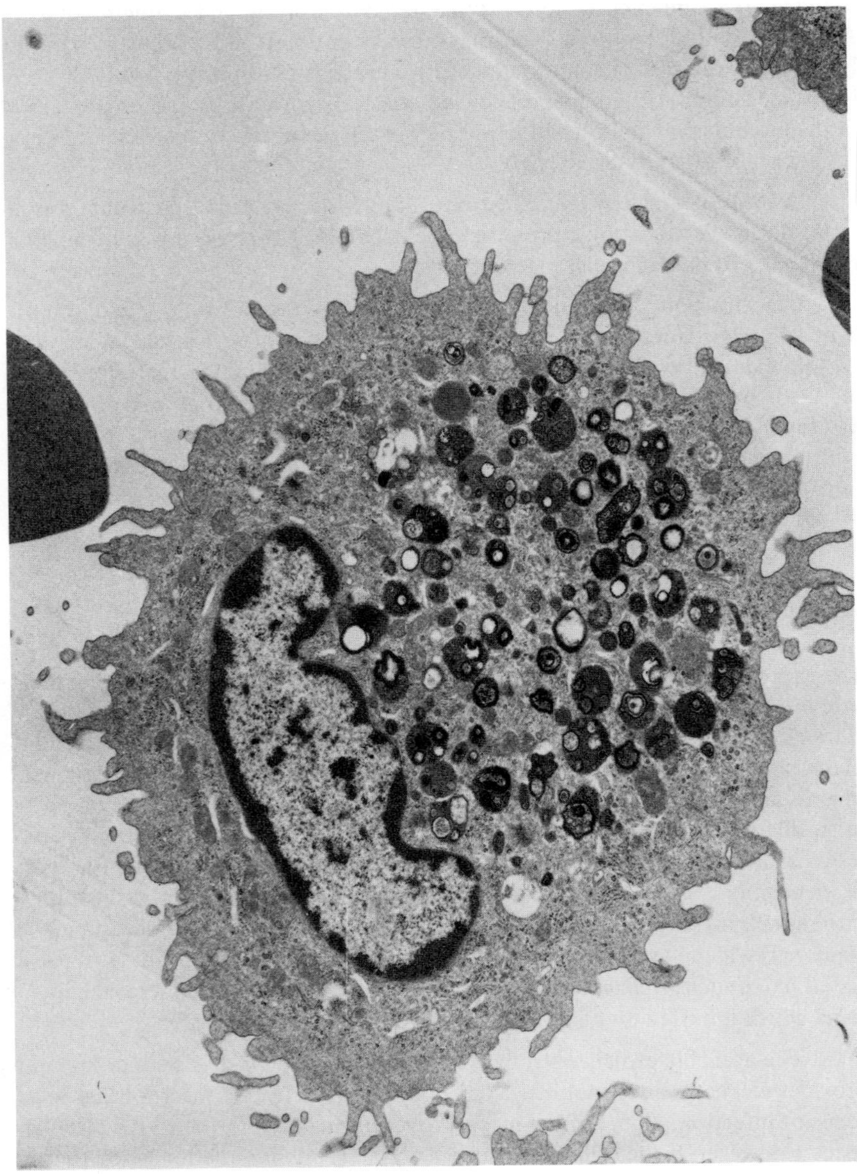

FIGURE 1 Multilamellar structures and myelin figures in a normal alveolar macrophage. Note the multilayered structures resembling old phagosomes. Uranyl acetate and lead citrate. ×5430.

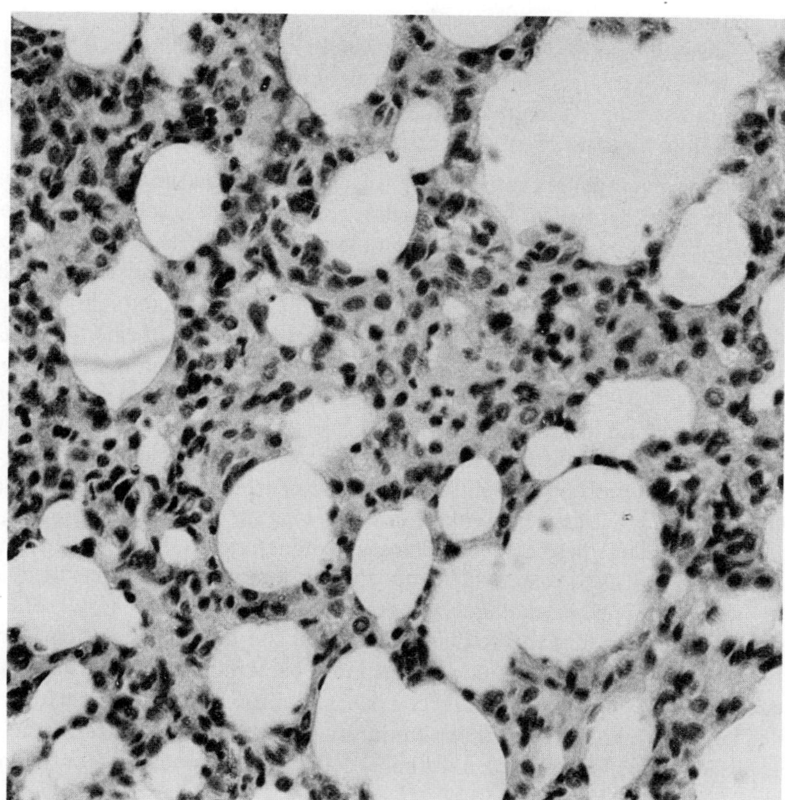

FIGURE 2 Interstitial granulomatous response. Rabbits were sensitized s.c. with 100 μg of killed BCG in 0.1 ml oil at the base of each ear. Three weeks after sensitization the animals were challenged i.t. with 3 mg of killed BCG in saline. The lungs were removed 2 days after challenge. Note the interstitial nature of the granulomatous response with lack of free cells in the alveolar spaces. Hematoxylin and eosin. ×280.

be made: (a) this population is usually MIF-positive if the corresponding Ag is added [23], (b) the macrophages have an enhanced capacity to kill bacteria [58], and (c) macrophages usually have increased metabolic activity as well as hydrolase levels [59,74]. The events of allergic granuloma formation can be readily observed by sensitizing a rabbit with 100 μg of killed BCG at the base of the ear; after 3 weeks, when the animal is tuberculin positive, a challenge dose of BCG given intratracheally will elicit a marked granulomatous response. In this case, the nonchallenged tuberculin positive animal has a normal appearing lung and the alveolar cells are usually MIF negative. In contrast, the sensitized-challenged animals exhibit a profound pulmonary granulomatous reaction resulting in a doubling of the lung weight within 48 hr after challenge. The granulomatous response is largely interstitial and exhibits marked consolidation of large areas of the lung. If the reaction is intense, necrosis is usually evident 3 to 4 weeks after administration of the challenge dose (Fig. 3).

Alveolar macrophages activated by this type of cellular immune reaction probably have a potential for killing which is greater than that which develops when macrophages become activated by nonimmunologic mechanisms. Although BCG-vaccinated mice are highly resistant to weakly pathogenic organisms such as *Lysteria monocytogenes,* they exhibit no detectable resistance to highly virulent organisms such as *Francisella tularensis* [10]. In contrast, specifically immunized animals are highly resistant to challenge with *F. tularensis,* which is a classical intracellular parasite. These observations suggest that for activated macrophages to be able to contain or kill a highly virulent bacterium, some specific mechanism is also involved. While this issue has not been resolved, a logical expectation might be that specific Ab (cytophilic Ab?) could neutralize some surface toxic moiety on a highly virulent bacterium, thus allowing the activated macrophage to kill. This principle has been convincingly demonstrated in the case of typhus rickettsia where virulent rickettsia disrupt the phagosome and grow in the cytoplasm of the macrophage leading to the demise of the phagocyte. However, specific Ab can neutralize this toxic manifestation and then the macrophage can kill the rickettsiae [24]. The toxic expression is bacterium-associated and not a secretion product. It is obvious how cellular immunity might interact with this type of humoral immunity. Cellular immunity would direct mobilization of macrophages to foci of infected endothelial cells and Ab would protect the macrophages from intoxication.

A relatively recent concept involves the possibility that immune lymphocytes and activated macrophages may secrete antimicrobial factors that can act extracellularly. Bast et al. [8] and Sethi et al. [71] have reported on extracellular killing of *L. monocytogenes* by a product of immunologically activated macrophages. Pearsall et al. [63] have observed lymphokine toxicity for certain yeast cells. These potential mechanisms could be important under conditions of reduced phagocytosis of the parasite.

IV. Antifungal Activities of Macrophages

The role alveolar macrophages play in the resistance to and recovery from fungal infections is less well defined than their role in bacterial systems. Peritoneal macrophages, blood monocytes or leukocytes have been used in most of the studies concerned with the fate of phagocytosed fungi. There are obvious limita-

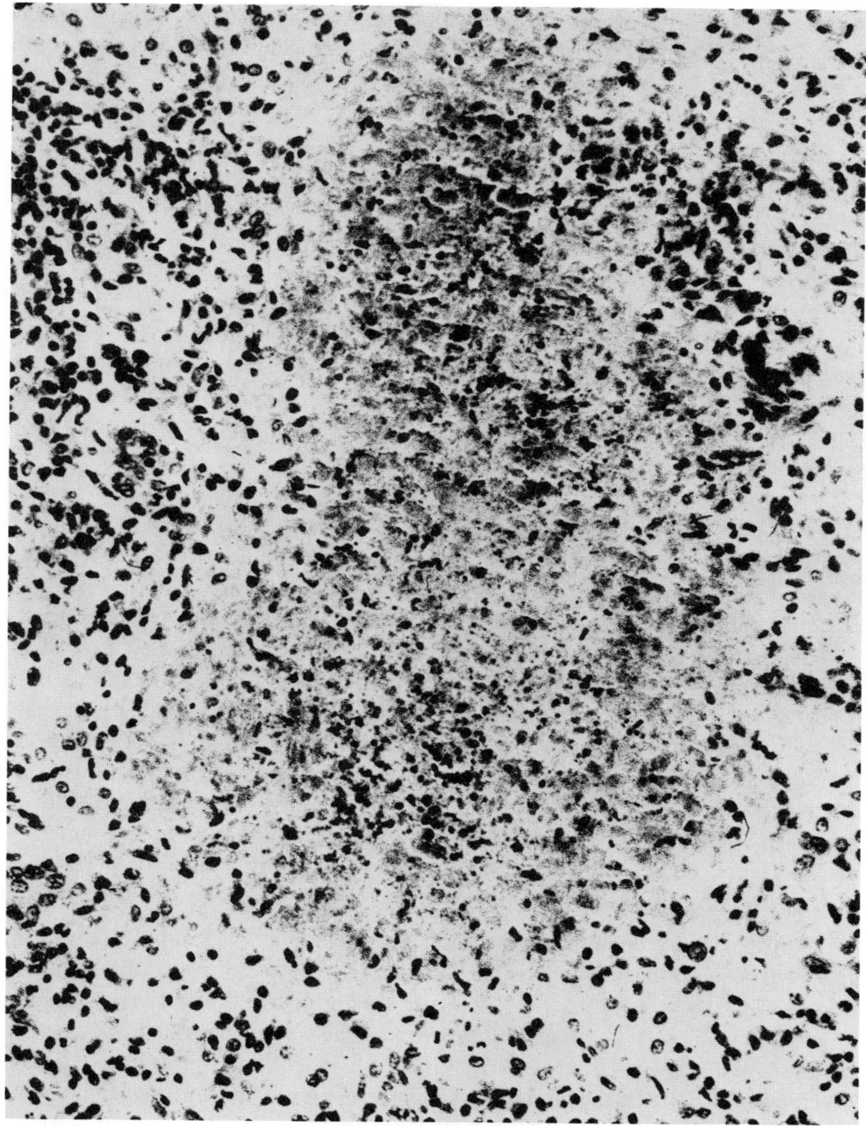

FIGURE 3 Section of lung illustrating a necrotic center in a BCG-induced allergic granuloma. The rabbit was sensitized with 100 μg of killed BCG in oil at the base of each ear by the s.c. route. Three weeks later the animal was challenged i.t. with 3 mg of killed BCG in saline. Necrosis is evident 3 weeks after giving the challenge dose. Hematoxylin and eosin. ×280.

tions in extrapolating results obtained in nonpulmonary systems to events which might occur in the lung; however, some of the major functions of phagocytes are probably similar. More importantly, this paucity of data focuses on the need for additional investigations on the function of alveolar macrophages in pulmonary mycoses.

It has been generally assumed that cell-mediated immune mechanisms are probably more important than humoral mechanisms in most fungal infections. There is some indirect evidence from experimental infections in animals that supports this assumption [20,36]. It has also been observed that certain mycotic infections are more prevalent in patients with impaired cell-mediated immunity than in patients with impaired humoral immunity [33,56]. Although available evidence suggests that macrophages may be important effector cells in resistance against some of the mycoses which involve the respiratory system, they may be relatively unimportant in others and, in some cases, may even contribute to the disease process.

Invasive fungal diseases represent an increasingly important cause of morbidity and mortality in patients whose host defenses have been altered by their primary disease or by immunosuppressive therapy [52]. Certain, but not all, fungi are responsible for this increase in fungal complications. Zimmerman [84] reported that the major increase in fungal complications was due to candidiasis, aspergillosis and mucormycosis and that these infections were clearly associated with modern cancer therapy. The incidence of cryptococcosis and histoplasmosis is also higher in patients with leukemia and lymphoma; however, the incidence does not appear to be increasing in these patients in spite of intensive chemotherapy. In contrast, there appears to be no increase in the frequency of two other important pulmonary mycoses, namely, blastomycosis and coccidioidomycosis. These observations suggest that different combinations of immune mechanisms are involved in the three groups of fungal infections. However, the role macrophages play in these diseases does not follow a single pattern.

In the case of candidiasis, macrophages are unable to contain the organism and have been implicated as possible vectors in the development of disseminated disease. Stanley and Hurley [75] observed that mouse peritoneal macrophages infected in vitro with *Candida albicans* were actively attracted to the yeasts and rapidly ingested the blastospores. Within 2 hr, 95% of the intracellular organisms developed germ tubes; the elongating germ tubes eventually ruptured the macrophage cell membranes. The infected macrophages aggregated to form infective foci as the emerging germ tubes attracted additional macrophages to the complex; however, the growth of the fungus was not inhibited. The results from these experiments suggest a mechanism by which *Candida* may be disseminated in vivo. The small mycelial-macrophage aggregate could act as infective emboli being transported and trapped in small blood vessels through which they could invade the cells of other tissues.

Gentry and Remington [25] reported that "activated" macrophages from mice chronically infected with *Besnoitia, Toxoplasma,* or *Listeria* showed no enhanced resistance to destruction by *C. albicans,* although such macrophages resisted destruction by *Cryptococcus.* In addition, these investigators observed that chronically infected mice were not protected against infection with *C. albicans* administered intravenously.

Since macrophages are unable to contain *Candida,* it is apparent that extracellular factors must be involved in resistance to this organism. The work of Pearsall et al. [63] indicates that supernatant fluids from phytohemagglutin-stimulated mouse lymphocytes are toxic for *C. albicans* in vitro. These observations are of considerable interest for, if lymphokines exert direct antimicrobial activity in vivo, a new concept may emerge with respect to the mechanisms by which cellular immunity is operative against some types of microorganisms.

In contrast to the inability of macrophages to inhibit the growth of *Candida,* Epstein et al. [20] reported that *Aspergillus* spores phagocytosed by alveolar macrophages in experimentally infected mice seldom germinate and the mice are highly resistant to pulmonary infections; however, macrophages from cortisone-treated mice show a diminished ability to kill or prevent germination of phagocytosed spores and, as a consequence, the mice develop overwhelming and fatal infections. The inability of macrophages from cortisone-treated mice to prevent spore germination appeared to be related, at least in part, to an inhibition of lysosome-phagosome fusion [64]. In these experiments, cortisone-treated and control mice were exposed to aerosolized *Aspergillus* spores, and fractionated alveolar macrophages were examined for distribution of acid phosphatase activity. Following phagocytosis of the spores, acid phosphatase activity was localized primarily in the supernatant fraction of alveolar macrophages in control mice. In contrast, the enzyme activity was mainly associated with the particulate fraction of alveolar macrophages obtained from cortisone-treated mice. These observations support the concept that cortisone either stabilizes lysosomal membranes or somehow suppresses the metabolic events necessary for fusion. As a consequence, it appears that alterations in alveolar macrophage lysosomes may be implicated in the pathogenesis of pulmonary aspergillosis. Thus, in two of the most common opportunistic fungal diseases, namely, candidiasis and aspergillosis, macrophages may contribute to the pathogenesis in the former and play a protective role in the latter.

Histoplasma capsulatum infections characteristically involve one or more organs of the reticuloendothelial system. In stained preparations of sputum or lung biopsy specimens, the fungus appears as small oval bodies primarily in large mononuclear cells (Fig. 4) but occasionally in polymorphonuclear cells. Histoplasmosis is seen more frequently in compromised patients but, as with cryptococcosis, does not appear to be increasing in frequency among such patients [52].

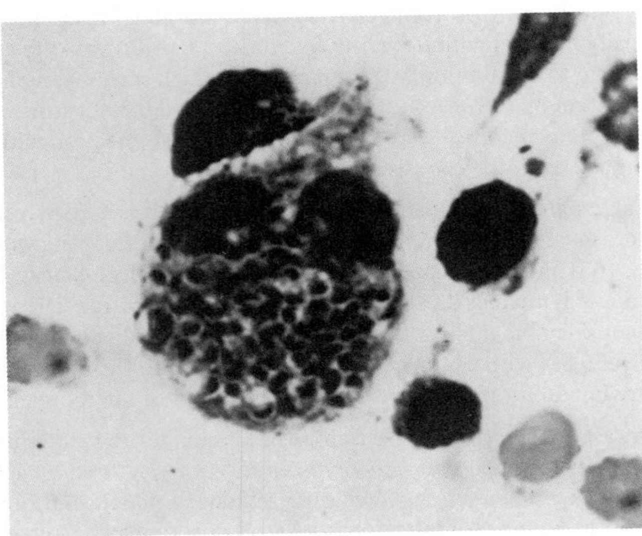

FIGURE 4 Histoplasmosis: Parasitized mononuclear cell in a peripheral blood smear. ×1300. (Reproduced with permission from Ref. 12.)

Dumont and Robert [18] studied the ultrastructural aspects of phagocytosis of *H. capsulatum* by unstimulated, unsensitized hamster peritoneal macrophages after i.p. injection of fungi. Fungi were observed in eosinophils and neutrophils as well as macrophages. Within macrophages, the organisms were present in two types of phagosomes, a "tight" and a "loose" type. The first host response to ingested organisms was the interaction of phagosomes and lysosomes to form phagolysosomes; however, no progressive alteration of fungi was observed in phagolysosomes. After 1 hr, fungi were most frequently observed in large clear vacuoles. The results of this study indicate that, although some fungi were possibly altered, most were well preserved and multiplied inside the different cytoplasmic vacuoles within the macrophages. Some of the macrophages containing fungi showed signs of cytoplasmic degeneration. Such macrophages, together with the fungi present in their cytoplasm, were observed to be phagocytosed by other macrophages. In addition, altered neutrophils, some of which contained fungi, were regularly observed in macrophages. Thus, the host response in this system was characterized by successive phagocytosis of the same fungi by different macrophages without concomitant destruction of the organisms.

Subsequently, Howard, Otto, and Gupta [36] compared the growth of *H. capsulatum* in peritoneal macrophages from immune and normal mice. They showed that the percentage of infected macrophages was approximately the same in tissue cultures from normal and immunized mice. However, it was observed that cells freshly harvested from immunized mice restricted the intracellular growth of *H. capsulatum;* the generation time of the fungus was prolonged threefold within the immune macrophages in comparison with normal macrophages. In contrast, when immune cells were maintained in culture for 48 hr before infection, the intracellular growth of the fungus was not inhibited. These observations suggested that some type of cell or labile factor did not persist during incubation of the cultures. When freshly harvested immune cells were allowed to attach onto coverslips and then were washed thoroughly before parasitization with *H. capsulatum,* most of the inhibitory activity was lost. Intracellular growth suppression was restored in part by the addition of partially purified lymphocytes from immunized mice. Since the immune lymphocytes did not affect the viability of yeast cells suspended in buffer, it was concluded that lymphocytes exerted their effect on the macrophage and not directly on the fungus. In another series of experiments, these investigators established that normal macrophages or 48 hr cultures of immune macrophages (which were no longer inhibitory) could restrict the intracellular growth of this facultative intracellular parasite after in vitro exposure to lymphocytes from immunized mice. Furthermore, the addition of immune lymphocytes to cultures of macrophages already parasitized by the fungus resulted in inhibition of intracellular growth. These observations indicate the importance of lymphocyte-macrophage interaction in the development of effective macrophage killing in this system.

Howard [35] examined the subsequent fate of intracellularly inhibited *H. capsulatum* by assessing staining characteristics, viability on subculture and radioisotopic techniques. No tinctorial distinction could be made between yeasts within normal or immune phagocytes. Yeast cells recovered from the cytoplasm of immune monocytes 24 hr after phagocytosis excluded the dye eosin-Y, germinated when incubated on appropriate medium, and initiated growth at a normal rate within phagocytes from normal animals. However, results from autoradiographic studies established that protein synthesis by fungi in residence within immune macrophages was substantially reduced. Collectively, these data clearly indicate that, although the growth of *H. capsulatum* was inhibited within immune macrophages, the fungus was not killed by the encounter. It is thus apparent that, in the case of histoplasmosis, as in tuberculosis [65], acquired immunity is not necessarily accompanied by death of the intracellular organisms. Howard suggests that the recovery and continued well-being of a host could depend on the continuous inhibition of the particular pathogen and that inhibited microorganisms may eventually be destroyed by the accumulated nonspecific factors associated with granulomatous lesions.

In contrast to *H. capsulatum, Cryptococcus neoformans* may exist in tissue for extended lengths of time without stimulating a significant inflammatory response; however, after a relatively long period of residence in the tissue, a chronic inflammatory response, rich in giant cells, macrophages and lymphocytes, may develop. Pulmonary nodules resected operatively are usually solid granulomas except for areas of central necrosis [12].

Diamond and Bennett [16] studied the interaction of *C. neoformans* with cultured macrophages derived from human peripheral blood monocytes. Although the organisms were actively phagocytized, there was no detectable intracellular killing by the macrophages. In fact, intracellular fungi grew more rapidly than a corresponding control culture of cryptococci growing in a tissue culture medium. These investigators were unable to produce activated macrophages in vitro that could inhibit the intracellular growth of cryptococci. Thus, although blood monocytes can kill *C. neoformans,* macrophages derived in vitro from these cells apparently cannot kill. Differentiation of monocytes into macrophages in other systems has been shown to be accompanied by a loss of detectable myeloperoxidase activity [11]. In view of the central role of the myeloperoxidase-H_2O_2-halide system in killing of *C. neoformans* by human neutrophils [17], Diamond and Bennett [16] speculate that the inability of macrophages to kill this organism may be related to the absence of these mechanisms.

Gentry and Remington [25] also studied the effect of *C. neoformans* on normal and activated macrophages. Monolayers of peritoneal macrophages from mice infected with *Besnoitia* or *Listeria* were not destroyed after phagocytosing *Cryptococcus;* however, normal control macrophages underwent necrosis. Killing of *C. neoformans* by these cells was not studied. Mice chronically infected with the *Besnoitia* or *Toxoplasma,* when challenged with a lethal dose of *C. neoformans,* showed decreased mortality compared to control animals. On the basis of these results, the authors suggested that persistent infection with these intracellular bacteria and protozoa confers resistance against *Cryptococcus* infection and that activated macrophages play a major role in this resistance. Diamond and Bennett [16] also observed that macrophages activated in vitro with small inocula of *C. neoformans* were resistant to destruction by cryptococcal infection. However, survival of macrophages was accompanied by increased survival and growth of the organism in culture as discussed above. Thus, they concluded that monocyte-derived macrophages are not of major importance in resistance to cryptococcosis in man and may even enhance the disease process by serving as a vehicle for dissemination in a manner similar to that observed in candidiasis.

In many of the experiments which have been performed with *Cryptococcus,* encapsulated forms of the organism have been used. However, it appears that the infectious particle, as it exists in nature, is a relatively small, nonencapsulated organism; Emmons [19] reported that *C. neoformans* in pigeon excreta usually does not possess a visible capsule. Farhi et al. [21] suggested that, in this form, the organism could be more readily disseminated by air currents and is more

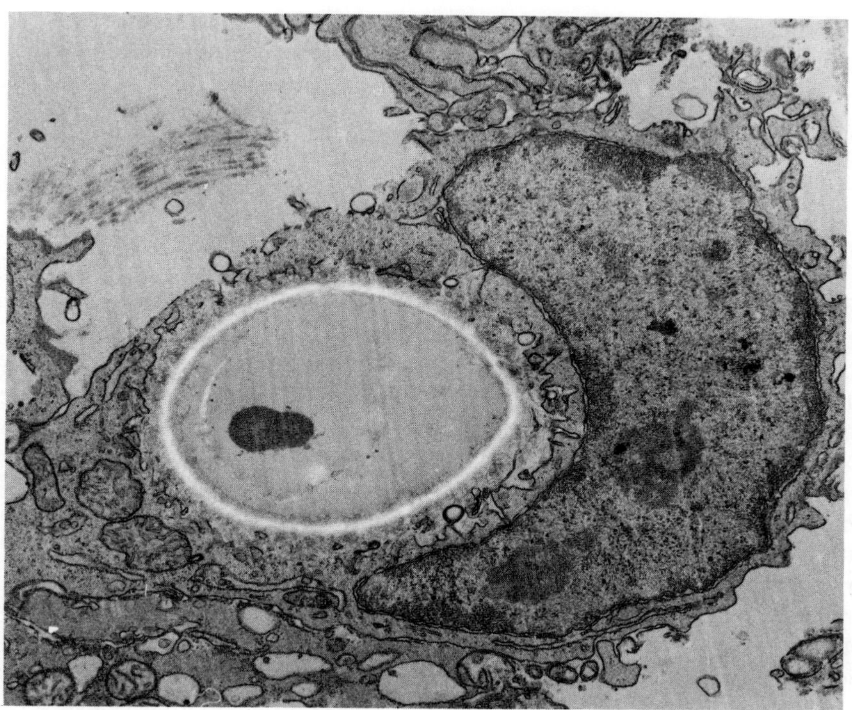

FIGURE 5 Human lung biopsy from a patient with cryptococcosis. Electron micrograph showing a highly degraded yeast inside an alveolar phagocyte. Uranyl acetate-lead citrate stain. ×13,500.

likely to be inhaled into the lungs than the large encapsulated yeast. An illustration of a human alveolar macrophage with *C. neoformans* possessing a small capsule is presented in Fig. 5. Nonencapsulated yeasts are readily phagocytosed and killed when incubated with neutrophils and serum [78]. When capsular material was added to the system, no killing of yeast cells could be attributed to phagocytosis. However, even in the presence of cryptococcal capsular material, normal serum was found to contain anticryptococcal activity. In the presence of serum from healthy individuals, leukocytes from patients with cryptococcosis phagocytized *C. neoformans* normally which suggests that there is no functional defect in the leukocytes. When patients' sera were tested with leukocytes from healthy subjects, phagocytosis was inhibited.

Diamond [15] found that, even when phagocytosis is blocked, human peripheral blood mononuclear cells can readily kill cryptococci if anticryptococcal Ab is present. In the absence of either Ab or leukocytes, killing was significantly reduced. The nature of the effector cell which operates to facilitate extracellular killing in this system is uncertain but it appears to be a cell which can adhere to surfaces. Thus, antibody-dependent cell-mediated killing, as well as other cellular nonphagocytic killing mechanisms, may be of major importance in the extracellular elimination of organisms which are not readily ingested by phagocytic cells.

V. Antiviral Activities of Alveolar Macrophages

Viral infections of the respiratory tract collectively constitute the major cause of morbidity due to infectious organisms. Mims [57] reviewed the evidence that viruses introduced into the lungs may be taken up by macrophages. Although the most common viral respiratory infections are relatively benign and are confined to the upper respiratory tract, early stages in a number of systemic virus diseases, such as smallpox, measles, and chickenpox, also involve the respiratory system. In spite of the frequency of respiratory infections, few definitive data are available on the interaction of viruses with alveolar macrophages. Virus particles entering the mucociliary region of the lower respiratory tract most likely are entrapped in mucus and carried upwards; those deposited distal to those regions are likely to have a primary encounter with pulmonary macrophages. These phagocytes thus present a potentially important barrier to the spread of infection to extrapulmonary sites.

Merigan [55] recently summarized the evidence that macrophages are indeed a major line of host defense against viruses. Macrophage phagocytic and digestive functions vary for different viruses; the virulence of certain viruses appears to be related directly to the ability of macrophages to deal with them. Genetic differences in susceptibility to some murine viruses have been correlated with the efficiency of virus replication in macrophages. In addition, the age-determined resistance of mice to herpes simplex virus has been attributed to the greater capacity of macrophages from adult animals to restrict the multiplication and spread of the virus. Furthermore, macrophages possess specific surface receptors for antibody [9] and, therefore, have an enhanced potential to clear and degrade virus and Ab-virus complexes. Interferon production represents another potentially important mechanism of macrophage antiviral activity. Alveolar macrophages are able to synthesize interferon which may participate in the containment of certain viruses [1], especially during the early stages of infection.

A. Macrophage Permissiveness and Viral Virulence

The early work of Liu [53] suggested the importance of alveolar macrophages in respiratory infections. He used fluorescein-labeled antibody to study the pathogenesis of influenza in ferrets following the intranasal administration of virus. The ferret-adapted PR-8 strain of influenza A virus produced a severe infection in less than 24 hr. Histologic examination of the lungs from animals with pneumonia revealed fluorescent macrophages in both the walls and lumina of alveoli; many fluorescent cells were also observed in the bronchial epithelium. The lungs contained large amounts of virus indicating that the agent had replicated in infected cells. In contrast, ferrets given the Lee strain of influenza B did not appear ill in spite of some pneumonia found at autopsy. Lung sections taken from pneumonic areas contained fluorescent macrophages in the pulmonary interstitium but the bronchial epithelium had no viral antigen. The presence of fluorescent material in macrophages most likely resulted from the phagocytosis of the inoculated virus, but infectivity titrations indicated no virus multiplication. Collectively, these results suggest that the capacity of alveolar macrophages to support virus replication may have been important in determining the outcome of these infections. Liu also observed fluorescent cells in the mediastinal lymph nodes of ferrets infected with influenza A virus. The size and distribution of the fluorescent cells suggested that they were probably macrophages and not lymphocytes. It is possible that free virus particles or viral Ags entered the bronchial, perivascular, or subpleural adventitiae and penetrated the connective tissue of the lung and were phagocytized by resident macrophages. Subsequently, the macrophages could transport the viral Ags to the lymph nodes. Accordingly, if macrophages allow virus replication, they may serve as a vehicle for dissemination of the infection.

Observations on mouse hepatitis virus (MHV) also emphasize the relationship between virulence and the capacity of viruses to multiply in macrophages; the avirulent MGV does not replicate in macrophages, whereas the virulent strain MHV_3 multiplies readily in mouse peritoneal macrophages [4].

Infection by inhalation is generally accepted as the primary means of natural transmission of a number of viruses, including the poxviruses. Roberts [69] studied the pathogenesis of airborne infectious ectromelia virus (mousepox) in mice by a combination of infectivity titrations and fluorescent antibody staining. After aerosol infection, ectromelia virus multiplication was first detected in the lungs and upper respiratory tract. Virus was taken up by alveolar macrophages and in some, multiplied. Infection also could be initiated in mucosal cells of respiratory bronchioles or in the upper respiratory tract. The first viral antigen that appeared in the pulmonary lymph nodes was in free macrophages rather than in the fixed phagocytic cells lining the sinuses of the node. It seems possible that ectromelia virus could have spread from the respiratory system to the viscera by the movement of infected macrophages, particularly if a lesion were present that disrupted the continuity of the alveolar spaces.

Johnson [39] investigated the role of macrophages in the spread of herpes simplex virus infections in mice. He demonstrated conclusively that the difference in susceptibility of different age groups of mice to herpes simplex virus correlated with a difference in the ability of macrophages to disseminate infections; infected macrophages derived from infant mice passed the infection to other cells while those from mature animals did not. In an extension of these studies, Zisman et al. [85] were able to increase susceptibility to herpetic hepatitis in adult mice by administering silica or antimacrophage serum to impair macrophage function. Furthermore, Hirsch et al. [34] could protect infant mice by adoptive transfer of macrophages derived from syngenetic adult mice. Stevens and Cook [76] studied the mechanisms involved in age-dependent resistance to herpes. They established that the herpes simplex genome is expressed in nonpermissive macrophages in that small amounts of virus were produced in the macrophages from adult mice. However, the infection appears to be primarily an abortive one in which all viral components are made but not efficiently assembled. In addition to the restrictive events concerned with assembly, most of the virions that are assembled in macrophages are destroyed, most likely by lysosomal hydrolases. As a consequence of expression of viral genes, both macrophage and virus are ultimately destroyed. It is apparent that such interactions could effectively alter the course of herpes infection in vivo.

B. Macrophages and Genetically Determined Resistance to Viral Infection

Genetically determined resistance to viral infection was first described by Webster [80] who found that strains of mice resistant to *Salmonella enteritidis* were also resistant to group B arboviruses. The factors which determined resistance or sensitivity were shown to follow the patterns of simple Mendelian inheritance and segregated independently as autosomal dominant genes. Goodman and Koprowski [28,29] subsequently examined the mechanisms responsible for resistance to West Nile encephalitis virus. The virus was rapidly cleared from the blood of both sensitive and resistant mice for the first 12 hr following intravenous inoculation; however, sensitive mice subsequently developed a secondary viremia. Resistance could be transferred by transplantation of spleen, bone marrow or lymph node cells from resistant to sensitive mice. The results from experiments using cultured peritoneal macrophages and kidney cells showed that macrophages from resistant mice supported West Nile virus replication poorly, whereas renal cells from the same animals supported viral growth equally as well as cells from susceptible animals.

More recently, Hanson et al. [32] reported that West Nile virus replicates in macrophages and embryonic fibroblasts of both susceptible and resistant mice;

however, the final yield of infectious virus is considerably less in cells from resistant strains than in those from sensitive strains. These investigators found that resistant animals as well as cell cultures from such animals were protected by concentrations of interferon which were less effective in susceptible mice. From these and other data, it was suggested that, in this system, the observed resistance resulted from increased sensitivity of cells to interferon. Further studies are needed to define the precise mechanisms operative in these genetically determined differences in viral susceptibility.

Additional evidence suggesting that macrophages may be the cells reflecting genetic resistance or sensitivity to viruses is provided by the results from studies with mouse hepatitis virus (MHV). Bang and Warwick [7] found that adult mice of the PRI strain are susceptible to lethal infection with the Nelson strain of MHV, whereas the C_3H strain is resistant. Mating experiments indicated that virus susceptibility segregates as a single Mendelian autosomal dominant gene. It was found that cultures of peritoneal or hepatic macrophages obtained from susceptible mice support multiplication of MHV, whereas macrophages from resistant mice do not. These observations support the concept that inherited resistance to some viral agents may be determined by the macrophage.

C. Fate of Antibody-Neutralized Virus in Macrophages

Specific antibody in many systems prevents virus adsorption to the host cell [77]. Macrophages represent a notable exception to this generalization. Berken and Benacerraf [9] demonstrated that IgG is cytophilic for macrophages; presumably antibody-neutralized virus can attach to macrophages by way of the Fc portion of the antibody and be phagocytosed. The results from studies with labeled vaccinia virus indicate that neutralized virus is ingested by macrophages more avidly than nonneutralized virus [72]. However, the presence of antibody on the virion surface prevents the sequence of events which normally leads to uncoating of the genome; the antibody-coated virus is unable to lyse the phagocytic vesicle and release its core into the cytoplasm where virus replication occurs. As a consequence, the neutralized virus is degraded to acid-soluble fragments, presumably by lysosomal hydrolases released into the phagocytic vesicle following fusion with primary or secondary lysosomes (Fig. 6).

The physiologic importance of the intracellular rerouting of neutralized virus is confirmed by the studies of Mims [57]. When ectromelia virus was injected intravenously into hyperimmune mice, the inoculum was taken up by the liver and spleen macrophages as in normal mice and could be located by the fluorescent Ab technique. However, the Ag disappeared from the cells from immune animals. Virus premixed with immune rabbit serum also was taken up in the same way in normal mice and could be demonstrated in liver macrophages by

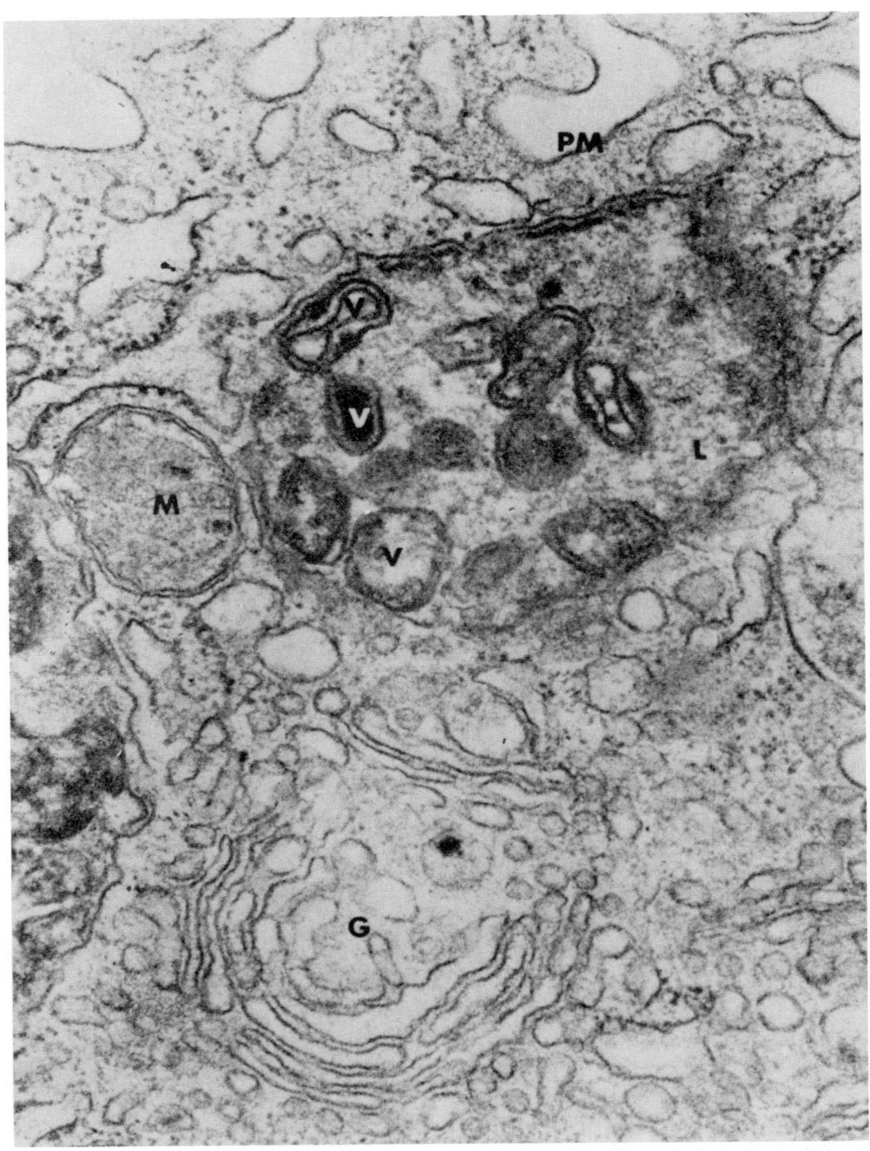

FIGURE 6 Partially degraded vaccinia virions within macrophage lysosomes 4 hr following addition of antibody-neutralized virus to culture. The virus-containing lysosomes lie adjacent to the Golgi complex. One vaccinia core appears intact, but remainder show empty cores, suggesting digestion of DNA. PM, plasma membrane; V, vaccinia virion; M, mitochondrion; L, lysosome; G, Golgi apparatus. ×60,000. (Reproduced with permission from Ref. 72.)

fluorescein-labeled Ab to rabbit gamma globulin. The fluorescent rabbit gamma-globulin slowly faded and the virus failed to replicate in the cells. Moreover, when macrophages from hyperimmune mice were thoroughly washed and infected with ectromelia virus in vitro, they were, if anything, more readily infected than normal macrophages. These observations suggest that, in this system, the macrophages are not specifically immune and that specific antibody is the major factor involved in the inhibition of virus replication in normally susceptible cells.

D. Interferon Production by Alveolar Macrophages

Interferon can be produced by and function in a large variety of cell types in vitro and in vivo. Gresser [31] was one of the first investigators to report that human white blood cells had the capacity to produce interferon. His finding suggested that cells of the reticuloendothelial system (RES) might contribute to the host's defense mechanisms against viral infection by producing interferon.

The work of Kono and Ho [45] supported the concept that the cells of the RES may be involved in interferon-mediated immunity. They demonstrated that normal rabbit tissue rich in reticuloendothelial cells appeared to produce interferon more efficiently in vitro and in vivo than tissues with lower populations of mononuclear phagocytes. Tissue cultures prepared from liver and spleen produced interferon more rapidly and in greater amounts than cells from other organs, such as the kidney or brain. Comparable results were obtained when rabbits were injected with virus intravenously and interferon levels in various tissues were determined 60-90 min after inoculation of virus. The tissues with the highest levels of interferon at these early intervals were those of the RES. The results from another series of experiments provide additional evidence that phagocytic cells are important sources of interferon, at least early in infection. When the RES was blocked with thorotrast prior to the intravenous injection of virus, serum interferon levels were significantly reduced during the first 3 hr after infection. However, at later intervals, interferon production was not consistently affected and peak titers were not diminished. These observations indicate that cells other than phagocytic cells most likely produce interferon later in infection.

Acton and Myrvik [1] reported that rabbit alveolar macrophages infected in vitro with parainfluenza-3 virus produced significant amounts of interferon 24-72 hr after infection. When normal alveolar macrophages were treated with the interferon preparations, there was a significant reduction in the yield of the challenge virus, rabbitpox virus. A corresponding reduction in the death of challenged macrophages treated with interferon was also observed. These results indicate that alveolar macrophages are capable of producing interferon which can passively protect other alveolar macrophages from infection with virulent virus. Subsequently, it was shown that monocytes harvested 1-3 days after the intratracheal injection of parainfluenza-3 virus exhibited a significant increase in resistance to rabbitpox virus when compared with monocytes from rabbits injected with an equal volume of control fluid [2]. In spite of the fact that macrophages acquired resistance in vivo following intratracheal injection of virus, no interferon activity could be detected in lung wash fluids or extracts of resistant macrophages. Thus, although the time of appearance of resistance in vivo correlates well with that required for the induction of interferon in vitro, the observed resistance cannot be unequivocally attributed to interferon.

Smith and Wagner [73] also studied interferon production in alveolar macrophages, as well as in glycogen-induced peritoneal macrophages and polymorphonuclear (PMN) leukocytes. They found that both macrophage populations produced large amounts of interferon after infection with Newcastle disease virus (NDV) in vitro. These investigators also observed that cells in macrophage-rich peritoneal exudates made significantly more interferon than cells in PMN-rich exudates. In fact, it was observed that the amount of interferon produced by cells in the PMN-enriched cultures was always related to the degree of contamination with macrophages. Yamada et al. [82] suggested that macrophages are the primary source of interferon in peritoneal exudates infected with NDV. They attempted to separate the macrophages from the PMN leukocytes in peritoneal cell preparations. Using NDV as the inducer, interferon production was high in the macrophage culture whereas it was relatively low in the lymphocyte and PMN leukocyte cultures.

The work of De Maeyer et al. [13] has provided additional insight into the question of which cells are responsible for the synthesis of circulating interferon. They observed that, after intravenous injection of virus, interferon originates in cell populations which possess quite different radiosensitivities depending upon which virus is inoculated. The cells which produced myxovirus-induced circulating interferon were highly radiosensitive, whereas the interferon response to other viruses was less sensitive or was unaltered. The animals' capacity to produce interferon in response to myxoviruses could be restored with bone marrow cells. Thus, it appeared that the cells involved could be either lymphocytes, granulocytes, or promonocytes, all of which are radiosensitive bone marrow-derived cells. In subsequent experiments, it was shown that the system induced by myxoviruses also was quite sensitive to antilymphocyte serum (ALS) [14]. Since the treatment with ALS reduced the circulating lymphocyte count by 93% and the granulocyte count by only 12%, it was concluded that the cells involved in myxovirus-induced interferon production in this system were probably lymphocytes. All that could be concluded about the origin of nonmyxovirus-induced interferon was that it came from cells more radioresistant than lymphocytes.

Jullien et al. [41] extended these studies and examined the nature of the radioresistant cell systems which produce interferon after the intravenous administration of poly I.C or encephalomyocarditis (EMC) virus in rat-to-mouse chimeras. Interferon induced by poly I.C becomes of donor type within 3 months after injecting Wistar rat bone-marrow cells into irradiated C3H/He mice. This observation indicates that the interferon is made in cells derived from the hemopoietic system. In contrast, EMC-induced interferon remains of the recipient type in xenogeneic chimeras; this observation indicates that most of this interferon originates from a cell population not derived from the hemopoietic system. In order to ascertain whether the respective radiosensitivity of the systems producing rat interferon in chimeras corresponded to that of normal mice, rat-to-mouse chimeras were subjected to a second x-irradiation, one month after the first irradiation and restoration. Circulating interferon production was studied 4 days later. The reirradiation strongly depressed NDV-induced interferon production but had no effect on rat interferon synthesis induced by poly I.C. These results point to a macrophage origin for much of the poly I.C.-induced circulating interferon. The authors stress that their results on the cellular origin of circulating interferon were obtained by administering the inducer intravenously. They suggest that other routes of administration might involve different cell types, since clearance of the inducer most likely would be different.

E. Cell-Mediated Immunity in Virus Infections

Allison [3] reviewed the mechanisms by which cell-mediated immunity may confer protection against viruses. There is evidence that viruses which stimulate cellular immunity induce the production of Ags which are incorporated into the plasma membrane of infected cells. These and other viral Ags may transform lymphocytes into blast cells which then can produce interferon, as well as substances which may be associated with nonspecific "activation" and sequestration of macrophages.

Host cells bearing viral Ags on their surfaces are recognized as foreign by sensitized lymphocytes which, in turn, can destroy the cells and interrupt virus multiplication. As indicated previously, alveolar macrophages may support the replication of certain viruses, such as influenza and poxviruses, and serve as a vehicle for virus dissemination. In these cases, sensitized lymphocytes, as well as Ab and complement, may lyse the infected macrophages and thus be major factors in containing the infection.

F. Interrelationship of Specific and Nonspecific Immunity During Viral Infections

It is apparent that the host response to virus infections encompasses nonspecific mechanisms of resistance as well as specific humoral and cell-mediated immunity. The nonspecific mechanisms include the anti-viral activities of activated macrophages and interferon; the specific mechanisms involve the viral-neutralizing capacity of Ab as well as specifically immune lymphocytes. Specific immunity acquired during the infection probably is the major factor involved in virus clearance even in a previously nonimmune host.

Evidence is accumulating which suggests that there is an intimate relationship between the specific and nonspecific immune mechanisms [26]. For example, cultures of peritoneal macrophages harvested from mice previously immunized with NDV produce significantly greater amounts of interferon than control cells when exposed to the homologous inducer [82]. The basis for this "immune induction" of interferon is not known, but it appears likely that IgG cytophilic for macrophages may help "fix" antigen to the cells. Support for this concept is provided by the observations of Azuma [6], who established that enhancement of interferon production in macrophages infected with underneutralized NDV was inhibited by procedures which blocked attachment of cytophilic antibody to the macrophages.

VI. Recapitulation

The alveolar macrophage system is a major component of a highly organized pulmonary defense system that can function in a steady state in the normal host or in a highly responsive manner when called into action by the events of cell-mediated immunity. Alveolar macrophages have their origin in the bone marrow and are replenished in a steady state process in the normal host. This phagocytic system is generally dependent on specific immunoglobulins (IgA and IgG) for its function; IgA probably functions mainly as an antitoxin and in the neutralization of viral infectivity, whereas, IgG, in addition, is important as the major opsonin. Although complement levels are low in the airways, complement can be an important participant in apparent infections when the inflammatory response promotes transduction of complement as well as serum Ig. Some of the lymphoid cells probably enter the airways from the bronchus-associated lymphoid tissue; the majority of these lymphoid cells are most likely B cells. The macrophages enter the interstitium of the lung and, after a pause that results in additional maturation, they continue their migration into the respiratory space; their main portal of exit is the gastrointestinal tract. Specifically sensitive T cells circulating through the lung or present in the lung parenchyma can be signaled by specific antigen to initiate the events of cell-mediated immunity by attracting, activating, and mobilizing macrophages to an infectious focus. Present evidence suggests that alveolar macrophages may utilize metabolically generated H_2O_2 in conjunction with some type of oxidase to kill microorganisms. The hydrolases in the lysosomes probably play a major role in digesting a phagocytized microbial carcass. It is also likely that mobilized and activated lymphocytes and macrophages can produce an exterior milieu which is inimical for at least some microorganisms. The various specific immunologic mechanisms probably act in concert with nonspecific factors in mucus such as lysozyme and other nonantibody antimicrobial agents; certain events of inflammation as well as the mucociliary apparatus also are important contributors to the overall defense of the lung.

References

1. J. D. Acton and Q. N. Myrvik, Production of interferon by alveolar macrophages, *J. Bacteriol.*, **91**:2300-2306 (1966).
2. J. D. Acton and Q. N. Myrvik, Resistance of alveolar monocytes to rabbit pox virus following intratracheal injection of parainfluenza-3 virus, *J. Reticuloendothel. Soc.*, **5**:68-78 (1968).
3. A. C. Allison, Immunity against viruses, *Scientific Basis of Medicine Annual Reviews.* University of London, The Athlone Press, 1972, pp. 50-73.
4. A. C. Allison and L. Mallucci, Histochemical studies of lysozymes and lysosomal enzymes in virus-infected cell cultures, *J. Exp. Med.*, **121**:463-476 (1965).
5. J. A. Armstrong and P. D. Hart, Response of cultured macrophages to *Mycobacterium tuberculosis,* with observations on fusion of lysosomes with phagosomes, *J. Exp. Med.*, **134**:713-740 (1971).
6. M. Azuma, Participation of cytophilic antibody in enhancement of interferon production in macrophages by underneutralized NDV, *Arch. Gesamte Virusforsch.*, **41**:11-19 (1973).
7. F. B. Bang and A. Warsick, Mouse macrophages as host cells for the mouse hepatitis virus and the genetic basis of their susceptibility, *Proc. Natl. Acad. Sci. USA*, **46**:1065-1075 (1960).
8. R. C. Bast, Jr., R. P. Cleveland, B. H. Littman, B. Zbar, and H. J. Rapp, Acquired cellular immunity: Extracellular killing of *Listeria monocytogenes* by a product of immunologically activated macrophages, *Cell. Immunol.*, **10**:248-259 (1974).
9. A. Berken and B. Benacerraf, Properties of antibodies cytophilic for macrophages, *J. Exp. Med.*, **123**:119-144 (1966).
10. J. L. Claflin and C. L. Larson, Infection-immunity in tularemia: Specificity of cellular immunity, *Infect. Immun.*, **5**:311-318 (1972).
11. Z. A. Cohn, The structure and function of monocytes and macrophages, *Adv. Immunol.*, **9**:163-214 (1968).
12. N. F. Conant, D. T. Smith, R. D. Baker, and J. L. Callaway, *Manual of Clinical Mycology*. Philadelphia, Pa., Saunders, 1971, p. 305.
13. E. De Maeyer, J. De Maeyer-Guignard, and P. Jullien, Interferon synthesis in x-irradiated animals. III. The high radiosensitivity of myxovirus-induced circulating interferon production, *Proc. Soc. Exp. Biol. Med.*, **131**:36-41 (1969).
14. J. DeMaeyer-Guignard and E. De Maeyer, Effect of antilymphocyte serum on circulating interferon in mice as a function of the inducer, *Nature [New Biol.]*, **229**:212-214 (1971).

15. R. D. Diamond, Antibody-dependent killing of *Cryptococcus neoformans* by human peripheral blood mononuclear cells, *Nature,* **247**:148-150 (1974).
16. R. D. Diamond and J. E. Bennett, Growth of *Cryptococcus neoformans* within human macrophages in vitro, *Infect. Immun.,* 7:231-236 (1973).
17. R. D. Diamond, R. K. Root, and J. E. Bennett, Factors influencing killing of *Cryptococcus neoformans* by human leukocytes in vitro, *J. Infect. Dis.,* **125**:367-376 (1972).
18. A. Dumont and A. Robert, Electron microscopic study of phagocytosis of *Histoplasma capsulatum* by hamster peritoneal macrophages, *Lab. Invest.,* **23**:278-286 (1970).
19. C. W. Emmons, Natural occurrence of opportunistic fungi, *Lab. Invest.,* **11**:1026-1032 (1962).
20. S. M. Epstein, E. Verwey, T. D. Miale, and H. Sidransky, Studies on the pathogenesis of experimental pulmonary aspergillosis, *Am. J. Pathol.,* **51**: 769-788 (1967).
21. F. Farhi, G. S. Bulmer, and J. R. Tacker, *Cryptococcus neoformans.* IV. The not-so-encapsulated yeast, *Infect. Immun.,* **1**:526-531 (1970).
22. R. E. Fowles, I. M. Fajardo, J. L. Leibowitch, and J. R. David, The enhancement of macrophage bacteriostasis by products of activated lymphocytes, *J. Exp. Med.,* **138**:952-964 (1973).
23. F. Galindo and Q. N. Myrvik, Migratory response of granulomatous alveolar cells from BCG-sensitized rabbits, *J. Immunol.,* **105**:227-237 (1969).
24. M. R. Gambrill and C. L. Wisseman, Jr., Mechanisms of immunity in typhus infections. III. Influence of human immune serum and complement on the fate of *Rickettsia mooseri* within human macrophages, *Infect. Immun.,* **8**:631-640 (1973).
25. L. O. Gentry and J. S. Remington, Resistance against *Cryptococcus* confined by intracellular bacteria and protozoa, *J. Infect. Dis.,* **123**:22-31 (1971).
26. L. A. Glasgow, Interrelationship of interferon and immunity during viral infections, *J. Gen. Physiol.,* **56**:212-226S (1970).
27. E. Goldstein, W. Lippert, and D. Warshauer, Pulmonary alveolar macrophage. Defender against bacterial infection of the lung, *J. Clin. Invest.,* **54**:519-528 (1974).
28. G. T. Goodman and H. Koprowski, Macrophages as a cellular expression of inherited natural resistance, *Proc. Natl. Acad. Sci. USA,* **48**:160-165 (1962).
29. G. T. Goodman and H. Koprowski, Study of the mechanism of innate resistance to virus infection, *J. Cell Comp. Physiol.,* **59**:333-373 (1962).
30. G. M. Green and E. H. Kass, The role of the alveolar macrophage in the clearance of bacteria from the lung, *J. Exp. Med.,* **119**:167-176 (1964).
31. I. Gresser, Production of interferon by suspensions of human leukocytes, *Proc. Soc. Exp. Biol. Med.,* **108**:799-803 (1961).
32. B. Hanson, H. Koprowski, S. Baron, and C. E. Buckler, Interferon-mediated natural resistance of mice to Arbor B virus infection, *Microbiol.,* **1B**:51-68 (1969).

33. P. D. Hart, E. Russell, Jr., and J. S. Remington, The compromised host and infection. II. Deep fungal infection, *J. Infect. Dis.*, **120**:169-191 (1969).
34. M. S. Hirsch, B. Zisman, and A. C. Allison, Macrophages and age-dependent resistance to herpes simplex virus in mice, *J. Immunol.*, **104**:1160-1165 (1970).
35. D. H. Howard, Further studies on the inhibition of *Histoplasma capsulatum* within macrophages from immunized animals, *Infect. Immun.*, **8**:577-581 (1973).
36. D. H. Howard, V. Otto, and R. K. Gupta, Lymphocyte-mediated cellular immunity in histoplasmosis, *Infect. Immun.*, **4**:605-610 (1971).
37. A. E. Jackson, P. M. Southern, A. K. Pierce, B. D. Fallis, and J. P. Sanford, Pulmonary clearance of Gram-negative bacilli, *J. Lab. Clin. Med.*, **69**:833-841 (1967).
38. C. R. Jenkin, The effect of opsonins on the intracellular survival of bacteria, *Br. J. Exp. Pathol.*, **44**:47-57 (1963).
39. R. T. Johnson, Pathogenesis of herpes virus encephalitis. II. Cellular basis for development of resistance with age, *J. Exp. Med.*, **120**:359-374 (1964).
40. T. C. Jones, Macrophages and intracellular parasitism, *J. Reticuloendothel. Soc.*, **15**:439-450 (1974).
41. P. Jullien, J. De Maeyer-Guignard, and E. De Maeyer, Interferon synthesis in x-irradiated animals. V. Origin of mouse serum interferon induced by poly I.C and encephalomyocarditis virus, *Infect. Immun.*, **10**:1023-1028 (1974).
42. E. H. Kass, G. M. Green, and E. Goldstein, Mechanisms of antibacterial action in the respiratory system, *Bacteriol. Ref.*, **30**:488-496 (1966).
43. S. J. Klebanoff, Myeloperoxidase-halide-hydrogen peroxide anti-bacterial system, *J. Bacteriol.*, **95**:2131-2138 (1968).
44. C. L. Klun and G. P. Youmans, The effect of lymphocyte supernatant fluids on the intracellular growth of virulent tubercle bacilli, *J. Reticuloendothel. Soc.*, **13**:263-274 (1973).
45. Y. Kono and M. Ho, The role of the reticuloendothelial system in interferon formation in the rabbit, *Virology*, **25**:162-166 (1965).
46. J. L. Krahenbuhl and J. S. Remington, In vitro induction of nonspecific resistance in macrophages by specifically sensitized lymphocytes, *Infect. Immun.*, **4**:337-343 (1971).
47. G. A. Laurenzi, L. Berman, M. First, and E. H. Kass, A quantitative study of the deposition and clearance of bacteria in the murine lung, *J. Clin. Invest.*, **43**:759-768 (1964).
48. G. A. Laurenzi and J. J. Guarneri, A study of the mechanisms of pulmonary resistance to infection: The relationship of bacterial clearance to ciliary and alveolar macrophage function, *Am. Rev. Respir. Dis.*, **93**:134-141 (1966).
49. G. A. Laurenzi, J. J. Guarneri, R. G. Endriga, and J. P. Carey, Clearance of bacteria by the lower respiratory tract, *Science*, **142**:1575-1573 (1963).
50. E. S. Leake, D. G. Evans, and Q. N. Myrvik, Ultrastructural patterns of bacterial breakdown in normal and granulomatous rabbit alveolar macrophages, *J. Reticuloendothel. Soc.*, **9**:174-199 (1971).

51. E. S. Leake, D. Gonzalez-Ojeda, and Q. N. Myrvik, Enzymatic differences between normal alveolar macrophages and oil-induced peritoneal macrophages, *Exp. Cell Res.*, **33**:553-561 (1964).
52. A. S. Levine, R. J. Graw, Jr., and R. Young, C. Management of infections in patients with leukemia and lymphoma: Current concepts and experimental approaches, *Semin. Hematol.*, **9**:141-179 (1972).
53. C. Liu, Studies on influenza infection in ferrets by means of fluorescein-labelled antibody. I. The pathogenesis and diagnosis of the disease, *J. Exp. Med.*, **101**:665-676 (1955).
54. R. J. Mason, T. P. Stossel, and M. Vaughan, Quantitative studies of phagocytosis by alveolar macrophages, *Biochim. Biophys. Acta*, **304**:864-870 (1973).
55. T. C. Merigan, Host defenses against viral disease, *N. Engl. J. Med.*, **290**: 323-329 (1974).
56. D. G. Miller, Patterns of immunological deficiency in lymphoma and leukemias, *Ann. Intern. Med.*, **57**:703-716 (1962).
57. C. A. Mims, Aspects of the pathogenesis of virus diseases, *Bacteriol. Rev.*, **28**:30-71 (1964).
58. Q. N. Myrvik, Function of the alveolar macrophage in immunity, *J. Reticuloendothel. Soc.*, **11**:459-468 (1972).
59. Q. N. Myrvik and D. G. Evans, Effect of bacillus Calmette-Guerin on the metabolism of alveolar macrophages. *The Reticuloendothelial System and Atherosclerosis.* New York, Plenum, 1967, pp. 203-213.
60. C. F. Nathan, H. G. Remold, and J. R. David, Characterization of a lymphocyte factor which alters macrophage functions, *J. Exp. Med.*, **137**:275-290 (1973).
61. R. Oren, A. E. Farnham, K. Saito, E. Milofsky, and M. L. Karnovsky, Metabolic patterns in three types of phagocytizing cells, *J. Cell Biol.*, **17**: 487-501 (1963).
62. B. B. Paul, R. R. Strauss, R. J. Selvaraj, and A. J. Sbarra, Peroxidase mediated anti-microbial activities of alveolar macrophage granules, *Science*, **181**: 849-850 (1973).
63. N. N. Pearsall, J. S. Sundsmo, and R. S. Weiser, Lymphokine toxicity for yeast cells, *J. Immunol.*, **110**:1444-1446 (1973).
64. R. H. Persellin and L. C. Ku, Effects of steroid hormones on human polymorphonuclear leukocyte lysosomes, *J. Clin. Invest.*, **54**:919-925 (1974).
65. R. J. W. Rees and P. D. Hart, Analysis of the host-parasite equilibrium in chronic murine tuberculosis by total and viable bacillary counts, *Br. J. Exp. Pathol.*, **42**:357-366 (1961).
66. H. Y. Reynolds and R. E. Thompson, Pulmonary host defenses I. Analysis of protein and lipids in bronchial secretions and antibody responses after vaccination with *Pseudomonas aeruginosa*, *J. Immunol.*, **111**:358-368 (1973).
67. H. Y. Reynolds and R. E. Thompson, Pulmonary host defenses II. Interaction of respiratory antibodies with *Pseudomonas aeruginosa* and alveolar macrophages, *J. Immunol.*, **11**:369-380.

68. J. B. Robbins, K. Kenny, and E. Suter, The isolation and biological activities of rabbit γM- and γG-anti-*Salmonella typhimurium* antibodies, *J. Exp. Med.*, **122**:385-402 (1965).
69. J. A. Roberts, Histopathogenesis of mousepox. I. Respiratory infection, *Br. J. Exp. Pathol.*, **43**:451-461 (1962).
70. D. Rowley, M. Thoni, and H. Isliker, Opsonic requirements for bacterial phagocytosis, *Nature*, **207**:210-211 (1965).
71. K. K. Sethi, M. Teschner, and H. Brandis, In vitro antilisterial activity of soluble product(s) released from *Listeria*-immune murine peritoneal macrophages, *Infect. Immun.*, **10**:960-962 (1974).
72. S. C. Silverstein, Macrophages and viral immunity, *Semin. Hematol.*, **7**:185-214 (1970).
73. T. J. Smith and R. R. Wagner, Rabbit macrophage interferons I. Conditions for biosynthesis by virus-induced and uninfected cells. II. Some physiochemical properties and estimations of molecular weights, *J. Exp. Med.*, **125**:559-577; 579-593 (1967).
74. W. A. Sorber, E. S. Leake, and Q. N. Myrvik, Comparative densities of hydrolase-containing granules from normal and BCG-induced alveolar macrophages, *Infect. Immun.*, **7**:86-92 (1973).
75. V. C. Stanley and R. Hurley, The growth of *Candida* species in cultures of mouse peritoneal macrophages, *J. Pathol.*, **97**:357-366 (1969).
76. J. G. Stevens and M. L. Cook, Restriction of herpes simplex virus by macrophages. An analysis of the cell-virus interaction, *J. Exp. Med.*, **133**:19-38 (1971).
77. S. E. Svehag, Formation and dissociation of virus-antibody complexes with special references to the neutralization process, *Prog. Med. Virol.*, **10**:1-63 (1971).
78. J. R. Tacker, F. Farhi, and G. S. Bulmer, Intracellular fate of *Cryptococcus neoformans*, *Infect. Immun.*, **6**:162-167 (1972).
79. G. L. Truitt and G. B. Mackaness, Cell-mediated resistance to aerogenic infection of the lung, *Am. Rev. Respir. Dis.*, **104**:829-843 (1971).
80. L. T. Webster, Inheritance of resistance of mice to enteric bacterial and neurotropic virus infections, *J. Exp. Med.*, **65**:261-286 (1937).
81. I. Dodd Wilson, Studies on the opsinic activity of human secretory IgA using an in vitro phagocytosis system, *J. Ummunol.*, **108**:726-730 (1972).
82. M. Yamada, M. Azuma, R. Hishioka, and T. Takehird, Relationship between immunity and interferon production in macrophages. I. Effect of immunity on interferon production, *Jpn. J. Microbiol.*, **14**:311-318 (1970).
83. H. I. Zeya and J. K. Spitznagel, Characterization of cationic protein-bearing granules of polymorphonuclear leukocytes, *Lab. Invest.*, **24**:229-236 (1971).
84. L. E. Zimmerman, Fatal fungus infections complicating other diseases, *Am. J. Clin. Pathol.*, **25**:46-65 (1955).
85. B. Zisman, M. S. Hirsch, and A. C. Allison, Selective effects of anti-macrophage serum, silica and anti-lymphocyte serum in pathogenesis of herpes virus infection of young adult mice, *J. Immunol.*, **104**:1155-1159 (1970).

25

The Relationship of the Alveolar Macrophage to the Immunologic Responses of the Lung

SORELL L. SCHWARTZ

Georgetown University School of Medicine
Washington, D.C.

JOSEPH A. BELLANTI

International Center for Interdisciplinary Studies of Immunology and
Georgetown University Medical Center
Washington, D.C.

I. General Concepts of Immunology Which May Apply to the Lung

It is clear that immunologic factors are important in the pathogenesis of lung diseases. They affect the organisms'response to exogenous agents and are subject to modification by exogenous factors. Specific immunological studies of the lung, in comparison to those of the other tissues and organs, are few. Little is known of the role of the alveolar macrophage in the immune response, but it is reasonable to hypothesize that some pulmonary diseases of unknown etiology have immunologic factors important in their pathogenesis. Consequently, the purpose of this chapter is to consider what the immune function of the alveolar macrophage *might* be. Furthermore, consideration will be given to the means by which such function might be altered.

For ease of discussion, we may consider the basic function of the immunologic system to be detection and elimination from the body of substances which are recognized as foreign [5]. The host employs a wide variety of cells and cell products, each interacting with one another in the removal of this foreignness. Such interactions are usually efficient, successful and without detriment to the host. However, an immunological imbalance may be created when either the type of antigen presented to the system or the reactivity of the host is inappropriate. In the human, these aberrant reactions can lead to the production of harmful sequelae; ranging from immunologically mediated diseases (e.g., bronchial asthma) to the initiation or exacerbation of chronic lung disease (e.g., emphysema, due to the inappropriate release of proteolytic enzymes from leukocytes).

The total immunologic capability of the host is represented schematically in Fig. 1. There are three types of responses to foreign substances, the progression of which depends upon the nature of the substance and the genetic constitution of the host. The *primary arm,*† the most primitive type, consists of those responses to a first encounter with a foreign substance, *endocytosis* and *inflammation.* If the substance is completely eliminated at this stage, the host response terminates. Protection from pathogenic organisms in primitive, unicellular forms rests solely on phagocytosis. This process, although efficient in simple life forms, provides inadequate protection in creatures whose organization and functions are more complex.

The primary encounter with a foreign substance may not always result in termination of the exposure of the lung to foreignness. For example, inert particles (e.g., silica) may be toxic to macrophages, leading to cytolysis and recirculation of the particle [2]. The more generally recognized recirculation of particles, however, is concerned with the release or transfer of immunogens which stimulate lymphocyte responsiveness. This is termed the *specific immune response* and consists of two effector mechanisms: (a) the production of antibody (IgE, IgM, IgG, IgA, IgD), by bone marrow-dependent (B) lymphocytes, and (b) lymphocyte-mediated antigen elimination (delayed hypersensitivity), manifestations of the thymus-dependent (T) lymphocytes. These mechanisms are enhanced through the action of complement, the coagulation sequence, and a bank of "memory" cells which can proliferate if a particular antigen is reencountered. These responses form the basis of antimicrobial immunity and are important in acute and chronic infectious diseases as well as in the surveillance against malignancy. In some clinical states, there may be exaggerated cell-mediated immunity (delayed hypersensitivity) or cell-mediated unresponsiveness (anergy). If antigen continues to persist, then tertiary responses may be initiated; these are not beneficial to the host (Fig. 1). Antigen persistence may be due to the nature of the antigen itself, or because of genetic or maturational defects of the host. Four immunological effector mechanisms may be elicited according to the classification of Gell and Coombs [19]: types I, II, III, IV (Table 1).

---

†In this chapter, the use of the terms "primary" and "secondary" refer to the entire system for handling foreignness. These should not be confused with the terms "primary" and "secondary" as they relate to the *specific* immune response.

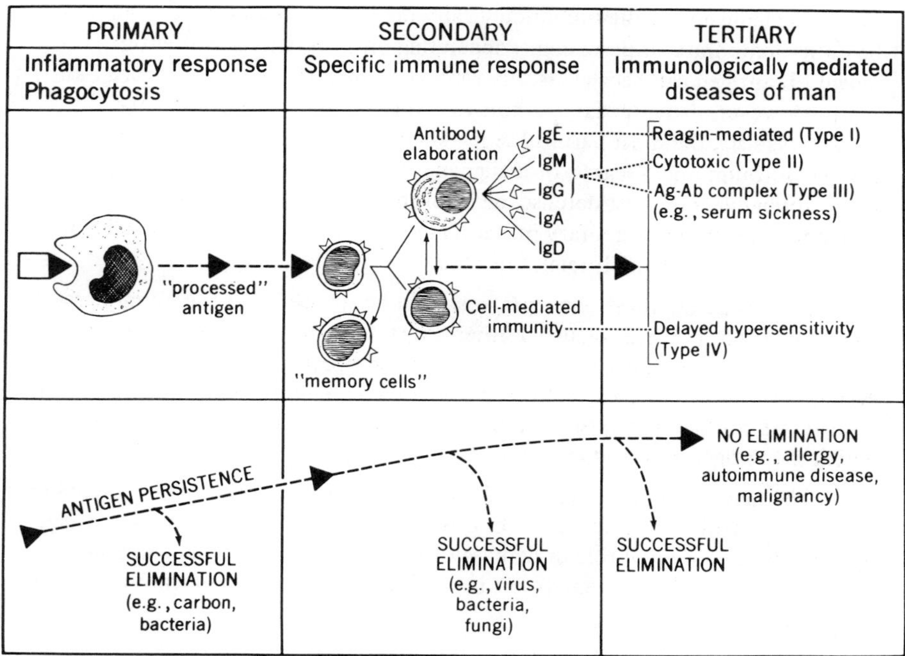

FIGURE 1 Schematic representation of the total immunological capability of the host based upon the efficiency of elimination of foreign matter. (From Ref. 4a.)

TABLE 1 Tertiary Arm of the Response to Foreignness; Immunologic Mechanisms of Tissue Injury

Type	Manifestation	Mechanism
I	Immediate hypersensitivity reactions	IgE and other immunoglobulins
II	Cytotoxic antibody	IgG and IgM
III	Antigen-antibody	Mainly IgG
IV	Delayed hypersensitivity (cell-mediated)	Sensitized lymphocytes

These mechanisms are the immunologically mediated diseases (IMD) and may be either temporary or permanent, depending on the efficiency of antigen removal. If antigen can be successfully removed, the tertiary responses are transient. However, if the tertiary responses, in effect, are overwhelmed and the antigen persists, the most harmful sequelae of the immune response emerge (e.g., allergy, autoimmune diseases, or malignancy). Thus, the impairment in processing of foreignness by host defense mechanisms may lead to pulmonary disease, which may be either temporary or permanent, depending upon the efficiency of the elimination of the foreign substance.

In considering these concepts, it should be stressed that the immune response does not occur in vacuo. Rather, every foreign substance may stimulate one or more immunologic system(s). Certain compartments of the immunologic system, however, may be selectively stimulated depending upon the nature of the antigen, its configuration, the degree of macrophage processing, and the route by which the antigen is introduced into the host [49].

The macrophage and lymphoid compartments constitute the major cellular defense mechanisms of the body. In this context, it is the alveolar macrophage which plays an essential role in defense of the lungs. Thus, any decrement in function of this cell type may result in serious consequences not only to the lung but to the entire system.

II. Primary Arm of Recognition of Foreignness

A. The Successful Response of the Alveolar Macrophage

It is generally recognized that the rate of removal of particles from alveolar surfaces by mechanical means is very slow, in contrast to the more rapid tracheobronchial mucociliary system [21]. Mechanical removal is too slow to allow the air sac to maintain sterility and to protect the lung against pneumoconiotic responses to particles. Therefore, the alveolar surface of the lung must have other strategies for dealing with particles deposited in alveoli. Of primary importance is the alveolar macrophage, which has been emphasized in other chapters in this section. Although macrophage activity may be enhanced by the secondary arm of immunity (e.g., opsonins or cytophilic antibody), it is the success of macrophage activity which determines the primary effectiveness of the immune response.

When considering how the alveolar macrophage responds to inhaled particles, living or inert, it is useful to consider three major actions of the cell: (a) the immediate removal of the particle (from the surface of the air sac); (b) alteration of the particle; and (c) transport of the particle. For the most part, these three activities involve one or more of the following: endocytosis, intracellular transport of endosomes, coalescence of endosomes with lysosomal organelles, and the release (e.g., exocytosis) of endocytosed material or its residue [11]. The removal of particles from the surface of the lung is accomplished by endocytic processes. Alteration of the particles may be a result of lysosomal enzyme activity. In addition, part of the efficacy of macrophage function, particularly as it concerns inert particles, rests with the ability of the cells to concentrate large numbers of these particles and for the macrophage to find its way to the mucociliary escalator for transport to the oropharynx [21].

Though the elimination of foreign substances is the basis of a successful primary response, there are other roles for the macrophage in immune function. More specifically, it may have a role in antigen-processing. Considerable information is available concerning antigen processing by macrophages from sites other than the lung [49]. However, "antigen processing" is a commonly used, but somewhat inaccurate, term. It is not certain that "processing" by macrophages does, in fact, result in the production of fragments which are more antigenic than native antigen. Although the participation of peripheral macrophages in stimulation of lymphocyte function has been described, there is a paucity of studies concerned with alveolar macrophage-lymphocyte interactions. This will be described later in the chapter.

B. Failure of Successful Elimination of Foreignness by the Macrophage

1. Changes in Macrophage Differentiation

The failure of the macrophage to successfully eliminate foreignness, has obvious theoretical implications, though many of these are still to be experimentally tested. Failure can be considered as due: (a) solely to the macrophage without environmental influence; (b) to the macrophage as influenced by exogenous agents, or (c) to the nature of the particle itself. Some degree of differentiation of the macrophage may be necessary to allow successful deployment against microbial organisms. For example, peritoneal macrophages cultured in the presence of sheep erythrocytes and engaged in erythrophagocytosis, eventually lose their ability to destroy *Salmonella* [36]. This may be related to qualitative or quantitative adaptation of lysosomal organelles to erythrocytes, but which is apparently inadequate for the destruction of *Salmonella* organisms. It would be of considerable interest to ascertain whether the alveolar macrophage can also be altered by other substances (living or inert) making it less effective in the destruction of pathogenic organisms.

2. Alterations in the Integrity of the Vacuolar Apparatus

The components of inhaled air cause perplexing toxicology problems to the lung in general, and to the alveolar macrophage in particular. This is especially true of particulate matter. In addition to direct cytotoxicity resulting from the ingestion of certain particles (e.g., silica and asbestos), the uptake of other particles may indirectly interfere with the "processing" of microorganisms and, thus, alter the antimicrobial state of the lung.

Jeunet and coworkers [24,25] suggested that reticuloendothelial blockade due to an overload of phagocytic activity may be related to exhaustion of available membrane sites for phagocytosis. North [34], exposing macrophages to large particle loads, found phagocytic activity to be pulsatile, presumably related to the regeneration of ATP. Although microtubules have not yet been unequivocally shown to be involved in intracellular transport of phagosomes within alveolar macrophages, it is reasonable to assume such participation, based upon data obtained from other macrophages and cells [20]. If so, particle loading may result in a "jamming" of pathways extending from the plasma membrane to the lysosomal organ organelles. Tobacco smoke, for example, provides a rich source of particles. A number of investigators have noted morphologic alterations in alveolar macrophages from smokers which indicate the presence of numerous inclusion bodies derived from tobacco or cigarette paper [22,30,38, 58]. Further, the suggestion has been made that smokers suffer an increased susceptibility to infections [15,35]. Whether or not smokers' alveolar macrophages have a decreased phagocytic activity is unclear [10,22]. But, it has been observed that *pinocytic* activity of smokers' cells is depressed [58].

The question of whether a blockade of activity of macrophages occurs must be approached with great caution since blockade may demonstrate selectivity. In the studies by Jeunet et al. [25], for example, blockade produced by *Salmonella typhosa* extended to *Brucella melitensis* but not to colloidal gold. It may be possible, in addition, that other factors (e.g., lung surfactant) play a role in the regulation of endocytosis by alveolar macrophages. Surfactant may, in turn, be affected by environmental contaminants. For example, Lentz and DiLuzio [28] reported that the acellular lung wash from normal rats enhanced phagocytosis by alveolar macrophages, whereas washes obtained from rats exposed to cigarette smoke did not. Possibly related to this are observations by Finley and Ladman [16], which showed a decrease in the lecithin content of lavage fluid from smokers compared to that of nonsmokers.

3. Nonspecific Membrane Alterations

Increasing evidence points to the importance of nonspecific physicochemical membrane characteristics in endocytic activity. Some of these data come from the study of the effect of nicotine on macrophage function. Nicotine inhibits endocytosis in mouse peritoneal macrophages [45] and rabbit alveolar macrophages [44] and stimulates exocytosis in mouse peritoneal macrophages [42]. All of these actions occur at concentrations of nicotine which were also vacuologenic to mouse peritoneal macrophages [43] and rabbit alveolar macrophages. The rate of vacuole formation is concentration-dependent, occurring as rapidly as 15 min after exposure to nicotine concentrations in excess of 5×10^{-3} M. Disappearance of vacuolation occurs within 15 min after removal of the alkaloid.

The possibility that nicotine-induced internalization of the membrane could result in a compromise of macrophage function is very intriguing. The rapid appearance and disappearance of vacuolation under the conditions described may be possibly related to the surfactant properties of nicotine [43]. Furthermore, another amine, procaine amide, has been shown to be surface active, vacuologenic, and to inhibit endocytosis [8].

This leads to a consideration of what effects exogenous agents might have on the macrophage membrane. Like other macrophages which have been studied, alveolar macrophages appear to possess both Fc and complement receptors. Reynolds and Thompson [39] demonstrated that *Pseudomonas* organisms opsonized with IgG, but not with IgM, antibody were phagocytosed by alveolar macrophages. Furthermore, opsonization of *Pseudomonas* with secretory IgA (cf. Ref. 40) also did not support phagocytosis by alveolar macrophages. Utilizing a variety of immune reagents, and red-cell rosette formation with human and rabbit alveolar macrophages, Reynolds et al. [40] verified the presence of IgG receptors and the absence of IgM receptors. They also obtained strong evidence for C3b and C3d receptors on alveolar macrophages. Rhodes [41] compared the IgG receptor activities of guinea pig peritoneal and alveolar macrophages. He found the slope of the dose-response curve of rosette forming cells vs. concentration of sensitizing IgG to be significantly greater for the peritoneal cells than for alveolar cells, indicating a greater degree of heterogeneity among the latter. The avidity of binding of IgG antibody to peritoneal and alveolar cells was enhanced by extended periods of exposure of the cells to 10% fetal calf serum.

That alveolar macrophages have specific receptors is of importance in any consideration of the immunological role of these cells in lung defense. The most obvious effect of specific receptors would be to enhance phagocytosis. Rhodes [41] highlights other roles of receptors and includes facilitation of presentation of antigen by alveolar macrophages to specific T lymphocytes; facilitation of IgG mediated macrophage cytotoxicity; and removal of the blocking effect of immune complexes during immune responses to tumors. Thus, the ready accessibility of inhaled materials to the alveolar macrophage may make the receptors and, consequently, critical macrophage function, vulnerable to alteration.

Based on the above considerations, changes induced in the surface of the alveolar macrophage, as opposed to changes in metabolism or lysosomal membrane stability, may result in altered macrophage function. Future research efforts on the alveolar macrophage should include studies of the availability of surface receptors. Some provocative theoretical and experimental considerations of surface phenomena in phagocytosis have been made by van Oss and his coworkers. They based their considerations on earlier hypotheses [14] that a correlation exists between the surface-free energies of particles and phagocytes, and the extent of phagocytosis. To estimate the surface-free energies, they measured the contact angles that sessile aqueous drops make with monolayers of phagocytes and particles. van Oss and Gillman [50] reported that phagocytosis of bacteria occurred more readily when the bacteria formed a more hydrophobic monolayer than that of the phagocytic cells. Moreover, encapsulated bacteria were found to be more hydrophilic and less readily phagocytosed but were made more hydrophobic and more readily phagocytosed by anticapsular antibody [54]. van Oss et al. [53] suggested that the Fc component of IgG is hydrophobic and provides the opsonized particle with a hydrophobic outer surface. Additional studies have demonstrated the potential contribution of other immunological factors to the requirement for phagocytosis that phagocytes be more hydrophilic than particles. Complement (C1, C4, C2, C3 sequence) increased the hydrophobicity of passively sensitized bacteria [51,52]; an apparent lymphokine caused an increase in the hydrophilicity of guinea pig alveolar macrophages [47].

Neumann et al. [33] have provided a theoretical model for phagocytosis based upon the fact that thermodynamic stability favors a reduction in surface-free energy. The model is based on the observations of the hydrophobicity relationships necessary between particle and phagocyte. It does not, however, take into account cellular metabolic factors and microfilament and microtubule function. The parameters have been suggested to be of importance in phagocytosis [1]. However, these studies may provide important clues to the *initial* events of phagocytosis. The surface-free energy changes on contact of the particle with the phagocytes may provide conditions favorable for thermal phase transition from a solid (gel) state to a liquid-crystal state which has been observed for lipids of biological membranes (e.g., Refs. 12,56). Since some membrane bound enzymes have been shown to be markedly activated when the membrane passes through this phase transition (e.g., Ref. 57), a triggering effect on membrane-bound enzymes may be initiated by particle contact.

Physicochemical considerations may also provide a useful basis for consideration of how exogenous agents may alter alveolar macrophage function. For example, consider the effects of nicotine on macrophage function.

It was suggested that nicotine-induced vacuolation might reflect an induction of membrane expansion and collapse [43]. That is, nicotine, acting like a surfactant within a surface film, induces membrane expansion. If this expansion follows known surface pressure/area relationships, then a point will be reached at which maximum surface pressure is attained (i.e., the greatest number of molecules which can be accommodated per unit area).

Following the procedures utilized by van Oss and his coworkers described above, it was found that when monolayers of rabbit alveolar macrophages were treated with nicotine, the contact angle between a sessile aqueous drop and the monolayer was decreased [44]. This increased spreading (decreased contact angle) of a sessile aqueous drop on a monolayer of nicotine-treated cells provides some evidence for membrane expansion. One means by which this could have occurred would have been for nicotine to have lowered the "critical surface tension" [59] of the monolayer. The surface tension of a monolayer is a reflection of its surface-free energy [18]. If the surface effects of the cell monolayer were a reflection of those of the cell membrane, then a reduction in surface-free energy would reflect an increase in surface pressure of the membrane. It should be emphasized that induction of membrane expansion by nicotine should be considered to be a nonspecific property of the compound. For example, the actions of nicotine and procaine amide on macrophages as well as the membrane expansion effect of surface-active local anesthetics and tranquilizers on erythrocytes [46] may all derive from a common physicochemical mechanism.

Before a strong case can be made for membrane surface pressure as a determinant in the efficacy of the handling of foreign material by the alveolar macrophage as well as for the mechanisms of the toxic activities of some substances, further investigation is required. However, the observations that physicochemical alterations of the macrophage membrane may play a role in toxicity, reemphasizes the myriad of possible nonspecific phenomena to which the lung defenses may fall prey. The result, as defined earlier in this chapter, can be immunological injury.

III. Secondary Arm of the Recognition of Foreignness: The Specific Immune Response

A. The Possible Role of the Alveolar Macrophage in the Successful Specific Immune Response of the Lung

Having considered how the lung responds to the foreign substances which impinge upon it, this section will deal with how the alveolar macrophage interrelates with the other major element of lung defense, the lymphoidal system.

The immune response to antigens, as pointed out earlier, involves the participation of at least two populations of lymphocytes, the thymic-dependent (T) and the bone marrow-dependent or bursal equivalent B cells. Unlike the macrophages which appear to respond to foreignness nonspecifically, the lymphocytes respond to antigen in a highly specific fashion by virtue of specific immunoglobulin (Ig) receptors on their surfaces [54]. Recently, Feldman and Nossal [13] suggested that the nature of the surface receptor on the T cell is a monomeric IgM molecule. For the production of an antibody response to antigens requiring T lymphocyte participation, he suggested that monomeric IgM-antigen complexes are released and captured by receptors on the macrophage surface. This would be followed by presentation of the complex to B lymphocytes for subsequent antibody production. Although there is general agreement that an interaction between antigen, macrophage, and lymphocytes occurs, the nature of the interaction differs, depending on the nature of the antigen and whether a B or T lymphocyte is involved [52].

1. Antigen-Macrophage-B Lymphocyte Interactions

The molecular basis of the uptake of antigen by the macrophage appears to be related to two main considerations: (a) whether the antigen can interact with the macrophage membrane directly, and (b) whether the antigen has interacted with or has been complexed with antibody or complement (e.g., opsonization).

Macrophages appear to play their most important role in antigenic stimulation of lymphocytes for those antigens which are not easily trapped by lymph nodes. Consequently, soluble antigens, as opposed to particulate antigens, are more dependent on macrophages as mediators of the immune response in nonimmune animals [49]. It is not clear whether alteration of antigen by the macrophage is a prerequisite for induction of immune responsiveness. One school of thought has ascribed the processing of antigens by macrophages to involve the production of immunogenic RNA-antigen complexes [17]. Confirmation for such a concept is still lacking. Although both macrophages and polymorphonuclear leukocytes are capable of phagocytosis, only the macrophage appears to be capable of enhancing the immune response. The greatest portion of material endocytosed by macrophages is lost by catabolism, although a smaller fraction usually escapes complete digestion. It is likely that antigen may be vesicular bound rather than surface bound, and may be directly transferred to lymphocytes. Uhr and Weissmann [48] have shown that immunogenic material can be extracted from the intracellular vacuoles of macrophages. In any event macrophages appear to be involved in concentrating antigen for presentation to the surface of the lymphocyte. This transfer requires contact or, at least, a close juxtaposition of the macrophage surface with that of the lymphocyte.

The concepts just discussed are derived from studies of nonpulmonary macrophages. The question is, therefore, whether the *alveolar* macrophage also participates in lymphoproliferative responses. This would require the alveolar macrophage to have access to the lymphatic system which, in turn, would require the movement of the macrophage across the epithelial barrier through the pulmonary interstitium. There is no convincing evidence at present to suggest that the alveolar macrophage can do this. To date, most of the evidence points to the continual movement of these cells in the opposite direction, i.e., the movement of particle-laden macrophages towards the tracheobronchial mucociliary blanket for transportation to the oropharynx [9]. The finding that particles such as carbon or silica [9] can be detected in lymph nodes may be used as prima facie case for movement of alveolar macrophages to regional lymph nodes as well. However, there is evidence for the anatomic pathway for the movement of free particles to the interstitial space of the lung [9]. If these particles are bacteria or allergens, then they would be able to interact directly with lymphocytes. e.g., via lymphatic drainage. It would appear therefore that an antigen-processing function cannot be presently assigned to the alveolar macrophage. Nevertheless, it is tempting to speculate that macrophages may, via their phagocytic activity, protect the lung against the access of allergenic materials to lymphocytes, and, conversely, a decrement in alveolar macrophage function may have a causal relationship in the pathogenesis of certain allergic diseases [5].

2. *Macrophage-T Lymphocyte Interactions*

Following interaction of antigen with a specifically sensitized T lymphocyte, there is the production of an array of low molecular weight proteins with a diversity of biologic function (Table 2). Some of these promote chemotaxis by attracting cells to an area of injury; others are cytotoxic for certain cells; still others can cause lymphocytes to proliferate. In terms of the lymphocyte macrophage interaction, one of these factors, migration inhibitory factor (MIF), has the unusual property of not only preventing the egress of macrophages, but also enhances their metabolic activity [32]. Such "activated macrophages" have an increased hexosemonophosphate pathway activity and also have enhanced bactericidal activity against a diversity of microorganisms [29]. This helps protect the lung against microbial agents which produce pulmonary infection. The possible failure of the macrophage to respond may be seen in such diseases where lymphocyte function is depressed, e.g., sarcoidosis, lymphoma, viral infection. In such clinical situations, a heightened degree of infection occurs, which may represent a breakdown in T cell-macrophage interactions.

B. The Unsuccessful Specific Immune Response

As described above, in many clinical situations a lack of T lymphocytes action, referred to as anergy, may be seen. In addition, infectious diseases, sarcoidosis and lymphoma, certain immunodeficiencies (either primary or acquired) can be

TABLE 2 Lymphokines[a]

Name	Abre-viation	Action
Those affecting macrophages		
Migration inhibition factor	MIF	Inhibits the migration of normal macrophages
Macrophage aggregation factor	MAF	Agglutinates macrophages in suspension
Macrophage chemotactic factor	MCF	Causes macrophages to migrate through micropore fiber along gradient
Macrophage resistance factor (postulated)		Renders macrophages non-specifically resistant to in-fection with certain bacteria and viruses
Those affecting lymphocytes		
Blastogenic or mitogenic factor	BF or MF	Induces blast transformation and tritiated thymidine in-corporation in normal lymphocytes
Potentiating factor	PF	Augments or enhances ongoing transformation in mixed lymphocyte culture or anti-gen stimulated cultures
Cell cooperation or helper factor		Produced by T cells, increases the number or rate of forma-tion of antibody producing cells in vitro
Suppressor factor (postulated)		Inhibits activation of, and/or antibody production by B cells
Those affecting granulocytes		
Inhibition factor		Inhibits the migration of human buffy coat cells or peripheral blood leukocytes from capillary tubes or wells in agar plates

TABLE 2 (continued)

Name	Abbre-viation	Action
Those affecting granulocytes		
Chemotactic factor		Causes granulocytes to migrate through a micropore fiber along a gradient
Those affecting cultured cells		
Lymphotoxin	LT	Cytotoxic for certain cultured cells, e.g., mouse L cells or HeLa cells
Proliferation inhibition factor and cloning inhibition factor	PIF, CIF	Inhibit proliferation of cultured cells without lysing them
Interferon		Protects cells against virus infection
Those producing effects in vivo		
Skin reactive factor	SRF	In normal guinea pig skin induces indurated skin reactions that are histologically similar to delayed type hypersensitivity reactions
Macrophage disappearance factor		Injected intraperitoneally, causes macrophages to adhere to peritoneal wall

[a]Adapted from Ref. 57a.

associated with a lack of T cell function [26]. In other types of immunodeficiency, a lack of immunoglobulin can be associated with a deficiency in opsonin function, which in turn can lead to impaired macrophages endocytosis. In all of these situations, unsuccessful response to antigen uptake is seen, which could lead to detrimental effects, referred to as the tertiary immune responses.

IV. The Tertiary Arm of the Recognition of Foreignness

The ultimate result of antigen persistence leads to immunologic responses, which no longer are beneficial to the host and lead to tissue injury. They become

TABLE 3 Allergic Diseases of the Respiratory Tract

Type	Example of disease	Example of antigen	Mechanism
I	Allergic rhinitis Bronchial asthma	Pollen	IgE antibody
II	Goodpasture's syndrome	Glomerular basement membrane (GBM) antigen	Anti-GBM
III	Farmer's lung	Dust of molding hay	Antigen-antibody complexes
IV	Tuberculosis	Tuberculoprotein	Sensitized lymphocytes

manifest immunologically mediated diseases. Examples of these types of diseases of the respiratory tract are shown in Table 3. The major localized anaphylactic categories of diseases which affect the respiratory tract include allergic rhinitis and asthma. Symptoms of these diseases are mediated through the harmful action of cytotrophic antibodies, primarily the IgE class [23]. Following interaction of antigen with cell-bound reagin, vasoactive amines are released which leads to vasodilatation, hypersecretion, edema and swelling of the respiratory mucosa.

Allergic disease of the lung in the atopic individual leads to bronchospasm, edema, and altered secretions which may obstruct the lumina of the lower respiratory tract. This leads to ventilatory insufficiency due to obstruction with wheezing and dyspnea.

The second manifestation of immunologically mediated disease of the respiratory tract occurs when specific antibody is directed towards constituents of the lung which may lead to tissue damage (type II). This is exemplified by such diseases as Goodpasture's syndrome in which antibodies to glomerular basement membrane (GMB) is seen. In this disease, the nature of the triggering event is uncertain, but, clearly, antibody to this type of antigen leads to tissue injury of the lung as well as the kidney.

Another response of the host to persistent antigen is caused by repeated inhalation of proteinaceous material resulting in extrinsic allergic alveolitis as described by Pepys [37]. In this type of disorder, the effect of such persistent antigen is to stimulate IgG precipitating antibody in the serum which then forms complexes with antigen in the lung and mediates type III injury. The antigens involved in these reactions include a wide variety of industrial and agricultural antigens such as fungus and moldy hay as well as a number of nonoccupational antigens such as *Micropolyspora faeni*. The primary effect of the antigen-antibody complexes with complement is to lead to deposition in tissues which then provokes an influx of inflammatory cells, e.g., polymorphonuclear leukocytes. Phagocytosis of immune complexes leads to the release of lysosomal enzymes and possibly the inflammatory sequelae [55]. The pathogenetic mechanism in this disorder includes both type III and type IV cell-mediated injury.

Allergic disease of the lung involving type IV responses is seen in many chronic inflammatory infectious diseases such as tuberculosis. In this disorder, the persistence of antigen is a function of the nature of the microorganism. Other types of examples include the persistence of nonreplicating antigen such as silica or beryllium. The responses to these inert materials may also present a simple inflammatory episode associated with direct cytotoxicity.

V. Implications of Unsuccessful Responses for Diseases of the Lung

Having presented some general concepts about macrophages and immunity, we may now proceed to a working hypothesis of how the alveolar macrophage responds to foreignness, what the fate of foreign substances is, and what the implications for diseases of the lung in humans may be. For ease of discussion, we may list five components in the host's encounter with foreignness: (a) environment, (b) target cell, (c) phagocytic cells, (d) mediator cells and their products (mediators), and (e) specific antigen-recognition cells (T and B cells) and their products, the lymphokines and immunoglobulins, respectively. These components and their interactions are shown schematically in Fig. 2.

A. The Environment

The environmental substances which impact upon the respiratory tract range from low molecular weight chemical substances to more complex macromolecules and particulate matter. The environmental agent may be directly injurious to a target cell such as a respiratory epithelial cell; the environmental agent may be directly endocytosed by the alveolar macrophage; in the case of the more complex immunogenic materials, the products of the macrophage interactions or the environmental agent itself may directly interact with cells of the specific antigen recognition system and lead to the production of specific immunity. Although most environmental agents which give rise to pulmonary disease enter through inhalation, it is important to point out that some may reach the respiratory tract by ingestion or injection. This may take the form of foods, drugs, pollutants, insecticides, food additives, and other toxic substances used in manufacturing processes. Thus, many varied routes of exposure to environmental agents occur and must be recognized for the possibility of production of immunologically

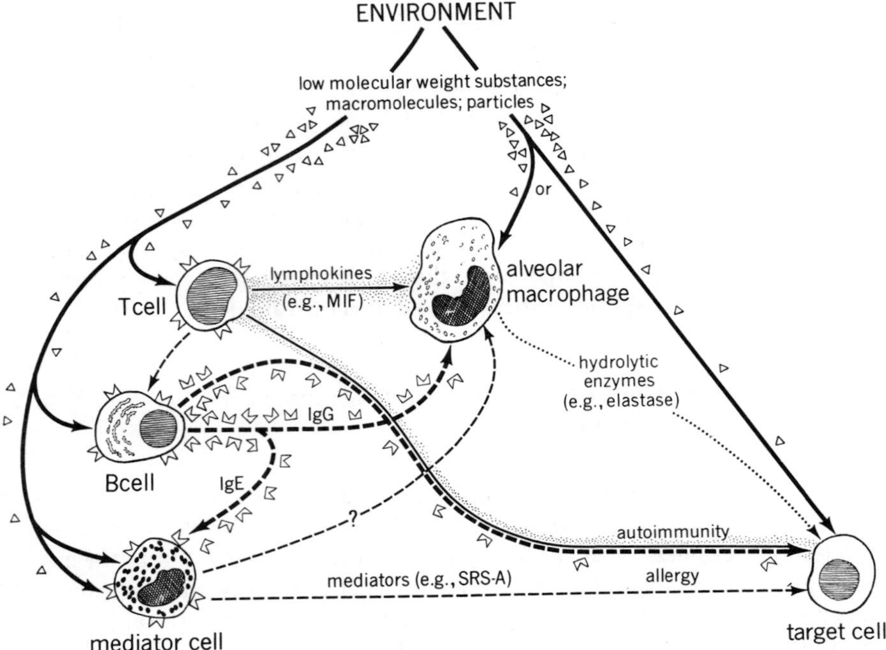

FIGURE 2 Schematic summary of the cellular and immunological interactions involved in the role of the alveolar macrophage in lung defense functions.

mediated disease of the lung which may take an unexpected form or masquerade as other entities. Bowden [9], among others, has reviewed a vast array of environmental agents with special reference to the alveolar macrophage.

B. Target Cells

There are a variety of target cells in the lung with which the environmental agent may have an impact. These include respiratory epithelial cells, which could sustain direct toxic injury, glandular cells, and smooth muscle cells. In the case of respiratory epithelial cells injury may lead to increased fluid transudation with pulmonary edema. Alternatively, the response of smooth muscle or glandular cell of the respiratory tract to antigen through the release of mediators as described below, may lead to increased contractility with bronchospasm and increased secretion of mucus characteristic of bronchoconstrictive disease.

C. Phagocytic Cells

Under ordinary circumstances, the primary phagocytic cells found within the air spaces of the lung are the alveolar macrophages. In cases of inflammation, the neutrophils may gain access to the air spaces and may actually surpass the number of alveolar macrophages. This movement of neutrophils, chemotaxis, occurs either in direct response to a stimulant, e.g., bacterial infection, through activation of certain components of the complement cascade or through the release of a variety of lymphokines with chemotactic properties released from sensitized T cells. In addition, a third class of phagocytic cells, the eosinophils, may gain entry to the respiratory passages as a result of the release of eosinophil chemotactic factor of anaphylaxis (ECF-A) from mast cells [27]. Collectively, the primary function of these phagocytic cells may be considered to be the uptake and ultimate destruction of foreign substances derived from the external environment (Fig. 2).

The environmental agent may directly or indirectly have an adverse effect on the alveolar macrophage. Endogenous agents such as amines and steroids which may be released in response to environmental influences also may affect the phagocytic, bactericidal, and locomotive functions of these cells.

D. Mediator Cells

Other cells in the respiratory tract contain pharmacologically active substances which can be released upon interaction with the environment. Although the mediator cells include a variety of cell types, the best studied are the mast cells. Mediator release can occur in a nonspecific manner as a direct consequence of cytolysis or membrane perturbation or through specific sensitization of the mast cell surface by an IgE antibody molecule. The mediators released include such substances as histamine, slow reactive substance of anaphylaxis (SRS-A), serotonin, kinins, prostaglandins, eosinophilic chemotactic factor of anaphylaxis (ECF-A), and platelet-activating factor (PAF). These mediators can lead to the bronchospasm of smooth muscle or to increased fluid exudation which may contribute to bronchospasm. Although not proven, the effect of the chemical agent may also adversely affect the activity of the alveolar macrophage (Fig. 2).

E. Specific Antigen Recognition Cells (ARC)

As described above, the lymphocyte system provides cells which have the capacity of reacting with immunogenic environmental agents either with the production of antibody or with the products associated with cell-mediated immunity.

1. B-Lymphocyte-Antigen Recognition System

The IgG antibodies are the most abundant and are found in significant concentrations in both the intravascular and extravascular spaces. This class of immunoglobulin provides the bulk of protective immunity to most infecting agents and is associated with the blocking antibodies of allergy that are produced in response to hyposensitization. These antibodies may also function as opsonins, as previously described, enhancing phagocytosis by alveolar macrophages (or other phagocytic cells) or may exert their effects by neutralizing the environmental agent (Fig. 2). In the respiratory tract, there appears to be a predominance of IgE and secretory IgA immunoglobulins. The IgA molecules are produced in relatively high concentrations by lymphoid cells contiguous with the respiratory tract. This class of immunoglobulin has been shown to be particularly beneficial in protecting against localized types of infections, e.g., respiratory viral infections [4]. Deficiencies in IgA are also apparently related to allergic and autoimmune diseases [3].

IgE antibodies have the unique ability to attach to receptors on various cell types such as the mast cell. Here they initiate various aspects of the immediate hypersensitivity reactions, (type I) through the release of vasoactive amines from these cells. The IgE antibodies, like the secretory IgA antibodies, are produced chiefly in cells lining the respiratory tract, and have been shown to be elevated in many patients with atopic diseases, e.g., atopic rhinitis and bronchial asthma.

2. T Lymphocyte Antigen-Recognition System

The net effects of the interaction of the environmental agent with the T cell may lead to a neutralization of the effect of the agent either through helper function of the T cell on antibody production by the B cell or alternatively through the release of some of the products of the T cell, e.g., lymphokines. It would be of considerable interest to study the effects of the lymphokines, e.g., MIF, MCF on *alveolar* macrophage function.

VI. Summary

The events involved in the interaction of environmental agents with the components of the immunologic system are complex; the steps involved in the generation of a complete immune response are interdependent. The outcome of this encounter can either be beneficial or detrimental. Although the focus of this chapter has been adult man, mention should also be made of the developmental aspects of immunity which can profoundly affect the responses to environmental agents. There is a congeries of evidence to suggest that all of the components of immunity are immature in the developing species; they attain increasing function with maturation. There is evidence to suggest that macrophage function in the developing host is quite different from that of the adult species. For example, phagocytic function as well as opsonizing function is quite deficient in the young infant owing to both immature cellular responses as well as deficiencies in opsonizing antibody and complement [7,31]. Moreover, there appears to be a maturational deficiency in certain biochemical functions of phagocytes associated with bactericidal killing, e.g., hexosemonophosphate activity [6]. Preliminary studies from our laboratory have provided evidence for morphological, functional, and biochemical maturation of the rabbit alveolar macrophage.

In summary, the implications of these findings for diseases of the lung in the human relate to the many pulmonary diseases which are encountered clinically, including allergy, hypersensitivity diseases, and many of the responses to chronic infectious disease agents. It is now clear that the role of the alveolar macrophage is central and of paramount importance in the initial recognition, disposal, and handling of all types of foreignness and that impairment of this cell type may be of crucial importance in the production of diseases of the lung.

References

1. A. C. Allison, The role of microfilaments and microtubules in cell movement, endocytosis and exocytosis, *CIBA Found. Symp.*, **14**:109-143 (1973).
2. A. C. Allison, J. S. Harington, and M. Birbeck, An examination of the cytotoxic effects of silica on macrophages, *J. Exp. Med.*, **124**:141-154 (1966).
3. A. J. Ammann and R. Hong, Selective IgA Deficiency. In *Immunologic Disorders in Infants and Children.* Edited by E. R. Stiehm and V. A. Fulginiti. Philadelphia, Pa., Saunders, 1973, pp. 199-214.
4. J. A. Bellanti, Biologic significance of the secretory αA immunoglobulins, *Pediatrics,* **48**:715-719 (1971).

4a. J. A. Bellanti, *Immunology*. Philadelphia, Pa., Saunders, 1971, p. 342.

5. J. A. Bellanti and R. E. Green, Immunological reactivity: Expression of efficiency in elimination of foreignness, *Lancet,* **1**:526-529 (1971).
6. J. A. Bellanti, B. E. Cantz, M. C. Yang, H. von Thadden, and R. J. Schlegel, Biochemical changes in human polymorphonuclear leukocytes during maturation. In *The Phagocytic Cell in Host Resistance.* Edited by J. A. Bellanti and D. H. Dayton. New York, Raven Press, 1975, pp. 321-329.
7. R. M. Blaese, Macrophages and the development of immunocompetence. In *The Phagocytic Cell in Host Resistance.* Edited by J. A. Bellanti and D. H. Dayton. New York, Raven Press, 1975, pp. 309-317.

8. J. C. Bond, J. E. Lundin, and S. L. Schwartz, Procaine amide-induced vacuolation in macrophages and effects on endocytic activity, *Toxicol. Appl. Pharmacol.*, **31**:93-99 (1975).
9. D. H. Bowden, The alveolar macrophage and its role in toxicology, *CRC Crit. Rev. Toxicol.*, **2**:95-122 (1973).
10. A. B. Cohen and M. J. Cline, The human alveolar macrophage. Isolation, cultivation in vitro and studies of morphologic and functional characteristics, *J. Clin. Invest.*, **50**:1390-1398 (1971).
11. C. De Duve and R. Wattiaux, Functions of lysosomes, *Ann. Rev. Physiol.*, **28**:435-492 (1966).
12. D. M. Engelman, The molecular structure of the membrane of *Acholeplasma laidlawii, Chem. Phys. Lipids,* **8**:298-302 (1972).
13. M. Feldmann and G. J. V. Nossal, Tolerance, enhancement and the regulation of interactions between T cells, B cells and macrophages, *Transplant. Rev.*, **13**:3-34 (1972).
14. W. O. Fenn, The theoretical response of living cells to contact with solid bodies, *J. Gen. Physiol.*, **4**:373-385 (1922).
15. J. F. Finklea, V. Hasselbald, S. H. Sandifer, D. I. Hammer, and G. R. Lowrimore, Cigarette smoking and acute non-influenzal respiratory disease, *Am. J. Epidemiol.*, **93**:457-462 (1971).
16. T. N. Finley and A. J. Ladman, Low yield of pulmonary surfactant in cigarette smokers, *N. Engl. J. Med.*, **286**:223-227 (1972).
17. M. Fishman and F. L. Adler, Antibody formation initiated in vitro, *J. Exp. Med.*, **117**:595-602 (1963).
18. H. W. Fox and W. A. Zisman, The spreading of liquids on low-energy surfaces. II. Modified tetrafluoroethylene polymers, *J. Colloid. Sci.*, **7**:109-121 (1952).
19. P. G. H. Gell and R. R. A. Coombs, *Clinical Aspects of Immunology.* Oxford, Blackwell, 1968, pp. 575-596.
20. S. Gordon and Z. A. Cohn, The macrophage, *Int. Rev. Cytol.*, **36**:171-214 (1973).
21. G. M. Green, Pulmonary clearance of infectious agents, *Ann. Rev. Med.*, **19**:315-336 (1968).
22. J. O. Harris, E. W. Swenson, and J. E. Johnson, Human alveolar macrophages. Comparison of phagocytic ability, glucose utilization and ultrastructure in smokers and nonsmokers, *J. Clin. Invest.*, **49**:2086-2096 (1970).
23. T. Ishizaka and K. Ishizaka, The biological function of Immunoglobulin E. In *The Biological Role of the Immunoglobulin E System.* DHEW Publication No. (NIH) 73-502, 1973, pp. 33-46.
24. F. S. Jeunet and R. A. Good, Reticuloendothelial function in the isolated perfused liver. II. Phagocytosis of heat-aggregated bovine serum albumin. Demonstration of two components in the blockade of the reticuloendothelial system, *J. Reticuloendothel. Soc.*, **6**:94-107 (1969).
25. F. S. Jeunet, N. A. Cain, and R. A. Good, Reticuloendothelial function in isolated perfused liver. III. Phagocytosis of *Salmonella typhosa* and

Brucella meliknsis and the blockade of the reticuloendothelial system, *J. Reticuloendothel. Soc.*, **6**:391-410 (1969).

26. F. S. Kantor, Infection anergy and cell-mediated immunity, *N. Engl. J. Med.*, **292**:629-634 (1975).
27. A. B. Kay and K. F. Austen, The IgE-mediated release of an eosinophil leukocyte chemotactic factor from human lung, *J. Immunol.*, **107**:889-902 (1971).
28. P. E. Lentz and N. R. DiLuzio, Functional alterations in alveolar macrophages exposed to cigarette smoke in vitro and in vivo, *J. Reticuloendothel. Soc.*, **10**:351 (1973).
29. G. B. Mackaness, The immunological basis of acquired cellular resistance, *J. Exp. Med.*, **120**:105-120 (1964).
30. R. R. Martin, Altered morphology and increased acid hydrolase content of pulmonary macrophages from cigarette smokers, *Am. Rev. Respir. Dis.*, **107**:596-601 (1973).
31. M. E. Miller, The immunodeficiencies of immaturity. In *Immunologic Disorders in Infants and Children.* Edited by E. R. Stiehm and V. A. Fulginiti. Philadelphia, Pa., Saunders, 1973, pp. 168-183.
32. C. F. Nathan, M. L. Karnovsky, and J. R. David, Alterations of macrophage functions by mediators from lymphocytes, *J. Exp. Med.*, **133**:1356-1376 (1971).
33. A. W. Neumann, C. F. Gillman, and C. J. van Oss, Phagocytosis and surface free energies, *Electroanal. Chem. Interfac. Electrochem.*, **49**:393-400 (1974).
34. R. J. North, The uptake of particulate antigens, *J. Reticuloendothel. Soc.*, **5**:203-229 (1968).
35. J. L. Parnell, D. O. Anderson, and C. Kinnis, Cigarette smoking and respiratory infections in a class of student nurses, *N. Engl. J. Med.*, **274**:979-984 (1966).
36. N. N. Pearsall and R. S. Weiser, *The Macrophage.* Philadelphia, Pa., Lea and Febiger, 1970, p. 65.
37. J. Pepys, *Hypersensitivity Diseases of the Lungs Due to Fungi and Organic Dusts.* New York, S. Karger, 1969, pp. 69-131.
38. S. A. Pratt, M. H. Smith, A. J. Ladman, and T. N. Finley, The ultrastructure of alveolar macrophages from human cigarette smokers and nonsmokers, *Lab. Invest.*, **24**:331-338 (1971).
39. H. Y. Reynolds and R. E. Thompson, Pulmonary host defenses. II. Interaction of respiratory antibodies with Pseudomonas aeruginosa and alveolar macrophages, *J. Immunol.*, **111**:369-380 (1973).
40. H. Y. Reynolds, J. P. Atkinson, H. H. Newball, and M. M. Frank, Receptors for immunoglobulin and complement on human alveolar macrophages, *J. Immunol.*, **114**:1813-1819 (1975).
41. J. Rhodes, Macrophage heterogeneity in receptor activity: The activation of Fc receptor function in vivo and in vitro, *J. Immunol.*, **114**:976-981 (1975).
42. S. L. Schwartz and J. C. Bond, Stimulation of release of pinolysosomal contents of macrophages by nicotine, *J. Pharmacol. Exp. Ther.*, **183**:378-384 (1972).

43. S. L. Schwartz and J. E. Lundin, Observations of the vaculogenic activity of nicotine in macrophages, *J. Pharmacol. Exp. Ther.*, **189**:293-302 (1974).
44. S. L. Schwartz, Interaction of nicotine and other amines with the endocytic and exocytic functions of macrophages, *Fed. Proc.*, **35**:85-88 (1976).
45. S. L. Schwartz, D. E. Evans, J. E. Lundin, and J. C. Bond, Inhibition of pinocytosis by nicotine, *J. Pharmacol. Exp. Ther.*, **183**:370-377 (1972).
46. P. Seeman, The membrane actions of anesthetics and tranquilizers, *Pharmacol. Rev.*, **24**:583-655 (1972).
47. S. G. Thrasher, T. Yoshida, C. J. van Oss, S. Cohen, and N. R. Rose, Alterations of macrophage interfacial tension by supernatants of antigen-activated lymphocyte cultures, *J. Immunol.*, **110**:321-326 (1973).
48. J. W. Uhr and G. Weissman, The sequestration of antigens in lysosomes, *J. Reticuloendothel. Soc.*, **5**:243-255 (1968).
49. E. R. Unanue, The regulatory role of macrophages in antigenic stimulation, *Adv. Immunol.*, **15**:95-165 (1972).
50. C. J. van Oss and C. F. Gillman, Phagocytosis as a surface phenomenon. Contact angles and phagocytosis of non-opsonized bacteria, *J. Reticuloendothel. Soc.*, **12**:283-292 (1972).
51. C. J. van Oss and C. F. Gillman, Phagocytosis as a surface phenomenon. II. Contact angles and phagocytosis of encapsulated bacteria before and after opsonization by specific antiserin and complement, *J. Reticuloendothel. Soc.*, **12**:497-502 (1972).
52. C. J. van Oss and C. F. Gillman, Phagocytosis as a surface phenomenon. III. Influence of C1423 on the contact angle and on the phagocytosis of sensitized encapsulated bacteria, *Immunol. Commun.*, **2**:415-419 (1973).
53. C. J. van Oss, C. F. Gillman, and A. W. Neumann, Phagocytosis as a surface phenomenon. IV. The minimum size and composition of antigen-antibody complexes that can become phagocytized, *Immunol. Commun.*, **3**:77-84 (1974).
54. N. L. Warner, Membrane immunoglobulins and antigen receptors on B and T lymphocytes, *Adv. Immunol.*, **19**:67-216 (1974).
55. G. Weissman, R. B. Zurier, and S. Hoffstein, Leukocytic proteases and the immunologic release of lysosomal enzymes, *Am. J. Pathol.*, **68**:539-564 (1972).
56. M. H. F. Wilkins, X-ray studies of membranes and model systems, *Ann. NY Acad. Sci.*, **195**:291-292 (1972).
57. G. Wilson and C. F. Fox, Biogenesis of microbial transport systems. Evidence for coupled incorporation of newly synthesized lipids and proteins into membranes, *J. Mol. Biol.*, **55**:49-60 (1971).
57a. World Health Organization, Cell-mediated immunity and resistance to infection, *WHO Tech. Rep. Ser.*, **519** Geneva, 1973.
58. H. Yeager, Jr., S. M. Zimmet, and S. L. Schwartz, Pinocytosis by human alveolar macrophages. Comparison of smokers and nonsmokers, *J. Clin. Invest.*, **54**:247-251 (1974).
59. W. A. Zisman, Relation of the equilibrium contact angle to liquid and solid constitution, *Adv. Chem. Ser.*, **43**:1-51 (1964).

26

Mechanisms of Macrophage Damage in Relation to the Pathogenesis of Some Lung Diseases

A. C. ALLISON

Clinical Research Centre
Harrow, Middlesex, England

I. Introduction

When analyzing the pathogenesis of lung diseases, alveolar macrophages must be considered in relation to other cell types and their secretions. Lymphocytes and the products which they release when activated have marked effects on the behavior of macrophages, and the latter probably collaborate with fibroblasts in fibrogenesis. Enzymes released from macrophages can degrade intercellular components of connective tissues, both fibers and matrix, and interact with constituents of serum such as complement components. Macrophage enzymes may also degrade pulmonary surfactant. In addition, macrophages, being the major phagocytic cells resident in alveoli, play an important role in maintaining the sterility or near sterility of the terminal airways under physiological conditions.

These are some of the many interactions of alveolar macrophages which have to be borne in mind. To facilitate analysis of the role of macrophages, three main groups of pathological reactions can be distinguished:

1. Predominantly fibrogenic reactions to inhaled dusts, notably silica and asbestos

2. Predominantly granulomatous reactions to inhaled organic materials or beryllium, or produced by diseases of unknown etiology such as sarcoidosis
3. Predominantly destructive reactions, resulting in emphysema

Several other activities of macrophages must be considered briefly, including the role of macrophages in defense against acute and chronic infections and the effects on these reactions of inhaled materials such as cigarette smoke or silica. The possible role of macrophages in limiting or delaying the growth of tumors is also of interest.

The interactions of macrophages with other cell types and their products in an organ such as the lung are so complex that analysis in vivo is difficult. It is therefore convenient to study the interactions of particles and other materials with cultures of macrophages, as well as to analyze the effects of products of activated macrophages on other systems. Concepts arising from cell biology, such as mechanisms of endocytosis and selective enzyme induction and release, are applicable to macrophages. Usually lysosomal enzymes are thought to act within cells: our recent observation that after exposure to various stimuli macrophages release these enzymes into the surrounding medium [1] has considerable relevance to their role in pathogenesis of diseases of the lung, as in other organs.

II. Inhaled Inorganic Dusts

Since the size and shape of inorganic dusts determine whether they are ingested by macrophages, these factors must be briefly discussed. With almost symmetric particles such as silica, nearly all the particles which remain airborne for long periods and can penetrate to the terminal respiratory tract are less than 5 μm in diameter. These can be taken up by macrophages within minutes of deposition. Some macrophages that have taken up particles migrate upward to the mucociliary escalator; others migrate into the walls of the alveoli and some probably carry ingested particles into the draining lymph nodes and elsewhere [2]. However, it is not excluded that some of the particles reaching the lymph node do so free in the lymph and are subsequently ingested.

The influence of length, diameter and shape is more complex in the case of fibers such as asbestos [3]. Deposition by sedimentation is controlled primarily by fiber diameter, as the falling speed of a fiber is mainly dependent on its diameter and is less affected by its length. In fine airways, however, interception becomes an important mechanism of deposition for long fibers, especially where airways branch. Fibers of chrysotile asbestos in particular, which resemble stretched coils, are readily deposited by interception, mainly at bifurcations, since their curvature increases the collision cross-section area. Timbrell and associates [4] have suggested that differences in the intrinsic diameter (and hence respirability) of the forms of crocidolite asbestos mined in the northwestern Cape and the northeastern Transvaal of South Africa and in Australia can account for the high incidence of mesotheliomas in the former as compared with the latter.

A. Fibrogenic Effects of Different Crystalline Forms of Silica

Next to oxygen, silica is the element most commonly found in the earth's crust. It forms an integral part of a wide range of geological materials of commercial importance, for example, the fibrous silicates, mainly asbestos. Silica itself is inhaled during other mining operations, notably for gold and coal. As a pure mineral, silica (silicon dioxide) occurs in three main crystal forms or isomers: quartz, tridymite, and cristobalite; other rare crystalline variants are coesite and stishovite, both found in meteorite craters [5-7]. Although the chemical reactivity of silica is low, most forms are fibrogenic in animals and highly cytotoxic to macrophages in culture [8-10]; the fibrogenic activities and cytotoxicity decrease in order from tridymite, cristobalite, and quartz to coesite. Stishovite is not fibrogenic in experimental animals [7] and not toxic to cells in culture [8]. The tetrahedral structure of silica appears to be essential for fibrogenic activity of the mineral; this structure is not found in stishovite which has a configuration similar to the rutile type of titanium dioxide which is also biologically inert [12]. Amorphous silica forms, produced by processing the mineral, are much less fibrogenic and cytotoxic than the crystalline forms (see Ref. 13).

B. Mechanism of Phagocytosis

It has long been known that macrophages are motile and can ingest particles and fluid, but only during the past few years has information been obtained about the underlying mechanisms. This has followed the recognition in a variety of cell types of microtubules consisting of the protein tubulin and of microfilaments composed of actin- and myosin-like proteins [14]. Allison and coworkers [15] showed that, in the peripheral cytoplasm of macrophages, beneath the plasma membrane, there is a network of microfilaments. These can be identified as actin-like by their capacity to bind heavy meromyosin, a derivative of myosin. Myosin indistinguishable from that in smooth muscle, but different from that in skeletal muscle, is also demonstrable in the cytoplasm of macrophages by immunofluorescence [14]. Movement of macrophages and phagocytosis of particles is strongly inhibited by cytochalasin, a fungal product that interferes with microfilament-mediated functions. Colchicine and other drugs that bring about disaggregation of cytoplasmic microtubules do not inhibit phagocytosis, although they affect the orderly directional movement of cells and of endocytic vacuoles in the cytoplasm. Microtubules appear to provide a framework and polarity for cytoplasmic movements but not the motive force itself.

On the basis of these and other observations, a mechanism for phagocytosis can be suggested [16]. The initial stage is attachment of a particle to the plasma membrane. Mammalian macrophages have on their plasma membrane receptors for antibody and complement, and it is likely that these are involved in the initial attachment of opsonized microorganisms. Latex particles and formalin-treated erythrocytes are attached in the absence of antibody, and it seems probable that their hydrophobic surface interacts with the plasma membrane [17]. Possibly, coating of inhaled particles with surfactant or other biological fluids, such as secretions containing immunoglobulin, facilitates phagocytosis by alveolar macrophages.

Certain types of attachment (e.g., of erythrocytes coated with IgG antibody) trigger phagocytosis, whereas others (of erythrocytes coated with IgM antibody and the C3 component of complement) do not [18]. It is believed [16] that attachment of a particle traps and immobilizes membrane proteins in the vicinity, allows them to form a cluster, and so increases the permeability of the membrane to sodium ions. Depolarization follows, and this allows entry of calcium ions from the extracellular environment and possibly also release from an intracytoplasmic store. An increase in the concentration of calcium ions in the cytoplasm triggers contraction of the microfilament system, moves the plasma membrane over attached particles and so produces phagocytosis. In the presence of concentrations of cytochalasin sufficient to inhibit phagocytosis completely, ferritin and other very small particles continue to be taken up in small vesicles of macrophages, a process which we have termed micropinocytosis [19]. This process, involving about 60% of the uptake of extracellular medium in macrophages, is also resistant to inhibitors of oxidative phosphorylation [20]. Macrophages therefore show three types of endocytosis: phagocytosis of particles greater than 1 μm in diameter; pinocytosis of fluid into small endocytic vacuoles visible by light microscopy (usually 500-1000 nm diam) and micropinocytosis into small vesicles about 70 nm diam. The first two processes appear to require the participation of actomyosin-like microfilaments beneath the plasma membrane, while the latter may be due to rearrangement of membrane constituents themselves.

Lysosomes become attached to endocytic vacuoles and discharge their content of hydrolytic enzymes into the vacuoles, which are then known as secondary lysosomes.

C. Cytotoxic Effects of Silica on Cultured Macrophages

Mouse peritoneal or rabbit alveolar macrophages have been cultivated in appropriate media, usually containing 5-20% decomplemented serum. Loss of viability has been assessed by rounding up and release from the substratum on which the cells have been cultured [10]; failure to exclude trypan blue, nigrosin or other dyes [21]; failure to split fluorescein esters [21,22]; failure to metabolize 2,3,5-triphenyltetrazolium chloride to the corresponding formazan [22]; and release of lysosomal and cytoplasmic enzymes into the medium [23,24]. Fluorescence microscopy of lysosomes stained vitally with acridine orange, histochemistry of lysosomal enzymes, and electron microscopy have also been useful [10]. These methods give results which are in acceptable agreement, so that only one or two need be used in any experiment.

Silica particles have two distinct types of cytotoxic effects on macrophages [16]. Rapid cytotoxicity occurs when relatively large amounts of silica are added to macrophages in a serum-free medium. Within 1 hr of exposure many cells are damaged, as shown by the criteria in the preceding paragraph. It is widely accepted that rapid cytotoxicity is mainly due to interaction of silica with the plasma membranes of the macrophages, and is the counterpart in nucleated cells of silica hemolysis. Not only lysosomal enzymes but also cytoplasmic enzymes such as lactate dehydrogenase are released within an hour of exposure. Rapid cytotoxicity can be inhibited by coating the silica particles with protein or phosphatidylcholine or in the presence of poly-2-vinylpyridine-1-oxide. Presumably inhaled particles are coated with surfactant or mucus, so that rapid cytotoxicity does not occur.

When moderate amounts of silica are added to macrophages in medium containing serum, delayed cytotoxicity is observed [10]. The particles are soon ingested, and time-lapse cine-photomicrographs show that the cells remain viable and continue to move for at least several hours. The lysosomes become clustered around phagocytic vacuoles containing silica, and discharge their contents into the vacuoles, as shown by histochemical studies for lysosomal enzymes [10].

In medium containing serum, serum proteins coat the silica particles at the time of ingestion, as can be shown by staining with fluorescent antibodies against the proteins [16]. This may explain why, in the presence of serum, cytotoxicity due to interaction with the plasma membrane is reduced. The particles coated with protein are taken up into lysosomes, and it is only when this coating is digested away (as shown by the disappearance of fluorescent staining) that the underlying silica surface is exposed to interact with the lysosomal membrane.

Thus far there is no difference between the uptake of toxic and nontoxic particles. After some hours of incubation, the interval depending on the concentration and nature of the particles, the concentration of serum in the medium and other factors, clear differences become apparent. Apart from discharge of many lysosomes, cells that have ingested nontoxic particles appear normal: they are fully extended and moving, whereas many of those that have ingested toxic particles become round and immobile. Histochemical staining for lysosomal enzymes shows that after ingestion of nontoxic particles, the reaction product is confined to secondary lysosomes, whereas after ingestion of silica diffuse cytoplasmic and even nuclear staining are seen [10]. Histochemical studies using as a marker ingested horseradish peroxidase [24] likewise show that in the presence of silica the enzyme is released from secondary lysosomes to produce diffuse staining. Electron micrographs of cells shortly after ingestion of silica show the particles of this material to be retained within the membranes of secondary lysosomes, and mitochondria and other cytoplasmic organelles to be normal [10]. Later the silica particles are widely scattered in the cytoplasm, mitochondria are swollen and other signs of cell damage are manifest.

It is therefore evident that silica particles, unlike those of nontoxic materials, can react with lysosomal membranes and make them permeable to hydro-

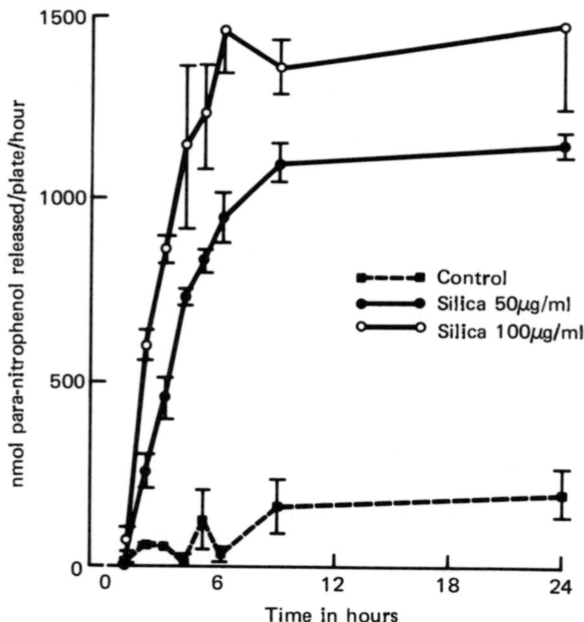

FIGURE 1 The appearance of a lysosomal enzyme, N-acetyl-β-D-glucosaminidase, in the culture medium at various times after incubating mouse peritoneal macrophages with silica (Dorentrup No. 12 quartz, <5 μm) and in the absence of silica. (Unpublished observations of P. Davies and A. C. Allison.)

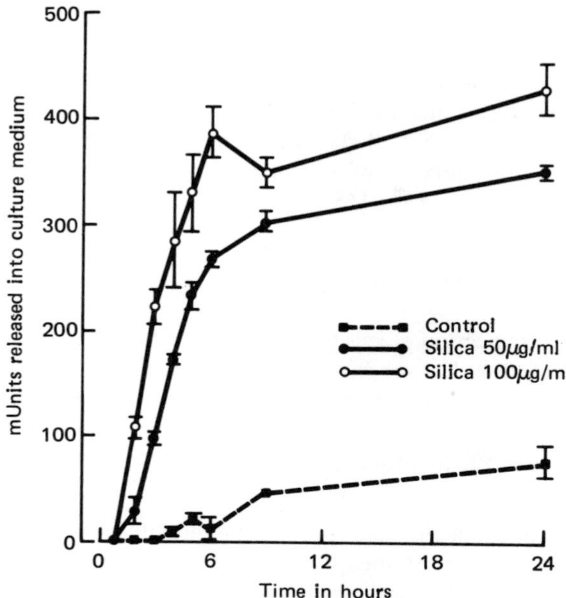

FIGURE 2 The appearance of a cytoplasmic enzyme, lactate dehydrogenase, in the culture medium at various times after incubating mouse peritoneal macrophages with silica (Dorentrup No. 12 quartz, $<5\ \mu m$) and in the absence of silica. (Unpublished observations of P. Davies and A. C. Allison.)

lytic enzymes. This appears to be the mechanism responsible for delayed silica cytotoxicity. If macrophages are exposed to poly-2-vinylpyridine-1-oxide at the same time as silica, or beforehand, or shortly afterward, silica cytotoxicity is markedly inhibited [10]. The polymer enters the same secondary lysosomes as silica particles, with which it can react as soon as the protein coat is digested away. The polymer cannot be degraded in macrophages and is retained in secondary lysosomes for long periods.

We [23] have recently compared the time course of release, from cultured macrophages that have ingested silica, of lysosomal and cytoplasmic marker enzymes (N-acetyl-β-D-glucosaminidase and lactate dehydrogenase, respectively). As shown in Figs. 1 and 2, release of the two marker enzymes is coincident, corresponding to cell death which begins about 2 hr after uptake of silica and reaches a maximum (80-90%) 6 hr later. When serum is absent from the medium, both enzymes appear in the medium within 1 hr of exposure to silica. Selective release of lysosomal enzymes from surviving macrophages, as occurs after exposure to asbestos, is not observed after addition of silica to macrophages.

Although incubation of macrophages with moderate doses of silica rapidly kills the cells, we have observed that uptake by macrophages of small amounts of silica (20 μg Dorentrup No. 12 quartz/ml) which do not cause detectable cell death result in significant increases in cell size and their content of nonlysosomal enzymes, such as leucine-2-naphthylamidase and lactate dehydrogenase. The possible role of such stimulation of macrophage metabolism by silica will be discussed in relation to fibrogenesis [25].

D. Effects of Asbestos Inhalation

After inhalation or injection of asbestos into the trachea or other sites, all asbestos fiber types can stimulate production of collagen in man and experimental animals [26]. Observations that fibers of similar dimensions composed of glass or other materials are also fibrogenic [27] draw attention to the importance of the fibrous nature of the inhaled particles as well as their physicochemical composition.

The deposition and clearance of UICC crocidolite asbestos made radioactive in a reactor has been studied [28]. Using brief "nose only" exposures, the distribution of deposited material between the upper and lower respiratory tract could be quantified. Clearance of material deposited in the lower respiratory tract was followed, either by serial killing or by integrating the long-term component of fecal excretion. The distribution of fiber within the conducting airways and the lung parenchyma was investigated by autoradiography. It proved possible to make these measurements with only a few milligrams of fiber, showing that comparative studies can be performed on dust samples collected from factories or mining operations. An average of 35% of inhaled asbestos was deposited, especially at bifurcations of smaller bronchioles. Fibers in the lung parenchyma tended to concentrate at the ends of alveolar ducts and at the entrances to alveolar sacs, although some fibers were found in the alveoli. These fibers were shorter and thinner (> 5 μm). After 30 days about 30% of deposited crocidolite remained in the lungs, the remainder having been excreted.

Epidemiological data show also a dose-related correlation of occupational exposure to all types of asbestos and bronchogenic cancer [26]. In addition, all commercial types of asbestos except anthophyllite may be responsible for the induction of mesotheliomas, the risk being greatest with crocidolite from the North-West Cape Province of South Africa. All types of asbestos injected into the pleural cavities of rats and other experimental animals have induced mesotheliomas [29]. After injection of asbestos into the pleural cavity, intramuscularly and at other sites, marked granulomatous reactions are observed. These may last for many months, and mesotheliomas tend to appear soon after the subsidence of the granulomatous reactions [30].

E. Effects of Asbestos on Cultures of Macrophages

Allison [31] examined the limit of the size of fibers that can be ingested by phagocytosis. Independently of the type of asbestos, short fibers (< 5 μm) were readily and completely taken up by phagocytosis, whereas long fibers (> 30 μm) were never completely ingested. The cells were closely attached to or enveloped the ends of the latter, but part of the asbestos fibers remained outside the cells. The reflection of the plasma membrane over the particles was demonstrable in stereoscan micrographs. With long fibers, two or more cells could be seen attached to a single fiber, sometimes with apparent continuity of cytoplasm, and the presence in the culture of multinucleate cells containing long fibers suggests that the process may lead to cell fusion. Particles of intermediate size (5-20 μm) were sometimes completely ingested and sometimes not. Asbestos differs from silica in that all the inhaled silica particles (which are nearly isometric) reaching the pulmonary alveoli can be ingested by macrophages, whereas some inhaled asbestos particles are not completely ingested. They can therefore interact with plasma membranes over a long period, and this may be relevant to their biological effects.

Earlier studies of the cytopathic effects of different types of asbestos on cultures of macrophages have been reviewed elsewhere [26]. In comparison with silica, cell death is delayed, although it is observed after exposure to moderate amounts of chrysotile. We have recently found a remarkable effect of chrysotile asbestos on cultured macrophage: it induces the selective release of lysosomal hydrolases from cells that are still viable, and indeed show marked increases of their content of lactate dehydrogenase [23]. The lack of cell death is confirmed by the failure to find lactate dehydrogenase in the culture medium.

The release of lysosomal enzymes into the medium is seen with concentrations of asbestos as low as 1 μg/ml, and is directly proportional to concentration up to 100 μg/ml (Fig. 3). The enzyme release is demonstrable within 4.5 hr and rises steeply so that by 28 hr, ~ 70% of the total enzyme activity is in the culture medium.

The role of enzyme release in the induction of granulomatous reactions and degradation of lung tissue is discussed below.

Electron micrographs [32] show that soon after ingestion small particles of asbestos are confined to phagocytic vesicles and secondary lysosomes. After 1 or more days in culture some particles are observed in the cytoplasm. The delayed cytotoxicity which is observed with all fiber types, but is most marked with chrysotile, is apparently analogous to that produced more acutely by silica, and the primary event is lysosomal damage.

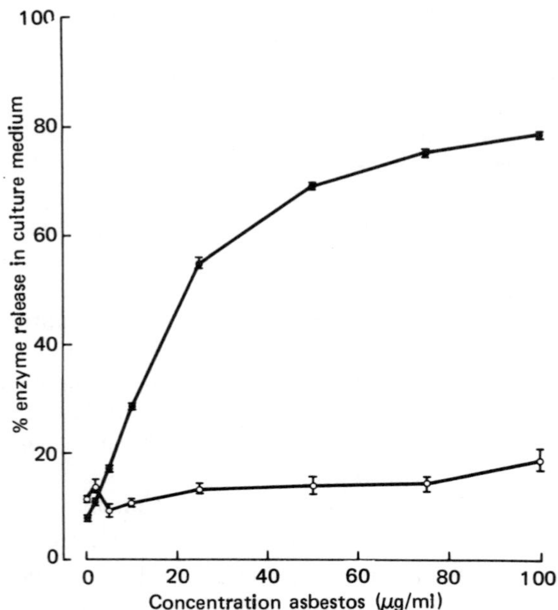

FIGURE 3 The release of a lysosomal enzyme, β-glucuronidase, (closed circles) and a cytoplasmic enzyme, lactate dehydrogenase, from mouse macrophages in culture incubated for 24 hr with various concentrations of UICC standard chrysotile A asbestos. (Unpublished observations of H. U. Schorlemmer, P. Davies, and A. C. Allison.)

F. Interactions of Silica and Asbestos with Natural and Artificial Membranes

Two of the major effects of silica and asbestos on macrophages, cytotoxicity and induced selective release of lysosomal enzymes, are attributable to interactions of the particles with membranes [33]. Early cytotoxicity follows an increase in the permeability of the plasma membrane and late cytotoxicity a similar interaction with the lysosomal membrane. Enzyme release is demonstrable after incubation of isolated lysosomes with silica particles [34]. Enzyme secretion from intact cells [23] follows induced fusion of lysosomal with plasma membranes. Interactions of silica and asbestos with natural and artificial membranes are therefore of interest.

A convenient model of interactions of particles with plasma membranes is hemolysis. The hemolytic activity of the several forms of crystalline silica and other dusts parallels their cytotoxicity and fibrogenicity, with stishovite being nearly inactive in all systems [35]. If silica particles are coated with aluminum hydroxide, phosphatidylcholine or protein, or the contact with erythrocytes occurs in the presence of poly-2-vinylpyridine-1-oxide, hemolysis is markedly inhibited [35]. Agents chelating calcium or magnesium have no demonstrable effect on silica hemolysis, nor does treatment of the erythrocytes with neuraminidase inhibit the reaction [31,36].

When analyzing the mechanism by which silica and asbestos exert these effects, two main types of cytolysis must be distinguished. The first is due to interaction of the lytic agent with membrane lipids, resulting in a disruption of the bilayer structure and rapid, nonosmotic lysis. Markers of low molecular weight—such as radioactive rubidium, a potassium analog which is not bound to protein—and markers of high molecular weight, such as hemoglobin or other cytoplasmic proteins or radioactive chromium bound to them, are nearly simultaneous. The presence of nonpenetrating solutes, such as sucrose, does not inhibit hemolysis. Hemolysis brought about by silica is of this type.

The phenolic hydroxyl groups of the sialic acid on the surface of silica particles can form hydrogen bonds with phosphate ester groups of phospholipids, as shown in model systems [37]. The interaction with phospholipids is also shown by observations that incubation with silica particles increases the permeability of liposomes composed of phosphatidylcholine and cholesterol, with no protein [38]. Poly-2-vinylpyridine-1-oxide preferentially forms hydrogen bonds with phenolic hydroxyl groups of silicic acid [37] and thereby prevents the interaction of the latter with membrane lipids.

In contrast, hemolysis by chrysotile asbestos is inhibited by agents preferentially chelating magnesium or by prior treatment of the target cells with neuraminidase to remove sialic acid groups [31,36]. Acid extraction of the surface magnesium groups from chrysotile fibers eliminates its hemolytic capacity. During the course of hemolysis by asbestos, markers of low molecular weight, such as rubidium, are released before those of high molecular weight, such as hemoglobin. The presence in the extracellular medium of nonpenetrating solutes, such as sucrose, does not affect increased rubidium permeability induced by asbestos but significantly inhibits hemoglobin release. All these observations suggest that asbestos is hemolytic because the surface magnesium groups of the fibers interact electrostatically with sialic acid groups of membrane glycoproteins [31]. As a result, the glycoproteins, which are free to diffuse within the plane of the membrane, are immobilized and crosslinked beneath the fiber. The resulting clusters of proteins form ion-conducting channels [39] which allow rapid efflux from the cell of potassium and, because of the osmotic pressure exerted by protein entrapped within the membrane, excess influx of sodium ions and water. The cells consequently swell and burst.

The capacity of asbestos to form clusters of membrane glycoproteins may also be a factor in fusion of lysosomal with plasma membranes, leading to release of lysosomal enzymes as discussed above. Elsewhere evidence has been summarized relating the clustering of membrane proteins to fusion [40].

G. Particle Ingestion and Phospholipid Metabolism

Ingestion of silica by macrophages leads to a breakdown of the diacylphosphatides, lecithin and cephalin, and to an increase of lysolecithin [41], and similar changes are found in hamster macrophages exposed to chrysotile asbestos [42]. However, it is not yet known whether the increase in lysolecithin contributes to or results from cell damage. Phospholipase A is present in relatively large quantities in macrophages [43]; the enzyme is localized in lysosomes [43,44] and could be activated or released as a result of interaction of silica or asbestos particles with the lysosomal membrane. Lysolecithin formation is not necessary for disruptive effects of silica or asbestos particles on membranes, as shown by the increased permeability of phospholipid-cholesterol liposomes exposed to silica [38] and the hemolytic effects of silica and asbestos particles; in neither case is phospholipase A action or lysolecithin formation demonstrable.

In the lung, release of phospholipase A from macrophages in the alveolar spaces could have serious consequences. The major constituent of surfactant, lecithin, could be converted by the enzyme into the highly surface-active lysolecithin. Experiments are in progress to determine whether inhalation of purified phospholipase A, or of the product of its activity, lysolecithin, affects the function of the lung. Conceivably it may impair the patency of the alveoli, in extreme cases resulting in atelectasis. Phospholipase A activity could also, through formation of arachidonic acid, increase the formation of prostaglandins, which are mediators of inflammation. Macrophages synthesize prostaglandins efficiently [45].

H. Macrophages and Fibrogenesis

Fibrogenesis is the process by which collagen is laid down as a structural or repair protein; metabolic turnover is usually slow. In diseases such as silicosis and asbestosis, fibrogenesis may continue progressively, long after the inhalation of excessive dust particles or fibers by man or experimental animals has stopped. The fibrosis which results from such exposures may be nodular in character, as in silicosis, or diffuse, as in asbestosis. In either case, such progressive accumulation of collagen eventually compromises pulmonary function.

Experiments with labeled cells provide no evidence that macrophages become collagen-synthesizing fibroblasts [46]. As already stated, nearly all inhaled silica particles are taken up by macrophages. Addition of silica particles to cultures of fibroblasts has no demonstrable effect on collagen biosynthesis or release [47]. Such observations are consistent with the two-stage theory of fibrogenesis by silica particles [10]. According to this view, ingestion of silica alters macrophage metabolism in such a way that a factor or factors are released which stimulate collagen biosynthesis by fibroblasts.

We have recently obtained experimental evidence in support of a two-stage theory of fibrogenesis (A. C. Allison, P. Davies, I. Clark, and H. U. Schorlemmer, unpublished observations). When peritoneal cells or silica particles were placed in diffusion chambers, limited by Millipore filters through which the cells were unable to migrate, and the chambers were left in the peritoneal cavities of mice, no fibrogenesis was observed after 1 month. However, when both peritoneal cells and silica were placed in the diffusion chambers, after 1 month marked thickening of the visceral and parietal pleura, with deposition of collagen beneath the mesothelial cells, was observed. The fibrogenesis was dose-dependent, being greatest when small doses of silica [which stimulate macrophage enzyme synthesis, but do not kill the cells (see above)] were used. Higher doses of silica resulted in death of most of the macrophages within the chamber and little fibrogenesis, so that it is unlikely that escape of particles or cells from the chambers could explain the observations. We conclude that a factor released from surviving macrophages stimulated by silica passes out of the diffusion chamber and stimulates collagen synthesis by fibroblasts. There is no chemotaxis, so that the fibrosis occurs in situ (where fibroblasts are already present) and not around the diffusion chamber as happens in fibrogranulomas of immunological origin.

Attempts to show the presence of a macrophage fibrogenic factor in culture have given discordant results. Heppleston and Styles [48] reported that mouse macrophages exposed to silica particles release a factor stimulating collagen synthesis by chick fibroblasts. Burrell and Anderson [49] obtained similar results with rabbit alveolar macrophages and human (WI38) fibroblasts. However, the rate at which cultures of fibroblasts synthesize and release collagen depends on many factors, including the presence of proline, vitamin C, and insulin in the medium and whether the cells are dividing; collagen is synthesized more slowly during the logarithmic phase of growth than when the cells are stationary. Hence slight toxic effects inhibiting cell division, or the provision of proline and other amino acids by protein degradation, might appear to stimulate collagen synthesis nonspecifically. Harington and his colleagues [50] found decreased rather than increased collagen biosynthesis in newborn hamster fibroblasts after addition of culture medium from hamster macrophages exposed to silica. Since the fibrogenic response of the hamster to silica and asbestos is slight, these discordant results may reflect differences in species or experimental protocol.

III. Other Pathogenetic Mechanisms

A. Lysosomal Enzyme Release and Granuloma Formation

Mononuclear phagocytes are the central cells in chronic inflammation [1]. In some types of chronic inflammation the mechanism is nonimmunological: the stimulating agent acts directly on mononuclear phagocytes. In others an immunological reaction, cell-mediated or humoral (or often both), participates and macrophages are involved secondarily. The first mechanism can result in the production of a granuloma in which nearly all the cells are mononuclear phagocytes, although collagen is broken down in the center and eventually collagen is synthesized by fibroblasts at the periphery [51]. The second type of chronic inflammatory reaction is mixed, with a substantial component of lymphocytes, usually of both the T and B lineage. The latter differentiate into plasma cells and secrete antibody which together with antigen forms immune complexes able to react with macrophages [52]. Stimulated T lymphocytes release products which can alter macrophage function in several ways [53].

Because in vivo interactions are complex, we have investigated the effects of granuloma-inducing agents on cultures of macrophages [1]. All those which have been examined so far have been found to induce the selective release of lysosomal hydrolases from macrophages. In contrast, inert particles of latex, carbon, and titanium dioxide do not have this effect. Hydrolase release may well be involved in the pathogenesis of the granuloma, and mechanisms underlying the reactions will be discussed below.

The constituents of pyogenic bacteria that induce acute inflammatory reactions are rapidly and completely digested, whereas bacteria or bacterial constituents that induce granulomas are incompletely degraded [54]. A thoroughly studied example is the group A streptococci which are involved in the pathogenesis of rheumatic fever. The cell walls of these bacteria consist of petptidoglycan and type-specific polysaccharide, and they are resistant to digestion by mononuclear phagocytes. When a suspension of the purified cell walls is injected into experimental animals, a chronic inflammatory lesion consisting almost exclusively of macrophages is induced [51]. Soon after cultures of macrophages are exposed to the cell wall preparations in low concentration, considerable increases in cellular enzymes, including lactate dehydrogenase, are found, and there is a marked selective release of lysosomal enzymes into the culture medium [21]. Similar results have been obtained with preparations of bacteria from the oral cavity that are involved in the pathogenesis of chronic inflammation of the gingiva [55].

It has already been mentioned that, unlike silica, chrysotile asbestos induces the release of lysosomal hydrolases from macrophages, and injection of chrysotile asbestos into the pleural cavity or skeletal muscle of experimental animals results in a marked chronic inflammatory infiltrate, demonstrable morphologically and by enzyme measurements. Another material that induces a substantial, pure macrophage infiltrate into the site of injection is the asbestiform mineral attapulgite, a type of Fuller's earth. Attapulgite likewise induces the selective release of hydrolases from cultures of macrophages. Inhalation of beryllium results in a chronic granulomatous reaction in the lung [56]. Incubation of macrophage cultures with small doses of beryllium sulfate (10 μg/ml) results in selective release of lysosomal hydrolases; higher doses of beryllium are cytotoxic (unpublished results of H. Schorlemmer and A. C. Allison). Since beryllium can induce delayed hypersensitivity the possible contribution of immunological reactions to the pathogenesis of berylliosis must also be borne in mind.

An opportunity to compare structure-activity relationships has been taken with several varieties of carrageenan, a mixture of sulfated D-galactose and 3,6-dehydro-D-galactose which induces chronic inflammation in experimental animals such as guinea pigs [57] and rats [58]. We found intramuscular injection of some varieties of carrageenan to induce marked chronic inflammatory responses, while others were much less active [59]. The capacity of different varieties of carrageenan to induce selective release of lysosomal enzymes from cultured macrophages paralleled their capacity to induce chronic inflammatory responses. Thus, λ-carrageenan, a linear polymer of D-galactose with α-1,3 linkages and sulfated on the fourth carbon, has the highest activity in both systems whereas κ-carrageenan, containing alternate units of 4-sulfated D-galactose and 3,6-anhydro-D-galactose with α-1,3 and β-1,4 linkages is much less active. Exposure of macrophages to a large variety of biologically inactive particles, including polystyrene latex, carbon, rutile, and anatase (titanium dioxide) does not induce selective enzyme release or provoke more than a very mild mononuclear (foreign body) reaction in vivo.

There is thus an excellent correlation between the capacity of different agents to induce lysosomal enzyme secretion from macrophages in culture and to induce granulomas in vivo. The next question to be answered is the underlying mechanism. When stimulated, macrophages secrete collagenase [60], plasminogen activator [61], and neutral proteinase [24]. Macrophage proteinases can cleave the C5 component of complement, generating C5a which is chemotactic for macrophages [62]. Thus release of proteinases could bring about accumulation of macrophages at the site of the granuloma. The proteinases could also affect the kinin-generating, blood coagulation, and fibrinolytic systems, as discussed below.

B. Immunological Reactions Producing Chronic Inflammation

1. *Humoral Immunity*

As pointed out elsewhere [64], acute inflammatory reactions of immunological origin (due to cell-bound antibodies or Arthus reactions) involve antibody which is synthesized elsewhere (in lymph nodes and spleen). The antibodies are carried to the site by the bloodstream, where they react with mast cells, polymorphonuclear leukocytes, and platelets to release preformed products. In chronic inflammatory reactions of immunological origin the lymphocytes have migrated into the reaction site, and are stimulated there to multiply and differentiate into T lymphoblasts, which release various products, and into antibody-secreting cells of B lymphocyte lineage. The antibody formed combines with antigen to form immune complexes, which can in turn interact with macrophages and induce selective release of hydrolases [52].

The hydrolase release is observed over a range of ratios of antigen to IgG antibody, from antigen excess through equivalence to antibody excess. The latter does not induce release of hydrolases from polymorphs [65]. Injection of immune complexes at equivalence induces Arthus reactions, in which after 72 hr polymorph immigration and destruction is followed by a predominantly macrophage-containing lesion. Injections of complexes in antibody excess induce macrophage granulomas [66]. As discussed in the previous section, induced release of enzymes from macrophages could recruit mononuclear cells into lesions induced by the complexes, thereby resulting in granuloma formation. This could be relevant to the induction of chronic pulmonary disease by foreign antigens (e.g., bird-fancier's disease; [67]). However, in the case of farmer's lung, another mechanism of pathogenesis is discussed below.

2. *Cell-Mediated Immunity*

Cell-mediated immune reactions regularly involve macrophages also. When T lymphocytes are stimulated by antigens or mitogens, they release factors chemotactic for and able to immobilize macrophages [53]. These could be responsible for the recruitment of macrophages into sites where cell-mediated immune reactions are in progress. The capacity of macrophages to limit the multiplication of intracellular organisms such as *Listeria* is increased by products of activated lymphocytes [68]. The latter also induce the selective release of lysosomal enzymes from macrophages [69], so that the sequence of events described above could be initiated. In the presence of persistent antigenic stimulation, e.g., by tubercle bacilli, cell-mediated immunity produces chronic reactions involving mainly macrophages and lymphocytes, but with some fibrogenic responses as well.

C. Responses to Particles Activating Complement by the Alternative Pathway

The most common of the diseases caused by inhalation of organic dust (extrinsic allergic alveolitis; Ref. 67) is farmer's lung, which follows inhalation of moldy hay (grain, straw, etc.). The active agent is the thermophilic fungus, *Micropolyspora faeni,* which is abundant in moldy hay [70]. Cellular events in pulmonary diseases following the inhalation of organic dusts have been studied using biopsy material from affected humans [71] and after intratracheal injection into sensitized [72] and unsensitized [73] experimental animals. Lung biopsies taken during the acute stage of the disease show noncaseating epithelioid granulomas, diffuse interstitial inflammatory changes, bronchiolitis and arterial lesions [71]. Later the granulomas resolve and residual lymphocytic infiltration becomes apparent. In the chronic form diffuse fibrosis with a variable degree of cystic change is seen. Focal collections of plasma cells and absence of granulomas in hilar nodes distinguish this form of the disease from sarcoidosis [71].

Patients with repeated exposure to moldy hay have precipitins reacting with *M. faeni* antigens, and it has been suggested that the disease is due to the formation of immune complexes. However, the acute disease observed in patients after inhalation of relatively large amounts of fungal material [74] resembles acute farmer's lung, and cases with clinical and radiological appearances typical of farmer's lung can occur without demonstrable precipitins [75]. Intratracheal injections into unsensitized rabbits and rats of respirable moldy hay dust or zymosan induced cellular changes similar to those observed in lung biopsies from farmer's lung cases [73].

These results suggest that farmer's lung may result from some mechanism other than immune complex formation, and Edwards and his colleagues [76] have found that moldy hay dust and *M. faeni* activate complement by the alternative pathway. Evidence that this may be relevant to the pathogenesis of the disease comes from the observation that intratracheal injection of zymosan particles, which are also able to activate complement by the alternative pathway, induces a similar sequence of cellular reactions in the lungs [73]. During the first few days both polymorphonuclear and mononuclear leukocytes are present; most of the dust particles are ingested by the mononuclears. The polymorphonuclear infiltrate disappears, leaving the mononuclear cells and, later, some lymphocytes and plasma cells. The latter are presumably mounting an immune response to the inhaled particulate antigens.

The cellular events can be explained by activation of complement by the alternative pathway, which would result in cleavage of C3 and C5, with the generation of factors chemotactic for polymorphonuclear leukocytes and monocytes [62,77]. This may result in the initial leukocytic infiltration into the lungs after inhalation of *M. faeni.* Moldy hay dust and zymosan particles are able, moreover, to induce selective release of lysosomal enzymes from macrophages (H.-U. Schorlemmer, P. Davies, A. C. Allison, and J. H. Edwards, unpublished). This effect is powerful: for example, more than half the lysosomal enzymes were released from mouse macrophages cultured with 200 μg/ml moldy hay dust for 24 hr, without detectable cell death. Activation of complement by the alternative pathway may well be involved since incubation of macrophages with the larger cleavage product of C3, namely, C3b, results in an increase in lysosomal enzymes in the cells and the selective release of these enzymes into the culture medium (H.-U. Schorlemmer and A. C. Allison, unpublished). For reasons already discussed, selective release of hydrolases from surviving macrophages could result in C3 activation and the perpetuation of a granulomatous lesion. Intramuscular injections of moldy hay dust, *M. faeni* spores and zymosan particles efficiently induce acute and then chronic inflammatory reactions demonstrable histologically and by measurements of lysosomal enzyme activity (M. de Gugig, H.-U. Schorlemmer, and A. C. Allison, unpublished).

The pulmonary reactions to other microorganisms may also be due, at least in part, to their interaction with the complement system. Thus, it has recently been shown by de Bracco and her colleagues [77] that extracts of *Aspergillus fumigatus* are able to activate complement by both the classical and alternative pathways. The heated extracts activated preferentially the alternative pathway. A comparison of the capacity of microorganisms to activate the complement system, and to induce inflammatory reactions is currently in progress in our laboratory.

D. Proteinase Release and Emphysema

The importance of proteinases in the pathogenesis of chronic obstructive pulmonary disease (COPD) is emphasized by the increased susceptibility to this condition in persons with inherited deficiency of plasma α_1-trypsin inhibitor (α_1-TI). The disease occurs in a majority of individuals homozygous for the Pi^Z allele, and appears in the third or fourth decade in contrast to the sixth or seventh decade as seen in those with normal levels of α_1-TI [79]. In COPD associated with α_1-TI deficiency there is a predominantly lower-zone emphysema with severely diminished forced expiratory flow resulting from loss of lung recoil mediated by elastic tissue [80].

Evidence has accumulated that proteinases administered through the airways can produce emphysema. This is true of papain [80], leukocytic homogenates [81], and purified elastase [82]. Porcine pancreatic elastase diluted with saline or human serum of α_1-TI phenotypes MM or ZZ (deficient) were administered intratracheally to Syrian hamsters [82]. In animals given elastase alone or with ZZ serum there was inflammation and loss of elastic fibers. The hemorrhage and inflammation subsided after 2 weeks, but destruction of alveolar walls progressed for many weeks, and was not reversed when specimens were examined after 4 months. Elastase administered in human serum containing α_1-TI of type MM did not cause any destructive lung changes.

These studies provide good evidence that, in the absence of adequate protection by plasma trypsin inhibitor, elastase can produce emphysema. The polymorphonuclear leukocyte (PMN) has usually been regarded as a probable source of elastase in the lungs. The ability of PMN homogenates to induce experimental emphysema in dogs has been reported by Marco et al. [81]. Two levels of neutral proteinase activity in human PMN have been described, one comparable to controls and the other significantly lower; it has been suggested that a combination of normal proteinase activity with α_1-TI deficiency may be associated with an infavorable course of COPD [83].

An alternative source of elastase is the macrophage. These cells, when stimulated, release substantial amounts of elastase as well as collagenase (Barrett and Gordon, unpublished). Since macrophages are normally present in the alveoli, which PMN are not, and macrophages accumulate in large numbers in chronic inflammation, the role of elastase or neutral proteinase released from these cells in the pathogenesis of emphysema should be investigated further. Enzyme release induced by bacterial cell walls, immune complexes, or other factors, as discussed above, could participate.

In view of the suggestion that macrophage products may be involved in fibrogenesis, it is of interest that infants with inherited α_1-TI deficiency are more prone than others to develop cirrhosis [84]. Moreover, levels of α_1-TI are low in the sera of infants with the idiopathic respiratory distress syndrome, especially those that fail to survive [85]. Whether enzymes released from macrophages contribute to the pathogenesis of this syndrome is still unknown.

Evidence has been summarized in this chapter suggesting that induced enzyme release from macrophages may result in granulomatous reactions or fibrogenesis in some cases and destruction of elastic fibers and other lung constituents (emphysema) on the other. The question arises how the reactions can lead to increased cellularity on the one hand and to decreased cellularity on the other. Although the underlying mechanisms are still unknown, it is possible from available evidence to make some suggestions. Thus, secretion of enzymes and its induction are selective [25]. Some enzymes, such as muramidase, are secreted in constant amounts by cultured macrophages, irrespective of whether they are stimulated. Other enzymes, including elastase, are observed only after certain types of stimulation. Moreover, selective inhibition of enzymes is clearly important. In both the inductive and inhibitory reactions, genetic factors are likely to play a part as well, and the presence of microorganisms and their products (e.g., bacterial endotoxins or cell walls). Concurrence of inherited and acquired factors probably determine the specific responses of the lungs in different individuals.

E. Effects of Oxidants and Metal Fumes on Macrophages

Effects on lung function of inhalation of pure oxygen, or of oxidants such as ozone or nitrogen dioxide, have been extensively investigated. One of the cell types affected is the alveolar macrophage. Ozone, administered in low concentrations to experimental animals or cultures of macrophages, decreases the levels of acid phosphatase, β-glucuronidase and lysozyme in these cells and increases the enzyme levels in extracellular fluid [86]. This may be at least partly due to cell death since macrophages washed out of lungs of animals exposed to ozone lyse spontaneously [87]. Macrophage lysis can be inhibited by fluid lavaged from rabbit lungs or by dipalmitoyllecithin; exposure of the protectant material to ozone in vivo or in vitro abolishes the protective effect [87]. The authors postulate that ozone and other environmental pollutants abolish the protective factor normally present in lung fluid, with secondary loss of alveolar macrophages and their defense against inhaled microorganisms (see Chap. 23 and 24). It is possible that pollutants also induce secretion of lysosomal enzymes from surviving alveolar macrophages: electron micrographs of these cells after ozone inhalation show few lysosomes and many large cytoplasmic vacuoles, together with swollen mitochondria [89]. Effects of hyperoxia on lysosomes of other cell types have been described [88].

Pulmonary macrophages have a relatively high rate of oxidative phosphorylation, which is inhibited by cadmium and other metals [84]. Since metal fumes are common air pollutants they may affect alveolar macrophage function. A high frequency of pulmonary emphysema and chronic bronchitis among workers exposed to cadmium fumes has long been known. Pulmonary emphysema is observed in experimental animals after inhalation of aerosols containing cadmium [90]. It has been reported that electron microscopy of lungs of animals poisoned by chronic cadium administration show also collagen and elastin deposition, without any polymorphonuclear leukocytic infiltration [91]. The macrophage could be a primary target, with secondary effects on fibroblasts.

F. Effects of Air Pollutants on Pulmonary Macrophage Microbicidal Capacity

The relationship between silicosis and susceptibility to tuberculosis has long been known in human patients and experimental animals [93]. All published studies of silicotic subjects have shown a much higher incidence of tuberculosis than in nonsilicotic subjects from the same areas. Before effective chemotherapy was available, tuberculosis was the major cause of death in silicosis. The response to chemotherapy of tuberculosis infections in subjects with pneumoconiosis was less satisfactory than in subjects without the latter. Infections with various strains of *Mycobacterium tuberculosis* in several experimental animals were aggravated by silica inhalation. Silica administration does not depress delayed hypersensitivity or antibody formation under most circumstances, so it seemed likely that silica was affecting recovery from tuberculosis by effects on macrophages themselves. Allison and Hart [92] found that even very small, sublethal doses of silica increased the growth of *M. tuberculosis* in macrophage cultures. Silica inhalation also impairs clearance of pyogenic bacteria [94].

Ozone and high oxygen inhalation decrease the capacity of alveolar macrophages to kill inhaled bacteria [95]. The same is true of cigarette smoke, which also inhibits the bactericidal capacity of alveolar macrophage cultures [94].

G. Macrophages and the Inhibition Tumor Cell Growth

The observation by Gorer [96] over twenty years ago that macrophages are prominent during rejection of tumor cells has recently been extended to analyze the role of macrophages in tumor immunity. Evidence has been presented that macrophages from immune animals can damage tumor cells in an immunologically specific fashion [94,98], and that supernatants of lymphocytes reacting with antigen can confer on normal macrophages the capacity to kill specific tumor cells [99]. Stimulation by infection or other means also enables macrophages in a nonspecific way to prevent tumor cell growth [100,101]. Details of the mechanism are discussed by Keller [101]. Stimulated macrophages may inhibit or delay appearance of tumors in the lungs.

IV. General Conclusions

Alveolar macrophages, like those in other sites, originate from the bone marrow. This has been shown by differential irradiation of the bone marrow and lungs and tritiated thymidine labeling [102], as well as the use of genetically controlled esterase [103] and histocompatibility antigen markers [104]. After passage through the bloodstream, mononuclear phagocytes reside in the lungs for about 3 days before they become mature alveolar macrophages with a substantial charge of lysosomal enzymes.

Three distinct mechanisms of endocytosis are now recognized, and the associated biochemical processes have been defined. Capacity for phagocytosis is the hallmark of the macrophage, and the associated bactericidal activity is important. It is impaired by silica, cigarette smoke, or other pollutants.

The phagocytic capacity of macrophages accounts also for their being prime targets for inhaled toxic particles such as silica and asbestos. Silica is rapidly cytotoxic to cultures of macrophages, and this is explained by the capacity of the particles to react with membrane phospholipids. Asbestos is less cytotoxic for cultures of macrophages, but, unlike silica, chrysotile asbestos induces secretion from the surviving cells of substantial amounts of hydrolytic enzymes. This may explain the formation of granulomas after injection of asbestos into the pleura and other sites. All the agents so far tested which induce nonimmunological granulomas (e.g., bacterial cell walls, carrageenan, and beryllium) likewise induce hydrolase release from macrophages, and this may generate macrophage chemotactic factors and other mediators of chronic inflammation. Inhalation of *M. faeni* probably produces farmer's lung by a pathogenetic mechanism depending on activation of complement by the alternative pathway, chemotaxis of polymorphonuclear and mononuclear cells, and stimulation of hydrolase secretion from the latter by C3b. Secretion by macrophages of hydrolytic enzymes, notably elastase, collagenase, and neutral proteinase, may contribute to the pathogenesis of emphysema. Organic and inorganic particulate air pollutants can impair the microbicidal function of macrophages. Stimulated macrophages can inhibit tumor cell growth, and this mechanism may be operative in the lungs.

References

1. A. C. Allison and P. Davies, Increased biochemical and biological activities of mononuclear phagocytes exposed to various stimuli, with special reference to secretion of lysosomal enzymes. In *The Mononuclear Phagocyte.* Edited by R. van Furth. Oxford, Blackwell, 1974, pp. 487-506.
2. W. Stöber, H. J. Einbrodt, and W. Klosterkotter, Quantitative studies of dust retention in animal and human lungs after chronic inhalation. In *Inhaled Particles and Vapours II. Proc. Int. Symp. Brit. Occup. Hyg. Soc., Cambridge, September-October, 1965.* Edited by C. N. Davies. Oxford, Pergamon, 1967, pp. 409-417.
3. V. Timbrell, Physical factors as aetiological mechanisms. In *Biological Effects of Asbestos, Proc. Working Conf. Int. Agency for Research on Cancer, Lyon, France, October, 1972.* Edited by P. Bogovski, J. D. Gilson, V. Timbrell, and J. C. Wagner. Lyon, IARC Scientific Publications No. 8, 1973, pp. 13-16.
4. V. Timbrell, D. M. Griffiths, and F. D. Pooley, Possible biological importance of fibre diameters of South African amphiboles, *Nature,* **232**:55-56 (1971).
5. L. Coes, A new dense silica, *Science,* **111**:131-132 (1953).

6. H. Brieger and P. Gross, On the theory of silicosis. I. Coesite, *Arch. Environ. Health,* **13**:38-43 (1966).
7. H. Brieger and P. Gross, On the theory of silicosis. III. Stishovite, *Arch. Environ. Health,* **15**:751-757 (1967).
8. W. Stöber, Silikotische Wirksamkeit und physich-chemische Eigenschaften verscheidener Silicon Dioxid Modifikationen, *Beitr. Silikoseforsch.,* **89**: 1-113 (1966).
9. J. Marks, The neutralization of silica cytotoxicity in vitro, *Br. J. Indust. Med.,* **14**:81 (1957).
10. A. C. Allison, J. S. Harington, and M. Birbeck, An examination of the cytotoxic effects of silica on macrophages, *J. Exp. Med.,* **124**:141-154 (1966).
11. K. Thomas, H. J. Einbrodt, and W. Schoedel, Vorwort, *Beitr. Silikoseforsch. (Sonderband),* **6**:13-18 (1965).
12. A. Preisinger, Structure of stishovite, a high-density SiO_2, *Naturwissenschaften,* **49**:345 (1962).
13. J. S. Harington and A. C. Allison, Tissue and cellular reactions to inhalants. In *Handbook of Physiology.* Edited by D. Lee. New York, Academic Press, 1976.
14. A. C. Allison, On the role of microfilaments and microtubules in cell movement, endocytosis and exocytosis, *Ciba Found. Symp.,* :109-143 (1973).
15. A. C. Allison, P. Davies, and S. de Petris, Role of contractile microfilaments in macrophage movement and endocytosis, *Nature [New Biol.],* **232**:153-156 (1971).
16. A. C. Allison, Pathogenic effects of inhaled particles and antigens, *Ann. NY Acad. Sci.,* **221**:199-308 (1974).
17. M. Rabinovitch and M. J. De Stafano, Interactions of red cells with phagocytes of the wax moth (*Galleria mellonella*) and mouse, *Exp. Cell Res.,* **59**:272-282 (1970).
18. H. Huber and M. Wiener, Binding of immune complexes to human macrophages: The role of membrane receptor sites. In *Activation of Macrophages.* Edited by W. H. Wagner and H. Hahn. Amsterdam, Excerpta Medica, 1974, pp. 54-61.
19. E. J. Wills, P. Davies, A. C. Allison, and D. Haswell, Cytochalasin fails to inhibit pinocytosis by macrophages, *Nature [New Biol.],* **240**:58-60 (1972).
20. A. C. Allison and P. Davies, Mechanisms of endocytosis and exocytosis, *Symp. Soc. Exp. Biol.,* **28**:419-446 (1974).
21. P. Davies, R. C. Page, and A. C. Allison, Changes in cellular enzyme levels and extracellular release of lysosomal acid hydrolases in macrophages exposed to streptococcal cell wall substance, *J. Exp. Med.,* **139**:1262-1282 (1974).
22. R. W. I. Kessel, L. Monaco, and M. A. Marchisio, The specificity of the cytotoxic action of silica. A study in vitro, *Br. J. Exp. Pathol.,* **44**:351-364 (1963).
23. P. Davies, A. C. Allison, J. Ackerman, A. Butterfield, and S. Williams,

Asbestos induces selective release of lysosomal enzymes from mononuclear phagocytes, *Nature,* **251**:423-425 (1974).

24. S. Nadler and S. Goldfischer, The intracellular release of lysosomal contents in macrophages that have ingested silica, *J. Histochem. Cytochem.,* **18**:368-371 (1970).
25. P. Davies and A. C. Allison, Secretion of macrophage enzymes in relation to the pathogenesis of chronic inflammation. In *Macrophages.* Edited by D. S. Nelson. New York, Academic Press, 1976, pp. 427-461.
26. J. S. Harington, A. C. Allison, and D. V. B. Badami, Mineral fibers—physicochemical and biological properties, *Adv. Pharmacol. Chemother.,* **12**:1-112 (1974).
27. J. M. G. Davies, The fibrogenic effects of mineral dusts injected into the pleural cavity of mice, *Br. J. Exp. Pathol.,* **53**:190-201 (1972).
28. A. Morgan, J. C. Evans, R. J. Evans, R. F. Houman, A. Homes, and S. G. Doyle, Studies on the Deposition of Inhaled Fibrous Material in the Respiratory Tract of the Rat and Its Subsequent Clearance Using Radioactive Tracer Techniques. II. Deposition of the UICC Standard Reference Samples of Asbestos, *Environ. Res.,* **10**:196-201 (1975).
29. J. C. Wagner and G. Berry, Information obtained from animal experiments. In *Biological Effects of Asbestos, Proc. Working Conf., Int. Agency for Research on Cancer, Lyon, France, October, 1972.* Edited by P. Bogovski, J. C. Gilson, V. Timbrell and J. C. Wagner. Lyon, IARC Scientific Publications No. 8, 1973, pp. 285-288.
30. J. C. Wagner, G. Berry, and V. Timbrell, Mesotheliomata in rats after inoculation with asbestos and other materials, *Br. J. Cancer,* **28**:173-185 (1975).
31. A. C. Allison, Experimental methods—cell and tissue culture: Effects of asbestos particles on macrophages, mesothelial cells and fibroblasts. In *Biological Effects of Asbestos, Proc. Working Conf. Int. Agency for Research on Cancer, Lyon, France, October, 1972.* Edited by P. Bogovski, J. C. Gilson, V. Timbrell, and J. C. Wagner. Lyon, IARC Scientific Publications No. 8, 1973, pp. 89-93.
32. A. C. Allison, Lysosomes and the toxicity of particulate pollutants, *Arch. Intern. Med.,* **128**:131-139 (1971).
33. A. C. Allison, Some effects of pharmacologically active compounds on membranes, *Br. Med. Bull.,* **24**:135-147 (1968).
34. W. Dehnen and J. Fetzer, Zur Wirkung von Quartz auf Lysosomen in vitro, *Naturwissenschaften,* **54**:23 only (1967).
35. K. Stalder and W. Stöber, Haemolytic activity of suspensions of different silica modifications and inert dusts, *Nature,* **207**:874-875 (1965).
36. J. S. Harington, K. Miller, and G. MacNab, Hemolysis by asbestos, *Environ. Res.,* **4**:95-117 (1971).
37. T. Nash, A. C. Allison, and J. S. Harington, Physico-chemical properties of silica in relation to its toxicity, *Nature,* **210**:259-261 (1966).
38. G. Weissman and G. A. Rita, Molecular basis of gouty inflammation: Interaction of monosodium urate crystals with lysosomes and liposomes, *Nature [New Biol.],* **240**:167-172 (1972).

39. A. C. Allison, Plasma membrane interactions and the control of cell division. In *Control of Proliferation in Animal Cells.* Edited by B. Clarkson and R. Baserga. New York, Cold Spring Harbor, 1970, pp. 447-459.
40. G. Poste and A. C. Allison, Membrane fusion, *Biochim. Biophys. Acta,* **300**:421-465 (1973).
41. P. G. Munder, M. Modolell, E. Ferber, and H. Fischer, The relationship between macrophages and adjuvant activity. In *Mononuclear Phagocytes, Int. Conf. Mononuclear Phagocytes, Leiden, September, 1969.* Edited by R. van Furth. Oxford, Blackwell, 1970, Chap. 27, pp. 445-459.
42. K. Miller and J. S. Harington, Some biochemical effects of asbestos on macrophages, *Br. J. Exp. Pathol.,* **53**:397-405 (1972).
43. R. C. Franson and M. Waite, Lysosomal phospholipase A1 and A2 of normal and bacillus Calmette-Guerin induced macrophages, *J. Cell Biol.,* **56**:621-627 (1973).
44. A. Mellors and A. L. Tappel, Hydrolysis of phospholipids by a lysosomal enzyme, *J. Lipid Res.,* **8**:479-485 (1967).
45. J. Morley, M. A. Bray, D. Gordon, and W. Paul, Interaction of prostaglandins and lymphokines in arthritis. In *The Immunological Basis of Connective Tissue Disorders.* Proc. of the 5th Lepetit Colloquium, Held in Madrid, Spain, 11-13 November, 1974. Edited by Luigi G. Silvestri. Amsterdam, North-Holland, 1975, pp. 129-140.
46. R. Ross, N. B. Everett, and R. Taylor, Prostaglandins and lymphokines in arthritis wound healing and collagen formation. VI. The origin of the wound fibroblast studied in parabiosis, *J. Cell Biol.,* **44**:645-654 (1970).
47. R. J. Richards and T. G. Morris, Collagen and mucopolysaccharide production in growing lung fibroblasts exposed to chrysotile asbestos, *Life Sci.,* **12**:441-451 (1973).
48. A. G. Heppleston and J. A. Styles, Activity of a macrophage factor in collagen formation by silica, *Nature,* **214**:521-522 (1967).
49. R. Burrell and M. Anderson, The induction of fibrosis by silica-treated alveolar macrophages, *Environ. Res.,* **6**:389-394 (1973).
50. J. S. Harington, M. Ritchie, P. C. King, and K. Miller, The in vitro effects of silica-treated macrophages on collagen production by hamster fibroblasts, *J. Pathol.,* **109**:21-37 (1973).
51. R. C. Page, P. Davies, and A. C. Allison, Pathogenesis of the chronic inflammatory lesions induced by group A streptococcal cell walls, *Lab. Invest.,* **30**:568-581 (1974).
52. C. Cardella, P. Davies, and A. C. Allison, Immune complexes induce selective release of lysosomal hydrolases from macrophages, *Nature,* **247**:46-48 (1974).
53. J. David and R. A. David, Cellular hypersensitivity and immunity. Inhibition of macrophage migration and the mediators, *Prog. Allergy,* **16**:300-449 (1972).
54. W. G. Spector, N. Reichhold, and G. B. Ryan, Degradation of granuloma-inducing organisms by macrophages, *J. Pathol.,* **101**:339-345 (1970).
55 R. C. Page, P. Davies, and A. C. Allison, Effects of dental plaque the

production and release of lysosomal hydrolases by macrophages in culture, *Arch. Oral. Biol.*, **18**:1481-1495 (1973).

56. H. Spencer, *Pathology of the Lung*, 2nd ed. Oxford, Pergamon, 1968.
57. W. van B. Robertson and B. Schwartz, Ascorbic acid and formation of collagen, *J. Biol. Chem.*, **201**:689-696 (1953).
58. K. F. Benitz and L. M. Hall, Local morphological response following a single subcutaneous injection of carrageenan in the rat, *Proc. Soc. Exp. Biol. Med.*, **102**:442-445 (1959).
59. P. Davies, A. C. Allison, M. Dym, and C. J. Cardella, The selective release of lysosomal enzymes for mononuclear phagocytes by immune complexes causing chronic inflammation. In *Infection and Immunology in the Rheumatic Diseases.* Edited by D. C. Dumonde. Oxford, Blackwell, 1976.
60. L. N. Wahl, S. M. Wahl, S. E. Mergenhagen, and G. R. Martin, Collagenase production by endotoxin-activated macrophages, *Proc. Nat. Acad. Sci. USA*, **71**:3598-3601 (1974).
61. J. C. Unkeless, S. Gordon, and E. Reich, Secretion of plasminogen activator by stimulated macrophages, *J. Exp. Med.*, **139**:834-850 (1974).
62. R. Snyderman, H. S. Shin, and A. M. Dannenberg, Macrophage proteinase and inflammation. The production of chemotactic activity from the fifth complement of complement by mactophage proteinase, *J. Immunol.*, **109**: 896-898 (1972).
63. A. C. Allison, Lysosomes and the responses of cells to toxic materials, *Sci. Basis Med.*, **1**:18-34 (1968).
64. A. C. Allison and P. Davies, Mechanisms underlying chronic inflammation. In *Future Trands in Inflammation.* Edited by G. P. Velo, D. A. Willoughby, and J. P. Giraud. Padua and London, Piccin, 1974, pp. 449-480.
65. P. M. Henson, Interaction of cells with immune complexes: Adherence, release of constituents and tissue injury, *J. Exp. Med.*, **1347** (suppl.): 1145-1250 (1971).
66. W. G. Spector and N. Heesom, The production of granulomata by antigen-antibody complexes, *J. Pathol.*, **98**:31-39 (1969).
67. J. Pepys, Immunologic approaches in pulmonary diseases caused by inhaled materials, *Ann. NY Acad. Sci.*, **221**:27-35 (1974).
68. G. B. Mackaness, P. H. Lagrange, T. E. Miller, and T. Ishibashi, The formation of activated T-cells. In *Activation of Macrophages.* Edited by W. H. Wagner and H. Hahn. Amsterdam, Excerpta Medica, 1974, pp. 193-209.
69. R. M. Pantalone and R. C. Page, Lymphokine-linked and production and release of lysosomal enzymes by macrophages, *Proc. Nat. Acad. Sci. USA*, **72**:2091-2094 (1975).
70. F. Wenzel, D. A. Emmanuel, B. R. Lawton, and E. G. Magnin, Isolation of the causative agent of farmer's lung, *Ann. Allergy*, **22**:533-540 (1965).
71. R. M. Seal, E. J. Hapke, G. O. Thomas, J. C. Meek, and M. Hayes, The pathology of acute and chronic stages of farmer's lung, *Thorax*, **23**:469-489 (1968).
72. B. Wilkie, B. Pauli, and M. Gygax, Hypersensitivity pneumonitis: Experimental production in guinea pigs with antigens of *Micropolyspora faeni*, *Pathol. Microbiol.*, **39**:393-411 (1973).

73. J. H. Edwards, J. C. Wagner, and R. M. E. Seal, Pulmonary responses to particulate materials capable of activating the alternative pathway of complement, *Clin. Allergy,* **6**:79-88 (1976).
74. D. A. Emmanuel, F. J. Wenzel, and B. R. Lawton, Pulmonary mycotoxicosis, *Chest,* **67**:293-304 (1975).
75. I. W. B. Grant, W. Blyth, V. E. Wardrop, R. M. Gordon, and A. Moir, Presence of farmer's lung in Scotland—A pilot survey, *Br. Med. J.,* **1**:530-534 (1972).
76. J. H. Edwards, J. T. Baker, and B. H. Davies, Preciptin test negative farmer's lung—activation of the alternative pathway of complement by mouldy hay dusts, *Clin. Allergy,* **4**:379-385 (1974).
77. C. V. De Shazo, M. T. McGrade, R. P. Henson, and C. G. Cochrane, The effect of complement depletion on neutrophil migration in acute immunologic arthritis, *J. Immunol.,* **108**:1414-1419 (1972).
78. M. M. E. De Bracco, D. B. Budzko, and R. Negroni, Mechanisms of activation of complement by extracts of *Aspergillus fumigatus, Clin. Immunol. Immunopathol.,* **5**:333-339 (1976).
79. C. Mittman (ed.), *Pulmonary Emphysema and Proteolysis,* New York and London, Academic Press, 1972.
80. P. Gross, E. A. Pfitzer, E. Talker, M. A. Babyak, and M. Kaschak, Experimental emphysema: Its production with papain in normal and silicotic rats, *Arch. Environ. Health,* **11**:50-58 (1965).
81. V. Marco, B. Mass, B. R. Meraneg, G. Weinbaum, and P. Kembel, Induction of experimental emphysema in dogs using leukocyte homogenates, *Am. Rev. Respir. Dis.,* **104**:595 (1971).
82. P. D. Kaplan, C. Kuhn, and J. A. Pierce, The induction of emphysema with elastase, *J. Lab. Clin. Med.,* **82**:349-365 (1973).
83. M. Galdston, A. Janoff, and A. L. David, Familial variation of leukocyte lysosome protease and serum α_1-antitrypsin determinants in chronic obstructive pulmonary disease, *Am. Rev. Respir. Dis.,* **107**:718-727 (1973).
84. H. L. Sharp, R. A. Bridges, W. Krivit, and G. F. Freier, Cirrhosis associated with α-1-antitrypsin deficiency: A previously unrecognized inherited disorder, *J. Lab. Clin. Med.,* **73**:934-939 (1959).
85. H. E. Evans, M. Levi, and I. Mandl, Serum enzyme inhibitor concentrations in the respiratory distress syndrome, *Am. Rev. Respir. Dis.,* **101**:359-363 (1970).
86. D. J. Hurst and D. L. Coffin, Ozone effect on lysosomal hydrolases of alveolar macrophages in vitro, *Arch. Intern. Med.,* **9**:125-134 (1971).
87. D. E. Gardner, E. A. Pfitzer, R. T. Christian, and D. L. Coffin, Loss of protective factor for alveolar macrophages when exposed to ozone, *Arch. Intern. Med.,* **9**:144-150 (1971).
88. A. C. Allison, Role of lysosomes in oxygen toxicity, *Nature,* **205**:141-142 (1965).
89. M. Mustafa, C. E. Cross, and W. S. Tyler, Interference of cadmium ion with oxidative metabolism of alveolar macrophages, *Arch. Intern. Med.,* **9**:116-124 (1971).
90. G. C. Snider, J. A. Hayes, A. L. Korthy, and G. P. Lewis, Centrilobular

emphysema experimentally induced by cadmium chloride aerosol, *Am. Rev. Respir. Dis.*, **108**:40-48 (1973).

91. M. L. Miller, L. Murthy, and J. R. J. Sorenson, Fine structure of connective tissue after ingestion of cadmium. Observations on the interstitium of the male rat lung, *Arch. Pathol.*, **98**:386-392 (1974).
92. A. C. Allison and P. D'A. Hart, Potentiation by silica of the growth of *Mycobacterium tuberculosis* in macrophage cultures, *Br. J. Exp. Pathol.*, **49**:465-476 (1968).
93. E. Goldstein, G. M. Green, and C. Seamans, The effect of silicosis on the defense mechanisms of the murine lung, *J. Infect. Dis.*, **120**:210-216 (1969).
94. E. Goldstein, W. S. Tyler, P. D. Hoeprich, and C. Eagle, Ozone and the antibacterial defense mechanisms of the murine lung, *Arch. Intern. Med.*, **9**:165-168 (1971).
95. G. M. Green and D. Carolin, The depressant effect of cigarette smoke on the in vitro antibacterial activity of alveolar macrophages, *N. Engl. J. Med.*, **276**:421 (1967).
96. P. A. Gorer, Some recent work on tumour immunity, *Adv. Cancer Res.*, **4**:149-169 (1956).
97. B. Bennett, L. J. Old, and E. A. Boyse, The phagocytosis of tumor cells in vitro, *Transplantation*, **2**:183-202 (1964).
98. G. A. Granger and R. S. Weiser, Homograft target cells: Contact destruction by immune macrophages, *Science*, **151**:97-99 (1966).
99. R. Evans and P. Alexander, Co-operation of immune lymphoid cells with macrophages in tumor immunity, *Nature*, **228**:620-622 (1972).
100. J. B. Hibbs, L. H. Lambert, and J. S. Remington, Possible role of macrophage mediated nonspecific cytotoxicity in tumor resistance, *Nature [New Biol.]*, **235**:48 (1972).
101. R. Keller, Mechanisms by which activated macrophages destroy syngeneic rat tumor cells in vitro. Cytokinetics, non-involvement of T-lymphocytes and effects of metabolic inhibitors, *Immunology*, **27**:285 (1974).
102. G. P. Velo and W. G. Spector, The origin and turnover of macrophages in experimental pneumonis, *J. Pathol.*, **109**:7-19 (1973).
103. M. A. Brunstetter, J. A. Hardie, R. Schiff, J. P. Lewis, and C. E. Cross, The origin of pulmonary alveolar macrophages, *Arch. Intern. Med.*, **9**:130 (1971).
104. J. J. Godleski and J. D. Brain, The origin of alveolar macrophages in mouse radiation chimeras, *J. Exp. Med.*, **136**:630-643 (1972).

AUTHOR INDEX

Numbers in brackets are reference numbers and indicate that an author's work is referred to although his name is not cited in the text. Italic numbers give the page on which the complete reference is listed.

Part I comprises pages 1-488
Part II comprises pages 489-1102

B

Part I comprises pages 1-488
Part II comprises pages 489-1102

Part I comprises pages 1-488
Part II comprises pages 489-1102

Part I comprises pages 1-488
Part II comprises pages 489-1102

Part I comprises pages 1-488
Part II comprises pages 489-1102

Part I comprises pages 1-488
Part II comprises pages 489-1102

D

Part I comprises pages 1-488
Part II comprises pages 489-1102

E

Part I comprises pages 1-488
Part II comprises pages 489-1102

F

Part I comprises pages 1-488
Part II comprises pages 489-1102

Part I comprises pages 1-488
Part II comprises pages 489-1102

Part I comprises pages 1-488
Part II comprises pages 489-1102

H

Part I comprises pages 1-488
Part II comprises pages 489-1102

Part I comprises pages 1-488
Part II comprises pages 489-1102

Part I comprises pages 1-488
Part II comprises pages 489-1102

Part I comprises pages 1-488
Part II comprises pages 489-1102

Part I comprises pages 1-488
Part II comprises pages 489-1102

Part I comprises pages 1-488
Part II comprises pages 489-1102

Part I comprises pages 1-488
Part II comprises pages 489-1102

Part I comprises pages 1-488
Part II comprises pages 489-1102

Part I comprises pages 1-488
Part II comprises pages 489-1102

O

Part I comprises pages 1-488
Part II comprises pages 489-1102

Part I comprises pages 1-488
Part II comprises pages 489-1102

Q

R

Part I comprises pages 1-488
Part II comprises pages 489-1102

Part I comprises pages 1-488
Part II comprises pages 489-1102

S

Part I comprises pages 1-488
Part II comprises pages 489-1102

Part I comprises pages 1-488
Part II comprises pages 489-1102

Part I comprises pages 1-488
Part II comprises pages 489-1102

T

Part I comprises pages 1-488
Part II comprises pages 489-1102

U

V

Part I comprises pages 1-488
Part II comprises pages 489-1102

Part I comprises pages 1-488
Part II comprises pages 489-1102

Y

Part I comprises pages 1-488
Part II comprises pages 489-1102

Z

SUBJECT INDEX

A

Part I comprises pages 1-488
Part II comprises pages 489-1102

Part I comprises pages 1-488
Part II comprises pages 489-1102

Part I comprises pages 1-488
Part II comprises pages 489-1102

Part I comprises pages 1-488
Part II comprises pages 489-1102

C

Part I comprises pages 1-488
Part II comprises pages 489-1102

Part I comprises pages 1-488
Part II comprises pages 489-1102

Part I comprises pages 1-488
Part II comprises pages 489-1102

E

Part I comprises pages 1-488
Part II comprises pages 489-1102

Part I comprises pages 1-488
Part II comprises pages 489-1102

F

Part I comprises pages 1-488
Part II comprises pages 489-1102

Part I comprises pages 1-488
Part II comprises pages 489-1102

Part I comprises pages 1-488
Part II comprises pages 489-1102

J

K

L

Part I comprises pages 1-488
Part II comprises pages 489-1102

Part I comprises pages 1-488
Part II comprises pages 489-1102

M

Part I comprises pages 1-488
Part II comprises pages 489-1102

Part I comprises pages 1-488
Part II comprises pages 489-1102

Part I comprises pages 1-488
Part II comprises pages 489-1102

N

Part I comprises pages 1-488
Part II comprises pages 489-1102

O

Part I comprises pages 1-488
Part II comprises pages 489-1102

Part I comprises pages 1-488
Part II comprises pages 489-1102

Part I comprises pages 1-488
Part II comprises pages 489-1102

Part I comprises pages 1-488
Part II comprises pages 489-1102

Part I comprises pages 1-488
Part II comprises pages 489-1102

Part I comprises Pages 1-488
Part II comprises Pages 489-1102

Part I comprises pages 1-488
Part II comprises pages 489-1102